Drinking Water Quality and Human Health

Drinking Water Quality and Human Health

Special Issue Editors

Patrick Levallois
Cristina Villanueva Belmonte

MDPI • Basel • Beijing • Wuhan • Barcelona • Belgrade

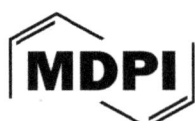

Special Issue Editors

Patrick Levallois
Institut national de santé publique du Québec (INSPQ)
Canada

Cristina Villanueva Belmonte
ISGlobal—Barcelona Institute for Global Health
Spain

Editorial Office

MDPI
St. Alban-Anlage 66
4052 Basel, Switzerland

This is a reprint of articles from the Special Issue published online in the open access journal *International Journal of Environmental Research and Public Health* (ISSN 1660-4601) from 2017 to 2019 (available at: https://www.mdpi.com/journal/ijerph/special_issues/drinking_water).

For citation purposes, cite each article independently as indicated on the article page online and as indicated below:

LastName, A.A.; LastName, B.B.; LastName, C.C. Article Title. *Journal Name* **Year**, *Article Number*, Page Range.

ISBN 978-3-03897-726-1 (Pbk)
ISBN 978-3-03897-727-8 (PDF)

Cover image of istock.com/Bartosz Hadyniak.

Contents

About the Special Issue Editors

Patrick Levallois, MD, MSc, full clinical professor at Université Laval (Québec, QC, Canada). He is a medical specialist in preventive medicine and public health and a medical adviser at Institut national de santé publique du Québec (INSPQ). He is presently the coordinator of the Water Scientific Group of this institution, dealing with water and health issues and advising different governmental bodies. He has worked for 40 years on issues related to drinking water and health. A tenured professor at Laval until 2017, he taught epidemiology and environmental health and led several important research projects on drinking water quality and health impacts. His work concerns mainly chemical quality (disinfection by-products, nitrates, arsenic, etc.) but also microbiological quality (related to farming activities and climate change). He has worked and conducted research mainly in Québec, QC (Canada) but has developed important international links, principally with US and European partners, researchers, and public health officers. During a sabbatical at the Centre for Research in Environmental Epidemiology (CREAL) (Barcelona), he organized with Cristiana M. Villanueva an international symposium on «Exposure and health effects of chemicals in drinking water». To date, he has published more than 100 papers in scientific journals. h-index: 27 (Scopus), >2400 citations by February 2019).

Cristina Villanueva Belmonte, PhD. Associate Research Professor at ISGlobal, Barcelona. She studied Environmental Sciences and completed a PhD in Environmental Epidemiology at the Universitat Autònoma de Barcelona (UAB), Spain. She did a post-doc at the National Institute of Health and Medical Research (INSERM) in Rennes (France), and since 2006, she has been a researcher at the Centre for Research in Environmental Epidemiology (CREAL)—now ISGlobal. She has been a lecturer of Environmental Epidemiology to students of Environmental Sciences (UAB), and at the Master of Public Health (UPF-UAB). Currently, she teaches Environmental Health course for the Global Health Master (UB). She is a world-famous expert on water contaminants and their impact on health, including exposure assessment to water contaminants through drinking water and swimming pools (disinfection by-products, nitrate, etc.), the evaluation of the association with health effects (cancer, reproductive outcomes, child health), the understanding of their underlying mechanisms, and the estimation of the burden of disease attributed to chemicals. She leads related research on trihalomethanes in drinking water and burden of disease, the working group on water exposures in the Multi Case Control Study (MCC)—Spain study and in the Infancia y Medio Ambiente (INMA) project, HELIX project, and is part of the research team in the EXPOSOMICS EU project. Her work has resulted in 91 publications in scientific journals (h-index: 30 (Scopus), >1900 citations by February 2019).

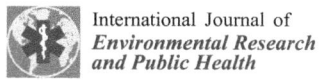

International Journal of
Environmental Research and Public Health

Editorial

Drinking Water Quality and Human Health: An Editorial

Patrick Levallois [1,2,*] and Cristina M. Villanueva [3,4,5,6]

[1] Direction de la santé environnementale et de la toxicologie, Institut national de la santé publique du Québec, QC G1V 5B3, Canada
[2] Département de médecine sociale et préventive, Faculté de médecine, Université Laval, Québec, QC G1V 0A6, Canada
[3] ISGlobal, 08003 Barcelona, Spain; cristina.villanueva@isglobal.org
[4] Universitat Pompeu Fabra (UPF), 08002 Barcelona, Spain
[5] Consortium for Biomedical Research in Epidemiology and Public Health (CIBERESP), Carlos III Institute of Health, 28029 Madrid, Spain
[6] IMIM (Hospital del Mar Medical Research Institute), 08003 Barcelona, Spain
* Correspondence: patrick.levallois@msp.ulaval.ca

Received: 12 February 2019; Accepted: 19 February 2019; Published: 21 February 2019

Drinking water quality is paramount for public health. Despite improvements in recent decades, access to good quality drinking water remains a critical issue. The World Health Organization estimates that almost 10% of the population in the world do not have access to improved drinking water sources [1], and one of the United Nations Sustainable Development Goals is to ensure universal access to water and sanitation by 2030 [2]. Among other diseases, waterborne infections cause diarrhea, which kills nearly one million people every year. Most are children under the age of five [1]. At the same time, chemical pollution is an ongoing concern, particularly in industrialized countries and increasingly in low and medium income countries (LMICs). Exposure to chemicals in drinking water may lead to a range of chronic diseases (e.g., cancer and cardiovascular disease), adverse reproductive outcomes and effects on children's health (e.g., neurodevelopment), among other health effects [3].

Although drinking water quality is regulated and monitored in many countries, increasing knowledge leads to the need for reviewing standards and guidelines on a nearly permanent basis, both for regulated and newly identified contaminants. Drinking water standards are mostly based on animal toxicity data, and more robust epidemiologic studies with an accurate exposure assessment are rare. The current risk assessment paradigm dealing mostly with one-by-one chemicals dismisses potential synergisms or interactions from exposures to mixtures of contaminants, particularly at the low-exposure range. Thus, evidence is needed on exposure and health effects of mixtures of contaminants in drinking water [4].

In a special issue on "Drinking Water Quality and Human Health" *IJERPH* [5], 20 papers were recently published on different topics related to drinking water. Eight papers were on microbiological contamination, 11 papers on chemical contamination, and one on radioactivity. Five of the eight papers were on microbiology and the one on radioactivity concerned developing countries, but none on chemical quality. In fact, all the papers on chemical contamination were from industrialized countries, illustrating that microbial quality is still the priority in LMICs. However, chemical pollution from a diversity of sources may also affect these settings and research will be necessary in the future.

Concerning microbiological contamination, one paper deals with the quality of well water in Maryland, USA [6], and it confirms the frequent contamination by fecal indicators and recommends continuous monitoring of such unregulated water. Another paper did a review of Vibrio pathogens, which are an ongoing concern in rural sub-Saharan Africa [7]. Two papers focus on the importance of global primary prevention. One investigated the effectiveness of Water Safety Plans (WSP) implemented in 12 countries of the Asia-Pacific region [8]. The other evaluated the lack of intervention to improve Water, Sanitation and Hygiene (WASH) in Nigerian communities and its effect on the frequency of common childhood diseases (mainly diarrhea) in children [9]. The efficacies of two types of intervention were also presented. One was a cost-effective household treatment in a village in South Africa [10], the other a community intervention in mid-western Nepal [11]. Finally, two epidemiological studies were conducted in industrialized countries. A time-series study evaluated the association between general indicators of drinking water quality (mainly turbidity) and the occurrence of gastroenteritis in 17 urban sites in the USA and Europe. [12] The other evaluated the performance of an algorithm to predict the occurrence of waterborne disease outbreaks in France [13].

On the eleven papers on chemical contamination, three focused on the descriptive characteristics of the contamination: one on nitrite seasonality in Finland [14], the second on geogenic cation (Na, K, Mg, and Ca) stability in Denmark [15] and the third on historical variation of THM concentrations in french water networks [16]. Another paper focused on fluoride exposure assessments using biomonitoring data in the Canadian population [17]. The other papers targeted the health effects associated with drinking water contamination. An extensive up-to-date review was provided regarding the health effects of nitrate [18]. A more limited review was on heterogeneity in studies on cancer and disinfection by-products [19]. A thorough epidemiological study on adverse birth outcomes and atrazine exposure in Ohio found a small link with lower birth weight [20]. Another more geographical study, found a link between some characteristics of drinking water in Taiwan and chronic kidney diseases [21]. Finally, the other papers discuss the methods of deriving drinking water standards. One focuses on manganese in Quebec, Canada [22], another on the screening values for pharmaceuticals in drinking water, in Minnesota, USA [23]. The latter developed the methodology used in Minnesota to derive guidelines—taking the enhanced exposure of young babies to water chemicals into particular consideration [24]. Finally, the paper on radioactivity presented a description of Polonium 210 water contamination in Malaysia [25].

In conclusion, despite several constraints (e.g., time schedule, fees, etc.), co-editors were satisfied to gather 20 papers by worldwide teams on such important topics. Our small experience demonstrates the variety and importance of microbiological and chemical contamination of drinking water and their possible health effects.

Author Contributions: P.L. wrote a first draft of the editorial and approved the final version. C.M.V. did a critical review and added important complementary information to finalize this editorial.

Funding: This editorial work received no special funding.

Acknowledgments: Authors want to acknowledge the important work of the IJERPH staff and of numbers of anonymous reviewers.

Conflicts of Interest: The authors declare no conflict of interest.

References

1. WHO/UNICEF Drinking-Water. Available online: https://www.who.int/news-room/fact-sheets/detail/drinking-water (accessed on 11 February 2019).
2. United Nations Clean Water and Sanitation. Available online: https://www.un.org/sustainabledevelopment/water-and-sanitation/ (accessed on 12 February 2019).
3. Villanueva, C.M.; Kogevinas, M.; Cordier, S.; Templeton, M.R.; Vermeulen, R.; Nuckols, J.R.; Nieuwenhuijsen, M.J.; Levallois, P. Assessing Exposure and Health Consequences of Chemicals in Drinking Water: Current State of Knowledge and Research Needs. *Environ. Health Perspect.* **2014**, *122*, 213–221. [CrossRef] [PubMed]
4. Villanueva, C.M.; Levallois, P. Exposure Assessment of Water Contaminants. In *Exposure Assessment in Environmental Epidemiology*; Nieuwenhuijsen, M.J., Ed.; Oxford University Press: New York, NY, USA, 2015; pp. 329–348. ISBN 978-0-19-937878-4.
5. IJERPH | Special Issue: Drinking Water Quality and Human Health. Available online: https://www.mdpi.com/journal/ijerph/special_issues/drinking_water (accessed on 11 February 2019).

6.   Murray, R.T.; Rosenberg Goldstein, R.E.; Maring, E.F.; Pee, D.G.; Aspinwall, K.; Wilson, S.M.; Sapkota, A.R. Prevalence of Microbiological and Chemical Contaminants in Private Drinking Water Wells in Maryland, USA. *Int. J. Environ. Res. Public Health* **2018**, *15*, 1686. [CrossRef] [PubMed]

7.   Osunla, C.A.; Okoh, A.I. Vibrio Pathogens: A Public Health Concern in Rural Water Resources in Sub-Saharan Africa. *Int. J. Environ. Res. Public Health* **2017**, *14*, 1188. [CrossRef] [PubMed]

8.   Kumpel, E.; Delaire, C.; Peletz, R.; Kisiangani, J.; Rinehold, A.; De France, J.; Sutherland, D.; Khush, R. Measuring the Impacts of Water Safety Plans in the Asia-Pacific Region. *Int. J. Environ. Res. Public Health* **2018**, *15*, 1223. [CrossRef] [PubMed]

9.   He, Z.; Bishwajit, G.; Zou, D.; Yaya, S.; Cheng, Z.; Zhou, Y. Burden of Common Childhood Diseases in Relation to Improved Water, Sanitation, and Hygiene (WASH) among Nigerian Children. *Int. J. Environ. Res. Public Health* **2018**, *15*, 1241. [CrossRef] [PubMed]

10.   Moropeng, R.C.; Budeli, P.; Mpenyana-Monyatsi, L.; Momba, M.N.B. Dramatic Reduction in Diarrhoeal Diseases through Implementation of Cost-Effective Household Drinking Water Treatment Systems in Makwane Village, Limpopo Province, South Africa. *Int. J. Environ. Res. Public Health* **2018**, *15*, 410. [CrossRef] [PubMed]

11.   Tosi Robinson, D.; Schertenleib, A.; Kunwar, B.M.; Shrestha, R.; Bhatta, M.; Marks, S.J. Assessing the Impact of a Risk-Based Intervention on Piped Water Quality in Rural Communities: The Case of Mid-Western Nepal. *Int. J. Environ. Res. Public Health* **2018**, *15*, 1616. [CrossRef] [PubMed]

12.   Beaudeau, P. A Systematic Review of the Time Series Studies Addressing the Endemic Risk of Acute Gastroenteritis According to Drinking Water Operation Conditions in Urban Areas of Developed Countries. *Int. J. Environ. Res. Public Health* **2018**, *15*, 867. [CrossRef] [PubMed]

13.   Mouly, D.; Goria, S.; Mounié, M.; Beaudeau, P.; Galey, C.; Gallay, A.; Ducrot, C.; Le Strat, Y. Waterborne Disease Outbreak Detection: A Simulation-Based Study. *Int. J. Environ. Res. Public Health* **2018**, *15*, 1505. [CrossRef] [PubMed]

14.   Rantanen, P.-L.; Mellin, I.; Keinänen-Toivola, M.M.; Ahonen, M.; Vahala, R. The Seasonality of Nitrite Concentrations in a Chloraminated Drinking Water Distribution System. *Int. J. Environ. Res. Public Health* **2018**, *15*, 1756. [CrossRef] [PubMed]

15.   Wodschow, K.; Hansen, B.; Schullehner, J.; Ersbøll, A.K. Stability of Major Geogenic Cations in Drinking Water—An Issue of Public Health Importance: A Danish Study, 1980–2017. *Int. J. Environ. Res. Public Health* **2018**, *15*, 1212. [CrossRef] [PubMed]

16.   Corso, M.; Galey, C.; Seux, R.; Beaudeau, P. An Assessment of Current and Past Concentrations of Trihalomethanes in Drinking Water throughout France. *Int. J. Environ. Res. Public Health* **2018**, *15*, 1669.

17.   Jean, K.J.; Wassef, N.; Gagnon, F.; Valcke, M. A Physiologically-Based Pharmacokinetic Modeling Approach Using Biomonitoring Data in Order to Assess the Contribution of Drinking Water for the Achievement of an Optimal Fluoride Dose for Dental Health in Children. *Int. J. Environ. Res. Public Health* **2018**, *15*, 1358. [CrossRef] [PubMed]

18.   Ward, M.H.; Jones, R.R.; Brender, J.D.; De Kok, T.M.; Weyer, P.J.; Nolan, B.T.; Villanueva, C.M.; Van Breda, S.G. Drinking Water Nitrate and Human Health: An Updated Review. *Int. J. Environ. Res. Public Health* **2018**, *15*, 1557. [CrossRef] [PubMed]

19.   Benmarhnia, T.; Delpla, I.; Schwarz, L.; Rodriguez, M.J.; Levallois, P. Heterogeneity in the Relationship between Disinfection By-Products in Drinking Water and Cancer: A Systematic Review. *Int. J. Environ. Res. Public Health* **2018**, *15*, 979. [CrossRef] [PubMed]

20.   Almberg, K.S.; Turyk, M.E.; Jones, R.M.; Rankin, K.; Freels, S.; Stayner, L.T. Atrazine Contamination of Drinking Water and Adverse Birth Outcomes in Community Water Systems with Elevated Atrazine in Ohio, 2006–2008. *Int. J. Environ. Res. Public Health* **2018**, *15*, 1889. [CrossRef] [PubMed]

21.   Chang, K.Y.; Wu, I.-W.; Huang, B.-R.; Juang, J.-G.; Wu, J.-C.; Chang, S.-W.; Chang, C.C. Associations between Water Quality Measures and Chronic Kidney Disease Prevalence in Taiwan. *Int. J. Environ. Res. Public Health* **2018**, *15*, 2726. [CrossRef] [PubMed]

22.   Valcke, M.; Bourgault, M.-H.; Haddad, S.; Bouchard, M.; Gauvin, D.; Levallois, P. Deriving A Drinking Water Guideline for A Non-Carcinogenic Contaminant: The Case of Manganese. *Int. J. Environ. Res. Public Health* **2018**, *15*, 1293. [CrossRef] [PubMed]

23. Suchomel, A.; Goeden, H.; Dady, J. A Method for Developing Rapid Screening Values for Active Pharmaceutical Ingredients (APIs) in Water and Results of Initial Application for 119 APIs. *Int. J. Environ. Res. Public Health* **2018**, *15*, 1308. [CrossRef] [PubMed]

24. Goeden, H. Focus on Chronic Exposure for Deriving Drinking Water Guidance Underestimates Potential Risk to Infants. *Int. J. Environ. Res. Public Health* **2018**, *15*, 512. [CrossRef] [PubMed]

25. Ahmed, M.F.; Alam, L.; Mohamed, C.A.R.; Mokhtar, M.B.; Ta, G.C. Health Risk of Polonium 210 Ingestion via Drinking Water: An Experience of Malaysia. *Int. J. Environ. Res. Public Health* **2018**, *15*, 2056. [CrossRef] [PubMed]

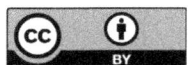

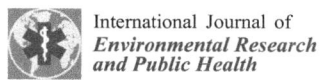

International Journal of
Environmental Research and Public Health

Article

Prevalence of Microbiological and Chemical Contaminants in Private Drinking Water Wells in Maryland, USA

Rianna T. Murray [1], Rachel E. Rosenberg Goldstein [1,2], Elisabeth F. Maring [3], Daphne G. Pee [4], Karen Aspinwall [4], Sacoby M. Wilson [1] and Amy R. Sapkota [1,*]

[1] Maryland Institute for Applied Environmental Health, University of Maryland School of Public Health, 4200 Valley Drive, College Park, MD 20742, USA; rmurray@umd.edu (R.T.M.); rerosenb@umd.edu (R.E.R.G.); swilson2@umd.edu (S.M.W.)
[2] Department of Agricultural & Resource Economics, College of Agriculture & Natural Resources, University of Maryland, 2200 Symons Hall, 7998 Regents Drive, College Park, MD 20742, USA
[3] Department of Family Science, University of Maryland School of Public Health, 4200 Valley Drive, College Park, MD 20742, USA; efmaring@umd.edu
[4] University of Maryland Extension, University of Maryland, 2200 Symons Hall, 7998 Regents Drive, College Park, MD 20742, USA; dpee@umd.edu (D.G.P.); Karen@cattailcompany.com (K.A.)
* Correspondence: ars@umd.edu; Tel.: +1-301-405-1772

Received: 16 July 2018; Accepted: 3 August 2018; Published: 7 August 2018

Abstract: Although many U.S. homes rely on private wells, few studies have investigated the quality of these water sources. This cross-sectional study evaluated private well water quality in Maryland, and explored possible environmental sources that could impact water quality. Well water samples (n = 118) were collected in four Maryland counties and were analyzed for microbiological and chemical contaminants. Data from the U.S. Census of Agriculture were used to evaluate associations between the presence of animal feeding operations and well water quality at the zip code level using logistic regression. Overall, 43.2% of tested wells did not meet at least one federal health-based drinking water standard. Total coliforms, fecal coliforms, enterococci, and *Escherichia coli* were detected in 25.4%, 15.3%, 5.1%, and 3.4% of tested wells, respectively. Approximately 26%, 3.4%, and <1% of wells did not meet standards for pH, nitrate-N, and total dissolved solids, respectively. There were no statistically significant associations between the presence of cattle, dairy, broiler, turkey, or aquaculture operations and the detection of fecal indicator bacteria in tested wells. In conclusion, nearly half of tested wells did not meet federal health-based drinking water standards, and additional research is needed to evaluate factors that impact well water quality. However, homeowner education on well water testing and well maintenance could be important for public health.

Keywords: private wells; groundwater; drinking water; animal feeding operation; fecal coliforms; enterococci; *E. coli*; Maryland

---

1. Introduction

An estimated 44.5 million people in 13 million households across the United States, 14% of the nation's population, rely on private domestic wells as their primary drinking water source [1,2]. The Safe Drinking Water Act (SDWA) was originally passed by Congress in 1974 to protect public health by regulating the nation's public drinking water supply and its sources, including rivers, lakes, reservoirs, springs, and groundwater wells [3]. However, private wells that serve less than 25 people or have less than 15 service connections are neither regulated by the SDWA nor monitored by local regulatory agencies for contaminants that may be associated with adverse human health outcomes [3].

The U.S. Environmental Protection Agency (U.S. EPA) and the National Groundwater Association provide guidance to homeowners and recommend testing private wells annually for a number of parameters including total coliform bacteria, nitrates, total dissolved solids (TDS), and pH [4,5]. As this testing is voluntary, little is known about the level or frequency of testing that is performed by private well owners, or about their knowledge and literacy regarding proper well maintenance, testing, and test results. Data on the microbiological and chemical quality of well water are also scarce. Additionally, many homeowners who utilize private water wells may lack the educational and/or financial resources necessary to address water quality issues associated with private water systems [6,7]. The U.S. Centers for Disease Control and Prevention (CDC) recently reported a significant decrease in the annual proportion of reported waterborne disease outbreaks between 1971 and 2006 in public drinking water systems; however, an increase was observed in the annual proportion of outbreaks associated with individual (private) water systems over the same time period [8]. More recently, a study in North Carolina found that between 2007 and 2013, 99% of emergency department visits for acute gastrointestinal illness caused by microbial contamination of drinking water were associated with private wells [9]. While the CDC report and the North Carolina study suggest a potential public health issue regarding private wells, the lack of information on private well water quality and monitoring makes it difficult to determine the specific contaminants causing these observed illnesses.

Recent studies conducted in Pennsylvania, Virginia, and Wisconsin reported that 40–50% of private wells exceed at least one SDWA health-based standard, most often for coliform bacteria [10–14]. These studies and others have demonstrated the influence of factors such as well construction characteristics, local geology, and climatic conditions on private well water quality [10,12,15–17]. Wallender et al. (2014) evaluated data from the CDC's Waterborne Disease and Outbreak Surveillance System (WBDOSS) and found that improper design, maintenance, or location of private wells and septic systems contributed to 67% of reported outbreaks from groundwater contamination from 1971 and 2008 [18]. In Maryland, approximately 19% of the population relies on private wells [2], however, only one previous study has investigated private well water quality in the state [19]. Additionally, previous studies have indicated that homeowners generally do not regularly test their private wells or seek technical assistance unless they perceive a water quality problem at the point of use [12,20,21], illustrating a need to educate well owners on the importance of monitoring their wells. To address this need, we developed safe drinking water clinics in several Maryland counties. The goals of the clinics were as follows: (1) to educate well owners on proper well maintenance practices and health risks of contaminated wells; (2) to provide well water quality testing in accordance with EPA guidelines; and (3) to characterize the prevalence of microbiological and chemical contaminants in tested wells.

After the clinics were completed, we recognized a need to evaluate potential environmental factors that could influence well water quality in Maryland. Recently, Li et al. (2015) investigated microbiological contamination of domestic and community supply wells in California's Central Valley, a region with intensive animal agriculture [22]. Approximately 5.9% and 10.3% of wells were positive for generic *E. coli* and *Enterococcus* spp., respectively, with significant associations observed between concentrations of enterococci and proximity of wells to animal feeding operations [22]. In Maryland, there are 12,200 registered farms, including a number of animal feeding operations [23]. In 2014, the state ranked ninth among U.S. states in broiler chicken production [23]. Maryland also has dairy and livestock farms, with 49,000 milk-producing cows and another 190,000 beef cattle and calves [23]. If wells are not properly constructed or maintained, there is potential for surface contaminants from agricultural operations to influence well water quality. As such, we leveraged the well water data collected during the safe drinking water clinics to investigate the possible association between the presence of animal feeding operations and well water quality.

2. Materials and Methods

2.1. Safe Drinking Water Clinics

Between 2012 and 2014, five safe drinking water clinics were held in four Maryland counties: Cecil (two clinics), Kent, Montgomery, and Queen Anne's (Figure 1, Table 1). Cecil, Kent, and Queen Anne's counties are located on Maryland's Eastern Shore (Figure 1), where a large number of homes rely on private wells. The Eastern Shore is highly agricultural and has the highest concentration of animal feeding operations (particularly broiler chicken operations) in the state [24–26]. Montgomery County is also characterized by a large number of homes that rely on private wells; however, there are fewer animal feeding operations in this county.

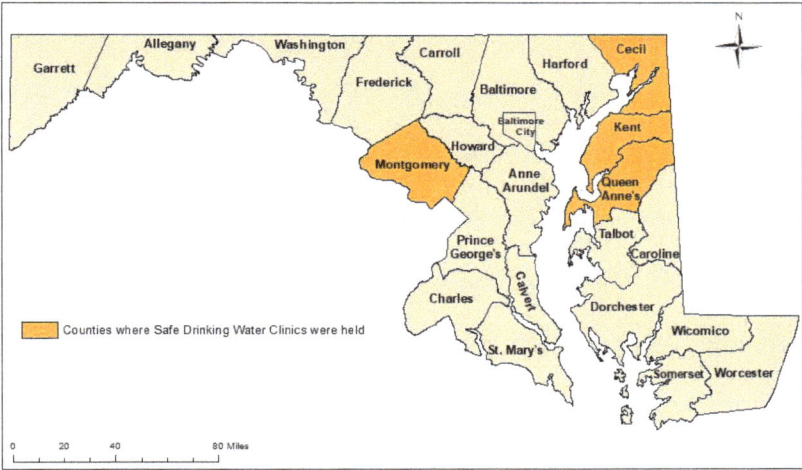

Figure 1. Maryland counties where safe drinking water clinics were held.

Table 1. Dates on which the safe drinking water clinics were held.

Maryland County	Kick-Off Meeting	Interpretation Meeting
Cecil County I	March 2012	May 2012
Kent County	October 2012	December 2012
Montgomery	February 2013	March 2013
Cecil II	September 2013	November 2013
Queen Anne's	February 2014	March 2014

Clinic participants (*n* = 150) were recruited at county health fairs, farmers' markets, and through promotional material on community email listservs and local newspapers. Participants were limited to homeowners in the aforementioned counties with private wells who were interested in participating in the clinics. The safe drinking water clinics were a multi-stage process (Figure 2) that began with a kick-off meeting where registered participants were told of the purpose and significance of the project, provided with water sampling instructions and kits (gloves, two 1 L sterile, polypropylene, wide-mouth Nalgene environmental sampling bottles (Nalgene, Lima, OH, USA) and a large Ziploc bag), and taught how to sample their well water from kitchen or bathroom faucets in accordance with standard protocols. A paper-based survey that was developed by our research and extension teams, and approved by the University of Maryland College Park Institutional Review Board, was also given to participants at the kick-off meetings. The survey included questions on well characteristics, homeowner well management practices, prior testing conducted (if any), demographic questions (age, sex, race/ethnicity, and income level), and general health-related questions, including, "In the past month, have you experienced diarrhea?" and "In the past month, have you experienced vomiting?"

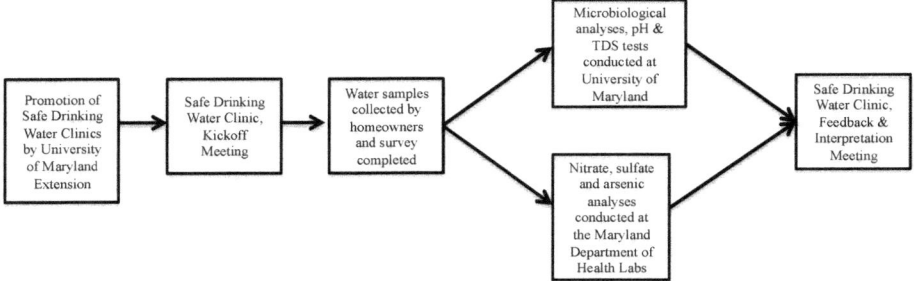

Figure 2. University of Maryland safe drinking water clinic approach. TDS—total dissolved solids.

Participants returned their water samples and completed surveys to their local University of Maryland (UMD) extension office. Samples were kept on ice and transported to the lab within 12 h. Following completion of laboratory analyses (described below), a second follow-up clinic was held where water quality results were returned to participants who provided water samples. The results were individually and confidentially interpreted for participants and potential solutions for wells that did not meet federal standards were discussed where necessary. A follow-up survey was sent to all participants within 12 months after the clinics were conducted to document actions taken by well owners to solve water quality problems or improve the management of their water supply as a result of attending our clinics (data not shown).

2.2. Laboratory Analyses

Water samples were analyzed within 24 h of collection for total coliforms, fecal coliforms, *E. coli*, *Enterococcus* spp., and *Salmonella* spp., according to standard U.S. EPA membrane filtration methods [27–30]. Briefly, 100 mL of each sample was filtered through 0.45-μm, 47-mm mixed cellulose ester filters. The filters were then placed on the appropriate selective media for each microorganism. Membrane-*Enterococcus* Indoxyl-β-D-Glucoside Agar (mEI) was used for the isolation and enumeration of *Enterococcus* spp.; MI Agar was used for the isolation and enumeration of both total coliforms and *E. coli*; and mFC was used for the isolation and enumeration of fecal coliforms. The mEI plates were incubated at 41 °C for 24 h, mFC plates were incubated at 44.5 °C for 24 h and MI plates were incubated at 37 °C for 24 h. For *Salmonella* detection, membranes were placed in lactose broth, vortexed vigorously for 3 min, and incubated for 24 h at 37 °C. An aliquot of this enrichment was transferred to TT (tetrathionate) broth base, Hajna; incubated at 37 °C for 24 h; plated on XLT4; and incubated at 37 °C for 24 h. Positive and negative controls were used during each test, and plate counts were performed immediately after incubations.

TDS (mg/L) and pH were analyzed using the Pocket Pal TDS Tester and the Stream Survey Test Kit, respectively (Hach Company, Loveland, CO, USA) [31,32]. For nitrate testing, 1 L of each sample was placed into a sterile 1 L polypropylene Nalgene environmental sampling bottle (Nalgene, Lima, OH, USA), 2 mL sulfuric acid solution was added, and the pH was adjusted to <2. For total arsenic testing, 1 L of each sample was placed into a sterile 1 L polypropylene Nalgene environmental sampling bottle (Nalgene, Lima, OH, USA), 2–3 mL of nitric acid solution was added, and the pH was adjusted to <2. The remainder of each water sample was used for sulfate testing. Nitrate and sulfate testing were completed at the Maryland Department of Health (MDH) Labs using an Agilent (Santa Clara, CA, USA) gas chromatograph-mass spectrometer. Nitrate analyses were performed according to U.S. EPA Method 353.2, while sulfate analyses were performed according to U.S. EPA Method 375.2 [33,34]. Total arsenic testing was also completed at the MDH Labs using an Agilent (Santa Clara, CA, USA) inductively-coupled plasma-mass spectrometer per U.S. EPA Method 200.8 [35]. All quality control/quality assurance approaches recommended by the U.S. EPA methods were employed, including analyses of quality control samples, as well as laboratory reagent blanks and fortified blanks [33–35].

2.3. Animal Feeding Operations Data

We obtained animal feeding operations data from the 2007 U.S. Census of Agriculture, National Agricultural Statistics Service [36]. Specifically, we obtained data on the number of animal feeding operations with sales by zip code for the following animal types: broiler chickens, turkeys, aquaculture, sheep or goats, hogs, dairy cattle, and beef cattle. The 2007 Census was used because it is the most recent U.S. Census of Agriculture that provides data at the zip code level.

2.4. Statistical Analyses

We performed descriptive statistics on all well water data. We also linked well water data and animal feeding operation data by zip code and used univariate logistic regression models to evaluate associations between the presence of each type of animal feeding operation and detection of indicator bacteria in well water samples. The presence of total coliform bacteria and fecal coliform bacteria were the dichotomous (presence/absence) outcome variables of interest. All statistical analyses were performed in SAS 9.4 (Cary, NC, USA) [37].

3. Results

3.1. Characteristics of Safe Drinking Water Clinic Participants

A total of 150 homeowners attended our safe drinking water clinics. However, only 118 participants returned both a water sample and a completed survey (Table 2). Only the 118 participants who returned both a water sample and a completed survey were included in this study's analyses. The Queen Anne's County clinic drew the most participants (n = 28; 23.1%), followed by the first clinic conducted in Cecil County (n = 25; 21.4%). A vast majority of participants were white (87.3%) and most were in the 60–69 age group (33.9%). Participants were also well-educated: 29.7% had obtained a Bachelor's degree and 39.8% had obtained a graduate degree. At the time of the clinics, a large number of participants had lived at their current residence for at least 10–20 years (39%). Twenty-nine (24.6%) participants indicated that they had never tested their well water quality, and 58 (49.2%) participants had only tested their water once. Approximately 12% and 0% of participants experienced diarrhea and vomiting, respectively, within 30 days prior to completing the survey.

Table 2. Characteristics of the safe drinking water clinic participants.

Characteristic	Category	Number (%) (n = 118)
County	Cecil (1)	25 (21.2)
	Kent	21 (17.8)
	Montgomery	25 (21.2)
	Cecil (2)	19 (16.1)
	Queen Anne's	28 (23.7)
Age	18–49	17 (14.4)
	50–59	29 (24.6)
	60–69	40 (33.9)
	70–79	23 (19.5)
	≥80	9 (7.6)

Table 2. *Cont.*

Characteristic	Category	Number (%) (n = 118)
Race/Ethnicity	African American	5 (4.2)
	Hispanic	1 (0.8)
	White	103 (87.3)
	Other or Unspecified	9 (7.6)
Level of formal education	<High school	1 (0.8)
	High School	10 (8.5)
	High school and some college	16 (13.6)
	Associate's degree	9 (7.6)
	Bachelor's degree	35 (29.7)
	Graduate degree	47 (39.8)
Number of years living at current home	1–10 years	34 (28.8)
	10–20 years	46 (39.0)
	More than 20 years	34 (28.8)
	Unknown	4 (3.4)
Previous testing of well water quality	Never	29 (24.6)
	Once	58 (49.2)
	Every few years	11 (9.3)
	Every year	4 (3.4)
	>Once per year	1 (0.8)
	Other or Unsure	12 (10.2)
Experienced diarrhea within the last 30 days	Yes	14 (11.9)
	No	104 (88.1)
Experienced vomiting within the last 30 days	Yes	0 (0%)
	No	118 (100%)

3.2. Well Water Quality

Overall, 43.2% of wells tested in this study did not meet at least one EPA health-based drinking water standard (Figure 3). Total coliform bacteria were the most common (25.4%) microbiological contaminant detected. Fecal coliforms (15.3%), Enterococcus spp. (5.1%), and E. coli (3.4%) were also detected. Salmonella was not detected in any of the private wells analyzed in this study. Regarding chemical contaminants, 26% of tested wells did not meet the recommended drinking water standard for pH (Figure 3), with most of these (83.8%) having a pH below the lower limit of 6.5. There were a few wells (16.2%) with a high pH above the recommended limit of 8.5. Nitrate occurred above the 10 mg/L drinking water standard in 3.4% of tested wells, and less than 1% of wells exceeded the recommended limit for total dissolved solids (TDS) of 500 mg/L. None of the wells had an arsenic level above the EPA maximum contaminant level (MCL) for arsenic (10 mg/L). Similarly, none of the wells tested exceeded the EPA MCL for sulfate of 250 mg/L. Although there were individual wells in each county that exceeded the EPA MCLs for some of the chemical water quality parameters investigated, the mean levels in each county were within EPA specifications (Figure 4).

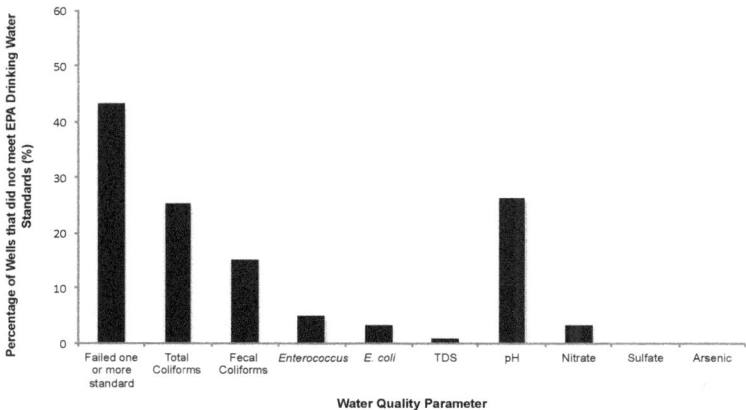

Figure 3. Percentage of tested private wells that did not meet U.S. Environmental Protection Agency (US EPA) drinking water standards.

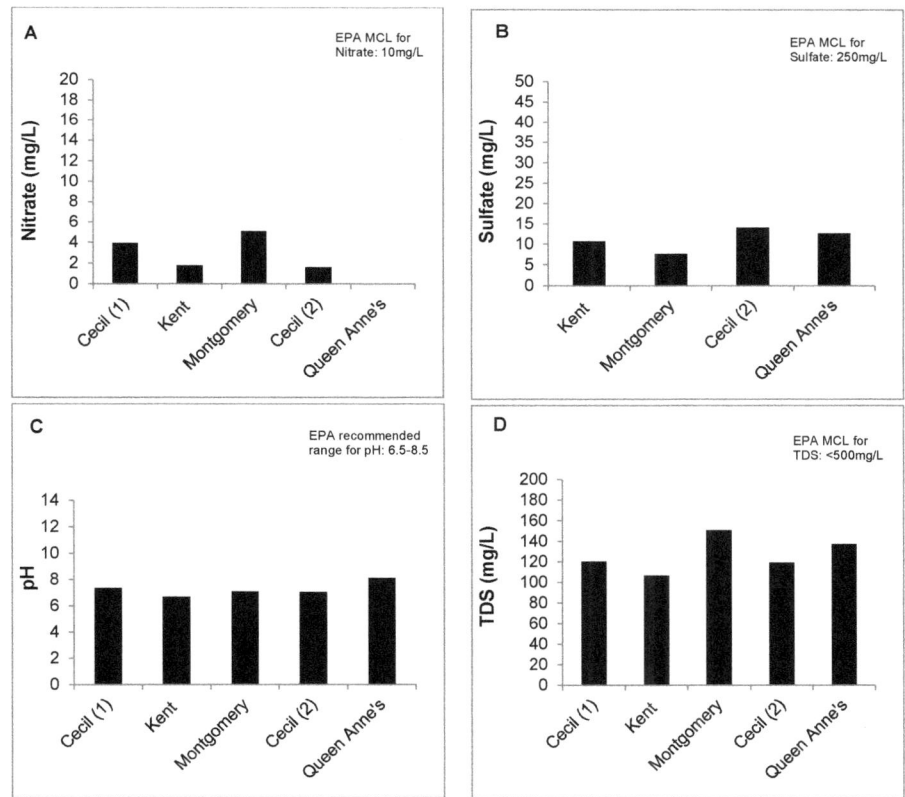

Figure 4. Mean levels of nitrate (Panel **A**), sulfate (Panel **B**), pH (Panel **C**) and total dissolved solids (TDS) (Panel **D**) detected in tested private wells by county [38]. MCL—maximum contaminant level.

Kent County had the highest percentage of wells that tested positive for fecal indicator bacteria, with 52.4% of wells testing positive for at least one type of indicator bacteria (Figure 5). *E. coli* was detected in wells sampled in every county with the exception of Cecil County. *Enterococcus* was detected in samples from all counties; however, it was not detected during the first clinic conducted in Cecil County.

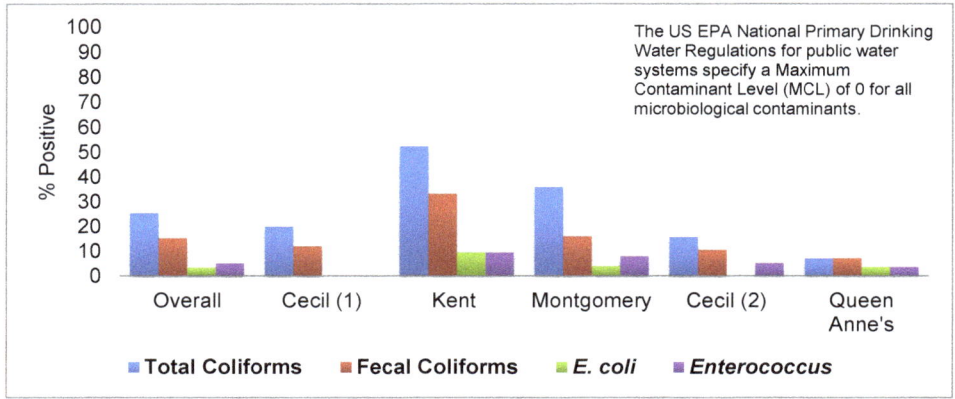

Figure 5. Percentage of tested private wells that were positive for fecal indicator bacteria by county.

3.3. Influence of Animal Feeding Operations on Well Water Quality

Our zip code-level analysis found no evidence that the presence of animal feeding operations influenced the occurrence of fecal indicator bacteria in tested wells (Table 3). In zip codes that contained cattle operations, the contamination of wells by total coliform bacteria was 1.23 times greater than in zip codes that did not contain cattle operations; however, this finding was not statistically significant (Odds Ratio (OR) = 1.23; 95% Confidence Interval (CI) = 0.89, 1.68). In zip codes that contained dairy and aquaculture operations, the contamination of wells by total coliform bacteria was more likely than in zip codes that did not contain one of these operations (dairy operations: OR = 1.12; 95% CI = 0.96, 1.31; aquaculture operations: OR = 1.32; 95% CI = 0.59, 2.93). However, these associations were not statistically significant (Table 3).

Table 3. Zip code-level analysis of the association between the presence of animal feeding operations and the occurrence of total and fecal coliforms in tested wells.

Zip Code Variable	Total Coliforms Odds Ratio (95% CI)	Fecal Coliforms Odds Ratio (95% CI)
Cattle operations	1.23 (0.89, 1.68)	1.19 (0.82, 1.73)
Broiler operations	0.93 (0.84, 1.03)	1.10 (0.41, 3.00)
Hog operations	0.76 (0.49, 1.17)	0.81 (0.48, 1.37)
Dairy operations	1.12 (0.96, 1.31)	1.11 (0.93, 1.33)
Turkey operations	0.92 (0.68, 1.24)	1.24 (0.44, 3.47)
Aquaculture operations	1.32 (0.59, 2.93)	1.33 (0.52, 3.40)

Similarly, in zip codes that contained broiler, cattle, dairy, turkey, and aquaculture operations, the contamination of wells by fecal coliform bacteria was more likely than in zip codes that did not contain one of these operations; however, none of these associations were significant. The presence of broiler, hog, and turkey operations in zip codes was slightly protective for total coliform bacteria, and the presence of hog operations in zip codes was slightly protective for fecal coliform bacteria (Table 3). However, these findings were not significant for any type of operation with either indicator bacterium.

4. Discussion

Our data demonstrate that a majority of private wells included in this study are contaminated with fecal indicator bacteria and/or chemical contaminants at levels that exceed the SDWA drinking water quality guidelines set forth by the U.S. EPA. These findings are consistent with previous studies of private water wells that have been conducted in other states. A recent study of private wells in Pennsylvania found that 41% of wells failed to meet at least one drinking water standard [10], comparable with the 43% of wells that failed to meet one or more standards in our study. Similarly, in Wisconsin, an analysis of private water wells in rural areas found that 47% of these wells exceeded one or more health-based water quality standards [12]. Total coliform bacteria was also the most common microbiological contaminant in the Pennsylvania study and was detected in 33% of wells [10], comparable with the 25% of tested wells contaminated with total coliforms in our study. A recent study of private wells in Virginia found that 46% tested positive for total coliform bacteria, with 10% testing positive for *E. coli* [11]. Meanwhile, a North Carolina study of private wells found that 49% tested positive for total coliform bacteria and 6.4% tested positive for *E. coli* [14]. Previous studies have also indicated that seasonality may play a role in well water quality. [12,39]. In our study, the county with the highest percentage of wells that tested positive for fecal indicator bacteria was Kent County, which was sampled in the Fall (Table 1). However, because our study was cross-sectional, we did not collect samples over multiple seasons and, therefore, we cannot evaluate whether seasonal trends influenced our results. Nevertheless, our study adds to the growing body of research nationwide on the water quality of private wells that illustrates the need for improved monitoring of these wells.

Monitoring of fecal indicator bacteria in private well water is important for assessing the potential health risks associated with these water sources. To improve understanding of environmental factors that may impact private well water quality, we also investigated whether proximity to animal feeding operations was associated with microbial contamination of wells. Our data showed that there were no statistically significant associations between the presence of an animal feeding operation within a zip code and microbial contamination of private wells within the same zip code; however, this may be due to the small number of well water samples obtained during this initial study. Given that exposure to well water has been shown as an important risk factor for gastrointestinal illnesses [40–42], such as campylobacteriosis, exploration of this potential association deserves further study involving a larger number of private wells.

In a case-control study conducted in Sweden, Carrique-Mas et al. (2005) demonstrated that living in a household with a private well was a risk factor for *Campylobacter* infection (OR = 2.6; 95% CI = 0.9–7.4), although that association was not statistically significant [40]. Another case-control study conducted in Norway also found that the risk of campylobacteriosis was higher for those who obtained their water from a private household well compared with those receiving water from a public system (OR = 2.0; 95% CI = 1.2, 3.2) [41]. Consumption of water from a private well was also identified as a significant risk factor for sporadic campylobacteriosis (OR = 1.92; 95% CI = 1.46, 2.53) in a second Norwegian study by MacDonald et al. [42]. The potential for private wells to influence gastrointestinal illnesses such as campylobacteriosis (that are traditionally thought to be foodborne) remains understudied in the United States and deserves further attention.

One major challenge of improving private well water quality and reducing the risk of adverse health outcomes associated with this water source is that the numbers and locations of U.S. private wells are poorly characterized. Neither individual counties nor states have a complete database with addresses and other contact information for private well homeowners. As such, regular communications to homeowners reminding them to test their wells annually and delivering interventions where necessary is challenging. While the U.S. Geological Survey developed a nationwide inventory on the private well population [2], it was created using data on the population served by public water supply systems by county in each state and lacks the specific geographic locations of private wells. Creating a nationwide database of private well owners that is regularly updated by states could allow for improved evaluation of the factors that may influence well contamination, enhanced communication with well owners, and potential improvements in levels of waterborne illness.

In this study, we demonstrated the presence of fecal indicator bacteria in private drinking water wells in Maryland. As the presence of these indicator bacteria suggests a potential human health risk, well owners are often left to mitigate these risks through system repair, enhancement, or decontamination. However, knowledge of the contamination source of the well would be helpful in selecting an appropriate remediation method. Microbial source tracking (MST) is a collection of methods used to determine the likely source of contamination associated with the presence of fecal indicator bacteria [43]. MST has been previously used in a variety of applications, including in the management of surface water contamination and watershed remediation [43,44]. Allevi et al. (2013) utilized MST techniques to characterize the magnitude and incidence of microbial contamination in private wells in Virginia, and to identify the likely sources of this contamination [45]. Similarly, Krolik et al. (2014, 2016) analyzed well water samples from southeastern Ontario using MST to elucidate whether human or bovine sources were responsible for well contamination [46,47]. Future work relating to our study could include the application of MST methods to help identify the source of microbial contamination in Maryland wells, and to elucidate potential relationships between microbial contamination and environmental characteristics, particularly those relating to land use.

Given the small, cross-sectional nature of our study, there are several limitations to be considered. Our sample size of 118 households was relatively small, representing only a small fraction of the estimated 1,070,000 people who rely on private wells in Maryland [2]. Another limitation is the possibility that study participants may have improperly collected the water sample in their homes, which could then influence our ability to accurately determine their water quality parameters. We sought to minimize this potential problem by training participants on water sampling techniques during the safe drinking water clinic kickoff meetings, and by providing instruction sheets (along with the water sampling kits) on how participants should collect their water samples. Another limitation of this study is the use of U.S. Census of Agriculture data from 2007 with results from well water samples that were collected between 2013 and 2014. As noted above, the Census of Agriculture data were only available at the zip code level for the 2007 Census, and not for subsequent years. However, it is unlikely that the number of animal feeding operations in Maryland changed significantly between 2007 and 2013.

Despite these limitations, this is the first study to assess the water quality of private wells across multiple counties in Maryland, and to investigate the influence of animal feeding operations on well water quality, thereby addressing an important research gap in the state. This study also demonstrated the value in partnerships between land grant university research faculty and county-based extension faculty. Finally, the study highlighted the need for more educational outreach to private well owners in Maryland in order to improve private drinking water quality in the state. Additional studies are needed to identify and confirm potential factors that can influence private well water quality in Maryland, such as animal feeding operations, septic tanks, well construction characteristics, soil geology, and climatic conditions.

5. Conclusions

Our findings suggest that there are a significant number of private domestic wells in Maryland that do not meet the guidelines for well water quality set forth by the SDWA. This finding is similar to studies conducted in other states, including the nearby states of Virginia and Pennsylvania. In addition, while other studies have reported associations between proximity to animal feeding operations and microbial contamination of private wells, this association was not observed in this cross-sectional study and may have been influenced by our limited sample size. Further studies are needed to identify and confirm possible sources of contamination of private wells in Maryland. The lack of regular monitoring of private wells makes periodic assessments at national, regional, and local scales important sources of information about this key source of drinking water throughout the United States. The presence of microbial contaminants at levels greater than human health-based standards in 43.2% of private wells tested in this study highlights the importance of education and routine monitoring regarding the water quality of domestic wells to protect public health.

Author Contributions: All authors contributed substantially to the work and approved the final version of the manuscript. Study Conceptualization, A.R.S., E.F.M., R.E.R.G., K.A., and D.G.P.; Methodology, A.R.S., E.F.M., R.E.R.G., K.A., and R.T.M.; Participant Recruitment and Engagement, A.R.S., E.F.M., R.E.R.G., K.A., and D.G.P.; Formal Analysis, A.R.S., R.E.R.G., and R.T.M.; Data Curation, A.R.S., R.E.R.G., and R.T.M.; Writing—Original Draft Preparation, R.T.M.; Writing—Review & Editing, A.R.S., E.F.M., R.E.R.G., K.A., D.G.P., R.T.M., and S.M.W.; Supervision, A.R.S. and S.M.W.; Project Administration, A.R.S.; Funding Acquisition, A.R.S., E.F.M., and K.A.

Funding: This study was funded by pilot grants from the USDA National Integrated Water Quality Program, the University of Maryland Extension, and the NSF-funded ADVANCE program at the University of Maryland. These grants were not used to cover publication costs.

Acknowledgments: The authors wish to thank Emma Claye for her help processing the water samples in the lab; Kate K. Manchisi who helped with data entry of surveys; and Andrew Lazur, Extension Specialist—Water Quality, for his review of the manuscript and helpful insights.

Conflicts of Interest: The authors declare no conflict of interest. The funders had no role in the design of the study; in the collection, analyses, or interpretation of data; in the writing of the manuscript; and in the decision to publish the results.

References

1. US Census Bureau American Housing Survey (AHS) for the United States. 2015. Available online: https://www.census.gov/programs-surveys/ahs.html (accessed on 27 August 2017).
2. Maupin, M.A.; Kenny, J.F.; Hutson, S.S.; Lovelace, J.K.; Barber, N.L.; Linsey, K.S. *Estimated Use of Water in the United States in 2010*; U.S. Geological Survey: Reston, VA, USA, 2014; p. 56.
3. U.S. Environmental Protection Agency. *Title XIV of the Public Health Service Act (The Safe Drinking Water Act)*; U.S. Environmental Protection Agency: Washington, DC, USA, 1974.
4. U.S. Environmental Protection Agency, Office of Water. Private Drinking Water Wells. Available online: https://www.epa.gov/privatewells (accessed on 27 March 2016).
5. National Groundwater Association (NGA). Schedule Your Annual Water Well Checkup. Available online: http://www.ngwa.org/Events-Education/awareness/Pages/Schedule-your-annual-water-well-checkup.aspx (accessed on 21 October 2017).
6. Gasteyer, S.P.; Vaswani, R. *Still Living without the Basics in the 21st Century: Analyzing the Availability of Water and Sanitation Services in the United States*; Rural Community Assistance Partnership: Washington, DC, USA, 2004.
7. Wescoat, J.L.; Headington, L.; Theobald, R. Water and poverty in the United States. *Geoforum* **2007**, *38*, 801–814. [CrossRef]
8. Craun, G.F.; Brunkard, J.M.; Yoder, J.S.; Roberts, V.A.; Carpenter, J.; Wade, T.; Calderon, R.L.; Roberts, J.M.; Beach, M.J.; Roy, S.L. Causes of Outbreaks Associated with Drinking Water in the United States from 1971 to 2006. *Clin. Microbiol. Rev.* **2010**, *23*, 507–528. [CrossRef] [PubMed]
9. DeFelice, N.B.; Johnston, J.E.; Gibson, J.M. Reducing Emergency Department Visits for Acute Gastrointestinal Illnesses in North Carolina (USA) by Extending Community Water Service. *Environ. Health Perspect.* **2016**, *124*. [CrossRef] [PubMed]
10. Swistock, B.R.; Clemens, S.; Sharpe, W.E.; Rummel, S. Water Quality and Management of Private Drinking Water Wells in Pennsylvania. *J. Environ. Health* **2013**, *75*, 60–66. [PubMed]
11. Pieper, K.J.; Krometis, L.-A.H.; Gallagher, D.L.; Benham, B.L.; Edwards, M. Incidence of waterborne lead in private drinking water systems in Virginia. *J. Water Health* **2015**, *13*, 897–908. [CrossRef] [PubMed]
12. Knobeloch, L.; Gorski, P.; Christenson, M.; Anderson, H. Private Drinking Water Quality in Rural Wisconsin. *J. Environ. Health* **2013**, *75*, 16–20. [PubMed]

13. Smith, T.; Krometis, L.-A.H.; Hagedorn, C.; Lawrence, A.H.; Benham, B.; Ling, E.; Ziegler, P.; Marmagas, S.W. Associations between fecal indicator bacteria prevalence and demographic data in private water supplies in Virginia. *J. Water Health* **2014**, *12*, 824–834. [CrossRef] [PubMed]

14. Stillo, F.; MacDonald Gibson, J. Exposure to Contaminated Drinking Water and Health Disparities in North Carolina. *Am. J. Public Health* **2017**, *107*, 180–185. [CrossRef] [PubMed]

15. DeSimone, L. *Quality of Water from Domestic Wells in Principal Aquifers of the United States, 1991–2004*; U.S. Geological Survey: Reston, VA, USA, 2009; p. 139.

16. Pieper, K.J.; Krometis, L.-A.H.; Benham, B.L.; Gallagher, D.L. Simultaneous Influence of Geology and System Design on Drinking Water Quality in Private Systems. *J. Environ. Health Denver* **2016**, *79*, E1–E9.

17. Swistock, B.R.; Sharpe, W.E.; Robillard, P.D. A survey of lead, nitrate and radon contamination of private individual water systems in Pennsylvania. *J. Environ. Health* **1993**, *55*, 6–13.

18. Wallender, E.K.; Ailes, E.C.; Yoder, J.S.; Roberts, V.A.; Brunkard, J.M. Contributing Factors to Disease Outbreaks Associated with Untreated Groundwater. *Groundwater* **2014**, *52*, 886–897. [CrossRef] [PubMed]

19. Tuthill, A.; Meikle, D.B.; Alavanja, M.C.R. Coliform bacteria and nitrate contamination of wells in major soils of Frederick, Maryland. *J. Environ. Health Denver* **1998**, *60*, 16–20.

20. Knobeloch, L. *Use of the Behavioral Risk Factor Surveillance Survey to Assess the Safety of Private Drinking Water Supplies*; Wisconsin Department of Health Services: Madison, WI, USA, 2010.

21. Krometis, L.-A. Associations between homeowner perceptions of water quality and measures of contamination in private drinking water supplies. In Proceedings of the 142nd APHA Annual Meeting and Exposition, New Orleans, LA, USA, 15–19 November 2014.

22. Li, X.; Atwill, E.R.; Antaki, E.; Applegate, O.; Bergamaschi, B.; Bond, R.F.; Chase, J.; Ransom, K.M.; Samuels, W.; Watanabe, N.; et al. Fecal Indicator and Pathogenic Bacteria and Their Antibiotic Resistance in Alluvial Groundwater of an Irrigated Agricultural Region with Dairies. *J. Environ. Qual.* **2015**, *44*, 1435–1447. [CrossRef] [PubMed]

23. Maryland State Archives Maryland at a Glance: Agriculture and Farming. Available online: http://msa.maryland.gov/msa/mdmanual/01glance/html/agri.html#poultry (accessed on 4 October 2016).

24. Dance, S. As chicken industry booms, Eastern Shore farmers face not-in-my-backyard activism. *The Baltimore Sun*, 2 April 2016.

25. Wheeler, T. Environmentalists call for moratorium on growth of Shore poultry industry. *The Baltimore Sun*, 8 September 2015.

26. Environmental Integrity Project More Phosphorus, Less Monitoring. Available online: http://www.environmentalintegrity.org/wp-content/uploads/2016/11/Poultry-report_2013.pdf (accessed on 19 November 2016).

27. U.S. Environmental Protection Agency. *Method 1604: Total Coliforms and Escherichia coli in Water by Membrane Filtration Using a Simultaneous Detection Technique (MI Medium)*; U.S. Environmental Protection Agency: Washington, DC, USA, 2002.

28. U.S. Environmental Protection Agency (USEPA). *Manual for the Certification of Laboratories Analyzing Drinking Water: Criteria and Procedures Quality Assurance*, 5th ed.; U.S. Environmental Protection Agency: Cincinnati, OH, USA, 2005.

29. U.S. Environmental Protection Agency. *Method 1600: Enterococci in Water by Membrane Filtration Using Membrane-Enterococcus Indoxyl-β-D-Glucoside Agar (mEI)*; U.S. Environmental Protection Agency: Washington, DC, USA, 2009.

30. U.S. Environmental Protection Agency. *Method 1603: Escherichia coli (E. coli) in Water by Membrane Filtration Using Modified Membrane—Thermotolerant Escherichia coli Agar (Modified mTEC)*; U.S. Environmental Protection Agency: Washington, DC, USA, 2009.

31. Hach USA Stream Survey Test Kit—Hach USA. Available online: https://www.hach.com/stream-survey-test-kit/product?id=7640219501 (accessed on 12 July 2018).

32. Hach USA Pocket Pro Low Range TDS Tester—Hach USA. Available online: https://www.hach.com/pocket-pro-low-range-tds-tester/product?id=17990686204&_bt=218809546514&_bk=&_bm=b&_bn=g&gclid=EAIaIQobChMIlN_F6Jua3AIVjYvICh1clwGYEAAYASAAEgIJ9_D_BwE (accessed on 12 July 2018).

33. U.S. Environmental Protection Agency. *Method 353.2, Revision 2.0: Determination of Nitrate-Nitrite Nitrogen by Automated Colorimetry*; Environmental Monitoring Systems Laboratory Office of Research and Development, U.S. Environmental Protection Agency: Cincinnati, OH, USA, 1993.

34. U.S. Environmental Protection Agency. *Method 375.2, Revision 2.0: Determination of Sulfate by Automated Colorimetry*; Environmental Monitoring Systems Laboratory Office of Research and Development, U.S. Environmental Protection Agency: Cincinnati, OH, USA, 1993.

35. U.S. Environmental Protection Agency. *Method 200.8: Determination of Trace Elements in Waters and Wastes by Inductively Coupled Plasma-Mass Spectrometry*; U.S. Environmental Protection Agency: Cincinnati, OH, USA, 1994.

36. United States Department of Agriculture (USDA). USDA NASS QuickStats Query Tool. Available online: https://quickstats.nass.usda.gov/ (accessed on 19 February 2018).

37. SAS Institute. *The SAS System for Windows Copyright © 2014*, version 9.4; SAS Institute Inc.: Cary, NC, USA, 2014.

38. U.S. Environmental Protection Agency (USEPA). *CFR Part 141: National Primary Drinking Water Implementation Regulations*; U.S. Environmental Protection Agency: Washington, DC, USA, 1974.

39. Richardson, H.Y.; Nichols, G.; Lane, C.; Lake, I.R.; Hunter, P.R. Microbiological surveillance of private water supplies in England—The impact of environmental and climate factors on water quality. *Water Res.* **2009**, *43*, 2159–2168. [CrossRef] [PubMed]

40. Carrique-Mas, J.; Andersson, Y.; Hjertqvist, M.; Svensson, Å.; Torner, A.; Giesecke, J. Risk factors for domestic sporadic campylobacteriosis among young children in Sweden. *Scand. J. Infect. Dis.* **2005**, *37*, 101–110. [CrossRef] [PubMed]

41. Kapperud, G.; Espeland, G.; Wahl, E.; Walde, A.; Herikstad, H.; Gustavsen, S.; Tveit, I.; Natås, O.; Bevanger, L.; Digranes, A. Factors Associated with Increased and Decreased Risk of Campylobacter Infection: A Prospective Case-Control Study in Norway. *Am. J. Epidemiol.* **2003**, *158*, 234–242. [CrossRef] [PubMed]

42. MacDonald, E.; White, R.; Mexia, R.; Bruun, T.; Kapperud, G.; Lange, H.; Nygård, K.; Vold, L. Risk Factors for Sporadic Domestically Acquired Campylobacter Infections in Norway 2010–2011: A National Prospective Case-Control Study. *PLoS ONE* **2015**, *10*, e0139636. [CrossRef] [PubMed]

43. Simpson, J.M.; Santo Domingo, J.W.; Reasoner, D.J. Microbial Source Tracking: State of the Science. *Environ. Sci. Technol.* **2002**, *36*, 5279–5288. [CrossRef] [PubMed]

44. Bradshaw, J.K.; Snyder, B.J.; Oladeinde, A.; Spidle, D.; Berrang, M.E.; Meinersmann, R.J.; Oakley, B.; Sidle, R.C.; Sullivan, K.; Molina, M. Characterizing relationships among fecal indicator bacteria, microbial source tracking markers, and associated waterborne pathogen occurrence in stream water and sediments in a mixed land use watershed. *Water Res.* **2016**, *101*, 498–509. [CrossRef] [PubMed]

45. Allevi, R.P.; Krometis, L.-A.H.; Hagedorn, C.; Benham, B.; Lawrence, A.H.; Ling, E.J.; Ziegler, P.E. Quantitative analysis of microbial contamination in private drinking water supply systems. *J. Water Health* **2013**, *11*, 244–255. [CrossRef] [PubMed]

46. Krolik, J.; Evans, G.; Belanger, P.; Maier, A.; Hall, G.; Joyce, A.; Guimont, S.; Pelot, A.; Majury, A. Microbial source tracking and spatial analysis of E. coli contaminated private well waters in southeastern Ontario. *J. Water Health* **2014**, *12*, 348–357. [CrossRef] [PubMed]

47. Krolik, J.; Maier, A.; Thompson, S.; Majury, A. Microbial source tracking of private well water samples across at-risk regions in southern Ontario and analysis of traditional fecal indicator bacteria assays including culture and qPCR. *J. Water Health* **2016**, *14*, 1047–1058. [CrossRef] [PubMed]

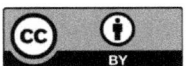

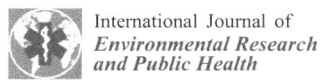

Review

Vibrio Pathogens: A Public Health Concern in Rural Water Resources in Sub-Saharan Africa

Charles A. Osunla [1,2,3,*] **and Anthony I. Okoh** [1,2]

1   SAMRC Microbial Water Quality Monitoring Centre, University of Fort Hare, Alice, Private Bag X1314, Alice 5700, South Africa; aokoh@ufh.ac.za
2   Applied and Environmental Microbiology Research Group (AEMREG), Department of Biochemistry and Microbiology, University of Fort Hare, Alice 5700, South Africa
3   Department of Microbiology, Adekunle Ajasin University, P. M. B, Akungba-Akoko 34211, Ondo-State, Nigeria
*   Correspondence: osunlacharles@gmail.com or charles.osunla@aaua.edu.ng

Received: 27 August 2017; Accepted: 4 October 2017; Published: 7 October 2017

Abstract: Members of the *Vibrio* genus are autochthonous inhabitants of aquatic environments and play vital roles in sustaining the aquatic milieu. The genus comprises about 100 species, which are mostly of marine or freshwater origin, and their classification is frequently updated due to the continuous discovery of novel species. The main route of transmission of *Vibrio* pathogens to man is through drinking of contaminated water and consumption inadequately cooked aquatic food products. In sub-Saharan Africa and much of the developing world, some rural dwellers use freshwater resources such as rivers for domestic activities, bathing, and cultural and religious purposes. This review describes the impact of inadequately treated sewage effluents on the receiving freshwater resources and the associated risk to the rural dwellers that depends on the water. *Vibrio* infections remain a threat to public health. In the last decade, *Vibrio* disease outbreaks have created alertness on the personal, economic, and public health uncertainties associated with the impact of contaminated water in the aquatic environment of sub-Saharan Africa. In this review, we carried out an overview of *Vibrio* pathogens in rural water resources in Sub-Saharan Africa and the implication of *Vibrio* pathogens on public health. Continuous monitoring of *Vibrio* pathogens among environmental freshwater and treated effluents is expected to help reduce the risk associated with the early detection of sources of infection, and also aid our understanding of the natural ecology and evolution of *Vibrio* pathogens.

Keywords: *Vibrio* pathogens; rural water resources; public health; sub-Saharan Africa

1. Introduction

Freshwater bodies serve as the main water resources in rural areas used for drinking, cooking, and irrigation for agriculture in most communities that have little or no access to potable, safe water. They easily become polluted as a result of fast population growth, land development along river banks, and urbanization [1]. Continuous pollution has resulted in various water-associated disease epidemics in both developed and developing countries [2,3]. More than 50% of the 663 million people worldwide who lack access to safe water reside in Sub-Saharan Africa, predominantly in rural areas [4]. This leads to poor health due to various water-related illnesses. However, access alone is not enough to guarantee better health. Insufficient hygienic practices can also lead to the contamination of safe water after it leaves the water point, making it unsafe to drink. Globally, 80% of wastewater flows back into the ecosystem without being treated or reused, contributing to a situation where around 1.8 billion people use a source of drinking water contaminated with faeces, putting them at risk of contracting cholera, dysentery, typhoid, and polio [5]. Mainly in low-income areas of cities and towns within developing countries, a large proportion of wastewater is discharged directly into the closest surface water drain or informal drainage channel, sometimes with very little or no treatment at all [5]. In addition to household effluent and human waste, urban-based hospitals and industries such as small-scale mining and motor garages often dump highly toxic chemicals and medical waste into the wastewater system. Even in developed countries where wastewater is collected and treated, several reports have established that most wastewater treatment plants (WWTPs) do not completely remove contaminants from sewage waters based on the system used [6], thus releasing effluents with varying matrices of contaminants at a specific point source into water bodies such as rivers, streams, and lakes. Despite recent advances in water quality and wastewater treatments, waterborne diseases still pose a major threat to public health worldwide [7]. As these receiving water bodies are the only available sources of potable water, their contamination has resulted in many waterborne diseases such as diarrhoea, gastroenteritis, and cholera in children, adults, and refugees in various developing countries such as Nigeria, Rwanda, Congo, Zimbabwe, Sudan, Afghanistan, Chile, and Brazil [8]. In rural areas of sub-Saharan countries like South Africa, rivers play an essential role in the life of the people for social, cultural, and religious purposes. The general public at large is directly affected by the prevailing poor quality of river water which has required the regulation of the biological quality of both effluents and the receiving waterbodies. The lack of policy and management of drinking water safety issues is an important issue which is believed to be a major factor causing the health and safety problems in developing countries. This calls for concerted efforts tailored towards ensuring that more researches are carried out for addressing the paucity of policies guiding the safety of drinking water in sub-Saharan Africa [9].

Over the years, several researchers have focused on the sternness of diseases caused by *Vibrio cholerae* leaving out relatively minor *Vibrio* species of medical interest, some of which are described as emerging pathogens able to cause mild to severe human diseases. The *Vibrio* species are aboriginal gram-negative bacilli that inhabit freshwater and estuarine water environments with a wide range of salinity and temperature values, where they predominantly persist in a culturable and non-culturable state [10,11]. They are considered to exhibit both fermentative and respiratory metabolisms. Several investigations have also shown the prevalence of *Vibrio* species in surface water throughout the world, and their prevalence in the environment is influenced by season, location, and the analytical methods employed [12]. Dozens of known species have been estimated to establish disease conditions in humans [13,14]. They are usually linked to eruptions of *Vibrio* infections as a result of consuming undercooked seafood and water contaminated with sewage or the exposure of skin wounds to aquatic environments and animals [15–17]. The pathogenic *Vibrio* species of health relevance which are generally transmitted through water and seafood include *Vibrio parahaemolyticus*, *V. cholerae*, *Vibrio vulnificus*, *V. tubiashi*, and *Vibrio fluvial* is [18,19]. The *Vibrio* genus comprises about 100 species which are mostly found in marine and surface water, and this is subject to continuous updates as a result of the discovery of new species [20]. *V. vulnifcus*, *V. parahaemolyticus*, and *Vibrio mimicus* are considered to be the toxigenic food-borne pathogens [21,22].

V. cholerae is an example of a non-invasive organism, which only affects the small intestine via the release of enterotoxin and is the etiological agent of cholera, whereas *V. parahaemolyticus* and *V. vulnificus* are considered as intrusive microorganisms largely affecting the colon. *V. fluvialis* and *V. vulnificus* are considered as emerging human and foodborne pathogens, respectively, and are linked with outbreaks and sporadic cases of severe diarrhea [23–25]. *V. vulnificus* symptoms include blistering gastroenteritis, skin wounds, or a disease condition known as primary septicemia and the infection is very dangerous to people who have long-term chronic liver disease [26]. Halophilic *Vibrio* species are known to cause mild infections in humans, but can also cause high morbidity, mortality, or infections in fish and other aquatic animals [27,28]. Generally, the outbreak of *Vibrio* species in aquaculture has a direct impact on the economy of a country and also serves as a threat to public health. In this review, we carried out an overview of pathogenic *Vibrio* species in rural water resources of Sub-Saharan Africa and its implications on public health.

2. *Vibrio* Species

The bacteria genus *Vibrio* is considered to be among the natural dwellers of aquatic environments which play essential roles in maintaining the aquatic ecosystem. Vibrios are characterized as gram-negative organisms, have straight or sometimes curved rod-like shapes, and are around 1.4–2.6 μm in length [29]. They can be motile or non-motile; motile species move about with the aid of three flagella at one end. *Vibrio* species usually produce many horizontal unsheathed flagella. They are chemoorganotrophic which are characterized as non-endospores formers and grow in the absence of molecular oxygen. They are different from pseudomonads in that they undergo fermentative as well as respiratory metabolism and are generally positive to an oxidase test [30]; oxygen is the actual final electron acceptor. They are not capable of fixing nitrogen; the usual source of nitrogen is ammonium salts. Nearly all *Vibrio* pathogens are positive to an oxidase test with the exception of *V. metschnikovii* [29].

Vibro-static agent 0/129 has been reported to have an effect on most *Vibrio* species and this serves as the diagnostic test [31]. They exhibit the unique capability to halt and absorb a broad range of carbon, phosphorus, and nitrogen substrates [32–34], as well as the ability to secrete exterior enzymes chitinase and laminarase, which make abundant nutrients available to the indigenous microbes [35,36]. Furthermore, they have developed an adaptive mechanism to the ever changing environmental conditions which includes the changing of size to an ultra-microbial morphology (<0.4 μm diameter) [37]. *Vibrio* species are halophilic in nature, requiring about 2–3% sodium chloride (NaCl) for optimum development [38,39]. *Vibrio* species apart from *V. mimicus* and *V. cholerae* are referred to as halophilic organisms because they do not grow on media that is void of the addition of sodium chloride [40]. The potential significance of salinity to *Vibrio* species growth shows the dynamics of abundance in the aquatic ecosystem [41,42].

The genus *Vibrio* has experienced various modifications in recent years. Many studies concentrate on cholera as a result of the havoc that the disease has inflicted on public health, but recently, ample studies have established some of the minor *Vibrio* species to be of important health concern. This minor species are termed as emerging pathogens capable of causing slight to serious diseases in man [43,44], marine vertebrates, and invertebrates [45–47]. The details of selected *Vibrio* pathogens that are of medical relevance are listed in Table 1. Over a hundred species are presently in this genus, twelve of which are regarded as human pathogens [48].

Table 1. Some disease conditions initiated by pathogenic *Vibrio* species.

Vibrio Species	Intestinal Syndromes		Extra-Intestinal Syndromes		
	Diarrhea	Cholera	Septicemia	Skin-infection	Others *
Vibrio cholerae O1/139	-	##	-	-	≠
Vibrio cholerae non O1/non 139	##		#	#	≠
Vibrio alginolyticus	-		≠	##	≠
Vibrio damsela	-		##	##	-
Vibrio fluvialis	##		-	-	-
Vibrio metschnikovi	≠		-	-	≠
Vibrio mimicus	##		-	-	≠
Vibrio parahaemolyticus	##		##	##	≠
Vibrio vuinificus	≠		##	##	≠

key infections; # minor infections; ≠ random infections. * includes otitis media cholesystitis, meningitis. Adapted from [49].

Pathogenic *Vibrio* species of human origin are broadly categorized based on the kinds of disease conditions that they exhibit, including one group causing extra-intestinal illnesses and the other group causing gastrointestinal diseases. *Vibrio* species-specific diagnostic tests have been long-established with the aid of biochemical techniques, which are given in Table 2 [31]. Some *Vibrio* species, which are known to emit light, also exhibit symbiotic relationships with squids and various aquatic organisms [50]. Other *Vibrio* species are known to be morbific to certain organisms which include fish, coral, and frogs [51–53].

Table 2. Biochemical characterization of some *Vibrio* species.

Caption	V. cholerae	V. parahaemolyticus	V. fluvialis	V. furnissi	V. vulnificus	V. alginolyticus	V. cincinnatiensis	V. damsela	V. hollisae	V. metchnikovii	V. mimicus
TCBC agar	YLW	GRN	YLW	YLW	GRE	YLW	YLW	GRE	ABS	GRE	GRE
mCPC agar	Purple	ABS	ABS	ABS	YLW	ABS	NOTD	ABS	ABS	ABS	ABS
AGS	AKa	AKa	AKAK	AKAK	AKa	AKa	NOTD	NAD	Aka	AKAK	AKa
Grth. NaCl (0%)	+	-	-	-	-	-	-	-	-	-	+
Grth. NaCl (3%)	+	+	+	+	+	+	+	+	+	+	+
Grth. NaCl (6%)	-	+	+	+	+	+	+	v	+	+	-
Grth. NaCl (8%)	-	+	v	+	-	+	+	-	-	v	-
Grth. NaCl (10%)	-	-	-	-	-	+	-	-	-	-	-
Grth at 42 °C	+	+	v	-	+	+	+	-	-	v	+
CA	NOTD	+	-	NOTD	+	+	NOTD	NOTD	NOTD	NOTD	NOTD
VP	NOTD	-	-	NOTD	-	+	NOTD	NOTD	NOTD	NOTD	NOTD
SU	-	-	+	+	-	+	+	-	-	-	-
CE	-	v	+	-	-	-	+	-	-	+	-
LA	-	-	-	-	+	-	+	-	-	-	-
AB	-	-	+	+	-	-	+	+	+	-	+
MA	+	+	+	+	+	+	+	-	+	+	+
MA	+	+	+	+	Va	+	-	+	+	+	+
OX	+	+	+	+	+	+	-	+	+	-	+
Ad	-	-	-	-	-	-	+	+	-	+	-
Ld	+	+	+	+	+	+	+	+	-	+	+
Od	+	+	-	-	+	+	+	-	-	-	+
SU/129 (10 μg)	SNTIVE	REST	REST	REST	SNTIVE	REST	SNTIVE	SNTIVE	NAD	SNTIVE	SNTIVE
SU/129 (150 μg)	SNTIVE	SNTIVE	SNTIVE	SNTIVE	SNTIVE	SNTIVE	SNTIVE	SNTIVE	NAD	SNTIVE	SNTIVE
GE	+	+	+	+	+	+	-	+	-	+	+
UR	-	v	-	-	-	-	-	+	-	-	-

Note: AGS—arginine-glucose slant; Grth—Growth; CA—Capsule; VP—Voges-Proskauer; SU—Sucrose; CE—Cellobiose; LA—Lactose; AB—Arabinose; MA—Mannitol; OX—Oxidase; Ad—Arginine dihydrolase; Ld—Lysine decarboxylase; Od—Ornithine decarboxylase; GE—Gelatinase; UR—Urease; AC—Acid; AK—Alkaline; Va—Variable reaction; a—slight acid; YEL—yellow; NOTD—Not determined; SNTIVE—Sensitive; REST—Resistant; GRE—green; ABS—Absence of growth. Adapted from [40,41].

3. Ecology of *Vibrio* Species

Vibrios are autochthonous to the oceanic, estuarine, and freshwater ecosystem [54]. They are found in sediments [55] and are known to produce biofilms on surfaces [56,57]. They either swim freely in the water column, [58] or adhere to/live associated with other organisms [20,59]. Moreover, ample numbers of *Vibrio* species have developed adaptive features that enable them to predominantly thrive in salty and even riverine environments [60]. The study of the ecology of *Vibrio* species has been in existence for a long time, owing to the fact that many species are of medical importance to both human and animals [61]. Naturally occurring Vibrios in aquatic environments are well documented considering their great importance in the mineralization of organic matter and other nutrients [62,63]. Because *Vibrio* species are selectively scraped by aquatic flagellates, it is believed that they facilitate the degradation of organic matter in water milieu [64].

They also have the ability to break down chitin, which has been reported as one of the major sources of amino sugars in aquatic environments [62]. In addition, *Vibrio harveyi* secretes an average of ten unique enzymes capable of degrading chitin [65,66]. Accordingly, this might justify the ubiquitous occurrence of *Vibrio* species in aquatic systems [62]. Previous studies have highlighted several *Vibrio* species that are resident in freshwaters which are being transferred through flood run-off to marine environments [67]. Members of the *Vibrio* genus are not always introduced into the aquatic ecosystem with faecal pollution, unlike enteric pathogens that are found in aquatic environments as a result of the indiscriminate discharge of wastewater. Some hypotheses have attempted to explain the prevalence of some pathogenic *Vibrio* species in coastal areas. Several studies have also proposed terrestrial and aquatic animals as reservoirs for virulent genes in the environment [68]. In particular, bivalves and other filter feeding marine animals have been reported to concentrate ample numbers of bacteria in their tissues [69,70]. During warm periods in temperate waters, almost 100% of oysters harbour *Vibrio* species, and an annual study on the Southwest coast of India shows that 57% of all oysters contained pathogenic Vibrios [71].

Numerous studies that have investigated the distribution of *Vibrio* species suggest that pathogenic subpopulations of the genus *Vibrio* are potential reservoirs for disease epidemics [72,73], mainly in sub-Saharan Africa, where access to potable water is lacking [63,74], and/or in countries where the eating of undercooked oysters is most prevalent [22,75]. Previous studies have established that it is almost impossible to understand the effect of single physicochemical parameters on *Vibrio* species since all parameters are interdependent and the influence of the environmental conditions varies from one species to another [67]. The incidence and the rate distribution of *Vibrio* species have been linked to a vast array of environmental factors, most notably organic matter, salinity, temperature, and the association with aquatic animals depending on the pathogen and its habitat, and the geographic location [76–78]. Dissolved oxygen [79,80], chlorophyll [81–83], and plankton [84–87] have also been found to be important in the ecology of the *Vibrio* species. However, the effects of these environmental parameters have been reported to be species dependent [88,89].

Globally, climate change is anticipated to have direct or indirect effects on environmental conditions. The noticeable increase in water temperatures, both in oceans and coastal waters, is dependent on higher atmospheric temperatures [90]. An increased temperature in freshwater tends to increase the densities of *Vibrio* species in aquatic animals and this has been implicated in diarrhea and gastroenteritis outbreaks in countries with previous epidemic cholera and temperature-based models [76,77]. A high atmospheric water temperature is one of the factors that suggest the presence of *Vibrio* species as many studies have documented their abundance in warmer waters above 15 °C [12,91,92]. Slight increases in water temperature have been found to greatly influence the microbial load of *Vibrio* species in the face of climate change [93]. Cases of disease outbreak were reported in Hurricane Katrina in the United States in 2005 as result of pathogens [94]. At certain temperatures above 15 °C, attachment to chitin increases considerably owing to an increase in the appearance of the mannose-sensitive haemagglutinin pilus and the colonization factor, an N-acetylglucosamine binding protein [95,96].

At microenvironment temperatures, irrespective of aerated medium uptake, *Vibrio fluvialis* has been shown to exhibit the innate ability to survive and proliferate in saltwater microcosms for almost two weeks [97]. Studies have shown that *Vibrio fluvialis* in aquatic environments can be viable for up to twelve months and still be capable of establishing an infection, and it was later recovered from sediments from a viable but nonculturable stage, after more than six years [98]. According to a study conducted by Scheldt [99], it was observed that runoff from rivers might affect the salinity level in the receiving water bodies, which in turn enhances the proliferation of *Vibrio* species. Similarly, [100] revealed that the densities of *Vibrio species* in the Chesapeake lagoon have a relationship with the rate at which the river flows. They were able to establish the direct impact of runoff on the salinity as a result of dilution. Moreover, climate change is considered to have a noticeable effect on the volume of nutrients in the water since variations in the introduction of nutrients such as through freshwater runoff, as well as the addition of organic carbon, brings about changes in precipitation forms [101].

Vibrio species have been reported to be capable of surviving in many different environmental conditions due to the development of a spectrum of adaptive responses to nutrient deficit, variations in salinity and temperature, and a resistance to predation by heterotrophic protists and bacteriophage. One such approach is to undergo a change into a dormant or viable but non-culturable (VBNC) state during harsh situations [102,103]. The significance of the viable but non-culturable state in cholera epidemiology was revealed by incubating a viable but non-culturable state of *V. cholerae* in freshwater microcosms which actively expressed virulence and colonization traits [104]. Likewise, the formation of a biofilm by *Vibrio* species on the exoskeletons of crustaceans and other marine organisms is a survival strategy during famishment and/or other environmental difficulties [105–107]. In biofilms, bacteria are believed to conserve and absorb nutrients, resist antibiotics, and create promising associations with other bacteria or hosts. In a conducive environment that is usually season reliant, they are known to revert to the active vegetative state for development and proliferation [108].

4. Pathogenicity of *Vibrio* Species

The clinical manifestation of *Vibrio* infections commences with the drinking of contaminated water or the eating of mishandled marine products [24]. After passing through the acidic wall of the stomach, it attaches itself to the thin tissue lining the small intestine with the aid of toxin-coregulated pili (TCP) [109] and with establishment factors like accessory colonization factor, diverse haemagglutinins, and core-encoded pilus. Human pathogenic species are known to produce several extracellular factors including haemolysin, cytotoxin, siderophore, phospholipase, collagenase, enterotoxin, and haemagglutinin [110,111]. Taking into account all of the virulence properties, haemolysin, enterotoxin, and cytosine have a direct link to the clinical manifestation; conversely, siderophore and haemagglutinin are involved in the establishment of *Vibrio* pathogen disease conditions [28]. One of the important means by which pathogens establish their pathogenicity is through the production of bacterial enzymes. Essential proteolytic enzymes that breakdown the amide bond in proteins and other short amino acids are vital for regulating homeostasis in prokaryotes and eukaryotes. Occasionally, the enzymes produced by virulent *Vibrio* species are found to be toxic to the infected human host [112]. As presented in Table 3, relevant *Vibrio* pathogens associated with human infections produce and form proteolytic enzymes; some of these enzymes are broadly classified as toxic factors processing other protein toxins [49].

Studies have shown that poor sanitation and overcrowding are important factors that promote the persistence of *Vibrio cholerae* in the environment, an etiological agent of cholera [113]. Also, *V. cholerae* is known to express two major virulence factors, namely the cholera toxin (CT), which is borne on filamentous cholera-causing toxin phage (CTX phage); and a colonization factor named toxin co-regulated pilus (TCP), which is one of the crucial intestinal establishment factors and the host receptor for the cholera toxin. The cholera toxin causes prolific squelchy diarrhoea, and the two subsets of the isolates are acquired by lateral gene transfer (LGT) [114]. Toxigenic *V. cholerae* growth phase requires two main stages: One entails the ability to cleave and grow on biotic surfaces in a fairly oligotrophic aquatic environment with low osmolarity; while the other requires the successful colonization of a eutrophic, biochemically challenging human intestine populated by a highly diverse commensal host flora [115]. The release of toxins in a living host leads to the discharge of copious squelchy diarrhea that releases the causative organism back into the environment where it is capable of further infecting additional individuals through the consumption of contaminated water, or having access to the environmental stage of its lifecycle. At the environmental stage, the environment avails *V. cholerae* with a substantial benefit to transform by obtaining different genes from other bacteria via lateral gene transfer (LGT). *Vibrio cholerae* is naturally found in aquatic environments and is believed to coexist with zooplankton. When growing on chitin, which is the basic unit of planktonic crustaceans, the organism initiates a growth pattern known as natural competence which enables *Vibrio cholerae* to absorb novel DNA that aids the virulence of the toxigenic strains, via competence-specific DNA uptake machinery.

Considering all the known *Vibrio* pathogens that have been well documented, the most significant of them are *V. cholerae* subgroups O1 and O139, which have been recognized to cause cholera [116]. Intensive study has been pursued for some of the O1 and O139 serotypes that are known to produce an array of virulence genes mostly of the TCP Pathogenicity Island, tcpA, tcpI, and acfB, encrypting the establishment of the coregulated pilus toxin, with cholera toxin (CT) [117,118]. Recently, *V. parahaemolyticus* has been the major cause of up to 20–30% of food poisoning human outbreaks of bacterial origin in Japan, seafood stomach disease in Asia, and gastroenteritis from the consumption of seafood in the United States [119–121]. On rare occasions, *V. parahaemolyticus* is associated with ear or wound infections which, at times, pose threats to individuals that are immunosuppressed, immunocompromised, or have underlying medical conditions [122].

Table 3. Some proteolytic enzymes produced by pathogenic *Vibrio* species. Adapted from [49,123].

Vibrio Species	Vibrolysin	Collagenase	Chymotrypsin-Like Protease	Haemolysin
Vibrio alginolyticus		Present	Present	
Vibrio parahaemolyticus		Present	Present	Present
Vibrio mimicus	Present			
Vibrio cholerae	Present			Present
Vibrio vulnificus	Present		Present	
Vibrio fluvialis	Present			Present
Vibrio metschnikovii			Present	
Vibrio anguillarium				Present
Vibrio tubiashii				Present

V. parahaemolyticus is also known to harbor different virulence factors such as TDH-related hemolysin (trh) and thermostable direct hemolysin (tdh), adhesins, and two other type III secretions systems, T3SS1 and T3SS2, with varying degree of pathogenicity [124]. They both display similar hemolytic activity in living cells and lead to the lysis of human erythrocytes, most especially in brackish medium [125]. Another known virulence factor found in *V. parahaemolyticus* is thermolabile haemolysin (TLH) and this is veiled by the TLH gene which is also potent in disrupting red blood cells [126,127]. Studies have shown that both environmental and clinical strains of *V. parahaemolyticus* are known to express TLH [128], and the gene is considerably coordinated under assumed intestinal infection settings [129]. In addition, *V. parahaemolyticus* possesses two separate kinds of flagella that are used for reeling, swarming, and producing capsules. These features are envisaged to ensure the survival of strains in the environment, as well as to thrive in the human host.

The mode of action used by *V. vulnificus* to establish its pathogenicity in a human is reliant on host vulnerability, and this bacterium is considered as an opportunistic pathogen [130]. Generally, *V. vulnificus* infection in humans arises as a result of consuming improperly cooked seafood or a wound infection from sea water or contaminated fish [130,131]. The invasive nature of *V. vulnificus* is attributed to its ability to harbor varying multiple virulence factors such as iron availability in the host, the capsular polysaccharide, and a short generation time [132].

Several studies have described the prominent virulence factor expressed by *V. fluvialis* as hemolysis, which manifested on sheep blood agar. Different acknowledged virulence factors of *V. fluvialis* are as follows: cell vacuolation, hemaglutination cell adherence [133,134], mannose sensitive [135], hemolysin [136], cytotonic [137], mucinase [138], heat-labile Cytotoxin [139,140], and cytolysin [141]. Reference [25] discovered that the ability possessed in expressing all the virulence factors by *V. fluvialis* is not uniform. Generally, *Vibrio* pathogens thermostable direct haemolysin and cholera toxin are used to define *V. parahaemolyticus* and *V. cholerae*, respectively, while within *V. vulnificus* strains, host proneness appears to be a crucial factor for virulence.

5. Epidemiological Features of *Vibrio* Species

Vibrio species comprise genetically and metabolically different collections of heterotrophic bacteria that grow naturally and are able to proliferate in marine ecosystems and freshwater with increased salinity [142]. Since 1817, up to seven major plagues and cholera outbreaks have been reported in Asia and Africa, with minor cases in Australia and America. Sub-Saharan Africa is broadly affected by many cholera epidemics [143], where the risk associated with cholera infection is high. The prevalence of *Vibrio* species in the aquatic environment has a direct correlation to the numerous physicochemical and biological features of the water ecosystem. *V. cholerae* is found in surface water in a potent state between one hour to 13 days, while the incessant pollution by healthy carriers and victims of cholera epidemics serves as the main means of sustaining its proliferation in aquatic environments for up to 15 months in receiving waterbodies [144]. Consequently *Vibrio* pathogen infections remain a significant health challenge in middle-income countries, notably in Africa and Asia, endangering the basic health of weak people in the society [145]. *Vibrio* species have been implicated in cases of bloody diarrhoea, necrotizing fasciitis, and primary septicemia in immunocompromised individuals, especially in developing countries with inadequate sanitation, socioeconomic conditions, and water supply systems [28]; however, this is responsible for the varying degree of ill health and death in all age groups worldwide [146]. Natural tragedies such as tsunami and floods also aid outbreaks by unsettling the normal balance of nature [147]. This results in varying health challenges, making food and water supplies prone to contamination by parasites and bacteria when vital systems like those for water and sewage are destroyed. An example of such is the current outbreak of cholera in Yemen that has claimed over 1500 lives with more than 246,000 new cases and this now affects 21 out of the 22 provinces in Yemen [148].

Developing countries are extremely affected because of their paucity of resources, infrastructure, and disaster awareness systems [149]. The spread of cholera within neighbouring countries has been attributed to cross-border practices which include the migration of fisherman and commercial trade. The outbreaks of cholera and associated deaths that occurred between 1994 and 2016 in ten selected countries in sub-Saharan Africa countries are listed in Table 4. This further establishes the vulnerability of the developing countries and most especially children. In 2014 alone, about 190, 549 cases, with 2231 deaths, were reported all over the world, though available modeling suggests that the cases of cholera outbreak may be far higher with almost 1–4 million occurring every year. The current outbreak of cholera in DR Congo is very disheartening, with reported cases of high fatality rates. This has subjected the DR Congo health system to intense pressure. Overall, the prevailing noticeable upsurge of the size of outbreaks can be partially described in part by the resistance developed by *Vibrio cholerae* O1 strains to ciprofloxacin and the different cholera toxin B (ctxBtt) genotype [150]. Recent studies carried out by [151] acknowledged that most environmental strains of *V. cholerae* recovered from the Apies river in South Africa haboured virulent-related genes (hlyA, ToxR, tcp, and zot). The prevalence of these strains in our environments presents hidden public health threats to rural dwellers of developing countries that have little or no access to safe water for household uses. In addition, the occurrence of the virulent-related genes in the absence of the ctx gene in isolated *V. cholerae* calls for further research in an attempt to unravel possible triggers of cholera epidemics in most developing countries where known toxigenic strains of the bacterium are not common.

Table 4. Epidemiological updates of cholera outbreaks from 10 selected countries in Sub-Saharan Countries between 1994 and 2016. Adapted from [152].

Name of Countries	Year	Cases between (1994–2013)			Cases in 2014			Cases in 2015			Cases in 2016		
		Cases	Death	CFR	Cases	Death	CFR	Cases	Death	CFR	Cases	Death	CFR
Nigeria	2004–2013	105,483	3913	3.7	35,996	755	02	5913	188	3.2	768	32	4.2
Cameroun	2004–2013	46,172	1817	3.9	3355	184	05	120	5	4.2	77	1	1.2
Niger	1994–3013	21,538	978	4.5	2059	80	04	51	4	7.8	38	5	13.2
Lake Chad Basin	2004–2013	31,918	996	3.2	41,188	994	2.4	6084	197	3.2	883	38	4.3
Ghana	1998–2013	55,784	1095	2	28,944	247	01	687	10	1.5	600	00	00
Benin	2004–2013	5432	48	0.9	874	14	02	00	00	00	874	13	1.5
Togo	2006–2013	2142	38	1.8	329	11	03	50	02	4.0	02	00	00
Cote d'Ivoire	2002–2013	7573	272	3.6	248	14	06	200	02	1.0	16	01	06
Guinea Bissau	1996–2013	74,031	1684	2.3	18	3	7	00	00	00	00	00	00
DR Congo	-	-	-	-	19,305	265	01	18,403	272	1.5	28,162	772	2.7

Note: The risk factors for cholera outbreaks in the 10 selected countries in sub-Saharan Countries between 1994 and 2016 are poor sanitation, lack of safe water and cross border.

Additionally, the recent findings that affirm the occurrence of *V. cholerae* in river sediments further confirm that the risk of infection associated through exposure to the river could increase under circumstances of sediment resuspension [153]. The possibility of isolating *V. cholerae* strains from river sediments may possibly increase the understanding of the possible sources of the *V. cholerae* strains involved in the cholera epidemics that have affected many developing and Sub-Saharan African countries for many years.

The absence of cholera enterotoxin was also reported in *V. cholerae* non O1/O139 isolated from the water of several reservoirs in Burkina Faso. The fact that the bacterium did not harbor the ctx gene does not exclude the threat associated with the presence of the *V. cholerae* non O1/O139 in environmental waters [154,155]. Some studies have earlier demonstrated the antigenic translation of *V. cholerae* non O1/O139 to *V. cholerae* O1 in favourable conditions [156–158].

Between 1976 and 1997, Bangladesh witnessed the most devastating outbreak of *V. fluvialis* [159]. Moreover, between 1997 and 2000, *Vibrio* observation statistics indicate that *V. fluvialis* was liable for 82 out of 1584 *Vibrio* infections in the report submitted to Centers for Disease Control and Prevention. In Kolkata in India, [160] reported the increase in the rate at which *V. fluvialis* is isolated from hospitalized patients with cholera-like symptoms. [161] revealed the survival of *V. fluvialis* in wastewater effluents in South Africa and there is a previous report linking this bacterium to causing food poisoning [162], especially due to the consumption of inadequately prepared shellfish [163]. Generally, recent studies have established the epidemiological relevance of *V. fluvialis* in several countries regardless of their economic circumstances [25,131].

Human infections caused by *V. vulnificus* occur virtually everywhere has and have been isolated from estuarine or coastal environments, which was first reported in the United States by the Centre for Disease Control in 1964. Though it was erroneously recognized as a virulent strain of *V. parahaemolyticus*, it was later understood in 1970. The disease conditions displayed include wound infections and septicemia, which were unique and different from other *Vibrio* species [164–166]. This bacterium is unique for a number of reasons, such as its exceptional pathogenicity, high case fatality rate, interesting and unusual epidemiology, hidden virulence potential, and the increasing incidence of disease. Indeed, this pathogen is strikingly interesting because recorded cases occur in males (~85%) and in patients with repressed illnesses resulting in raised serum iron levels, primarily hepatitis and alcohol-related liver cirrhosis. Oestrogen appears to reduce the ability of this pathogen to elicit endotoxic shock in women; however, the molecular basis of this protective role remains unclear. Besides foodborne disease, *V. vulnificus* causes potent fatal wound infections. Generally, *V. vulnificus* wound infections are categorized by swelling, erythema, and acute pain. Significantly, as compared to other vibrios, *V. vulnificus* needs only minute portals of entry to initiate wound infections, and often initially appears as an insect bite [167]. *V. vulnificus* is heterogeneous and the basic features—genetic, biochemical, serological, as well as host range—are used to categorize it into three biotypes. Biotypes 1 and 2 are known to cause infections in human and aquatic animals, respectively. However, the third biotype is a hybrid of biotype 1 and 2. This was first discovered in 1996 from *V. vulnificus* infections at a fish market in Israel [168]. Recent studies have further revealed the complication surrounding the virulence process of *V. vulnificus* as biotype 1 has been discovered to habour two distinct genotypes termed C (clinical) and E (environmental). In addition, the genotype strains C are mostly associated with human septicaemia, while the genotype E is encountered in wound infections caused by *V. vulnificus*. [28] revealed the occurrence of *V. vulnificus* in effluents from wastewater treatment plants even after chlorination in South Africa. Several discrete genes are believed to be important in pathogenesis, as well as those involved in cytotoxicity, haemolysins, iron sequestration pathways, secretion systems, and acid neutralization pathways. Up to date, there has been no record of any single molecular target that has been documented which is capable of differentiating pathogenic and non-pathogenic *V. vulnificus* strains and this calls for more research in an attempt to unravel the differences that exist within these strains.

Vibrio parahaemolyticus, a halophilic bacterium, has gained global brutality, having being linked to an emergence of gastroenteritis throughout the world, including Africa, Europe, and Asia [169]. Several studies have tried to establish that this human pathogen resides in different geographical locations. *Vibrio parahaemolyticus* was first isolated and recognized as the causative agent of seafood-borne infections in Japan in 1950, which accounted for over 272 illnesses and 20 deaths after the consumption of shirasu, a local delicacy [170]. From 1996 to 1998, the Infectious Disease Surveillance Centre in Japan declared *V. parahaemolyticus* as the main cause of food poisoning [171]. Lethal *V. parahaemolyticus* is spread via the consumption of partially, undercooked, or contaminated marine products, and is capable of initiating acute gastroenteritis [172,173]. The disease condition caused by *V. parahaemolyticus* is associated with three major clinical manifestations which include gastroenteritis, wound infections, and septicemia. The most prominent of these syndromes is gastroenteritis, with symptoms such as watery diarrhea (occasionally bloody diarrhoea) with abdominal pains, nausea, spewing, headaches, and fever [171,174]. The mean period of *V. parahaemolyticus* illness is 15 h (range: 4–96 h) [175]. *V. parahaemolyticus* infection in immunocompetent folks is self-limiting, mild, and of moderate severity, lasting an average of three days [176,177]. About 45,000 annual cases of food-borne disease associated with *V. parahaemolyticus* infections are reported in the United States, and this is a public health threat because the incidence keeps increasing in spite of control measures; this is attributed to the impact of climate change on pathogen abundance and distribution. Almost 20 to 30% of all reported food poisoning cases in Japan are caused by *V. parahaemolyticus* [178] and it is considered as one of the major causes of seafood and marine products-borne illness [179,180]. Furthermore, several cases of gastroenteritis which result from the consumption of contaminated seafood, as well as cholera outbreaks, were also reported in Nigeria [181].

6. Treatment and Antibiotic Resistance of *Vibrio* Species

The frequency of *Vibrio* species infections, which cause illnesses that vary from acute diarrhea, septicemia, and gastroenteritis to primary sepsis and necrotizing fasciitis, continues to increase particularly in developing and middle-income countries where infectious diseases and poverty are endemic [182]. The treatment of the cholera disease condition is centered on the physiological ideology of replacing water and electrolytes and maintaining the intravascular volume. The main goal is to replenish potassium and bicarbonate, which were discharged along with choleric stool. For severely ill patients, the Centre for Disease and Control (CDC) recommends the use of antibiotics along with fluid replacement. The application of this physiological principle is primarily made available to patients who are sternly dehydrated and who continue to discharge large volumes of stool throughout the rehydration treatment. The use of antibiotic treatment is also recommended for all patients who are hospitalized. Antimicrobial agents are useful in aiding the rehydration treatment of cholera, because their use reduces the duration of diarrhoea (which in turn reduces the spread of the disease), and treats acute illnesses (by reducing the volume of diarrhoea). CDC recommends that the class of antibiotics used for treating any infection should be based on indigenous antibiotic susceptibility patterns. The first line of treatment for adults in most countries as recommended is doxycycline; however, azithromycin is recommended as the primary treatment for pregnant women and children. For the period of an epidemic, an antibiogram must be observed by carrying out regular tests on all sample isolates from different geographic regions [73].

Ever since the discovery of antibiotics and other antimicrobial therapies, they have always been used to treat both old and new emerging infections, subsequently leading to disease management and control [183,184]. However, treating antibiotic resistant infections with existing antibiotics has become more challenging, giving the rise in infections that result in higher morbidity and mortality [185,186]. In sub-Saharan Africa, the prevalence of the high burden of infectious diseases, which are mainly of bacterial origin, has increased the demand for antimicrobial remedies for treatment [182]. Furthermore, in the healthcare environment, shortfalls ranging from the inadequate diagnostic capacity and resources, high out of pocket cost of antimicrobial drugs, and lack of free access to antibiotics, to constrained access to health services and poor orientation with respect to antibiotic use [187–189], have gradually fueled the demand for antibiotics. Every year, quite a large number of *Vibrio* species are documented to harbour high resistance genes towards commonly used antibiotics. Drug resistance is one of the most alarming public health concerns that advances rapidly and threatens the advancement of disease management and control [190,191].

The upward trend of antibiotics resistance by microbial pathogens portends to weaken the idealistic hope of public health gains made since the widespread use of antibiotics was adopted. The emergence of antibiotics resistance among various species of *Vibrio* pathogens is a well-established phenomenon [192] and with the ongoing challenges of producing potent and effective new antibiotics [193], the management of communicable diseases has become a dire need in less industrialized countries where poor sanitation and malnutrition are prevalent. The indiscriminate use of antibiotics and chemotherapeutic agents as feed additives or immersion baths to establish preventive measures in farming and aquaculture environments has also been implicated in the emergence of multidrug resistance in aquatic microorganisms such as the *Vibrio* species [194].

Recent studies have established the role played by municipal and industrial wastewater and aquaculture as drivers of resistance genes in the aquatic ecosystem. A sizeable portion of the clinically used antibiotics consumed by humans is released in an active biological form through urine and faeces [195–197]. The residual portion of the antibiotics excreted by humans is discharged into wastewater treatment plants, with one of three fates: (1) biodegradation [198], (2) absorption to sewage sludge [199,200], or (3) exit as inadequately treated effluent [201,202]. Furthermore, 16 selected United Kingdom wastewater treatment plants (WWTPs) showed the existence of erythromycin, ofloxacin, and oxytetracycline residues in each of the WWTPs [203].

Moreover, about 30–90% of antibiotics ingested by animals are found in their faeces and urine [204]. Animal excreta are also known to pollute the environment with antibiotic resistant bacteria and antibiotics [205,206]. This phenomenon was recently verified in a study conducted in the Netherlands using 20 salable swine and 20 calf farms. The result revealed antibiotics in 55% of the swine faeces out of the 80% of the swine farms considered, and in 75% of the calf faeces from 95% of the cattle farms [204]. Among the antibiotics residues recovered, oxytetracycline, doxycycline, and sulfadiazine remained the most recurrent. This is in line with some noteworthy reports affirming that the use of antibiotics and biocides in fish farms tends to increase the circulation, which in turn contributes to the wide range of resistance genes within our environment.

Antibiotic resistance is known as the enhanced ability of an organism to withstand the effect of antibiotics to which it was previously vulnerable. In the treatment of different Vibrios infections, antibiotics such as Amoxicillin, Ampicillin, Chloramphenicol, Cotrimoxazole, Ciprofloxacin, Doxycycline, Erythromycin, Fluoroquinolone, Furazolidone Gentamicin, Kanamycin, Nalidixic acid, Neomycin, Norfloxacin, Polymyxin B, Quinolone, Streptomycin, Spectinomycin, sulfamethoxazole–trimethoprim, Sulphonamides, Tetracycline, Trimethoprim, and Vancomycin are generally drugs of choice [73,207–209]. Several reports have established that both clinical and environmental *Vibrio* strains harbor antibiotic resistance genes [210–212]. The presence of this bacterium in the aquatic environment increases human fright on food safety owing to the latter possibly causing disease epidemics depending on the environmental conditions [213]. The advent of antibiotics resistance is a challenging process repeatedly linking human, environmental, and pathogen-related features [184,187,192]. In general, the antibiotic routine in humans and animals conveys an intrinsic threat of opting for antimicrobial resistance genes (ARGs). The predominance of resistance genes in the environment is the outcome of an intricate combination of dynamics, which reveals an active balance of fitness costs and aids: costs of transporting the ARGs in the framework of the host genome and environment [214,215], relative to the sternness and recurrence of risk [216], pertinent to some physical environmental features, such as temperature [217] and microbial ecology [218], among others.

7. Mechanism of Antibiotics Resistance in *Vibrio* Species Infection

Several antibiotic resistance mechanisms in bacteria are usually enabled by exporting drugs through efflux pumps, chromosomal mutations, or developing genetic resistance via the exchange of conjugative plasmids, conjugative transposons, integrons, or self-transmissible chromosomally integrating SXT elements [209,219]. Some antibiotic-resistant *Vibrio* species in sub-Saharan Africa, as well as their resistance mechanisms, are listed in Table 5. *Vibrio* species are known to employ multi-drug efflux pumps to establish resistance against antimicrobial agents and other toxic compounds by a mechanism that prevents the accumulation of drugs inside the bacterial cells. *V. cholerae* has shown its ability in using multidrug efflux pumps to export a wide range of antibiotics, detergents, and dyes that are chemically and structurally unrelated [220]. Collectively, multi-drug efflux pumps are not employed only for drug resistance, but have also been implicated in the expression of important virulence genes in *Vibrio* pathogens. The spread of antibiotic-resistant pathogens in *V. cholerae* is known to be facilitated by horizontal gene transfer through self-transmissible mobile genetic elements, including SXT elements—mobile DNA elements belonging to the class of integrative conjugating elements (ICEs). The SXT genetic mobile element ICE conferring resistance to sulfamethoxazole-trimethoprim was first documented in *V. cholerae* O139 or a closely related ICE in Madras, India, owing to its ability to harbor resistance to trimethoprim, sulfamethoxazole, and streptomycin. The relationship between self-transmissible elements and multidrug resistance has been well documented in *Vibrio* species [221]. A recent study in Cameroun revealed that *Vibrio cholerae* O1 of environmental origin harbours heterogeneous multidrug resistance towards Amoxicillin (AML), Ampicillin (AMP), Tetracycline (TE), Chloramphenicol (C), Doxycycline (DXT), and Cotrimoxazole (SXT) [222]. The frequent usage of antibiotics as part of the *Vibrio* infection treatment regimen has resulted in the development of multidrug resistance in *V. cholerae* and seafood pathogens such as pathogenic *Vibrio* species [194].

Table 5. Selected drug-resistant *Vibrio* species strains reported in Sub-Saharan Africa. Adapted from [209] with slight modification.

Year	Country	Strain	Antibiotic Resistance	Mechanism	Reference
2006	Accra, Ghana	O1	SXT	SXT element, Class 2 integron, Class 1 integron.	[223]
2011–2014	Ghana	O1 biotype El Tor	Am, Cpr, NA, SXT.	ND	[224]
Nov. 2002–April 2004	Mozambique	O1 El Tor Ogawa	Cm, Co, Tet, Qu.	ND	[225]
1994	Rwanda	O1 EL Tor	Co	ND	[226]
Oct. 2004–Mar. 2006	Senegal	O1 El Tor	Co	ND	[227]
2009–2010	Nigeria	atypical El Tor	SXT, Spec	ND	[154]
2004–2005	Cameroun	O1	SXT, Amp	ND	[228]
Aug. 2006–Sep. 2008	North-west Ethiopia	O1 Inaba	Co, Cm, Amp, Ery, Tet, Cpr.	ND	[229]
2011–2012	DR Congo	Ogawa and Inaba	NA, Am, Cm, Tet, Do, Nf, SXT, Ery.	ND	[230]
Dec. 2006–Feb. 2007	Namibia	O1 El Tor Inaba	SXT, Sm.	ND	[231]
1998–1999	Kenya	O1	Spec, Cm, Co, Tet	ND	[232]
2006	Angola	O1 and *Vibrio parahaemolyticus*	Am, Cm, Tri, SXT, Tet.	Plasmid located Class 1 integrons.	[233]
2010	South Africa	*Vibrio fluvialis*, *Vibrio* species	Vf (Tri, Pen, Co, Spec). V spp. (Am and SXT).	ND	[28]
2008–2009	South Africa	O1 Inaba	Co, NA, Am, Tet, Cm, Ery, Ce.	Tet A gene, SXT element-integrase	[234]

Note: Am: amoxicillin; Amp: ampicillin; Cm: chloramphenicol; Co: cotrimoxazole; Cpr: ciprofloxacin; Ery: erythromycin; Spec: spectinomycin; SXT: sulfamethoxazole–trimethoprim; Tet: tetracycline; Tri: trimethoprim; NA: nalidixic acid; Qu: quinolone; Sm: streptomycin; pen: penicillin; Ce: cephalosporin.

As an environmental organism, *V. cholerae* has the means to acquire resistance genes from intimate contact with indigenous resistant environmental bacteria [235] through mobilizable genetic elements. The persistent discharge of antibiotics into WWTPs is associated with the release of resistance genes. These resistance genes in wastewater primarily originate from the gastrointestinal tracts of humans [236–238]. However, most of the genetic determinants that confer resistance to antibiotics are located on plasmids. Acquired antibiotic resistance in bacteria is generally mediated by extrachromosomal plasmids and is transferable to other bacteria within the environment [239]. The co-location of antibiotics and ARGs in WWTPs can select for novel combinations of AMR that can be shared between microorganisms by horizontal gene transfer (HGT) on mobile genetic elements (MGEs), such as plasmids, thereby increasing the prevalence and combination of multiple drug resistance in the microbial community [240,241]. Plasmid-mediated multidrug resistance is one of the most pressing problems in the treatment of infectious diseases. In the last decade, the emergence of antibiotic resistant genes in *Vibrio* species has been on the increase compared to previous years, and these genes include penicillin resistant genes penA, blaTEM-1 and Beta-lactam [242,243], chloramphenicol resistant genes [244], and tetracycline resistant genes [245]. There has been little or no regulation of the choice of antibiotics administered to animals, with overlaps in the classes of antibiotics used for farming and human therapy in most of the sub-Saharan countries. The risk of multiple drug resistance found in environmental microorganisms being transferred to other pathogens is of significant public health concern that calls for concerted efforts in tackling the threat posed to disease control and management [246–248]. These animals, animal products, farm workers, and the farming environment itself are potential reservoirs for resistance determinants. Antimicrobial resistance has been detected in farms; however, the extent of resistance and spill over in the country remains largely unknown. Hence, the transmission of resistance between animal feed and humans is important and requires investigation, as this has been linked to increasing clinical resistance in human medicine.

8. Strategic Recommendations for High-Risk Cholera Outbreak Areas

High-risk cholera areas along the coastline are regions that serve as pathways for exchange with neighbouring countries. The neighbouring areas that are prone to cholera outbreaks with high incidences call for cross-border collaboration needs for preparedness and early detection [249]. The priority strategic actions to be taken in the above onset regions include: (i) consolidating timely uncovering and prompt response schemes with community-based surveillance and cross-border alerts; (ii) establishing coordination machineries through the sectors and borders; (iii) building the capacity for outbreak management; (iv) targeted the pre-positioning of supplies; and (v) preparing communication messages and plans. Sustainable Water, Sanitation, and Hygiene activities should be of main concern in rural areas that are often affected by long outbreaks. An integrated WASH-epidemiological study has been steered by UNICEF in the West Africa region and proposes to (i) institute support with concerned Water Company Limited to advance the water quantity and quality delivered to the rural areas; (ii) reinforce post-chlorination of the network by mounting dosing chlorine pumps at premeditated points along the network; (iii) advocate the use of GIS technology during an outbreak to ascertain any strategic hotspots; and (iv) when hotspots are known, implement WASH and Health development programs targeting identified communities, and consider the use of Oral Cholera Vaccine [250].

9. Conclusions

The concerns about public health risks from *Vibrio* pathogens, most especially when rural waters, wastewater effluents, and mishandled sea products remain the means of transmission of *Vibrio* species infections, are expected to remain in the future. Every year, there has been an emergence of at least one new pathogenic *Vibrio* species which could be transferred through the environment as a new public health menace. This is as a result of a number of factors which include: (i) the impact of global climate change on environmental conditions; (ii) the indiscriminate use of chemotherapeutic agents and antibiotics in aquaculture environments and agriculture; (iii) the enhanced ability of the *Vibrio* species to transfer acquired resistance genes; (iv) the evolution of pathogens; and (v) the application of a global effective surveillance system to ascertain the risks of environmentally transmitted pathogenic

Vibrio species and the indiscriminate use of antibiotics for treatment and prophylaxis measures. The observed transmission of antibiotic-resistant bacteria and genes from animals to humans highlights the importance of biosecurity and the need to separate animals being treated for infection from the herd (where feasible), and not to re-use beddings from infected and treated animals. The use of an effective global surveillance system to monitor factors such as ecological modifications and climate change that enhance *Vibrio* species as significant human pathogens demands quantitative assessments rather than assumptions. There is a dire need of information on the indiscriminate traditional use of antibiotics in farming and aquaculture environments as immersion baths or feed additives, which is believed to contribute to the prevalence of antibiotic resistance in humans within sub-Saharan Africa. Furthermore, to reduce the proliferation and survival of emerging and currently recognized pathogens in the final effluent being discharged into receiving water bodies, there is an urgent need to adopt advanced treatment methods and maintenance strategies. The implementation of adequate surveillance management protocols to reduce the possibility of infections caused by pathogenic *Vibrio* species is also proposed. Finally, the use of advanced molecular techniques and the integration of skills from related fields (e.g., microbiology, biotechnology, and ecology) will promote a better understanding of the state and possible causes of pollution which can, in turn, help in developing long-term policies to improve water quality.

Acknowledgments: We are grateful to the Water Research Commission of South Africa and the South Africa Medical Research Council for financial support.

Author Contributions: Both authors contributed to the work presented in this paper. Both authors read and approved the final manuscript.

Conflicts of Interest: The authors declare no conflict of interest.

Abbreviations:

VBNC	Viable but non-culturable
TCP	Toxin coregulated pili
CT	Cholera toxin
CTX	Cholera causing toxin phage
LGT	Lateral gene transfer
DNA	Deoxyribonucleic acid
TDH	Thermostable direct haemolysin
TLH	Thermolabile haemolysin
CDC	Centres for Disease control
WWTPs	Wastewater treatment plants
ARGs	Antibiotic resistance genes
SXT	Self-transmissible chromosomally integrating SXT elements
ICE	Integrative conjugating elements
AMR	Antimicrobial resistance
HGT	Horizontal gene transfer
MGEs	Mobile genetic elements
GIS	Geographical information system
WASH	Water Sanitation and hygiene
UNICEF	The United Nations Children's fund

References

1. Ashton, P.J.; Hardwick, D.; Breen, C.M. Changes in water availability and demand within South Africa's shared river basins as determinants of regional social-ecological resilience. In *Exploring Sustainability Science: A Southern African Perspective*; Burns, M.J., Weaver, A., Eds.; Stellenbosch University Press: Stellenbosch, South Africa, 2008; pp. 279–310.
2. Cabral, J.P.S. Water microbiology. Bacterial pathogens and water. *Int. J. Environ. Res. Pub. Health* **2010**, *7*, 3657–3703. [CrossRef] [PubMed]

3. Chigor, V.N.; Sibanda, T.; Okoh, A.I. Studies on the bacteriological qualities of the Buffalo River and three source water dams along its course in the Eastern Cape Province of South Africa. *Environ. Sci. Pollut. Res.* **2013**, *20*, 4125–4136. [CrossRef] [PubMed]

4. ECOA (Equal Credit Opportunity Act). *European Union Development Assistance for Drinking Water Supply and Basic Sanitation in Sub-Saharan Countries*; European Court of Auditors, rue Alcide De Gasperi: Luxembourg, 2012.

5. UNESCO (The United Nations Educational, Scientific and Cultural Organization). *Water Quality and Wastewater*; The United Nations Educational, Scientific and Cultural Organization: Paris, France, 2017.

6. Rodriguez-Mozaz, S.; Chamorro, S.; Marti, E.; Huerta, B.; Gros, M.; SànchezMelsió, A.; Borrego, C.M.; Barceló, D.; Balcázar, J.L. Occurrence of antibiotics and antibiotic resistance genes in hospital and urban wastewaters and their impact on the receiving river. *Water Res.* **2015**, *69*, 234–242. [CrossRef] [PubMed]

7. Zhou, H.; Smith, D.W. Advanced technologies in water and wastewater treatment. *J. Environ. Eng. Sci.* **2002**, *1*, 247–264. [CrossRef]

8. Thapar, N.; Sanderson, I.R. Diarrhoea in children: An interface between developing and developed countries. *Lancet* **2004**, *363*, 641–653. [CrossRef]

9. Li, Z.; Jennings, A. Worldwide Regulations of Standard Values of Pesticides for Human Health Risk Control: A Review. *Int. J. Environ. Res. Public Health* **2017**, *14*, 7. [CrossRef] [PubMed]

10. Ramalingam, K.; Ramarani, S. Pathogenic changes due to inoculation of gram-negative bacteria Pseudomonas aeruginosa (MTCC 1688) on host tissue proteins and enzymes of the giant freshwater prawn, Macrobrachium rosenbergii (De Man). *J. Environ. Biol.* **2006**, *27*, 199–205.

11. Alam, M.; Chowdhury, W.B.; Bhuiyan, N.A.; Islam, A.; Hasan, N.A.; Nair, G.B.; Watanabe, H.; Siddique, A.K.; Huq, A.; Sack, R.B.; et al. Serogroup, virulence, and genetic traits of Vibrio parahaemolyticus in the estuarine ecosystem of Bangladesh. *Appl. Environ. Microbiol.* **2009**, *75*, 6268–6274. [CrossRef] [PubMed]

12. Johnson, C.N.; Bowers, J.C.; Griffitt, K.J.; Molina, V.; Clostio, R.W.; Pei, S.; Laws, E.; Paranjpye, R.N.; Strom, M.S.; Chen, A.; et al. Ecology of *Vibrio parahaemolyticus* and *Vibrio vulnificus* in the coastal and estuarine waters of Louisiana, Maryland, Mississippi, and Washington (United States). *Appl. Environ. Microbiol.* **2012**, *78*, 7249–7257. [CrossRef] [PubMed]

13. Austin, B.; Austin, D.; Sutherland, R.; Thompson, F.; Swings, J. Pathogenicity of vibrios to rainbow trout (Oncorhynchus mykiss, Walbaum) and Artemia nauplii. *Environ. Microbiol.* **2005**, *7*, 1488–1495. [CrossRef] [PubMed]

14. Scallan, E.; Hoekstra, R.; Angulo, F.J.; Tause, R.V.; Widdowson, M.A.; Roy, S.L. Foodborne illness acquired in the United States—Major pathogens. *Emerg. Infect. Dis.* **2011**, *17*, 7–15. [CrossRef] [PubMed]

15. Lee, S.K.; Wang, H.Z.; Law, S.H.; Wu, R.S.; Kong, R.Y. Analysis of the 16S-23S rDNA intergenic spacers (IGSs) of marine vibrios for species-specific signature DNA sequences. *Mar. Pollut. Bull.* **2002**, *44*, 412–420. [CrossRef]

16. Todar, K. *Vibrio cholerae* and Asiatic Cholera. Available online: http://textbookofbacteriology.net/cholera.html (accessed on 11 October 2015).

17. Dechet, A.M.; Yu, P.A.; Koram, N.; Painter, J. Non-foodborne Vibrio infections: An important cause of morbidity and mortality in the United States, 1997–2006. *Clin. Infect. Dis.* **2008**, *46*, 970–976. [CrossRef] [PubMed]

18. Hassan, Z.H.; Zwartkruis-Nahuis, J.T.M.; de Boer, E. Occurrence of Vibrio parahaemolyticus in retailed seafood in the Netherlands. *Int. Food Res. J.* **2012**, *19*, 39–43.

19. Hoffmann, M.; Brown, E.W.; Feng, P.C.; Keys, C.E.; Fischer, M.; Monday, S.R. PCR-based method for targeting 16S-23S rRNA intergenic spacer regions among Vibrio species. *BMC Microbiol.* **2010**, *10*, 90. [CrossRef] [PubMed]

20. Pruzzo, C.; Huq, A.; Colwell, R.R.; Donelli, G. Pathogenic Vibrio species in the marine and estuarine environment. In *Ocean and Health Pathogens in the Marine Environment*; Belkin, S., Colwell, R.R., Eds.; Springer: New York, NY, USA, 2005; pp. 217–252.

21. Cazorla, C.; Guigon, A.; Noel, M.; Quilici, M.L.; Lacassin, F. Fatal *Vibrio vulnificus* Infections associated with Eating Raw Oysters, New Caledonia. *Emerg. Infect. Dis.* **2011**, *17*, 136–137. [CrossRef] [PubMed]

22. Newton, A.; Kendall, M.; Vugia, D.J.; Henao, O.L.; Mahon, B.E. Increasing rates of vibriosis in the United States, 1996–2010: Review of surveillance data from 2 systems. *Clin. Infect. Dis.* **2012**, *54*, S391–S395. [CrossRef] [PubMed]

23. Bhattacharjee, S.; Bal, B.; Pal, R.; Niyogi, S.K.; Sarkar, K. Is *Vibrio fluvialis* emerging as a pathogen with epidemic potential in coastal region of eastern India following cyclone Aila? *J. Health Popul. Nutr.* **2010**, *28*, 311–317. [PubMed]

24. Centers for Disease Control and Prevention. Cholera in Africa. Available online: https://www.cdc.gov/cholera/africa/index.html (accessed on 27 August 2017).

25. Liang, P.; Cui, X.; Du, X.; Kan, B.; Liang, W. The virulence phenotypes and molecular epidemiological characteristics of *Vibrio fluvialis* in China. *Gut Pathog.* **2013**, *5*, 6. [CrossRef] [PubMed]

26. Farmer, J.J., III; Hickman-Brenner, F.W. The genera *Vibrio* and Photobacterium. In *The Prokaryotes. A Handbook on the Biology of Bacteria: Ecophysiology, Isolation, Identification, and Applications*, 2nd ed.; Balows, A., Trüper, H.G., Dworkin, M., Harder, W., Schleifer, K.H., Eds.; Springer: Berlin, Germany, 1992; pp. 2952–3011.

27. Cano-Gómez, A.; Goulden, E.F.; Owens, L.; Høj, L. *Vibrio owensii* sp. nov., isolated from cultured crustaceans in Australia. *FEMS Microbiol. Lett.* **2010**, *302*, 175–181. [CrossRef] [PubMed]

28. Igbinosa, E.O.; Okoh, A.I. *Vibrio fluvialis*: An unusual enteric pathogen of increasing public health concern. *Int. J. Environ. Res. Public Health* **2010**, *7*, 3628–3643. [CrossRef] [PubMed]

29. Farmer, J.J., III; Janda, J.M.; Brenner, F.W.; Cameron, D.N.; Birkhead, K.M. Genus 1. *Vibrio* Pacini 1854, 411AL. In *Bergey's Manual of Systematic Bacteriology*, 2nd ed.; The Proteobacteria Part B The Gammaproteobacteria ed.; Brenner, D.J., Krieg, N.R., Staley, J.T., Eds.; Springer: New York, NY, USA, 2005; Volume 2, pp. 494–546.

30. Farmer, J.J.; Janda, J.M.; Birkhead, K. "*Vibrio*". In *Manual of Clinical Microbiology*; Murray, P.R., Ed.; ASM Press: Washington, DC, USA, 2003; pp. 706–718.

31. Ripabelli, G.; Sammarco, M.L.; Grasso, G.M.; Fanelli, I.; Caprioli, A.; Luzzi, I. Occurrence of *Vibrio* and other pathogenic bacteria in Mytilus galloprovincialis (mussels) harvested from Adriatic Sea, Italy. *J. Food Microbiol.* **1999**, *49*, 43–48. [CrossRef]

32. Dryselius, R.; Kurokawa, K.; Iida, T. Vibrionaceae, a versatile bacterial family with evolutionarily conserved variability. *Res. Microbiol.* **2007**, *158*, 479–486. [CrossRef] [PubMed]

33. Lai, C.J.; Chen, S.Y.; Lin, I.H.; Chang, C.H.; Wong, H.C. Change of protein profiles in the induction of the viable but nonculturable state of Vibrio parahaemolyticus. *Int. J. Food Microbiol.* **2009**, *135*, 118–124. [CrossRef] [PubMed]

34. Salter, I.; Zubkov, M.V.; Warwick, P.E.; Burkill, P.H. Marine bacterioplankton can increase evaporation and gas transfer by metabolizing insoluble surfactants from the air-seawater interface. *FEMS Microbiol. Lett.* **2009**, *294*, 225–231. [CrossRef] [PubMed]

35. Alderkamp, A.C.; Van Rijssel, M.; Bolhuis, H. Characterization of marine bacteria and the activity of their enzyme systems involved in degradation of the algal storage glucan laminarin. *FEMS Microbiol. Ecol.* **2007**, *59*, 108–117. [CrossRef] [PubMed]

36. Murray, A.E.; Arnosti, C.; De La Rocha, C.L.; Grossart, H.P.; Passow, U. Microbial dynamics in autotrophic and heterotrophic seawater mesocosms. II. Bacterioplankton community structure and hydrolytic enzyme activities. *Aquat. Microb. Ecol.* **2007**, *49*, 123–141. [CrossRef]

37. Denner, E.B.M.; Vybiral, D.; Fischer, U.R.; Velimirov, B.; Busse, H.J. *Vibrio calviensis* sp. nov., a halophilic, facultatively oligotrophic 0.2 micron-filterable marine bacterium. *Int. J. Syst. Evol. Microbiol.* **2002**, *52*, 549–553. [CrossRef] [PubMed]

38. Sridhar, M.; Sridhar, N.; Robertson, P.A.W.; Austin, B. Role of gut probionts in enhancing growth and disease resistance in rainbow trout (Oncorhynchus mykiss, Walbaum) fingerlings. *Asian Fisher. Sci.* **2006**, *19*, 1–13.

39. Tortora, G.J.; Funke, B.R.; Case, C.L. *Microbiology an Introduction 11th Edition*; Pearson Education, Inc.: London, UK, 2013.

40. Elliot, E.L.; Kaysner, C.A.; Jackson, L.; Tamplin, M.L. *V. cholerae, V. parahaemolyticus, V. vulnificus*, and other *Vibrio* spp. Ch. 9. In *Food and Drug Administration Bacteriological Analytical Manual*, 8th ed.; (revision A), (CD-ROM version); Merker, R.L., Ed.; AOAC International: Gaithersburg, MD, USA, 1998.

41. Tantillo, G.M.; Fontanarosa, M.; Di Pinto, A.; Musti, M. A Review Updated perspectives on emerging vibrios associated with human infections. *Lett. Appl. Microbiol.* **2004**, *39*, 117–126. [CrossRef] [PubMed]

42. Bryan, P.J.; Steffan, R.J.; DePaola, A.; Foster, J.W.; Bej, A.K. Adaptive response to cold temperatures in *Vibrio vulnificus. Curr. Microbiol.* **1999**, *38*, 168–175. [CrossRef] [PubMed]

43. Spira, W.M.; Huq, A.; Ahmed, Q.S.; Saeed, Y.A. Uptake of *V. cholerae* biotype El Tor from contaminated water by water hyacinth (Eichhornia crassipes). *Appl. Environ. Microbiol.* **1981**, *42*, 550–553. [PubMed]

44. Tracz, D.M.; Backhouse, P.G.; Olson, A.B.; McCrea, J.K.; Walsh, J.A.; Ng, L.K.; Gilmour, M.W. Rapid detection of *Vibrio* species using liquid microsphere arrays and real-time PCR targeting the ftsZ locus. *J. Med. Microbiol.* **2007**, *56*, 56–65. [CrossRef] [PubMed]

45. Tendencia, E.A. The first report of *Vibrio harveyi* infection in the sea horse Hippocampus kuda Bleekers 1852 in the Philippines. *Aquac. Res.* **2004**, *3*, 1292–1294. [CrossRef]

46. Qin, Y.X.; Wang, J.; Su, Y.Q.; Wang, D.X.; Chen, X.Z. Studies on the pathogenic bacterium of ulcer disease in Epinephelus awoara. *Acta Oceanol Sin.* **2006**, *25*, 154–159.

47. Cam, D.T.V.; Hao, N.V.; Dierckens, K.; Defoirdt, T.; Boon, N.; Sorgeloos, P.; Bossier, P. Novel approach of using homoserine lactone-degrading and poly-b-hydroxybutyrate-accumulating bacteria to protect Artemia from the pathogenic effects of *Vibrio harveyi*. *Aquaculture* **2009**, *291*, 23–30.

48. Summer, J.; De Paola, A.; Osaka, K.; Karunasager, I.; Walderhaug, M.; Bowers, J. Hazard Identification, Exposure Assessment and Hazard Characterization of *Vibrio* spp. in Seafood. In *Joint FAO/WHO Activities on Risk Assessment of Microbiological Hazards in Foods*; WHO: Geneva, Switzerland, 2001; pp. 1–105.

49. Miyoshi, S. Extracellular proteolytic enzymes produced by human pathogenic *Vibrio* species. *Front. Microbiol.* **2013**, *4*, 339. [CrossRef] [PubMed]

50. Ruby, E.G. Lessons from a cooperative bacterial-animal association: The *Vibrio fischeri*—Euprymna scolopes light organ symbiosis. *Annu. Rev. Microbiol.* **1996**, *50*, 591–624. [CrossRef] [PubMed]

51. Ben-Haim, Y.; Rosenberg, E. A novel *Vibrio* sp. pathogen of the coral Pocillopora damicronis. *Mar. Biol.* **2002**, *141*, 47–55.

52. Sussman, M.; Mieog, J.C.; Doyle, J.; Victor, S.; Willis, B.; Bourne, D.G. *Vibrio* zinc-metalloprotease causes photoinactivation of coral endosymbionts and coral tissue lesions. *PLoS Biol.* **2009**, *4*, 4511. [CrossRef] [PubMed]

53. Akram, N.; Palovaara, J.; Forsberg, J.; Lindh, M.V.; Milton, D.L.; Luo, H.; Gonzalez, J.M.; Pinhassi, J. Regulation of proteorhodopsin gene expression by nutrient limitation in the marine bacterium *Vibrio* sp. AND4. *Environ. Microbiol.* **2013**, *15*, 1400–1415. [CrossRef] [PubMed]

54. Kaneko, T.; Colwell, R.R. Ecology of *Vibrio parahaemolyticus* in Chesapeake Bay. *J. Bacteriol.* **1973**, *113*, 24–32. [PubMed]

55. Vezzulli, L.; Pezzati, E.; Moreno, M.; Fabiano, M.; Pane, L.; Pruzzo, C. The *Vibrio* Sea Consortium. Benthic ecology of *Vibrio* spp. and pathogenic Vibrio species in a coastal Mediterranean environment (La Spezia Gulf, Italy). *Microb. Ecol.* **2009**, *58*, 808–818. [CrossRef] [PubMed]

56. Hood, M.A.; Winter, P.A. Attachment of *Vibrio cholerae* under various environmental conditions and to selected substrates. *FEMS Microbiol. Ecol.* **1997**, *22*, 215–223. [CrossRef]

57. Grau, B.L.; Henk, M.C.; Pettis, G.S. High-frequency phase variation of *Vibrio vulnificus* 1003: Isolation and characterization of a rugose phenotypic variant. *J. Bacteriol.* **2005**, *187*, 2519–2525. [CrossRef] [PubMed]

58. McCarter, L. The multiple identities of *Vibrio parahaemolyticus*. *J. Mol. Microbiol. Biotechnol.* **1999**, *1*, 51–57. [PubMed]

59. Lipp, E.K.; Huq, A.; Colwell, R.R. Effects of global climate on infectious disease: The cholera model. *Clin. Microbiol. Rev.* **2002**, *15*, 757–770. [CrossRef] [PubMed]

60. Thompson, J.R.; Randa, M.A.; Marcelino, L.A.; Tomita-Mitchell, A.; Lim, E.; Polz, M.F. Diversity and dynamics of a north Atlantic coastal Vibrio community. *Appl. Environ. Microbiol.* **2004**, *70*, 4103–4110. [CrossRef] [PubMed]

61. Thompson, F.L.; Gevers, D.; Thompson, C.C.; Dawyndt, P.; Naser, S.; Hoste, B.; Munn, C.B.; Swings, J. Phylogeny and molecular identification of Vibrios on the basis of multilocus sequence analysis. *Appl. Environ. Microbiol.* **2005**, *71*, 5107–5115. [CrossRef] [PubMed]

62. Riemann, L.; Azam, F. Widespread N-acetyl-D-glucosamine uptake among pelagic marine bacteria and its ecological implications. *Appl. Environ. Microbiol.* **2002**, *68*, 5554–5562. [CrossRef] [PubMed]

63. Guerrant, R.L.; Carneiro-Filho, B.A.; Dillingham, R.A. Cholera, diarrhea, and oral rehydration therapy: Triumph and indictment. *Clin. Infect. Dis.* **2003**, *37*, 398–405. [CrossRef] [PubMed]

64. Beardsley, C.; Pernthaler, J.; Wosniok, W.; Amann, R. Are readily culturable bacteria in coastal North Sea waters suppressed by selective grazing mortality? *Appl. Environ. Microbiol.* **2003**, *69*, 2624–2630. [CrossRef] [PubMed]

65. Svitil, A.L.; Chadhain, S.M.; Moore, J.A.; Kirchman, D.L. Chitin degradation proteins produced by the marine bacterium Vibno harveyi growing on different forms of chitin. *Appl. Environ. Microbiol.* **1997**, *63*, 408–413. [PubMed]
66. Sugita, H.; Matsuo, N.; Hirose, Y.; Iwato, M.; Deguchi, Y. *Vibrio* sp. strain NM10, isolated from the intestine of a Japanese coastal fish, has an inhibitory effect against Pasteurella piscicida. *Appl. Environ. Microbiol.* **1997**, *63*, 4986–4989. [PubMed]
67. Cavallo, R.A.; Stabili, L. Presence of vibrios in seawater and Mytilus galloprovincialis (Lam) from the Mar Piccolo of Taranto (Ionian Sea). *Water Res.* **2002**, *36*, 3719–3726. [CrossRef]
68. West, P.A. The human pathogenic vibrios—A public health update with environmental perspectives. *Epidemiol. Infect.* **1989**, *103*, 1–34. [CrossRef] [PubMed]
69. Hernroth, B.; Larsson, A.; Edebo, L. Influence on uptake, distribution and elimination of *Salmonella typhimurium* in the blue mussel, Mytilus edulis. *J. Shellfish Res.* **2000**, *19*, 167–174.
70. Canesi, L.; Gavioli, M.; Pruzzo, C.; Gallo, G. Bacteria-hemocyte interactions and phagocytosis in marine bivalves. *Microsc. Res. Tech.* **2002**, *57*, 469–476. [CrossRef] [PubMed]
71. Parvathi, A.; Kumar, H.S.; Karunasagar, I. Detection and enumeration of *Vibrio vulnificus* in oysters from two estuaries along the southwest coast of India, using molecular methods. *Appl. Environ. Microbiol.* **2004**, *70*, 6909–6913. [CrossRef] [PubMed]
72. Lutz, S.; Anesio, A.M.; Villar, S.E.J.; Benning, L.G. Variations of algal communities cause darkening of a Greenland glacier. *FEMS Microbiol. Ecol.* **2014**, *89*, 402–414. [CrossRef] [PubMed]
73. CDC. Recommendations for the Use of Antibiotics for the Treatment of Cholera. Available online: https://www.cdc.gov/cholera/treatment/antibiotic-treatment.html (accessed on 27 August 2017).
74. Harris, J.B.; LaRocque, R.C.; Qadri, F.; Ryan, E.T.; Calderwood, S.B. Seminar: Cholera. *Lancet* **2012**, *379*, 2466–2476. [CrossRef]
75. Chen, Y.C.; Chang, M.C.; Chuang, Y.C.; Jeang, C.L. Characterization and virulence of hemolysin III from *Vibrio vulnificus*. *Curr. Microbiol.* **2004**, *49*, 175–179. [CrossRef] [PubMed]
76. Janelidze, N.; Jaiani, E.; Lashkhi, N.; Tskhvediani, A.; Kokashvili, T.; Gvarishvili, T.; Jgenti, D.; Mikashavidze, E.; Diasamidze, R.; Narodny, S.; et al. Microbial water quality of the Georgian coastal zone of the Black Sea. *Mar. Pollut. Bull.* **2011**, *62*, 573–580. [CrossRef] [PubMed]
77. Jaiani, E.; Kokashvili, T.; Mitaishvili, N.; Elbakidze, T.; Janelidze, N.; Lashkhi, N.; Kalandadze, R.; Mikashavidze, E.; Natroshvili, G.; Whitehouse, C.A.; et al. Microbial water quality of recreational lakes near Tbilisi, Georgia. *J. Water Health* **2013**, *11*, 333–345. [CrossRef] [PubMed]
78. Arunagiri, K.; Jayashree, K.; Sivakumar, T. Isolation and identification of Vibrios from marine food resources. *Int. J. Curr. Microbiol. App Sci.* **2013**, *2*, 217–232.
79. Ramirez, G.D.; Buck, G.W.; Smith, A.K.; Gordon, K.V.; Mott, J.B. Incidence of *Vibrio vulnificus* in estuarine waters of the south Texas Coastal Bend region. *J. Appl. Microbiol.* **2009**, *107*, 2047–2053. [CrossRef] [PubMed]
80. Igbinosa, E.O.; Obi, C.L.; Okoh, A.I. Seasonal abundance and distribution of Vibrio species in the treated effluent of wastewater treatment facilities in suburban and urban communities of Eastern Cape Province, South Africa. *J. Microbiol.* **2011**, *49*, 224–232. [CrossRef] [PubMed]
81. Hsieh, J.L.; Fries, J.S.; Noble, R.T. Dynamics and predictive modelling of *Vibrio* spp. in the Neuse River Estuary, North Carolina, USA. *Environ. Microbiol.* **2008**, *10*, 57–64. [CrossRef] [PubMed]
82. Neogi, S.B.; Koch, B.P.; Schmitt-Kopplin, P.; Pohl, C.; Kattner, G.; Yamasaki, S.; Lara, R.J. Biogeochemical controls on the bacterial populations in the eastern Atlantic Ocean. *Biogeosciences* **2011**, *8*, 3747–3759. [CrossRef]
83. Oberbeckmann, S.; Fuchs, B.M.; Meiners, M.; Wichels, A.; Wiltshire, K.H.; Gerdts, G. Seasonal dynamics and modeling of a *Vibrio* community in coastal waters of the North Sea. *Microb. Ecol.* **2012**, *63*, 543–551. [CrossRef] [PubMed]
84. Lizárraga-Partida, M.L.; Mendez-Gómez, E.; Rivas-Montaño, A.M.; Vargas-Hernández, E.; Portillo-López, A.; González-Ramírez, A.R.; Huq, A.; Colwell, R.R. Association of Vibrio cholerae with plankton in coastal areas of Mexico. *Environ. Microbiol.* **2009**, *11*, 201–208. [CrossRef] [PubMed]
85. Lara, R.J.; Neogi, S.B.; Islam, S.; Mahmud, Z.H.; Islam, S.; Paul, D.; Demoz, B.B.; Yamasaki, S.; Nair, G.B.; Kattner, G. *Vibrio cholerae* in waters of the Sunderban mangrove: Relationship with biogeochemical parameters and chitin in seston size fractions. *Wetl. Ecol. Manag.* **2011**, *19*, 109–119. [CrossRef]

86. Kokashvili, T.; Elbakidze, T.; Jaiani, E.; Janelidze, N.; Kamkamidze, G.; Whitehouse, C.; Huq, A.; Tediashvili, M. Comparative phenotypic characterization of Vibrio cholerae isolates collected from aquatic environments of Georgia. *Georgian Med. News* **2013**, *224*, 55–62.

87. Kokashvili, T.; Whitehouse, C.A.; Tskhvediani, A.; Grim, C.J.; Elbakidze, T.; Mitaishvili, N.; Janelidze, N.; Jaiani, E.; Haley, B.J.; Lashkhi, N.; et al. Occurrence and diversity of clinically important Vibrio species in the aquatic environment of Georgia. *Front. Public Health* **2015**, *3*, 232. [CrossRef] [PubMed]

88. Banakar, V.; Constantin de Magny, G.; Jacobs, J.; Murtugudde, R.; Huq, A.; Wood, R.J.; Colwell, R.R. Temporal and spatial variability in the distribution of *Vibrio vulnificus* in the Chesapeake Bay: A hindcast study. *EcoHealth* **2012**, *8*, 1–12. [CrossRef] [PubMed]

89. Caburlotto, G.; Bianchi, F.; Gennari, M.; Ghidini, V.; Socal, G.; Aubry, F.B.; Bastianini, M.; Tafi, M.; Tafi, M.M. Integrated evaluation of environmental parameters influencing Vibrio occurrence in the coastal Northern Adriatic Sea (Italy) facing the Venetian lagoon. *Microb. Ecol.* **2012**, *63*, 20–31. [CrossRef] [PubMed]

90. Schijven, J.F.; de Roda Husman, A.M. Effect of climate changes on waterborne disease in the Netherlands. *Water Sci. Technol.* **2005**, *5*, 79–87.

91. Paz, S.; Bisharat, N.; Paz, E.; Kidar, O.; Cohen, D. Climate change and the emergence of *Vibrio vulnificus* disease in Israel. *Environ. Res.* **2007**, *103*, 390–396. [CrossRef] [PubMed]

92. Lama, J.R.; Seas, C.R.; León-Barúa, R.; Gotuzzo, E.; Sack, R.B. Environmental temperature, cholera, and acute diarrhoea in adults in Lima, Peru. *J. Health Popul. Nutr.* **2011**, *22*, 399–403.

93. Rodo, X.; Pascual, M.; Fuchs, G.; Faruque, A.S. ENSO and cholera: A nonstationary link related to climate change? *Proc. Natl. Acad. Sci. USA* **2002**, *99*, 12901–12906. [CrossRef] [PubMed]

94. CDC. *Vibrio Outbreak Summaries*; US Department of Health and Human Services: Atlanta, GA, USA, 2003.

95. Turner, J.W.; Good, B.; Cole, D.; Lipp, E.K. Plankton composition and environmental factors contribute to Vibrio seasonality. *ISME J.* **2009**, *3*, 1082–1092. [CrossRef] [PubMed]

96. Stauder, M.; Vezzulli, L.; Pezzati, E.; Repetto, B.; Pruzzo, C. Temperature affects *Vibrio cholerae* O1 El Tor persistence in the aquatic environment via an enhanced expression of GbpA and MSHA adhesins. *Environ. Microbiol. Rep.* **2010**, *2*, 140–144. [CrossRef] [PubMed]

97. Munro, P.D.; Barbour, A.; Birkbeck, T.H. Comparison of gut bacterial flora of start-feeding larval turbot under different conditions. *J. Appl. Bacteriol.* **1994**, *77*, 560–566. [CrossRef]

98. Amel, B.K.; Amine, B.; Amina, B. Survival of *Vibrio fluvialis* in seawater under starvation conditions. *Microbiol. Res.* **2008**, *163*, 323–328. [CrossRef] [PubMed]

99. Struyf, E.; Damme, S.V.; Meire, P. Possible effects of climate change on estuarine nutrient fluxes: A case study in the highly nitrified Schelde estuary (Belgium, The Netherlands). *Estuar. Coast. Shelf Sci.* **2004**, *52*, 131–142.

100. Constantin de Magny, G.; Mozumder, P.K.; Grim, C.J.; Hasan, N.A.; Naser, M.N.; Alam, M.; Bradley Sack, R.; Huq, A.; Colwell, R.R. Role of zooplankton diversity in *Vibrio cholerae* population dynamics and in the incidence of cholera in the Bangladesh Sundarbans. *Appl. Environ. Microbiol.* **2011**, *77*, 6125–6132. [CrossRef] [PubMed]

101. Whitehead, P.G.; Wilby, R.L.; Battarbee, R.W.; Kernan, M.; Wade, A.J. A review of the potential impacts of climate change on surface water quality. *Hydrol. Sci. J.* **2009**, *54*, 101–123. [CrossRef]

102. Colwell, R.R. Viable but nonculturable bacteria: A survival strategy. *J. Infect. Chemother.* **2000**, *6*, 121–125. [CrossRef] [PubMed]

103. Colwell, R.R. Predicting the distribution of Vibrio spp. in the Chesapeake bay: A *Vibrio cholerae* case study. *EcoHealth* **2009**, *6*, 378–389.

104. Mishra, M.; Mohammed, F.; Akulwar, S.L.; Katkar, V.J.; Tankhiwale, N.S.; Powar, R.M. Re-emergence of El Tor *Vibrio* in outbreak of cholera in and around Nagpur. *Indian J. Med. Res.* **2004**, *120*, 478–480. [PubMed]

105. White, P.A.; Rasmussen, J.B. The genotoxic hazards of domestic wastes in surface waters. *Mutat. Res.* **1998**, *460*, 223–236. [CrossRef]

106. Akselman, R.; Jurquiza, V.; Costagliola, M.C.; Fraga, S.G.; Pichel, M.; Hozbor, C.; Peressutti, S.; Binsztein, N. *Vibrio cholerae* O1 found attached to the dinoflagellate Noctiluca scintillans in Argentine shelf waters. *Mar. Biodivers. Rec.* **2010**, *3*, 120. [CrossRef]

107. Shikuma, N.J.; Hadfield, M.G. Marine biofilms on submerged surfaces are a reservoir for *Escherichia coli* and *Vibrio cholerae*. *Biofouling* **2010**, *26*, 39–46. [CrossRef] [PubMed]

108. Hall-Stoodley, L.; Costerton, J.W.; Stoodley, P. Bacterial biofilms: From the natural environment to infectious diseases. *Nat. Rev. Microbiol.* **2004**, *2*, 95–108. [CrossRef] [PubMed]

109. Faruque, S.M.; Islam, M.J.; Ahmad, Q.S.; Faruque, A.S.G.; Sack, D.A.; Nair, G.B.; Mekalanos, J.J. Self-limiting nature of seasonal cholera epidemics: Role of host-mediated amplification of phage. *Proc. Natl. Acad. Sci. USA* **2005**, *102*, 6119–6124. [CrossRef] [PubMed]

110. Janda, J.M.; Powers, C.; Bryant, R.G.; Abbott, S. Current perspectives on the epidemiology and pathogenesis of clinically significant *Vibrio* spp. *Clin. Microbiol. Rev.* **1988**, *1*, 245–267. [CrossRef] [PubMed]

111. Austin, B.; Austin, D.A.; Blanch, A.R.; Cerda, M.; Grimont, P.A.D.; Jofre, J.; Koblavi, S.; Larsen, J.L.; Pedersen, K.; Tiainen, T.; et al. A comparison of methods for the typing of fish-pathogenic *Vibrio* spp. *Syst. Appl. Microbiol.* **1997**, *20*, 89–101. [CrossRef]

112. Harrington, D.J. Bacterial collagenases and collagen-degrading enzymes and their role in human disease. *Infect. Immun.* **1996**, *64*, 1885–1891. [PubMed]

113. Huq, A.; Grim, C.; Taylor, R. Detection, Isolation, and Identification of *Vibrio cholerae* from the Environment. In *Current Protocols in Microbiology*; John Wiley & Sons: New York, NY, USA, 2006.

114. Karaolis, D.K.; Johnson, J.A.; Bailey, C.C.; Boedeker, E.C.; Kaper, J.B.; Reeves, P.R. A *Vibrio cholerae* pathogenicity island associated with epidemic and pandemic strains. *Proc. Natl. Acad. Sci. USA* **1998**, *95*, 3134–3139. [CrossRef] [PubMed]

115. Heymann, D. *Vibrio cholerae* serogroups 01 and 0139. In *Control of Communicable Diseases Manual*, 19th ed.; Am Pub Health Ass: Washington, DC, USA, 2008; pp. 120–128.

116. Vezzulli, L.; Guzmán, C.A.; Colwell, R.R.; Pruzzo, C. Dual role colonization factors connecting Vibrio cholerae's lifestyles in human and aquatic environments open new perspectives for combating infectious diseases. *Curr. Opin. Biotechnol.* **2008**, *19*, 254–259. [CrossRef] [PubMed]

117. Hang, L.; John, M.; Asaduzzaman, M.; Bridges, E.A.; Vanderspurt, C.; Kirn, T.J.; Taylor, R.K.; Hillman, J.D.; Progulske-Fox, A.; Handfield, M.; Ryan, E.T.; Calderwood, S.B. Use of in vivo-induced antigen technology (IVIAT) to identify genes uniquely expressed during human infection with *Vibrio cholerae*. *Proc. Natl. Acad. Sci. USA* **2003**, *100*, 8508–8513. [CrossRef] [PubMed]

118. Faruque, S.M.; Nair, G.B.; Mekalanos, J.J. Genetics of stress adaptation and virulence in toxigenic *Vibrio cholerae*. *DNA Cell Biol.* **2004**, *11*, 723–741. [CrossRef] [PubMed]

119. Daniels, N.A.; MacKinnon, L.; Bishop, R.; Altekruse, S.; Ray, B.; Hammond, R.M.; Thompson, S.; Wilson, S.; Bean, N.H.; Griffin, P.M.; et al. *Vibrio parahaemolyticus* infections in the United States, 1973–1998. *J. Infect. Dis.* **2000**, *181*, 1661–1666. [CrossRef] [PubMed]

120. Broberg, C.A.; Calder, T.J.; Orth, K. *Vibrio parahaemolyticus* cell biology and pathogenicity determinants. *Microbes Infect.* **2011**, *13*, 992–1001. [CrossRef] [PubMed]

121. Paranjpye, R.; Hamel, O.S.; Stojanovski, A.; Liermann, M. Genetic diversity of clinical and environmental *Vibrio parahaemolyticus* strains from the Pacific Northwest. *Appl. Environ. Microbiol.* **2012**, *78*, 8631–8638. [CrossRef] [PubMed]

122. Zhang, L.; Orth, K. Virulence determinants for *Vibrio parahaemolyticus* infection. *Curr. Opin. Microbiol.* **2013**, *16*, 70–77. [CrossRef] [PubMed]

123. Zhang, X.H.; Austin, B. A Review Haemolysins in *Vibrio* species. *J. Appl. Microbiol.* **2005**, *98*, 1011–1019. [CrossRef] [PubMed]

124. Makino, K.; Oshima, K.; Kurokawa, K.; Yokoyama, K.; Uda, T.; Tagomori, K.; Iijima, Y.; Najima, M.; Nakano, M.; Yamashita, A.; et al. Genome sequence of *Vibrio parahaemolyticus*: A pathogenic mechanism distinct from that of *V. cholerae*. *Lancet* **2003**, *361*, 743–749. [CrossRef]

125. Liu, H. Analysis of the collective food poisoning events in Shanghai from 1990 to 2000. *Chin. J. Nat. Med.* **2003**, *5*, 17–20.

126. McCarthy, S.A.; DePaola, A.; Cook, D.W.; Kaysner, C.A.; Hill, W.E. Evaluation of alkaline phosphatase- and digoxigenin-labelled probes for detection of the thermolabile hemolysin (tlh) gene of *Vibrio parahaemolyticus*. *Lett. Appl. Microbiol.* **1999**, *28*, 66–70. [CrossRef] [PubMed]

127. Wang, L.; Shi, L.; Su, J.Y.; Ye, Y.X.; Zhong, Q.P. Detection of *Vibrio parahaemolyticus* in food samples using in situ loop-mediated isothermal amplification method. *Gene* **2013**, *515*, 421–425. [CrossRef] [PubMed]

128. Bej, A.K.; Patterson, D.P.; Brasher, C.W.; Vicker, M.C.L.; Jones, D.D.; Kaysner, C.A. Detection of total and hemolysin-producing *Vibrio parahaemolyticus* in shellfish using multiplex PCR amplification of tl, tdh and trh. *J. Microbiol. Methods* **1999**, *36*, 215–225. [CrossRef]

129. Gotoh, K.; Kodama, T.; Hiyoshi, H.; Izutsu, K.; Park, K.S.; Dryselius, R.; Akeda, Y.; Honda, T.; Iida, T. Bile acid-induced virulence gene expression of Vibrio parahaemolyticus reveals a novel therapeutic potential for bile acid sequestrants. *PLoS ONE* **2010**, *5*, 13365. [CrossRef] [PubMed]

130. Gulig, P.A.; Bourdage, K.L.; Starks, A.M. Molecular pathogenesis of *Vibrio vulnificus*. *J. Microbiol.* **2005**, *43*, 118–131. [PubMed]

131. Chowdhury, G.; Pazhani, G.P.; Dutta, D.; Guin, S.; Dutta, S.; Ghosh, S.; Izumiya, H.; Asakura, M.; Yamasaki, S.; Takeda, Y.; et al. *Vibrio fluvialis* in patients with diarrhea, Kolkata, India. *Emerg. Infect. Dis.* **2012**, *18*, 1868–1871. [CrossRef] [PubMed]

132. Strom, M.S.; Paranjpye, R.N. Epidemiology and pathogenesis of *Vibrio vulnificus*. *Microb. Infect.* **2000**, *2*, 177–188. [CrossRef]

133. Scoglio, M.E.; Di Pietro, A.; Picerno, I.; Delia, S.; Mauro, A.; Lagana, P. Virulence factors in Vibrios and Aeromonads isolated from seafood. *New Microbiol.* **2001**, *24*, 273–280. [PubMed]

134. Di Pietro, A.; Picerno, I.; Visalli, G.; Chirico, C.; Scoglio, M.E. Effects of "host factor" bile on adaptability and virulence of vibrios, foodborne potential pathogenic agents. *Ann. Ig.* **2004**, *16*, 615–625. [PubMed]

135. Rahman, M.M.; Qadri, F.; Albert, M.J.; Hossain, A.; Mosihuzzaman, M. Lipopolysaccharide composition and virulence properties of clinical and environmental strains of *Vibrio fluvialis* and *Vibrio mimicus*. *Microbiol. Immunol.* **1992**, *36*, 327–338. [CrossRef] [PubMed]

136. Wong, H.C.; Ting, S.H.; Shieh, W.R. Incidence of toxigenic vibrios in foods available in Taiwan. *J. Appl. Bacteriol.* **1992**, *73*, 197–202. [CrossRef] [PubMed]

137. Venkateswaran, K.; Kiiyukia, C.; Takak, M.; Nakano, H.; Matsuda, H.; Kawakami, H.; Hashimoto', H. Characterization of toxigenic vibrios isolated from the freshwater environment of Hiroshima, Japan. *Appl. Environ. Microbiol.* **1989**, *55*, 2613–2618. [PubMed]

138. Janda, J.M. Mucinase activity among selected members of the family Vibrionaceae. *Microb. Lett.* **1986**, *33*, 19–22.

139. Han, J.H.; Lee, J.H.; Choi, Y.H.; Park, J.H.; Choi, T.J.; Kong, I.S. Purification, characterization and molecular cloning of *Vibrio fluvialis* hemolysin. *Biochim. Biophys. Acta* **2002**, *1599*, 106–114. [CrossRef]

140. Kothary, M.H.; Lowman, H.; McCardell, B.A.; Tall, B.D. Purification and characterization of enterotoxigenic El Tor-like hemolysin produced by Vibrio fluvialis. *Infect. Immun.* **2003**, *71*, 3213–3220. [CrossRef] [PubMed]

141. Lockwood, D.E.; Kreger, A.S.; Richardson, S.H. Detection of toxins produced by *Vibrio fluvialis*. *Infect. Immun.* **1982**, *35*, 702–708. [PubMed]

142. Thompson, J.R.; Polz, M.F. Dynamics of Vibrio populations and their role in environmental nutrient cycling. In *The Biology of Vibrios*; Thompson, F.L., Austin, B., Swings, J., Eds.; ASM Press: Washington, DC, USA, 2006; pp. 190–203.

143. Igomu, T. Cholera Epidemic: Far from Being over. NBF News. Available online: www.nigerianbestforum. com/blog/?p=60321 (accessed on 23 August 2011).

144. Nevondo, T.S.; Cloete, T.E. Bacterial and chemical quality of water supply in the Dertig village settlement. *Water S. Afr.* **1999**, *25*, 215–220.

145. Mackintosh, G.; Colvin, C. Failure of rural schemes in South Africa to provide potable water. *Environ. Geol.* **2003**, *44*, 101–105.

146. Obi, C.L.; Bessong, P.O.; Momba, M.N.B.; Potegieter, N.; Samie, A.; Igumbor, E.O. Profile of antibiotic susceptibilities of bacterial isolates and physicochemical quality of water supply in rural Venda communities of South Africa. *Water SA* **2004**, *30*, 515–520. [CrossRef]

147. Qadri, F.; Chowdhury, N.R.; Takeda, Y.; Nair, G.B. Vibrio parahaemolyticus—Seafood safety and associations with higher organisms. In *Oceans and Health: Pathogens in the Marine Environment*; Springer: Berlin, Germany, 2005; pp. 277–295.

148. WHO. *Yemen Cholera Situation Report no. 4 19 JULY, 2017*; World Health Organization: Geneva, Switzerland, 2017.

149. Sur, D. Severe cholera outbreak following floods in a northern district of West Bengal. *Indian J. Med. Res.* **2000**, *112*, 178–182. [PubMed]

150. Quilici, M.L. *Vibrio cholerae* O1 Variant with Reduced Susceptibility to Ciprofloxacin, Western Africa. *Emerg. Infect. Dis.* **2010**, *16*, 1804–1805. [CrossRef] [PubMed]

151. Abia, A.L.K.; Ubomba-Jaswa, E.; Momba, M.N.B. Riverbed Sediments as Reservoirs of Multiple Vibrio cholerae Virulence-Associated Genes: A Potential Trigger for Cholera Outbreaks in Developing Countries. *J. Environ. Public Health* **2017**, *2017*, 9. [CrossRef] [PubMed]

152. UNICEF. *WCAR Epidemiological Updates*; The United Nations Children's Fund: New York, NY, USA, 2016.

153. Abia, A.L.K.; Ubomba-Jaswa, E.; Genthe, B.; Momba, M.N.B. Quantitative microbial risk assessment (QMRA) shows increased public health risk associated with exposure to river water under conditions of riverbed sediment resuspension. *Sci. Total Environ.* **2016**, *566*, 1143–1151. [CrossRef] [PubMed]

154. Marin, M.A.; Thompson, C.C.; Freitas, F.S.; Fonseca, E.L.; Aboderin, A.O.; Zailani, S.B.; Quartey, N.K.E.; Okeke, I.N.; Vicente, A.C.P. Cholera outbreaks in Nigeria are associated with multidrug resistant atypical El Tor and non-O1/non-O139 Vibrio cholerae. *PLoS Negl. Trop. Dis.* **2013**, *7*, 2049. [CrossRef] [PubMed]

155. Engel, M.F.; Muijsken, M.A.; Mooi-Kokenberg, E.; Kuijper, E.J.; van Westerloo, D.J. Vibrio cholerae non-O1 bacteraemia: Description of three cases in The Netherlands and a literature review. *Eur. Surveill.* **2016**, *21*, 30197. [CrossRef] [PubMed]

156. Li, M.; Shimada, T.; Morris, J.G.; Sulakvelidze, A.; Sozhamannan, S. Evidence for the emergence of non-O1 and non-O139 Vibrio cholerae strains with pathogenic potential by exchange of O-antigen biosynthesis regions. *Infect. Immun.* **2002**, *70*, 2441–2453. [CrossRef] [PubMed]

157. Montilla, R.; Chowdhury, M.A.; Huq, A.; Xu, B.; Colwell, R.R. Serogroup conversion of *Vibrio cholerae* non-O1 to *Vibrio cholerae* O1: Effect of growth state of cells, temperature and salinity. *Can. J. Microbiol.* **1996**, *42*, 87–93. [CrossRef] [PubMed]

158. Blokesch, M.; Schoolnik, G.K. Serogroup conversion of Vibrio cholerae in aquatic reservoirs. *PLoS Pathog.* **2007**, *3*, 2007. [CrossRef] [PubMed]

159. Huq, A.; Colwell, R.R.; Rahman, R.; Ali, A.; Chowdhury, M.A.; Parveen, S.; Sack, D.A.; Russek-Cohen, E. Detection of *Vibrio cholerae* O1 in the aquatic environment by fluorescent-monoclonal antibody and culture methods. *Appl. Environ. Microbiol.* **1990**, *56*, 2370–2373. [PubMed]

160. Srinivasan, V.B.; Virk, R.K.; Kaundal, A.; Chakraborty, R.; Datta, B.; Ramamurthy, T.; Mukhopadhyay, A.K.; Ghosh, A. Mechanism of drug resistance in clonally related clinical isolates of *Vibrio fluvialis* isolated in Kolkata, India. *Antimicrob. Agents Chemother.* **2006**, *50*, 2428–2432. [CrossRef] [PubMed]

161. Igbinosa, E.O.; Obi, L.C.; Okoh, A.I. Occurrence of potentially pathogenic vibrios in final effluents of a wastewater treatment facility in a rural community of the Eastern Cape Province of South Africa. *Res. Microbiol.* **2009**, *160*, 531–537. [CrossRef] [PubMed]

162. Kobayashi, K.; Ohnaka, T. Food poisoning due to newly recognized pathogens. *Asian Med. J.* **1989**, *32*, 1–12.

163. Levine, W.C.; Griffin, P.M. *Vibrio* infections on the Gulf Coast: Results of first year of regional surveillance Gulf Coast Vibrio Working Group. *J. Infect. Dis.* **1993**, *167*, 479–483. [CrossRef] [PubMed]

164. Hollis, D.G.; Weave, R.E.; Baker, C.N.; Thornsberry, C. Halophilic *Vibrio* species isolated from blood cultures. *J. Clin. Microbiol.* **1976**, *3*, 425–431. [PubMed]

165. Blake, P.A.; Weaver, R.E.; Hollis, D.G. Diseases of humans (other than cholera) caused by vibrios. *Annu. Rev. Microbiol.* **1980**, *34*, 341–367. [CrossRef] [PubMed]

166. Morris, J.G., Jr.; Black, R.E. Cholera and other vibrioses in the United States. *New Engl. J. Med.* **1985**, *312*, 343–350. [CrossRef] [PubMed]

167. Baker-Austin, C.; McArthur, J.V.; Tuckfield, R.C.; Najarro, M.; Lindell, A.H.; Gooch, J.; Stepanauskas, R. Antibiotic resistance in the shellfish pathogen Vibrio parahaemolyticus isolated from the coastal water and sediment of Georgia and South Carolina, USA. *J. Food Prot.* **2008**, *71*, 2552–2558. [CrossRef] [PubMed]

168. Zaidenstein, R.; Sadik, C.; Lerner, L.; Valinsky, L.; Kopelowitz, J.; Yishai, R.; Agmon, V.; Parsons, M.; Bopp, C.; Weinberger, M. Clinical characteristics and molecular subtyping of *Vibrio vulnificus* illnesses, Israel. *Emerg. Infect. Dis.* **2008**, *14*, 1875–1882. [CrossRef] [PubMed]

169. Okuda, J.; Ishibashi, M.; Abbott, S.; Janda, J.; Nishibuchi, M. Analysis of the thermostable direct hemolysin (tdh) gene and the tdh-related hemolysin (trh) genes in urease-positive strains of *Vibrio parahaemolyticus* isolated on the West Coast of the United States. *J. Clin. Microbiol.* **1997**, *35*, 1965–1971. [PubMed]

170. Fujino, T.; Okuno, Y.; Nakada, D.; Aoyama, A.; Fukai, K.; Mukai, T.; Ueho, T. On the bacteriological examination of shirasu-food poisoning. *Med. J. Osaka Univ.* **1953**, *4*, 299–304.

171. Su, Y.C.; Liu, C.C. *Vibrio parahaemolyticus*: A concern of seafood safety. *Food microbiol.* **2007**, *24*, 549–558. [CrossRef] [PubMed]

172. Letchumanan, V.; Chan, K.; Lee, L. *Vibrio parahaemolyticus*: A review on the pathogenesis, prevalence and advance molecular identification techniques. *Front. Microbiol.* **2014**, *5*, 705. [CrossRef] [PubMed]

173. Wang, L.P.; Chen, Y.W.; Huang, H.; Huang, Z.B.; Chen, H.; Shao, Z.Z. Isolation and identification of *Vibrio campbellii* as a bacterial pathogen for luminous vibriosis of Litopenaeus vannamei. *Aquac. Res.* **2015**, *46*, 395–404. [CrossRef]

174. Kaysner, C.A.; DePaola, A. *Vibrio* . In *Bacteriological Analytical Manual*, 8th ed.; Revision, A., Ed.; U.S. Food and Drug Administration: Arlington, VA, USA, 2001; Chapter 9.

175. Joseph, S.W.; Colwell, R.R.; Kaper, J.B. *Vibrio parahaemolyticus* and related halophilic Vibrios. *Crit. Rev. Microbiol.* **1982**, *10*, 77–124. [CrossRef] [PubMed]

176. Yeung, M.; Boor, K. Epidemiology, Pathogenesis, and Prevention of Foodborne *Vibrio parahaemolyticus* Infections. *Foodborne Pathog. Dis.* **2004**, *1*, 74–88. [CrossRef] [PubMed]

177. Nair, G.B.; Ramamurthy, T.; Bhattacharya, S.K.; Dutta, B.; Takeda, Y.; Sack, D.A. Global dissemination of Vibrio parahaemolyticus serotype O3:K6 and its serovariants. *Clin. Microbiol. Rev.* **2007**, *20*, 39–48. [CrossRef] [PubMed]

178. Alam, M.J.; Tomochika, K.I.; Miyoshi, S.I.; Shinoda, S. Environmental investigation of potentially pathogenic *Vibrio parahaemolyticus* in the Seto-Inland Sea, Japan. *FEMS Microbiol. Lett.* **2002**, *208*, 83–87. [CrossRef] [PubMed]

179. Koralage, M.; Alter, T.; Pichpol, D.; Strauch, E.; Zessin, K.; Huehn, S. Prevalence and molecular characteristics of *Vibrio* spp. isolated from preharvest shrimp of the North Western Province of Sri Lanka. *J. Food Prot.* **2012**, *75*, 1846–1850. [CrossRef] [PubMed]

180. Yu, W.T.; Jong, K.J.; Lin, Y.R.; Tsai, S.E.; Tey, Y.H.; Wong, H.C. Prevalence of *Vibrio parahaemolyticus* in oyster and clam culturing environments in Taiwan. *Int. J. Food Microbiol.* **2013**, *160*, 185–192. [CrossRef] [PubMed]

181. Adeleye, I.A.; Daniels, F.V.; Enyinnia, V.A. Characterization and pathogenicity of *Vibrio* spp. contaminating seafoods In Lagos, Nigeria. *Int. J. Food Saf.* **2010**, *1*, 1–9.

182. CDC. *National Enteric Disease Surveillance: COVIS Annual Summary*; Centers for Disease Control and Prevention. Department of Health and Human Services: Atlanta, GA, USA, 2014.

183. Saga, T.; Kaku, M.; Onodera, Y.; Yamachika, S.; Sato, K.; Takase, H. *Vibrio parahaemolyticus* chromosomal qnr homologue VPA0095: Demonstration by transformation with a mutated gene of its potential to reduce quinolone susceptibility in Escherichia coli. *Antimicrob. Agents Chemother.* **2005**, *49*, 2144–2145. [CrossRef] [PubMed]

184. Aminov, R.I. Horizontal gene exchange in environmental microbiota. *Front. Microbiol.* **2011**, *2*, 158. [CrossRef] [PubMed]

185. Carlet, J.; Collignon, P.; Goldmann, D.; Goossens, H.; Gyssens, I.C.; Harbarth, S.; Jarlier, V.; Levy, S.B.; N'Doye, B.; Pittet, D.; et al. Society's failure to protect a precious resource: Antibiotics. *Lancet* **2011**, *378*, 369–371. [CrossRef]

186. Finley, R.L.; Collignon, P.; Larsson, J.D.G.; McEwen, S.A.; Li, X.Z.; Gaze, W.H.; Reid-Smith, R.; Timinouni, M.; Graham, D.W.; Topp, E. The scourge of antibiotic resistance: The important role of the environment. *Clin. Infect. Dis.* **2013**, *57*, 704–710. [CrossRef] [PubMed]

187. Shears, P. Recent developments in cholera. *Curr. Opin. Infect. Dis.* **2001**, *14*, 553–558. [CrossRef] [PubMed]

188. CLSI. Clinical and laboratory standards institute. In *Methods for Antimicrobial Dilution and Disk Susceptibility Testing of Infrequently Isolated or Fastidious Bacteria; Approved Guideline-Second Edition. CLSI Document M45-A2*; Clinical and Laboratory Standards Institute: Wayne, PA, USA, 2010; pp. 1087–1898.

189. Crowther-Gibson, P.; Govender, N.; Lewis, D.A.; Bamford, C.; Brink, A.; von Gottberg, A.; Klugman, K.; du Plessis, M.; Fali, A.; Harris, B.; et al. Part IV. GARP: Human infections and antibiotic resistance. *SAM J.* **2011**, *101*, 567–578.

190. Slama, T.G.; Amin, A.; Brunton, S.A. A clinician's guide to the appropriate and accurate use of antibiotics: The Council for Appropriate and Rational Antibiotic Therapy (CARAT) criteria. *Am. J. Med.* **2005**, *118*, 1–6. [CrossRef] [PubMed]

191. Ansari, M.; Raissy, M. In vitro susceptibility of commonly used antibiotics against *Vibrio* spp. isolated from Lobster (*Panulirus homarus*). *Afr. J. Microbiol. Res.* **2010**, *4*, 2629–2631.

192. Saga, T.; Yamaguchi, K. History of antimicrobial agents and resistant bacteria. *JMJA* **2009**, *52*, 103–108.

193. World Health Organization (WHO). Cholera, Wkly. *Epidemiol. Rec.* **2013**, *89*, 345–356.

194. Sudha, S.; Mridula, C.; Silvester, R.; Hatha, A.A.M. Prevalence and antibiotic resistance of pathogenic Vibrios in shellfishes from Cochin market. *Indian J. Mar. Sci.* **2014**, *43*, 815–824.

195. Singer, A.C.; Colizza, V.; Schmitt, H.; Andrews, J.; Balcan, D.; Huang, W.E.; Keller, V.D.J.; Vespignani, A.; Williams, R.J. Assessing the ecotoxicologic hazards of a pandemic influenza medical response. *Environ. Health Perspect.* **2011**, *119*, 1084–1090. [CrossRef] [PubMed]

196. Zhang, Q.Q.; Ying, G.G.; Pan, C.G.; Liu, Y.S.; Zhao, J.L. Comprehensive evaluation of antibiotics emission and fate in the river basins of China: Source analysis, multimedia modeling, and linkage to bacterial resistance. *Environ. Sci. Technol.* **2015**, *49*, 6772–6782. [CrossRef] [PubMed]

197. Verlicchi, P.; Zambello, E. Predicted and measured concentrations of pharmaceuticals in hospital effluents. Examination of the strengths and weaknesses of the two approaches through the analysis of a case study. *Sci. Total Environ.* **2016**, *565*, 82–94. [CrossRef] [PubMed]

198. Chen, C.E.; Zhang, H.; Ying, G.G.; Zhou, L.J.; Jones, K.C. Passive sampling: A cost-effective method for understanding antibiotic fate, behaviour and impact. *Environ. Int.* **2015**, *85*, 284–291. [CrossRef] [PubMed]

199. Li, B.; Zhang, T. Biodegradation and adsorption of antibiotics in the activated sludge process. *Environ. Sci. Technol.* **2010**, *44*, 3468–3473. [CrossRef] [PubMed]

200. Ahmed, M.B.; Zhou, J.L.; Ngo, H.H.; Guo, W. Adsorptive removal of antibiotics from water and wastewater: Progress and challenges. *Sci. Total Environ.* **2015**, *532*, 112–126. [CrossRef] [PubMed]

201. Rivera-Utrilla, J.; Sánchez-Polo, M.; Ferro-García, M.Á.; Prados-Joya, G.; Ocampo-Pérez, R. Pharmaceuticals as emerging contaminants and their removal from water. *Rev. Chemosphere* **2013**, *93*, 1268–1287. [CrossRef] [PubMed]

202. Luo, Y.; Guo, W.; Ngo, H.H.; Nghiem, L.D.; Hai, F.I.; Zhang, J.; Liang, S.; Wang, X.C. A review on the occurrence of micropollutants in the aquatic environment and their fate and removal during wastewater treatment. *Sci. Total Environ.* **2014**, *47*, 619–641. [CrossRef] [PubMed]

203. Gardner, M.; Jones, V.; Comber, S.; Scrimshaw, M.D.; Coello-Garcia, T.; Cartmell, E.; Lester, J.; Ellor, B. Performance of UK wastewater treatment works with respect to trace contaminants. *Sci. Total Environ.* **2013**, *45*, 359–369. [CrossRef] [PubMed]

204. Berendsen, B.J.A.; Wegh, R.S.; Memelink, J.; Zuidema, T.; Stolker, L.A.M. The analysis of animal faeces as a tool to monitor antibiotic usage. *Talanta* **2015**, *132*, 258–268. [CrossRef] [PubMed]

205. Udikovic-Kolic, N.; Wichmann, F.; Broderick, N.A.; Handelsman, J. Bloom of resident antibiotic-resistant bacteria in soil following manure fertilization. *Proc. Natl. Acad. Sci. USA* **2014**, *111*, 15202–15207. [CrossRef] [PubMed]

206. Wichmann, F.; Udikovic-Kolic, N.; Andrew, S.; Handelsman, J. Diverse antibiotic resistance genes in dairy cow manure. *MBio* **2014**, *5*, 01017. [CrossRef] [PubMed]

207. Lima, A.A. Tropical diarrhea: New developments in traveler's diarrhea. *Curr. Opin. Infect. Dis.* **2001**, *14*, 547–552. [CrossRef] [PubMed]

208. Laganà, P.; Caruso, G.; Minutoli, E.; Zaccone, R.; Santi, D. Susceptibility to antibiotics of *Vibrio* spp. and Photobacterium damsela ssp. Piscicida strains isolated from Italian aquaculture farms. *New Microbiol.* **2011**, *34*, 53–63. [PubMed]

209. Kitaoka, M.; Miyata, S.T.; Unterweger, D.; Pukatzki, S. Antibiotic resistance mechanisms of *Vibrio cholerae*. *J. Med. Microbiol.* **2011**, *60*, 397–407. [CrossRef] [PubMed]

210. Cabello, F.C.; Godfrey, H.P.; Tomova, A.; Ivanova, L.; Dölz, H.; Millanao, A.; Buschmann, A.H. Antimicrobial use in aquaculture re-examined: Its relevance to antimicrobial resistance and to animal and human health. *Appl. Eviron. Microbiol.* **2013**, *15*, 1917–1942. [CrossRef] [PubMed]

211. Letchumanan, V.; Chan, K.G.; Lee, L.H. An insight of traditional plasmid curing in *Vibrio* species. *Front. Microbiol.* **2015**, *6*, 735. [CrossRef] [PubMed]

212. Shrestha, T.U.; Adhikari, N.; Maharjan, R.; Banjara, M.R.; Rijal, K.R.; Basnyat, S.R.; Agrawal, V.P. Multidrug resistant *Vibrio cholerae* O1 from clinical and environmental samples in Kathmandu city. *BMC Infect. Dis.* **2015**, *15*, 104. [CrossRef] [PubMed]

213. Ceccarelli, D.; Hasan, N.A.; Huq, A.; Colwell, R.R. Distribution and dynamics of epidemic and pandemic *Vibrio parahaemolyticus* virulence factors. *Front. Cell Infect. Microbiol.* **2013**, *3*, 97. [CrossRef] [PubMed]

214. Maher, M.C.; Alemayehu, W.; Lakew, T.; Gaynor, B.D.; Haug, S.; Cevallos, V.; Keenan, J.D.; Lietman, T.M.; Porco, T.C. The fitness cost of antibiotic resistance in Streptococcus pneumoniae: Insight from the field. *PLoS ONE* **2012**, *7*, 29407. [CrossRef] [PubMed]

215. Roux, D.; Danilchanka, O.; Guillard, T.; Cattoir, V.; Aschard, H.; Fu, Y.; Angoulvant, F.; Messika, J.; Ricard, J.D.; Mekalanos, J.J.; et al. Fitness cost of antibiotic susceptibility during bacterial infection. *Sci. Transl. Med.* **2015**, *7*, 297ra114. [CrossRef] [PubMed]

216. Gullberg, E.; Albrecht, L.M.; Karlsson, C.; Sandegren, L.; Andersson, D.I. Selection of a multidrug resistance plasmid by sublethal levels of antibiotics and heavy metals. *MBio* **2014**, *5*. [CrossRef] [PubMed]

217. Gifford, D.R.; Moss, E.; MacLean, R.C. Environmental variation alters the fitness effects of rifampicin resistance mutations in Pseudomonas aeruginosa. *Evolution* **2016**, *70*, 725–730. [CrossRef] [PubMed]

218. Amini, S.; Hottes, A.K.; Smith, L.E.; Tavazoie, S. Fitness landscape of antibiotic tolerance in Pseudomonas aeruginosa biofilms. *PLoS Pathog.* **2011**, *7*, 1002298. [CrossRef] [PubMed]

219. Burrus, V.; Marrero, J.; Waldor, M.K. The current ICE age: Biology and evolution of SXT-related integrating conjugative elements. *Plasmid* **2006**, *55*, 173–183. [CrossRef] [PubMed]

220. Paulsen, I.T.; Brown, M.H.; Skurray, R.A. Proton dependent multidrug efflux systems. *Microbiol. Rev.* **1996**, *60*, 575–608. [PubMed]

221. Waldor, M.K.; Mekalanos, J.J. Lysogenic conversion by a filamentous phage encoding cholera toxin. *Science* **1996**, *272*, 1910–1914. [CrossRef] [PubMed]

222. Akoachere, J.F.T.K.; Masalla, T.N.; Njom, H.A. Multi-drug resistant toxigenic *Vibrio cholerae* O1 is persistent in water sources in New Bell-Douala Cameroon. *BMC Infect. Dis.* **2013**, *13*, 366. [CrossRef] [PubMed]

223. Opintan, J.A.; Newman, M.J.; Nsiah-Poodoh, O.A.; Okeke, I.N. *Vibrio cholerae* O1 from Accra, Ghana carrying a class 2 integron and the SXT element. *J. Antimicrob. Chemother.* **2008**, *62*, 929–933. [CrossRef] [PubMed]

224. Eibach, D.; Herrera-Leon, S.; Gil, H.; Hogan, B.; Ehlkes, L.; Adjabeng, M.; Kreuels, B.; Nagel, M.; Opare, D.; Fobil, J.N.; et al. Molecular Epidemiology and Antibiotic Susceptibility of *Vibrio cholerae* Associated with a Large Cholera Outbreak in Ghana in 2014. *PLoS Negl. Trop. Dis.* **2016**, *10*, 4751. [CrossRef] [PubMed]

225. Mandomando, I.; Espasa, M.; Valles, X.; Sacarlal, J.; Sigau que, B.; Ruiz, J.; Alonso, P. Antimicrobial resistance of *Vibrio cholerae* O1 serotype Ogawa isolated in Manhica District Hospital, southern Mozambique. *J. Antimicrob. Chemother.* **2007**, *60*, 662–664. [CrossRef] [PubMed]

226. O'Shea, Y.A.; Reen, F.J.; Quirke, A.M.; Boyd, E.F. Evolutionary genetic analysis of the emergence of epidemic Vibrio cholerae isolates on the basis of comparative nucleotide sequence analysis and multilocus virulence gene profiles. *J. Clin. Microbiol.* **2004**, *42*, 4657–4671. [CrossRef] [PubMed]

227. Manga, N.M.; Ndour, C.T.; Diop, S.A.; Dia, N.M.; Ka-Sall, R.; Diop, B.M.; Sow, A.I.; Sow, P.S. Cholera in Senegal from 2004 to 2006: Lessons learned from successive outbreaks. *Med. Trop. (Mars)* **2008**, *68*, 589–592. [PubMed]

228. Ngandjio, A.; Tejiokem, M.; Wouafo, M.; Ndome, I.; Yonga, M.; Guenole, A.; Lemee, L.; Quilici, M.L.; Fonkoua, M.C. Antimicrobial resistance and molecular characterization of *Vibrio cholerae* O1 during the 2004 and 2005 outbreak of cholera inCameroon. *Foodborne Pathog. Dis.* **2009**, *6*, 49–56. [CrossRef] [PubMed]

229. Abera, B.; Bezabih, B.; Dessie, A. Antimicrobial susceptibilityof *V. cholerae* in north west, Ethiopia. *Ethiop. Med. J.* **2010**, *48*, 23–28. [PubMed]

230. Miwanda, B.; Moore, S.; Muyembe, J.J.; Nguefack-Tsague, G.; Kabangwa, I.K.; Ndjakani, D.Y.; Mutreja, A.; Thomson, N.; Thefenne, H.; Garnotel, E.; et al. Antimicrobial drug resistance of Vibrio cholerae, Democratic Republic of the Congo. *Emerg. Infect. Dis.* **2015**, *21*, 847–851. [CrossRef] [PubMed]

231. Smith, A.M.; Keddy, K.H.; De Wee, L. Characterization of cholera outbreak isolates from Namibia. *Epidemiol. Infect.* **2008**, *136*, 1207–1209. [PubMed]

232. Mwansa, J.C.L.; Mwaba, J.; Lukwesa, C.; Bhuiyan, N.A.; Ansaruzzaman, M.; Ramamurthy, T.; Alam, M.; Nair, G.B. Multiply antibiotic-resistant *Vibrio cholerae* O1 biotype El Tor strains emerge during cholera outbreaks in Zambia. *Epidemiol. Infect.* **2007**, *135*, 847–853. [CrossRef] [PubMed]

233. Ceccarelli, D.; Salvia, A.M.; Sami, J.; Cappuccinelli, P.; Colombo, M.M. New Cluster of plasmid-located class 1 integrons in *Vibrio cholerae* O1 and a dfrA15 cassette-containing integrin in *Vibrio parahaemolyticus* isolated in Angola. *Antimicrob. Agents Chemother.* **2006**, *50*, 2493–2499. [CrossRef] [PubMed]

234. Ismail, H.; Smith, A.M.; Archer, B.N.; Tau, N.P.; Sooka, A.; Thomas, J.; Prinsloo, B.; Keddy, K.H. Group for Enteric, Respiratory and Meningeal Disease Surveillance in South Africa (GERMS-SA). Case of imported *Vibrio cholerae* O1 from India to South Africa. *J. Infect. Dev. Ctries* **2012**, *6*, 897–900. [CrossRef] [PubMed]

235. Martinez-Urtaza, J.; Lozano-Leon, A.; Varela-Pet, J.; Trinanes, J.; Pazos, Y.; Garcia-Martin, O. Environmental determinants of the occurrence and distribution of Vibrio parahaemolyticus in the rias of Galicia, Spain. *Appl. Environ. Microbiol.* **2008**, *74*, 265–274. [CrossRef] [PubMed]

236. Hu, Y.; Yang, X.; Qin, J.; Lu, N.; Cheng, G.; Wu, N.; Pan, Y.; Li, J.; Zhu, L.; Wang, X.; et al. Metagenome-wide analysis of antibiotic resistance genes in a large cohort of human gut microbiota. *Nat. Commun.* **2013**, *4*, 2151. [CrossRef] [PubMed]

237. Chang, H.H.; Cohen, T.; Grad, Y.H.; Hanage, W.P.; O'Brien, T.F.; Lipsitch, M. Origin and proliferation of multiple-drug resistance in bacterial pathogens. *Microbiol. Mol. Biol. Rev.* **2015**, *79*, 101–116. [CrossRef] [PubMed]

238. Newton, R.J.; McLellan, S.L.; Dila, D.K.; Vineis, J.H.; Morrison, H.G.; Eren, A.M.; Soqin, M.L. Sewage reflects the microbiomes of human populations. *MBio* **2015**, *6*, 02574. [CrossRef] [PubMed]

239. Manjusha, S.; Sarita, G.B. Plasmid associated antibiotic resistance in *Vibrio* isolated from coastal waters of Kerala. *Int. Food Res. J.* **2011**, *18*, 1171–1181.

240. Szczepanowski, R.; Krahn, I.; Linke, B.; Goesmann, A.; Pühler, A.; Schlüter, A. Antibiotic multiresistance plasmid pRSB101 isolated from a wastewater treatment plant is related to plasmids residing in phytopathogenic bacteria and carries eight different resistance determinants including a multidrug transport system. *Microbiology* **2004**, *150*, 3613–3630. [CrossRef] [PubMed]

241. Xu, J.; Xu, Y.; Wang, H.; Guo, C.; Qiu, H.; He, Y.; Zhang, Y.; Li, X.; Meng, W. Occurrence of antibiotics and antibiotic resistance genes in a sewage treatment plant and its effluent-receiving river. *Chemosphere* **2015**, *119*, 1379–1385. [CrossRef] [PubMed]

242. Srinivasan, V.; Nam, H.M.; Nguyen, L.T.; Tamilselvam, B.; Murinda, S.E.; Oliver, S.P. Prevalence of antimicrobial resistance genes in Listeria monocytogenes isolated from dairy farms. *Foodborne Pathog. Dis.* **2005**, *2*, 201–211. [CrossRef] [PubMed]

243. Zhang, X.X.; Zhang, T.; Fang, H.H.P. Antibiotic resistance genes in water environment. *Appl. Microbiol. Biotech.* **2009**, *82*, 397–414. [CrossRef] [PubMed]

244. Dang, H.Y.; Ren, J.; Song, L.S.; Sun, S.; An, L.G. Dominant chloramphenicol-resistant bacteria and resistance genes in coastal marine waters of Jiazhou Bay, China. *World J. Microbiol. Biotech.* **2008**, *24*, 209–217. [CrossRef]

245. Kim, M.; Kwon, T.H.; Jung, S.M.; Cho, S.H.; Jin, S.Y.; Park, N.H.; Kim, C.; Kim, J. Antibiotic resistance of bacteria isolated from the internal organs of edible snow crabs. *PLoS ONE* **2013**, *8*, 70887. [CrossRef] [PubMed]

246. Forsberg, K.J.; Reyes, A.; Wang, B.; Selleck, E.M.; Sommer, M.O.A.; Dantas, G. The shared antibiotic resistome of soil bacteria and human pathogens. *Science* **2012**, *337*, 1107–1111. [CrossRef] [PubMed]

247. Cox, G.; Wright, G.D. Intrinsic antibiotic resistance: Mechanisms, origins, challenges and solutions. *Int. J. Med. Microbiol.* **2013**, *303*, 287–292. [CrossRef] [PubMed]

248. O'Neill, J. The Review on Antimicrobial Resistance Antimicrobials in Agriculture and the Environment: Reducing Unnecessary Use and Waste. Available online: https://www.noah.co.uk/wp-content/uploads/2016/06/Critique-ONeill-Report-Final.pdf (accessed on 27 August 2017).

249. Oger, P.Y.; Sudre, B. *Water, Sanitation and Hygiene and Cholera Epidemiology: An Integrated Evaluation in the Countries of the Lake Chad Basin*; UNICEF WCAR: Dakar, Senegal, 2011.

250. WASH and Cholera in Ghana, positioning paper, UNICEF. Available online: http://www.plateformecholera.info/attachments/article/221/UNICEF-Factsheet-Ghana-EN-FINAL.pdf (accessed on 27 August 2017).

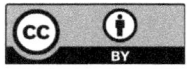

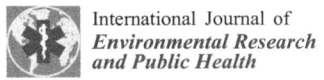

Article

Measuring the Impacts of Water Safety Plans in the Asia-Pacific Region

Emily Kumpel [1,2,†], Caroline Delaire [2,*,†], Rachel Peletz [3], Joyce Kisiangani [2], Angella Rinehold [4], Jennifer De France [4], David Sutherland [5] and Ranjiv Khush [3]

1   Department of Civil and Environmental Engineering, University of Massachusetts,
    Amherst, MA 01003, USA; ekumpel@umass.edu
2   The Aquaya Institute, P.O. Box 21862-00505, Nairobi, Kenya; joyce@aquaya.org
3   The Aquaya Institute, P.O. Box 5502, Santa Cruz, CA 95063, USA; rachel@aquaya.org (R.P.);
    ranjiv@aquaya.org (R.K.)
4   World Health Organization, 1211 Geneva, Switzerland; angella27@gmail.com (A.R.);
    defrancej@who.int (J.D.F.)
5   World Health Organization, Regional Office for South East Asia, New Delhi 110002, India;
    dcsuth@gmail.com
*   Correspondence: caroline@aquaya.org; Tel.: +254-701-178-714
†   These authors contributed equally to this work.

Received: 24 April 2018; Accepted: 7 June 2018; Published: 10 June 2018

Abstract: This study investigated the effectiveness of Water Safety Plans (WSP) implemented in 99 water supply systems across 12 countries in the Asia-Pacific region. An impact assessment methodology including 36 indicators was developed based on a conceptual framework proposed by the Center for Disease Control (CDC) and before/after data were collected between November 2014 and June 2016. WSPs were associated with infrastructure improvements at the vast majority (82) of participating sites and to increased financial support at 37 sites. In addition, significant changes were observed in operations and management practices, number of water safety-related meetings, unaccounted-for water, water quality testing activities, and monitoring of consumer satisfaction. However, the study also revealed challenges in the implementation of WSPs, including financial constraints and insufficient capacity. Finally, this study provided an opportunity to test the impact assessment methodology itself, and a series of recommendations are made to improve the approach (indicators, study design, data collection methods) for evaluating WSPs.

Keywords: water safety plans; drinking water quality; risk management; impact assessment; Asia-Pacific region

1. Introduction

Diarrheal diseases resulting from inadequate drinking water are estimated to cause 502,000 deaths per year [1]. Providing safe drinking water is essential to prevent water-related diseases. However, monitoring and maintaining water safety in piped systems and point sources around the world is challenging [2–4]. In 2004, the World Health Organization (WHO) formally introduced Water Safety Plans (WSPs) as a preferred management approach for ensuring the safety of drinking water supply [5]. WSPs provide a comprehensive methodology to assess and mitigate risks in all steps of the water supply system from catchment to consumer. Specifically, the approach includes the formation of a dedicated WSP team; a system assessment phase during which risks, existing control measures, and gaps are identified to inform the development and implementation of an improvement plan; routine monitoring and evaluation; and periodic review of the entire process (Figure S1). This methodology is applicable to both large piped systems and small community water supplies [6,7].

WSPs are considered "the most effective means of consistently ensuring the safety of a drinking-water supply" [8] and have been implemented in at least 93 countries [9]. However, despite growing literature on WSPs, there is no established and validated process to evaluate WSP impacts, and robust scientific evidence for the benefits of WSPs is limited.

A number of studies have documented the benefits of WSPs and the lessons learned from their implementation [10–16]. However, as shown in a recent literature review, there are very few examples of rigorous systematic assessments of WSP impacts [17]. Two studies in Iceland, France, and Spain assessed the outcomes of WSPs using before/after comparisons [18,19], but they included only seven and five utilities, respectively, and focused on developed countries. The US Center for Disease Control and Prevention (CDC) proposed a conceptual framework to evaluate the impacts of WSPs [19], which distinguishes shorter-term system-level changes ("outcomes") from longer-term service delivery and societal improvements ("impacts") and provides a comprehensive evaluation lens covering institutional, operational, financial, policy, water supply, health, and socioeconomic aspects. However, the CDC conceptual framework has not been comprehensively operationalized through field-testing of specific indicators and data collection methods. Validating an operationalized form of the CDC evaluation framework across a wide range of contexts (urban/rural, large/small systems, etc.) and geographic settings remains to be done.

Establishing a process to evaluate the effectiveness of WSPs is important in order to (1) compare WSPs with more targeted (i.e., less comprehensive) interventions to improve safe water supply, such as infrastructure upgrades, regulatory reforms, or capacity building; (2) strengthen support for WSPs among governments and sector stakeholders and (3) help strengthen WSP implementation through better understanding of the practices that are most challenging to change. At the water system level, an evaluation process can also be useful to managers for regular monitoring of WSP progress and evidence-based decision-making.

This study developed and tested methods for assessing the effectiveness of WSPs in 12 countries in the Asia-Pacific region. Specifically, it allowed for the investigation of the three following questions: (1) What types of data can be collected to evaluate WSP impacts? (2) How should these data be collected? (3) What study design should be applied depending on the context and objective of the evaluation? Using an operational impact assessment framework that was developed based on the CDC conceptual framework [20], before/after data were collected on 36 performance indicators along with qualitative information at 99 sites between November 2014 and June 2016. After presenting findings on WSP outcomes and impacts, this paper draws on the data obtained and the collection process to reflect on the challenges in evaluating WSPs and recommends study designs for future impact assessments.

2. Materials and Methods

2.1. Study Sites

This impact assessment was undertaken through the Water Quality Partnership for Health (WQP), a program launched in 2005 by the Australian Department of Foreign Affairs and Trade (DFAT) and WHO to introduce and institutionalize WSPs in the Asia-Pacific region. Sixteen countries receiving WQP support were invited by WHO Regional Offices to participate in the impact assessment. Among these countries, 12 were able to collect both baseline and follow-up data: Bangladesh, Bhutan, Cambodia, Cook Islands, Lao PDR, Mongolia, Nepal, Philippines, Samoa, Sri Lanka, Timor-Leste, and Vanuatu (Figure 1).

Overall, 99 sites participated in the study (Figure 1). Institutions responsible for selecting study sites varied between countries and included national-level government agencies (e.g., departments/ministries of health and water), national water suppliers, heads of local government units, and WHO country or regional staff. Site selection was non-random. Selection criteria varied between countries (Table S1), but generally reflected an attempt to capture the diversity of settings (according to system size, management type, geography, performance, challenges, etc.), while also prioritizing sites with longer-running WSPs and readily available data.

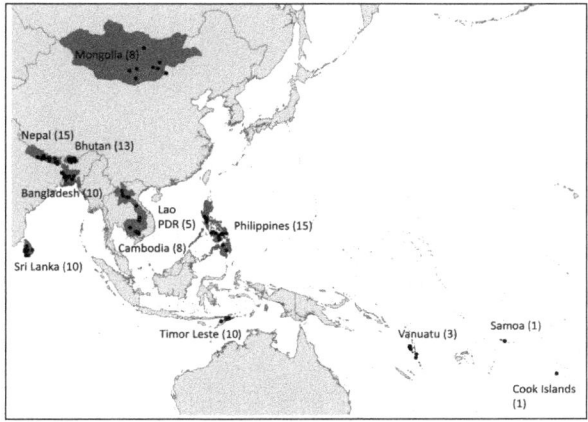

Figure 1. Twelve countries that participated in the WSP impact assessment, with number of participating sites indicated between parentheses.

Piped systems represented 90% of the study sites (89 out of 99), with approximately two-thirds (58) of these operated by public/private utilities or local government units, and a third (31) managed by communities (Table 1). Point sources, representing 10% of the study sites (10 out of 99), included water-refilling stations and groundwater sources (Table 1). In most countries (all except Sri Lanka, Cook Islands, Samoa, and Vanuatu), sites represented a mix of rural and urban settings. Overall, 62% of the sites (61) were urban and 38% (38) were rural (Table 1). The populations served by the water systems varied widely between 22 people (a small community-managed piped system in Bhutan) to 8.9 million people (a large urban utility in the Philippines) (Figure 2a). The median population served across all the sites was 7140 people. Eight of the 10 smallest systems were in Bhutan; the 10 largest systems were in the Philippines, Mongolia, Sri Lanka, and Bangladesh (Figure 2a).

Table 1. Number of sites that participated in the WSP impact assessment by country, type of water system, context (urban/rural), and WSP age.

| Country | Total Sites | Type of System | | | Context | | Age | |
| | | Piped Systems | | Point Sources | Urban | Rural | <2 years | >2 years |
		Utility/LGU [a]	Community-Managed [b]					
Bangladesh	10	8	2	0	8	2	7	3
Bhutan	13	6	7 [b]	0	7	6	10	3
Cambodia	8	4	0	4 [c]	4	4	0	8
Cook Islands	1	1	0	0	1	0	0	1
Lao PDR	5	3	0	2 [c]	3	2	1	4
Mongolia	8	7	0	1 [c]	3	5	5	3
Nepal	15	1	14	0	11	4	9	6
Philippines	15	12	0	3 [d]	8	7	11	4
Samoa	1	0	1	0	0	1	1	0
Sri Lanka	10	10	0	0	10	0	4	6
Timor-Leste	10	6	4	0	6	4	10	0
Vanuatu	3	0	3	0	0	3	3	0
Total	99	58	31	10	60	39	61	38

[a] Private or public utility or Local Government Unit (LGU); [b] three systems managed by schools; [c] groundwater sources; [d] water refilling stations.

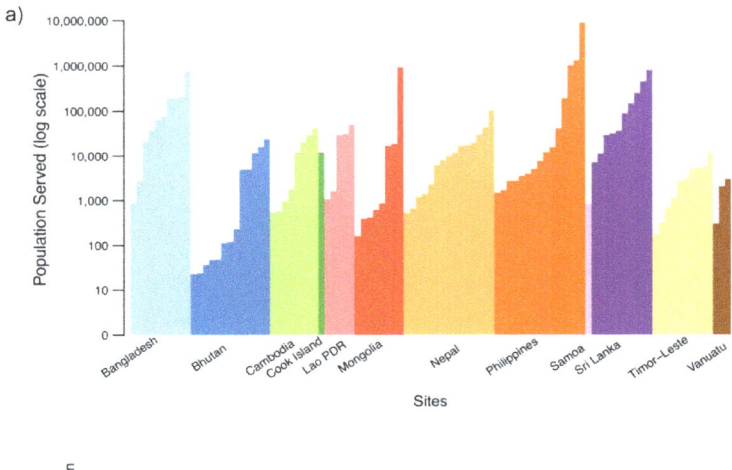

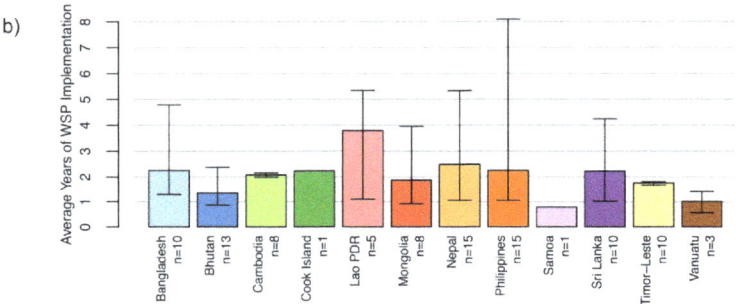

Figure 2. Description of sites: (**a**) Populations served by sites; (**b**) Mean age of WSP at time of follow-up data collection. The upper and lower bounds show the maximum and minimum ages in each country, respectively.

The age of WSPs implemented in the study sites varied considerably within and between countries (Figure 2b). At follow-up, the youngest WSP was 7 months (in Vanuatu) and the oldest was 8 years and 1 month (in the Philippines), with an overall mean WSP age of 25.2 months (Figure 2b).

2.2. Evaluation Framework

WHO developed an operational impact assessment framework for this study based on the CDC's conceptual framework [19], which distinguishes between shorter-term (occurring on the order of months) system-level changes, called "outcomes", and longer-term (occurring on the order of years) service delivery and societal improvements, called "impacts" (Figure 3). Outcomes explored in the study include changes in communication and knowledge (institutional outcomes); infrastructure and operation/management procedures (operational outcomes); revenue collection, cost recovery, and investment (financial outcomes); norms and regulations (policy outcomes); and inclusion of disadvantaged groups (equity outcomes, which were added to the CDC conceptual framework) (Figure 3). Impacts include changes in water service delivery such as coverage, continuity, quality, and potential health impacts (e.g., reduction in waterborne illness) (Figure 3). Eventual socioeconomic changes (e.g., reductions in medical expenses and coping costs) included in the CDC conceptual framework were not considered in this study due to concerns related to the practicality of data collection and because these impacts are expected to occur over longer time scales.

The operational impact assessment framework used for this study comprised 36 performance indicators, listed in Table 2, defined to measure the outcomes and impacts of WSPs. These indicators were developed in consultation with WSP stakeholders in participating countries in 2013, prior to the publication of the CDC indicators presented in Lockhart et al. [21]. Therefore, the two sets of indicators, although similar, are not identical. The operational impact assessment framework also included open-ended questions to help interpret the quantitative indicator data and gather additional information on the challenges of WSP implementation.

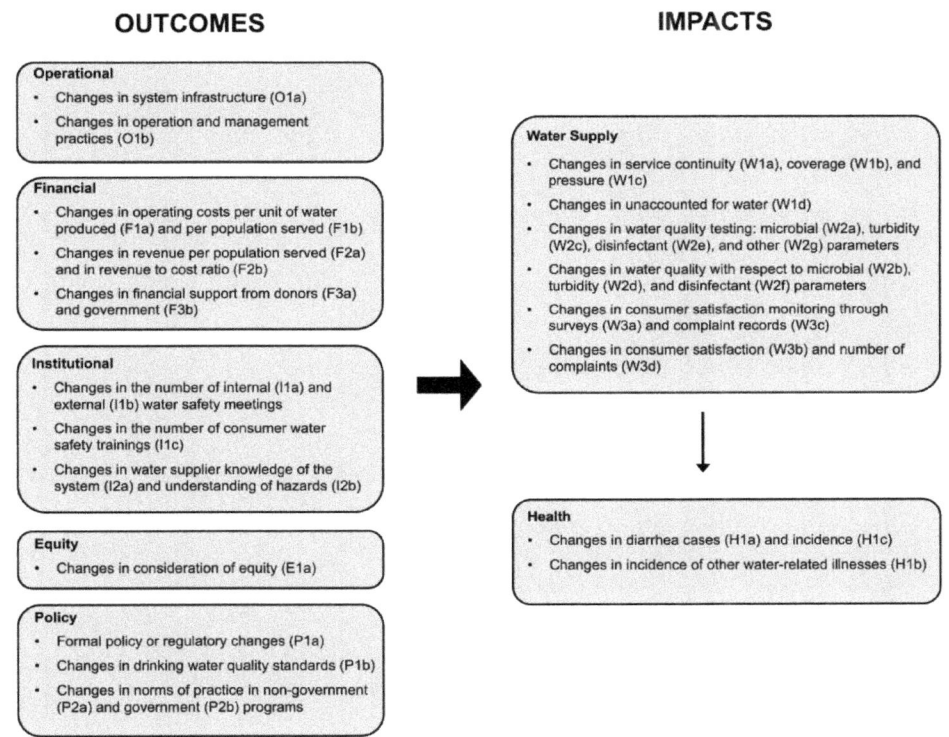

Figure 3. Operational impact assessment framework and indicators used in this study. More details on indicators, including units and sub-indicators, are presented in Table 2.

2.3. Study Design and Data Collection

An uncontrolled before-after study design was applied. Baseline data were collected between November 2014 and February 2016 and were intended to capture conditions at a site prior to WSP implementation. At 65% of sites, baseline data were collected retrospectively, i.e., after the start of the WSP. Follow-up data were collected between December 2015 and June 2016 (Figure S2, Table S2).

Data collection was undertaken by various organizations, including government agencies, national water utilities, universities, WHO country offices, and independent consultancies (Table S2). Data collection teams interviewed key personnel of the water supply systems (i.e., managing directors, water quality managers, operations staff) in their local language. For approximately half of the sites, data collectors received some form of training, while the rest relied solely on the data collection forms for guidance.

Table 2. Outcome and impact indicators (all are site-level, except policy indicators, which are country-level). For each indicator, data availability (at both baseline and follow-up), data quality, and suggestions for revising the impact assessment framework are reported. On the basis of these recommendations and other inputs, WHO will publish a separate document detailing revised indicators and associated data collection guidance.

Code	Indicator	Data Format	Availability (% of Sites)[5]	Data Quality	Category[6]	Comments on Suggested Revisions
O	**Operational Outcomes**					
O1a	Infrastructure change as a result of WSP[1]	Y/N, description	95	Good	A	Retain
O1b	Level of operations and management practices	Score of 8–40 (score of 1–5 each)	93	Good		
	(1) Operational monitoring plan				A	Retain
	(2) Compliance monitoring plan				A	Retain
	(3) Consumer satisfaction monitoring				D	Exclude because redundant with W3b
	(4) Standard operating procedures				A	Retain
	(5) Emergency response plan				A	Retain
	(6) Operator or caretaker training programs				A	Retain
	(7) Consumer education programs				D	Exclude because redundant with I1c
	(8) Equipment maintenance/calibration schedules				C	Reconsider including as addressing such maintenance schedules is not emphasized in the WSP process
F	**Financial Outcomes**					
F1a	Operating costs per unit water[2]	$/m^3	72	Poor	D	Exclude to simplify; revenue to cost ratio will suffice
F1b	Operating costs per population[2]	$/pop	71	Poor	D	Exclude to simplify; revenue to cost ratio will suffice
F2a	Revenue per population[2]	$/pop	71	Poor	D	Exclude to simplify; revenue to cost ratio will suffice
F2b	Revenue to cost ratio[2]	%	66	Poor	B	Retain but provide a step-by-step calculation guide to avoid mistakes and standardize the definitions of operating costs and revenue
F3a	Financial support as a direct result of WSP[1]	Y/N, description	89	Good	A	Retain
F3b	Funds from government for water supply	$/description	59	Poor	B	Retain but combine with indicator F3a and provide more guidance to clarify indicator and to improve reliability of data
I	**Institutional Outcomes**					
I1a	Internal water safety meetings[2]	Number	92	Good	A	Retain
I1b	External water safety meetings[2]	Number	92	Good	A	Retain
I1c	Consumer water safety trainings[2]	Number	85	Good	A	Retain
I2a	Understanding of system[3]	Score of 5–25	19	Poor	C	Reconsider including due to lack of meaningful measurements (unless a more effective and systematic measurement approach can be designed)
I2b	Understanding of hazards[3]	Number	19	Poor	C	

Table 2. *Cont.*

Code	Indicator	Data Format	Availability (% of Sites)[5]	Data Quality	Category[6]	Comments on Suggested Revisions
E	**Equity Outcomes**					
	Equity[4]					
E1a	(1) Participation	Score of 6–30 (score of 1–5 each)	88	Poor	C	Reconsider including due to widespread misinterpretation until explicit consideration of equity through the WSP process is widely promoted
	(2) Groups identified and documented					
	(3) Hazards/issues prioritized					
	(4) Improvements benefit equitably					
	(5) Monitoring data disaggregated					
	(6) Emergency response and communication programs reflect needs					
W	**Water Supply Impact**					
W1a	Continuity	Hours/week	93	Good	B	Retain but consider refining guidance to avoid rough estimates of continuity
W1b	Service coverage	%	76	Good	C	Reconsider including as expanding service coverage is often not a core priority or key outcome of WSPs
W1c	Pressure	atm/bar/m	22	Poor	C	Reconsider including due to data quality concerns (variable measurement methods and tendency to provide rough estimates)
W1d	Unaccounted-for Water (UFW)	%	30	Good	B	Retain but revise guidance to better distinguish between UFW and non-revenue water (NRW)
W2a	Microbial tests[2]	Number	89	Good	A	Retain
W2b	Microbial compliance[2]	%	60	Good	A	Retain
W2c	Turbidity tests[2]	Number	87	Good	A	Retain
W2d	Turbidity compliance[2]	%	37	Good	A	Retain
W2e	Disinfectant residual tests[2]	Number	74	Good	A	Retain
W2f	Disinfectant compliance[2]	%	21	Good	A	Retain
W2g	Other water quality parameter compliance[2]	%, description	0	Poor	B	Retain but standardize list of parameters and formatting
W3a	Consumer satisfaction surveys conducted	Y/N	92	Good	A	Retain

Table 2. Cont.

Code	Indicator	Data Format	Availability (% of Sites)[5]	Data Quality	Category[6]	Comments on Suggested Revisions
W	**Water Supply Impact**					
W3b	Consumers satisfied[2]	%	10	Good	B	Retain but consider recommending a household survey where suppliers do not have standardized data
W3c	Consumer complaint records kept	Y/N	92	Good	A	Retain
W3d	Number of consumer complaints[2]	%	22	Poor	B	Retain but standardize reporting
H	**Health Impact**					
H1a	Cases of diarrhea[2]	Number	43	Poor	B	Retain but revise guidance to highlight/address common discrepancies between health center and WSP coverage areas
H1b	Other water-related illnesses[2]	Number	31	Poor	B	Retain but revise guidance to highlight/address common discrepancies between health center and WSP coverage areas and combine with indicator H1a
H1c	Diarrheal incidence[2]	%	5	Poor	B	Retain but change to primary household data collection rather than review of existing household data available
P	**Policy Outcomes**					
P1a	Proactive water quality risk management approaches are/were included in formal water sector policies or regulations at time of follow-up assessment	Y/N, description	92	Poor	B	Retain but provide a standardized definition of risk management
P1b	Activity to develop or revise national drinking water quality standards has been undertaken	Y/N, description	92	Poor	D	Exclude because difficult to obtain information in a standardized and meaningful way and link to WSP implementation
P2a	Proactive water quality risk management approaches have been adopted by other water-sector stakeholders (e.g., NGOs, UNICEF)	Y/N, description	83	Poor	D	Exclude because difficult to obtain information in a standardized and meaningful way
P2b	Proactive water quality risk management approaches are promoted in national or sub-national programs	Y/N, description	83	Poor	C	Reconsider including this indicator reflects drivers of WSPs as opposed to outcomes

[1] Only asked at follow-up; [2] cumulative value over the 12-month period before data collection; [3] only asked if baseline data collection was prospective; [4] all elements refer to women and/or disadvantaged groups; [5] except for Policy Outcomes, where the unit is "% of countries"; [6] suggestions regarding each indicator fall into four categories: A. Retain without changes. Indicators are important and reliable data were easily collected; B. Retain but modify to standardize answers and avoid calculation mistakes. Indicators are important but were associated with data quality and/or availability challenges that can be easily overcome; C. Retention requires further consideration. Indicators were associated with significant data quality and/or availability challenges that may be difficult to overcome (except at higher capacity sites). If retained, modifications will be needed; D. Do not retain. Indicators are not core to the WSP process, are redundant and/or are not sufficiently important to warrant addressing data quality and/or availability challenges experienced.

Two data collection forms were used at each site (Figure S2): (1) an impact assessment form to collect data on the 36 indicators listed in Table 2 and (2) an audit form to evaluate the WSP level of development and stage of implementation, used only during follow-up data collection. Two versions of the audit form were available: one for urban and one for rural systems. The audit forms used are included in Appendix B of *A practical guide to auditing water safety plans* [22]. Sites were defined as rural or urban by country institutions themselves and definitions varied between countries. In addition to quantitative data, qualitative data were collected using the impact assessment form through (1) explanations provided by data collectors regarding quantitative responses and (2) open-ended questions to interviewees about the impacts and challenges of WSPs.

2.4. Data Processing and Analysis

Data from the forms were collated and cleaned in Excel. Inconsistencies between data provided and qualitative explanations were checked, as well as those between baseline and follow-up data, and clarifications were sought with country officials and data collection teams. Data that were missing, indicated to be only estimates, clear outliers, or obviously incorrect calculations were excluded. To evaluate the reliability of the indicators involving subjective scoring (operations and management (O1b) and equity (E1a), Table 2), an Aquaya staff member performed an independent scoring for 25% of sites using the available qualitative data. To assess how the operational impact assessment framework "performed," the quality and availability of the data collected for each of the 36 indicators were analyzed. To assess data quality, each indicator was examined in depth to see whether data were presented in a consistent way before and after WSP implementation and between countries, reflected adequate understanding of the question, and could be verified using contextual information. This allowed for the identification of indicators that were prone to confusion, challenging to quantify, or inappropriate in specific settings. Indicators for which data errors or inconsistencies were common were defined as being of poor quality, and indicators that were missing in over 75% of sites were defined as insufficiently available.

We selected 25 sites representing all 12 countries for qualitative data analysis based on the following criteria: (1) inclusion of all countries (at least one and not more than three sites per country); (2) availability of qualitative data in the data collection form and (3) representation (e.g., urban and rural settings, range of water supply systems, and range of population served). Qualitative data analysis was performed using the NVivo software [23]. Baseline and follow-up data were inductively coded using codes such as "complaints", "testing", and "lack of documentation". Coding queries and intersections between codes then allowed themes to emerge, such as "water quantity issues" or "operational costs".

Statistical before-after comparisons were performed for indicators meeting two inclusion criteria: (1) both baseline and follow-up data were available from at least 25% of sites and (2) there were no substantial concerns with data quality. Out of 36 indicators, twenty did not meet these inclusion criteria (see Section 3.2). In addition, two indicators did not lend themselves to before-after comparisons because they only applied to follow-up (O1a and F3a). Statistical analysis was thus performed on fourteen indicators. The statistical significance of before-after differences was analyzed using the paired Wilcox rank-sum test for continuous indicators or the chi-square test for binary indicators. Correlations between audit scores and impact/outcome indicators were also investigated.

2.5. Ethics Statement

Written government approval for the study was obtained from Bangladesh, Cambodia, Lao PDR, Mongolia, Philippines, Sri Lanka, and Vanuatu. Government approval was implicit for Bhutan, Cook Islands, Nepal, Timor-Leste, and Samoa, where data collection was done by government agencies. The study protocol was submitted to the Western Institutional Review Board (WIRB, wirb.com, Olympia, WA, USA) for ethical review and received a determination of exemption from full review under 45 CFR §46.101(b)(2) of the Common Rule in the USA.

3. Results

3.1. WSP Audit Scores

The WSP audit scores varied substantially between sites (Figure 4). No statistically significant relationships were found between audit scores and WSP age or population served ($p > 0.05$). The audit scores showed similar distributions for urban and rural sites, with the "average" category being the largest for both groups (Figure 4). The study generally did not find statistically significant relationships between audit scores and the outcomes or impacts measured. The absence of direct correlation between WSP implementation quality and outcomes/impacts suggests that WSP benefits result from a complex interplay of factors not limited to implementation rigor.

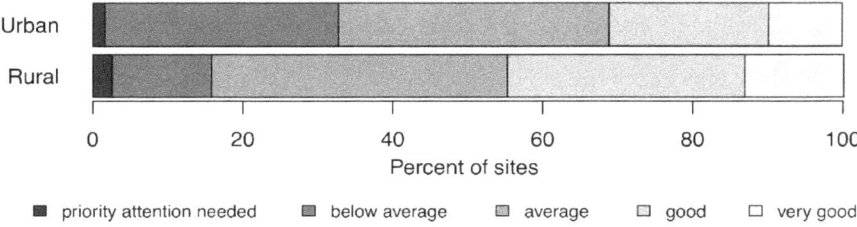

Figure 4. Distribution of qualitative audit scores assessing the quality of WSP implementation.

3.2. Evaluation Process: Analysis of the Indicators

Overall, 20 indicators suffered from substantial data quality issues (18), insufficient data availability (8), or both (6) (Table 2). Data were rarely available (i.e., in less than 25% of sites) for knowledge indicators (I2a-b), pressure (W1c), disinfectant residual compliance (W2f), "other" water quality parameters (W2g), consumer satisfaction (W3b), number of consumer complaints (W3d), and diarrheal incidence (H1c) (Table 2). In addition, financial (F1a-b, F2a-b, F3b), knowledge (I2a-b), equity (E1a), pressure (W1c), "other" water quality parameters (W2g), number of consumer complaints (W3d), health (H1a-c) and policy (P1a-b, P2a-b) indicators suffered from poor data quality (Table 2). With respect to financial indicators, the concerns included calculation mistakes, incomplete operating costs (missing line items), and misinterpretation of "revenue" (expected versus actually collected). For knowledge indicators, there were instances where different water system staff were interviewed at baseline and follow-up, limiting the ability to rigorously assess progress in knowledge. For equity indicators, the qualitative data revealed variability in the interpretation of "disadvantaged groups" and "explicit considerations of equity" between data collectors. For pressure, estimates were often provided, as opposed to actual measurements. Data on "other" water quality parameters and customer complaints suffered from inconsistent reporting, either between baseline and follow-up or between sites. With respect to health indicators, the primary concern was that information on disease incidence was collected from hospitals whose service areas did not necessarily align with that of water systems. Policy indicators were undermined by different interpretations of risk management between countries.

The remaining 16 indicators had both sufficient data availability and quality for analysis. Data from 14 of these indicators were quantitative and suitable for statistical analysis: operations and management (O1b), stakeholder communication (I1a-c), service (W1a-b and W1d), water quality (W2a-e), and consumer feedback (W3a and W3c) indicators. The two qualitative indicators—infrastructure improvements (O1a) and financial support received (F3a)—were assessed at follow-up only and were therefore considered outside of the statistical analysis.

Finally, for the two indicators relying on subjective scoring—level of operations and management practices (O1b) and equity (E1a)—scores assigned by data collection teams and by Aquaya staff were not significantly different ($p > 0.1$, except for 3 sub-indicators for which the discrepancies were small, Table S3), suggesting that such subjective indicators do not constitute a weakness of the impact assessment framework.

Disparities were observed in data availability between urban and rural sites, especially for financial and water supply indicators. Many rural sites did not have data on operating costs and revenue (F1a-b, F2a-b) because they distributed water for free, relied on volunteer management, or did not hold official records. For example, a rural site in Timor Leste reported: *"Two technicians [are] working as volunteers for operation and for maintenance with the support of [donor] and community ... There is no system for collecting revenue from consumers as of now"*. A rural site in Samoa stated: *"The caretaker . . . is not paid on monetary terms but by other means"*. According to a rural site in Mongolia, *"Revenue collected from users is spent on incentives and salaries for the well operator. However, no records are kept"*. Similarly, indicators on water quality testing and compliance (W2a-e) were, on average, available at only 57% of rural sites (compared to 76% of urban sites), due to a lack of water quality testing at many sites. As a rural site in Mongolia stated, *"Laboratory testing is expensive; therefore, testing cannot be performed regularly"*. In Nepal, a rural site reported not having its own test kit: *"[We are] dependent on [the] District headquarter test kit and it seems [a] little bit impossible [to do] frequent tests"*. In Lao PDR, a rural site stated: *"Someone else [has] collected water samples and tested, but not sure whether it was for microbial indicators or not. No records of water quality testing results [are] available at the village"*. In addition, no rural site could provide data on unaccounted-for water (W1d) at both baseline and follow-up, primarily due to the absence of bulk and/or consumer meters. These results illustrate the challenges of evaluating lower-capacity sites where data are less available than at higher-capacity sites. These challenges were even more apparent for the four non-piped water sources in Cambodia, where data were available for only five performance indicators (O1b, I1a-c, and W2a).

3.3. Outcomes and Impacts of WSPs in the Asia-Pacific Region

The vast majority of the sites (83%, 54 urban and 28 rural) reported infrastructure improvements as a direct result of WSP implementation (O1a). These improvements targeted various stages of the water supply system, including the catchment/source (e.g., toilet construction, flood protection), the treatment plant (e.g., capacity increase, automatic chlorination, new reservoirs), the distribution system (e.g., network expansion, new pumps, meter installation), the energy supply (e.g., purchase of generators), and monitoring activities (e.g., laboratory construction). Qualitative data indicated that infrastructure improvements were generally focused on water quality rather than water quantity. Several factors were cited as having facilitated these improvements, including recommendations by WSP teams, the enhanced authority of water quality divisions, and changes in management mindsets with respect to water safety risks. In addition, over a third of the sites (37) reported that WSP implementation was linked to financial support from donors or NGOs (other than DFAT) (F3a).

Aggregated results for the 14 quantitative performance indicators that met the inclusion criteria are presented in Table 3. Between baseline and follow-up, statistically significant improvements were observed in operations and management practices (O1b), the number of water safety-related meetings (I1a, I1b, I1c), unaccounted-for water (W1d), water quality testing activities (W2a, W2c, W2e), and monitoring of consumer satisfaction (W3a, W3c) (Table 3). The median score for the level of operations and management practices increased from 9% to 44% ($p < 0.01$, $n = 93$) (Table 3), showing greater attention to proactive risk management practices. The proportion of sites reporting internal, external, and consumer water safety meetings increased from 16% to 60% ($p < 0.01$, $n = 92$), 25% to 48% ($p < 0.01$, $n = 92$), and 16% to 53% ($p < 0.01$, $n = 85$), respectively (Table 3). The median level of unaccounted-for water (UFW) decreased from 25% to 20% ($p = 0.01$, $n = 30$) (Table 3). The median number of microbial, turbidity, and disinfectant residual tests performed increased from 3 to 12 ($p < 0.01$, $n = 89$), 0 to 4 ($p < 0.01$, $n = 87$), and 0 to 10 tests per year ($p < 0.01$, $n = 74$), respectively (Table 3). Between baseline and follow-up, the number of sites that conducted consumer satisfaction surveys and kept records of consumer complaints increased from 13% to 33% ($p < 0.01$, $n = 92$), and 41% to 61% ($p < 0.01$, $n = 92$), respectively (Table 3). In contrast, there were no significant changes in service continuity (W1a), service coverage (W1b), or in the compliance of test results with national standards (W2b and W2d) (Table 3). For the latter, the absence of observed changes may be due to the unavailability of data in a large number of sites and to reports of 100% compliance at baseline for the remaining sites (Table 3). All improvements in WSP outcomes and impacts observed in this study are summarized in Table 4.

Table 3. Comparisons of WSP outcome and impact indicators between baseline and follow-up. The analysis includes the number of sites (*n*), the percentage of sites reporting any given activity, median values across all sites at baseline and follow-up, and the statistical significance of the change between baseline and follow-up (*p*-value). *p*-values were determined using the paired Wilcox rank-sum test for all except the binary W3a and W3c indicators, which were determined using the chi-squared test. Results for each indicator, except O1b, are reported for 12-month periods.

Code	Indicator	*n*	Unit	% of Sites		Median Values		*p*-Values
				Base-Line	Follow-Up	Base-Line	Follow-Up	
	Operational Outcomes							
O1a	Infrastructure changes due to WSP	95	yes/no	-	86	-	-	-
O1b	Level of operations and management practices	93	%	-	-	9	44	<0.01
	Financial Outcomes							
F3a	Financial support due to WSP	89	yes/no	-	42	-	-	-
	Institutional Outcomes							
I1a	Internal meetings	92	number	16	60	0	2	<0.01
I1b	External water safety meetings	92	number	25	48	0	0	<0.01
I1c	Consumer water safety trainings	85	number	16	53	0	1	<0.01
	Water Supply Impact							
W1a	Continuity	93	h/week	34 [a]	37 [a]	97	104	0.59
W1b	Service coverage	76	%	-	-	85	81	0.75
W1d	Unaccounted-for water (UFW)	30	%	-	-	25	20	0.01
W2a	Microbial tests	89	number	73	85	3	12	<0.01
W2b	Microbial compliance	60	%	-	-	99	98	0.24
W2c	Turbidity tests	87	number	45	70	0	4	<0.01
W2d	Turbidity compliance	37	%	-	-	100	100	0.5
W2e	Disinfectant residual tests	74	number	39	57	0	10	<0.01
W3a	Consumer satisfaction surveys	92	%	13	33	-	-	<0.01
W3c	Consumer complaint records	92	%	41	61	-	-	<0.01

[a] Sites reporting continuous supply.

Table 4. Summary of observed WSP outcomes and impacts.

Indicators	Observed WSP Outcomes and Impacts	% of Sites Showing Improvements [1] (and Number of Countries)
O1a	Infrastructure improvements	86% (10 countries)
O1b	Improvement in operation and management	95% (12 countries)
F3a	Leveraging of donor funds	39% (9 countries)
I1a, b, c	Increased stakeholder communication and collaboration	66% (10 countries)
W1d	Reduction in unaccounted-for water (UFW)	21% (7 countries)
W2a, c, e	Increased water quality testing	65% (11 countries)
W3a, c	Increased monitoring of consumer satisfaction	33% (11 countries)

[1] For groups of indicators, the % of sites showing improvements in at least one indicator are reported.

The qualitative data indicated that knowledge and training obtained by water system staff through WSP implementation increased their attention to water quality, and that increased testing in turn improved their understanding of the system and their motivation to ensure water quality. Qualitative data also indicated that consumer complaints at follow-up were more often focused on water quantity (e.g., reliability, pressure) than on water quality.

The qualitative data analysis also revealed a number of challenges in the implementation of WSPs. Many sites reported that they were unable to implement risk mitigation measures due to financial constraints. Several sites noted that staff transfers or insufficient staffing levels impeded WSP implementation. Although statistically significant improvements were observed in operations and management practices (O1b), a number of sites reported persisting challenges related to operations and management, reflected in a lack of written procedures, poor record keeping, reactive (as opposed to proactive) maintenance, and discrepancies between planned and actual water quality testing. Some sites noted challenges in convening water safety meetings, especially when WSP team members were from different local government departments. These accounts are consistent with the generally low levels of operations and management practices (O1b) and number of meetings (I1a-b-c) reported in Table 3.

4. Discussion

4.1. How to Improve the WSP Impact Evaluation Process

This study, which was the first to use a comprehensive impact assessment framework to assess the effectiveness of WSPs across multiple countries and regions, identified a number of challenges relating to performance indicators, data collection, and the broader approach to WSP impact assessments. This section provides suggestions to address these challenges and better adapt the evaluation process to its context and objective. A revised impact assessment framework will be developed by WHO based in part on these suggestions and published as a separate document.

Based on the experiences with data collection across a wide range of sites, the 36 indicators have been categorized into four groups according to recommendations for future impact assessments (Table 2):

A. Retain without changes. Indicators are important and reliable data were easily collected.
B. Retain but modify to standardize answers and avoid calculation mistakes. Indicators are important but were associated with data quality and/or availability challenges that can be easily overcome.
C. Retention requires further consideration. Indicators were associated with significant data quality and/or availability challenges that may be difficult to overcome (except at higher-capacity sites). If retained, modifications will be needed.
D. Do not retain. Indicators are not core to the WSP process, are redundant and/or are not sufficiently important to warrant addressing data quality and/or availability challenges experienced.

Indicators in categories B and C should only be retained when they can yield standardized and comparable data across sites. To achieve this, data collection methods should take into consideration the capacity of water systems and provide step-by-step guidance where needed. Finally, although knowledge and health indicators were particularly challenging to quantify and did not yield useful results, they represent core target aspects of WSPs. Therefore, more robust and standardized methods to measure these indicators are needed so that these indicators can be included in future impact assessment frameworks.

The results also suggest that some indicators in categories A and B may need different data collection methods to ensure better data quality. Firstly, three indicators—service continuity (W1a), consumer satisfaction (W3b), and diarrheal incidence (H1c)—would likely yield more accurate data if evaluated through household surveys as opposed to questionnaires to the water supplier (W1a and W3b) and review of existing household data (H1c). In addition, if diarrheal incidence is to be evaluated, it needs to be appropriately sampled and statistically powered [24]. Secondly, for low-capacity systems that lack data, external measurements of water quality may be needed (e.g., to establish baseline data). For these water systems, data collectors may also need to clarify and assist with financial calculations when information on revenue or cost recovery is not readily available.

More generally, this study revealed two important challenges inherent to WSP impact assessments. Firstly, a relationship between the performance of a water system and the availability of data was observed. The sites for which data were most available were higher-capacity sites with high indicator levels at baseline. By contrast, lower-capacity sites with the most room for improvement often lacked reliable data at baseline, limiting the ability to detect changes. Therefore, to assess the extent to which WSPs can improve lower-capacity systems, data collection methods tailored to such systems (such as those recommended above for water quality and financial issues) are needed. Secondly, the diversity in system types (piped/point sources, urban/rural, small/large) and WSP age can be expected to lead to heterogeneities in the results achieved through WSP implementation. For example, a favorable WSP outcome for a low-capacity rural system may have been an increase in microbial water testing activities due to prioritization of monitoring practices, whereas a high-capacity urban system may have reduced the number of microbial tests due to improved efficiencies and risk management procedures. Looking for average effects in the entire sample would not reveal such case-specific outcomes. Therefore, limiting sample heterogeneity or selecting a sample size large enough to investigate sub-categories is recommended.

The design of future impact assessments should be selected according to their context and objective. Table 5 describes study designs falling under two categories: controlled and uncontrolled. On one hand, research studies aiming to rigorously determine the impacts of WSPs will require a "control" group comparable to the "intervention" group, as well as consistent and independent data collection. The intervention and control groups should be either randomly selected (randomized controlled trial) or methodically matched on a variety of relevant factors such as water system size, geographic setting, and/or revenue (matched controls trial). Such methodical study designs will ensure that observed changes in indicators can be attributed to WSP implementation, and will thus increase the generalizability and policy-relevance of the findings. On the other hand, country- or site-level monitoring and evaluation do not necessarily require controlled study designs. Although they cannot rigorously establish causality between WSP implementation and changes in indicators, uncontrolled designs such as before-after comparisons can be valuable to support advocacy and encourage better monitoring practices. Where resources are available, a before-after comparison can be made more robust by using historical data on indicators (as opposed to single "before" and "after" data points) and looking for changes in trends that coincide with WSP implementation (interrupted time series design). For all study designs, it is important to note that external validity (i.e., the generalizability of findings to an entire country or region) will depend on the extent to which study sites are representative of water systems in this country or region. Evaluators should thus select study sites using deliberate criteria to ensure representativeness. Random selection of water systems within the country or region of interest would ensure the highest degree of representativeness.

Finally, we recommend that future impact assessments include WSP audits as part of the methodology. Audits help ensure that interventions are implemented sufficiently well, i.e., that key intervention outputs are delivered, without which further assessments of outcomes and impacts may not be relevant. Audits can also help identify aspects of WSP implementation that need to be improved or adapted, which is key for programmatic improvements [25].

Table 5. Possible study designs for future WSP impact assessments, with advantages and challenges.

	Uncontrolled Study Designs Context: Site- or Country-Level Monitoring and Evaluation		Controlled Study Designs Context: Research and Rigorous Impact Assessments	
	Before-after Comparison	**Interrupted Time Series**	**Matched Controls**	**Randomized Controlled Trial**
Control group	No control group; for each site, relevant indicators are compared before and after WSP implementation	No control group; for each site, historical time series of relevant indicators are investigated to detect potential changes in slope coinciding with WSP implementation	Before WSP implementation, sites are manually assigned to a "control" or "intervention" group by matching a number of selected parameters between the two groups (e.g., system size, age, revenue, geographic setting)	Before WSP implementation, sites are randomly assigned to a "control" or "intervention" group. The randomization ensures that all possible confounding factors are equally distributed amongst the two groups.
WSP implementation	To all sites	To all sites	Only to "intervention" group	Only to "intervention" group
Data needed	Baseline and follow-up data	Historical data (pre- and post-WSP) on all relevant indicators (i.e., time series, not just baseline and follow-up data)	Inventory of all eligible study sites with data on parameters for matching Baseline and follow-up data	Inventory of all eligible study sites, ideally with data on some key parameters to confirm comparability between intervention and control groups Baseline and follow-up data
Advantages	Simplest study design (does not require a control group and only two data points per indicator: before and after) Results can be valuable for national advocacy and to encourage better monitoring/data collection practices Two rounds of data collection	Does not require a control group Provides more confidence than a simple before-after comparison that the changes observed may be associated with WSP implementation	A rigorous study design to examine associations between WSP implementation and outcomes/impacts, as long as all key parameters potentially affecting a water system's performance (i.e., confounding factors) are used for matching Two rounds of data collection	The only study design able to establish causality, i.e., the differences between the control and intervention groups can be attributed to WSP implementation because confounding factors are equally distributed amongst the two groups Two rounds of data collection
Challenges and limitation	Causality cannot be established from a simple before-after comparison, i.e., the changes observed cannot be attributed to WSP implementation	Limitations in establishing causality (i.e., the change in slope observed cannot be rigorously attributed to WSP implementation) Multiple (>2) rounds of data collection Difficult to obtain time series of all relevant indicators, especially in low-capacity sites that do not keep rigorous records. Where available data are limited, data collection could be limited to those indicators that are most likely to show changes (as identified by prior rigorous impact assessments conducted at other sites)	Difficult to obtain data on matching parameters, especially for small water systems Risk that confounding factors may be unevenly distributed between the two groups (especially if an insufficient number of parameters are selected for matching), limiting ability to establish causality	Randomizing WSP implementation may cause ethical concerns or political frictions. To mitigate these, WSPs could be implemented in the control group at the end of data collection (i.e., staggered implementation).

4.2. Achievements of WSPs in the Asia-Pacific Region

Despite the challenges described above, this study provided important insights into the implementation of WSPs in the Asia-Pacific region. A number of improvements in management procedures (levels of operations and management practices, number of water safety-related meetings, water quality testing activities, monitoring of consumer complaints), infrastructure, and finance were associated with WSP implementation. Given that most WSPs were only 1–3 years old, these indicators were the most likely to show significant improvements. The study also identified changes that are expected to occur over longer time periods related to water service delivery, including a reduction in unaccounted-for water. Although a previous literature review found limited evidence for institutional effects driven by WSPs [16], this study did identify institutional changes, such as an increase in the number of water-safety meetings and a greater attention to water quality reflected in the qualitative data. However, the qualitative data identified a number of challenges in the implementation of WSPs, including financial barriers and obstacles to the improvement of management procedures. This study also found that infrastructure improvements prioritized water quality rather than quantity while consumer complaints were primarily focused on water quantity, highlighting the importance of balancing water quality and quantity considerations through water safety planning.

4.3. Study Limitations

This impact assessment had several limitations. Firstly, the study design did not include a comparison ("control") group; therefore, although the observed changes were associated with WSPs, it is not possible to attribute causality to WSP implementation. Secondly, the site selection was not random, which may have led to the selection of "best-case" scenarios. Thirdly, data were frequently unavailable; therefore many relationships could not be tested. For example, the data did not allow us to investigate differences in outcomes and impacts between small and large, or between low- and high-capacity systems. Fourthly, the wide range of training and experience among data collectors led to issues with data consistency and quality. However, the analysts have attempted to address some of these limitations by carefully cleaning the data and checking for inconsistencies, and by only analyzing trends for indicators without data quality concerns and available at >25% of sites. Lastly, baseline data collection was retrospective at approximately two-thirds of the sites, which reduced the ability to measure knowledge indicators and may have led to recall errors. These limitations should be carefully addressed in future WSP impact assessments. Specifically, it is recommended to improve training of data collectors and assistance to lower-capacity water systems to collect and report data. Finally, this study showed the importance of collecting qualitative data to substantiate the quantitative indicators.

5. Conclusions

This study was the first attempt to conduct a comprehensive impact evaluation of WSPs on a regional scale. A number of positive outcomes and impacts from WSP development and implementation were identified, as were challenges. In addition, substantial heterogeneities between sites were observed, especially in data availability and record keeping. Therefore, increased efforts by water suppliers and regulators to improve data collection and recording practices are needed.

The study found that the process of assessing the impact of WSPs can be improved, and a number of suggestions have been made to refine the study design and the data collection process. A revised impact assessment framework will be developed by WHO based in part on these suggestions and published as a separate document. In addition, it is recommended that future research investigate the drivers and barriers for WSP success. More systematic monitoring of WSPs is needed to improve their implementation process, guide their scale-up, and build political support around them.

Supplementary Materials: The following are available online at http://www.mdpi.com/1660-4601/15/6/1223/s1, Figure S1: Description of the WSP process, Figure S2: Flowchart of data collection and analysis process,

Table S1: Number of sites participating in the impact assessment in each country and criteria used for their selection, Table S2: Description of data collection teams in each country, training processes, dates of baseline and follow-up data collection, and proportion of sites where baseline data were collected retrospectively, Table S3: Comparison of data collectors' scores with independently assigned scores by Aquaya staff.

Author Contributions: A.R., J.D.F. and D.S. conceived the study and developed the impact assessment framework. E.K., J.K., R.P. and R.K. developed the data analysis plan and did the quantitative and qualitative data analysis. C.D., A.R., E.K., R.P., R.K., J.D.F. and D.S. wrote the paper. The authors alone are responsible for the views expressed in this publication and they do not necessarily represent the views, decisions or policies of the World Health Organization.

Funding: This research was funded by the Australian Department of Foreign Affairs and Trade grant number 50078/60.

Acknowledgments: National colleagues led the considerable task of data collection in the 12 participating countries, with technical support from country, regional, and headquarters levels of WHO.

Conflicts of Interest: The authors affiliated with WHO in this publication declare that WHO received funding for WSP implementation.

References

1. Prüss-Ustün, A.; Bartram, J.; Clasen, T.; Colford, J.M.; Cumming, O.; Curtis, V.; Bonjour, S.; Dangour, A.D.; De France, J.; Fewtrell, L.; et al. Burden of Disease from Inadequate Water, Sanitation and Hygiene in Low- and Middle-Income Settings: A Retrospective Analysis of Data from 145 Countries. *Trop. Med. Int. Health* **2014**, *19*, 894–905. [CrossRef] [PubMed]

2. Bain, R.; Cronk, R.; Wright, J.; Yang, H.; Slaymaker, T.; Bartram, J. Fecal Contamination of Drinking-Water in Low- and Middle-Income Countries: A Systematic Review and Meta-Analysis. *PLoS Med.* **2014**, *11*, e1001644. [CrossRef] [PubMed]

3. Peletz, R.; Kumpel, E.; Bonham, M.; Rahman, Z.; Khush, R. To What Extent Is Drinking Water Tested in Sub-Saharan Africa? A Comparative Analysis of Regulated Water Quality Monitoring. *Int. J. Environ. Res. Public Health* **2016**, *13*, 275. [CrossRef] [PubMed]

4. Kumpel, E.; Peletz, R.; Mateyo, B.; Khush, R. Assessing Drinking Water Quality and Water Safety Management in Sub-Saharan Africa Using Regulated Monitoring Data. *Environ. Sci. Technol.* **2016**, *50*, 10869–10876. [CrossRef] [PubMed]

5. World Health Organization (WHO). *Guidelines for Drinking Water Quality*, 3rd ed.; World Health Organization: Geneva, Switzerland, 2004. Available online: http://www.who.int/water_sanitation_health/publications/gdwq3/en/ (accessed on 28 May 2018).

6. Bartram, J.; Corrales, L.; Davison, A.; Deere, D.; Drury, D.; Gordon, B.; Howard, G.; Rinehold, A.; Stevens, M. *Water Safety Plan Manual: Step-by-Step Risk Management for Drinking-Water Suppliers*; World Health Organization: Geneva, Switzerland, 2009.

7. World Health Organisation (WHO). *Water Safety Planning for Small Community Water Supplies: Step-by-Step Risk Management Guidance for Drinking-Water Supplies in Small Communities*; World Health Organisation: Geneva, Switzerland, 2012. Available online: http://www.who.int/water_sanitation_health/publications/small-comm-water_supplies/en/ (accessed on 28 May 2018).

8. World Health Organization (WHO). *Guidelines for Drinking-Water Quality*, 5th ed.; World Health Organisation: Geneva, Switzerland, 2011. Available online: http://www.who.int/water_sanitation_health/publications/2011/dwq_guidelines/en/ (accessed on 28 May 2018).

9. World Health Organization (WHO)/International Water Association (IWA). *Global Status Report on Water Safety Plans: A Review of Proactive Risk Assessment and Risk Management Practices to Ensure the Safety of Drinking-Water*; World Health Organisation: Geneva, Switzerland, 2017. Available online: http://www.who.int/water_sanitation_health/publications/global-status-report-on-water-safety-plans/en/ (accessed on 28 May 2018).

10. Byleveld, P.; Leask, S.; Jarvis, L.; Wall, K.; Henderson, W.; Tickell, J. Safe Drinking Water in Regional NSW, Australia. *Public Health Res. Pract.* **2016**, *26*, 2621615. [CrossRef] [PubMed]

11. Hubbard, B.; Gelting, R.; del Carmen Portillo, M.; Williams, T.; Torres, R. Awareness, Adoption and Implementation of the Water Safety Plan Methodology: Insights from Five Latin American and Caribbean Experiences. *J. Water Sanit. Hyg. Dev.* **2013**, *3*, 541–548. [CrossRef]

12. Kot, M.; Castleden, H.; Gagnon, G.A. The Human Dimension of Water Safety Plans: A Critical Review of Literature and Information Gaps. *Environ. Rev.* **2014**, *23*, 24–29. [CrossRef]
13. Mahmud, S.G.; Shamsuddin, S.A.J.; Feroze Ahmed, M.; Davison, A.; Deere, D.; Howard, G. Development and Implementation of Water Safety Plans for Small Water Supplies in Bangladesh: Benefits and Lessons Learned. *J. Water Health* **2007**, *5*, 585–597. [CrossRef] [PubMed]
14. Ncube, M.; Pawandiwa, M.N. Water Safety Planning and Implementation: Lessons from South Africa. *J. Water Sanit. Hyg. Dev.* **2013**, *3*, 557–563. [CrossRef]
15. Omar, Y.Y.; Parker, A.; Smith, J.A.; Pollard, S.J.T. Risk Management for Drinking Water Safety in Low and Middle Income Countries–Cultural Influences on Water Safety Plan (WSP) Implementation in Urban Water Utilities. *Sci. Total Environ.* **2017**, *576*, 895–906. [CrossRef] [PubMed]
16. Tibatemwa, S.; Godfrey, S.; Niwagaba, C.; Kizito, F. Implementing Water-Safety Plans in Urban Piped-Water Supplies in Uganda. *Waterlines* **2005**, *23*, 8–10. [CrossRef]
17. String, G.; Lantagne, D. A Systematic Review of Outcomes and Lessons Learned from General, Rural, and Country-Specific Water Safety Plan Implementations. *Water Sci. Technol. Water Supply* **2016**, *16*, 1580–1594. [CrossRef]
18. Gunnarsdottir, M.J.; Gardarsson, S.M.; Elliott, M.; Sigmundsdottir, G.; Bartram, J. Benefits of Water Safety Plans: Microbiology, Compliance, and Public Health. *Environ. Sci. Technol.* **2012**, *46*, 7782–7789. [CrossRef] [PubMed]
19. Setty, K.E.; Kayser, G.L.; Bowling, M.; Enault, J.; Loret, J.-F.; Serra, C.P.; Alonso, J.M.; Mateu, A.P.; Bartram, J. Water Quality, Compliance, and Health Outcomes among Utilities Implementing Water Safety Plans in France and Spain. *Int. J. Hyg. Environ. Health* **2017**, *220*, 513–530. [CrossRef] [PubMed]
20. Gelting, R.J.; Delea, K.; Medlin, E. A Conceptual Framework to Evaluate the Outcomes and Impacts of Water Safety Plans. *J. Water Sanit. Hyg. Dev.* **2012**, *2*, 103–111. [CrossRef]
21. Lockhart, G.; Oswald, W.E.; Hubbard, B.; Medlin, E.; Gelting, R.J. Development of Indicators for Measuring Outcomes of Water Safety Plans. *J. Water Sanit. Hyg. Dev.* **2014**, *4*, 171–181. [CrossRef] [PubMed]
22. World Health Organisation (WHO). Auditing Water Safety Plans. 2016. Available online: http://www.who.int/water_sanitation_health/publications/auditing-water-safety-plans/en/ (accessed on 28 May 2018).
23. QSR International Pty Ltd. *NVivo Qualitative Data Analysis Software*; QSR International Pty Ltd.: Burlington, MA, USA, 2014.
24. Schmidt, W.-P.; Arnold, B.F.; Boisson, S.; Genser, B.; Luby, S.P.; Barreto, M.L.; Clasen, T.; Cairncross, S. Epidemiological Methods in Diarrhoea Studies—An Update. *Int. J. Epidemiol.* **2011**, *40*, 1678–1692. [CrossRef] [PubMed]
25. Benjamin-Chung, J.; Sultana, S.; Halder, A.K.; Ahsan, M.A.; Arnold, B.F.; Hubbard, A.E.; Unicomb, L.; Luby, S.P.; Colford, J.M. Scaling Up a Water, Sanitation, and Hygiene Program in Rural Bangladesh: The Role of Program Implementation. *Am. J. Public Health* **2017**, *107*, 694–701. [CrossRef] [PubMed]

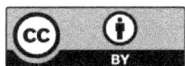

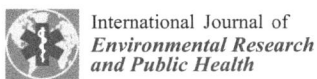

International Journal of
Environmental Research and Public Health

Article

Burden of Common Childhood Diseases in Relation to Improved Water, Sanitation, and Hygiene (WASH) among Nigerian Children

Zhifei He [1], Ghose Bishwajit [2], Dongsheng Zou [1], Sanni Yaya [2], Zhaohui Cheng [3] and Yan Zhou [1,*]

[1] School of Politics and Public Administration, Southwest University of Political Science & Law, Chongqing 401120, China; houis123@163.com (Z.H.); mrzds023@163.com (D.Z.)
[2] School of International Development and Global Studies, University of Ottawa, Ottawa, ON K1N 6N5, Canada; brammaputram@gmail.com (G.B.); sanni.yaya@uOttawa.ca (S.Y.)
[3] Health Information Center, Chongqing 401120, China; czhbtx@163.com
* Correspondence: mszhouyan023@163.com

Received: 25 April 2018; Accepted: 7 June 2018; Published: 12 June 2018

Abstract: Having access to improved water, sanitation, and hygiene (WASH) facilities constitute a key component of healthy living and quality of life. Prolonged exposure to insanitary living conditions can significantly enhance the burden of infectious diseases among children and affect nutritional status and growth. In this study we examined the prevalence of some common infectious diseases/disease symptoms of childhood among under-five children in Nigeria, and the association between the occurrence of these diseases with household's access to WASH facilities. Types of diseases used as outcome variables included diarrheal, and acute respiratory infections (fever and cough). Access to WASH facilities were defined by WHO classification. The association between diarrhoea, fever and chronic cough with sanitation, and hygiene was analyzed by logistic regression techniques. Results showed that the prevalence of diarrhoea, fever and cough was respectively 10.5% (95% CI = 9.7–2.0), 13.4% (95% CI = 11.9–14.8), and 10.4% (95% CI = 9.2–11.5). In the regression analysis, children in the households that lacked all three types of facilities were found to have respectively 1.32 [AOR = 1.329, 95% CI = 1.046–1.947], 1.24 [AOR = 1.242, 95% CI = 1.050–1.468] and 1.43 [AOR = 1.432, 95% CI = 1.113–2.902] times higher odds of suffering from diarrhea, fever and cough. The study concludes that unimproved WASH conditions is an important contributor to ARIs and diarrheal morbidities among Nigerian children. In light of these findings, it is recommended that programs targeting to reduce childhood morbidity and mortality from common infectious diseases should leverage equitable provision of WASH interventions.

Keywords: diarrhea; fever; cough; Nigeria; infant health

1. Introduction

As one of the fastest urbanizing country in the continent, Nigeria is experiencing significant challenges to provide access to improved Water, sanitation, and hygiene (WASH) to the population. Uncontrolled urbanization affects sanitation mainly through overcrowding of communities, constraints to quality housing, and reduced freshwater availability due to increasing consumption of water and water-intensive goods and pollution. The situation is exacerbated by poor environmental management and regulation which are failing to prevent the pollution of fresh water resources by accumulation of household and industrial waste water effluents [1]. Water crisis is looming large in the rural areas as well which is felt especially during the dry seasons, leaving as high as 70% of the households in serious water insecurity [2]. Nigeria's sanitation and water poverty have raised concerns among many and has been reported by numerous national and international agencies. As of 2015, respectively 69% and 57% of the population in the urban and rural areas faced chronic water shortage [3] with about another 100 million living without access to adequate sanitation facilities [4]. In contrast, findings from a multi-country study by the joint monitoring program of WHO and UNICEF reported that 75% of the population had improved water and 59% that had improved sanitation [5]. Lack of access to WASH has important implications for population health especially among children who are more susceptible to infection and higher risk of illness due to their underdeveloped immune system [6]. Water and sanitation induced illnesses among under-5 children is considered as a serious public health concern in Nigeria [4,7].

The importance of WASH on infant nutrition and health status, and early childhood development cannot be overemphasized. WASH, referred to as improved quantity and quality of water, sanitation, and hygiene is widely acknowledged as the most cost-effective strategy to reduce the burden of infant morbidity and mortality by limiting the vectors of transmission through multiple food, water and environmental routes [8–10]. Inadequate access to clean water, basic sanitation and poor hygiene practices cause nearly 90% of all deaths from diarrhea in children [11]. Promoting access to safe excreta disposal, basic hygiene practices such as hand washing with soap, and provision of safe water supply are regarded as key strategies to limit the burden of infectious diseases among children including soil-transmitted health infections and diarrhea [6]. According to some estimates, globally an estimated 2.4 million deaths (4.2% of all deaths) could have been averted a year through optimum use of WASH [12]. Results from a WHO analysis maintained that promoting access to safe water and better environmental conditions could prevent about 94% of all diarrheal diseases [13]. The poor WASH infrastructure in resource-poor settings e.g., sub-Saharan Africa is reflected through the indiscriminately high burden of diarrhea and acute respiratory infections or ARI (common cold, cough, fever) [14]. In Nigeria, for instance, about 130,000 deaths among children are attributable to water-borne infections [15]. The burden of diarrhea attributable deaths among under-5 children have been reported to be 150,000 per year [16].

During past few decades there has been an escalating healthcare concern regarding the rise of non-communicable chronic diseases in the Nigeria, accompanied by reduced attention and budgetary capacity for the persistently high child-mortality and poor WASH conditions. Nigeria has been a signatory of the United Nations Declaration of the Right to Water and regulates its WASH activities through the Federal Ministry of Water Resources (FMWR). In recent years FMWR has been strengthening its policy efforts for scaling up the water and sanitation sector, and have launched several comprehensive projects in joint collaboration with UNICEF WASH [16] and USAID [17]. Some of these projects are working with ambitious targets of reaching the entire population and help meet the water and sanitation related Sustainable Development Goals or SDGs (Goal 6) in the country. However, it is notable that despite being a large country (largest in Africa), and having large scale programs on child health and WASH, there remains the lack of comprehensive population based studies on their association, and thus potentially limiting the scope for informed policy making and programmatic approaches. Therefore, to address this gap we conducted the present study using a nationally representative data drawn from the Nigeria Demographic and Health Survey. Although the survey was conducted few years back (in 2013), it is expected that the present study can provide important insights for the ongoing projects on WASH and child health related projects in Nigeria as well as for other countries in sub-Saharan Africa.

2. Materials and Methods

2.1. The Survey and Sampling Design

Nigeria Demographic and Health Survey (NDHS) 2013 was the fourth of the kind in Nigeria which was implemented by the National Population Commission with the financial and technical assistance by Inner City Fund (ICF) International provisioned through the USAID-funded MEASURE DHS program.

DHS surveys are cross-sectional, nationally representative that collect information on a wide range of public health related topics such as anthropometric, demographic, socioeconomic, family planning and domestic violence to name a few. The survey covered men and women aged between 15–49 years and under-5 children residing in non-institutional settings. For sampling, a three-staged stratified cluster design was employed which was based on a list enumeration area from the 2006 Population Census of the Federal Republic of Nigeria. Enumeration areas are systematically selected units from the localities, which constitute the local government areas. Local government areas are subdivisions of each of the 36 administrative states (including the Federal Capital Territory called Abuja) and classified under six developmental zones in the country. Enumeration areas were used to form the survey clusters called primary sampling units. NDHS 2013 consisted of 904 clusters (372 in urban areas and 532 in rural areas) encompassing a total of 40,320 households from which 38,948 women were successfully interviewed with a response rate of 98%. Fieldwork lasted from 15 February 2013 to the end of May of the same year, and was carried out by 36 interviewing teams in each state plus one in the Federal Capital Territory of Abuja. A more detailed version of the survey was published elsewhere [18].

2.2. Variables

The outcome variables were prevalence of self-reported in commonly occurring Acute Respiratory Infections (ARIs) e.g., diarrhea, fever and cough. Mothers were asked whether or not the child suffered from these conditions during the past two weeks, and had the options to answer as- 'Yes' or 'No'. Diarrhoea refers to the passage of three or more loose or liquid stools per day (or more frequent passage than is normal for the individual [19].

The explanatory variables of interest were access to improved (1) water; (2) sanitation and hygiene practices. We used WHO guidelines to classify the type of water and sanitation facilities as improved/unimproved (Table 1). The dataset did not contain any hygiene related variable. As a proxy indicator we used the information on disposal of child's excreta which was also assessed by WHO guidelines.

Table 1. WHO classification of improved sanitation and water supply.

	Unimproved	Improved
Sanitation + Child's excreta disposal facilities	Unimproved sanitation facilities: do not ensure hygienic separation of human excreta from human contact. Unimproved facilities include pit latrines without a slab or platform, hanging latrines and bucket latrines.	Improved sanitation facilities: ensure hygienic separation of human excreta from human contact. They are use of the following facilities: Flush/pour flush to: piped sewer system, septic tank, pit latrine; Ventilated improved pit (VIP) latrine, Pit latrine with slab, Composting toilet.
Water	Unimproved drinking-water sources: Unprotected dug well, unprotected spring, cart with small tank/drum, surface water (river, dam, lake, pond, stream, canal, irrigation channels), and bottled water.	Other improved drinking-water sources: Public taps or standpipes, tube wells or boreholes, protected dug wells, protected springs or rainwater collection. Piped water on premises: Piped household water connection located inside the user's dwelling, plot or yard.

Source: WHO/UNICEF Joint Monitoring Programme for Water Supply and Sanitation. ISBN 978 92 4 156395 6 (NLM classification: WA 670).

A set of confounding variables were included in the analysis as well based on their relevance in light of previous studies such as Sex (Female, Male), Age in months (1–12, 13–24, 25–36, 37–48, 49–59), Birthweight are low birth-weight (LBW) and normal birth-weight (NBW), Stunting (No/Yes), Type of residency (Urban/Rural), Parents education (No education/Primary/Secondary/Higher), Household wealth status (Poor/Non-Poor) and presence of other infants in the household ($\leq$2/3–4/>4) [4,16–18].

For the calculation household wealth status, instead of direct income the volume of durable goods (e.g., TV, radio and bicycle) possessed by the household as well as and housing quality (e.g., type of floor, wall, and roof) are taken into consideration. Each item is assigned a factor score generated through principal component analysis (PCA) which are then summed and standardized for the households. The scores thus obtained from a continuous scale and subsequently categorized into quintiles to rank the household as poorest/poorer/middle/richer/richest to richest [20]. For the present study, households in lowest two categories were merged and categorized as poor, and those from middle to richest were merged as non-poor.

2.3. Data Analysis

Before the analysis we checked the dataset for presence of outliers, and potential multi-collinearity. Following that, the dataset was converted to a plan file as complex samples by adjusting for the sampling strata, primary sampling unit and sampling weight. This is because DHS surveys employ cluster sampling methods for sample selection which needs to be taken into consideration for all analyses. As the initial analysis, the basic socio-demographic characteristics of participants were presented in terms of frequencies and percentages. Prevalence rate were shown as percentages with 95% CIs. Following descriptive analysis, Chi square bivariate tests were performed to check for the significant associations between disease status and the indicators of WASH along with the covariates. Variables that were found to be significantly associated in the Chi square tests ($p < 0.25$) were retained for final regression analysis. In the final step, binary logistic regression model was used to calculate the odds ratios of the associations between diarrhoea, fever and cough with WASH indicators. Precisely, individual disease status was modelled as a function of the three WASH indicators and to the binary logistic regression, while adjusting for various demographic and socioeconomic parameters which were found (based on literature review) empirically and theoretically pertinent to the outcome and exposure variables. Results of regression analysis were presented as odds ratios along with their 95% CIs as in indicator of significance as well as precision of the OR values. For all associations *p*-value of < 0.05 was considered statistically significant. All analyses were performed with SPSS version 24.

Ethical Approval

The protocol of DHS surveys was approved by the Ethics Committee of ORC Macro Inc., Calverton, MD, USA. The study was based on analysis of anonymized secondary data available in the public domain of DHS, therefore no additional approval was necessary. However, approval for the reuse of the data was obtained by authors from DHS.

3. Results

3.1. Description of the Sample

As shown in Table 2, the study included a total of 24,802 infants with a mean age of 28 months ($\pm$17.28). Most of the infants were aged 1 year of below (21.7%), normal birth-weight (96.8%), located in the north-west region (36%), of rural origin (64.5%). Literacy rate was higher among fathers (61.2%) compared with mothers (51.6%). Over half (54.8%) of the households were non-poor and about two-third had a maximum of two children (66.4%).

Regarding household characteristics, respectively 49% and 44.2% of the households were lacking access to sanitary toilet and pure clean water facilities, and 35.2% households did not practice proper methods for disposal of child's excreta. Significant variations were observed in the rate of access to the three types of facilities across various individual (birthweight and stunting), geographical and household level factors (parents' educational attainment, wealth status and presence of other infants in the household).

Table 2. Description of the sample children in NDHS 2013.

Variables	Total	Households Lacking Improved		
	(*N* = 24,802)	Toilet Facilities %	Water Facilities %	Child's Excreta Disposal Facilities %
	N (%)	49.0	44.2	35.2
Demographics				
Sex				
Female	12,333 (49.9)	50.1	50.4	50.1
Male	12,469 (50.1)	49.9	49.6	49.9
		NS	NS	NS
Age (28/17.28)				
1–12 months	6131 (21.7)	24.7	25.1	25.0
13–24 months	5189 (20.5)	21.2	20.6	21.9
25–36 months	4616 (19.1)	18.6	18.7	17.7
37–48 months	4764 (19.6)	18.9	18.8	19.1
49–59 months	4102 (19.1)	16.7	16.8	16.3
		NS	NS	NS
Birthweight				
LBW	532 (3.2)	4.9	4.7	5.9
NBW	24,270 (96.8)	95.1	95.3	94.1
p		<0.0001	0.003	<0.0001
Stunted				
No	6909 (28.3)	31.7	31.3	25.3
Yes	17,893 (71.7)	68.3	68.7	74.7
p		<0.0001	<0.0001	<0.0001
Geographic factors				
Type of place of residence				
Urban	8342 (35.5)	17.9	20.6	25.8
Rural	16,460 (64.5)	82.1	79.4	74.2
p		<0.0001	<0.0001	<0.0001
Household socioeconomic details				
Mother's education				
No education	11,365 (48.4)	56.4	58.5	43.8
Primary	5084 (19.3)	21.8	18.7	23.9
Secondary/Higher	8353 (32.3)	21.8	22.8	32.4
p		<0.0001	<0.0001	<0.0001
Father's education				
No education	9142 (38.8)	45.9	47.4	36.3
Primary	4888 (19.1)	21.9	19.3	21.7
Secondary/Higher	10,772 (42.1)	32.2	33.3	42.0
p		<0.0001	<0.0001	<0.0001
Wealth status				
Poor	10,986 (45.2)	63.2	63.2	52.1
Non-Poor	13,816 (54.8)	36.8	36.8	47.9
p		<0.0001	<0.0001	0.063
Infants in household				
≤2	16,473 (66.4)	64.6	65.0	68.5
3–4	6981 (28.1)	29.1	28.7	27.2
>4	1348 (5.4)	6.3	6.3	4.3
p		0.014	0.039	0.001

N.B. NDHS = Nigeria Demographic and Health Survey, CI = Confidence interval.

Table 3 indicates that fever was the most common of all three illness types with a prevalence of fever 13.4% (95% CI = 11.9–14.8) followed by diarrhoea 10.5% (95% CI = 9.7–12.0) and cough 10.4% (95% CI = 9.2–11.5). The prevalence rates of diarrhoea, fever and cough were higher among those who were normal birth-weight, stunted, of rural origin, born to parents with no formal education (except for fever), and from households with poor wealth status and had more than four infants (except for fever).

Figure 1 illustrates the prevalence rates of diarrhoea, fever and chronic cough among households with and without access to improved sanitation, water and child excreta disposal facilities. It revealed that household that had improved facilities also had lower rates of prevalence of all three types of diseases.

Table 3. Weighted prevalence of self-reported Diarrhoea, Fever and Cough during last two-weeks among under-five children, NDHS 2013.

Variables	Diarrhoea	Fever	Cough
	10.5 (9.7–12.0)	**13.4 (11.9–14.8)**	**10.4 (9.2–11.5)**
Sex			
Female	49.8 (47.6–52.0)	48.7 (46.6–50.9)	49.7 (47.4–52.1)
Male	50.2 (48.0–52.4)	51.3 (49.1–53.4)	50.3 (47.9–52.6)
p	0.049	NS	Ns
Age			
1–12 months	23.4 (21.5–25.4)	25.0 (23.4–26.8)	24.5 (22.5–26.6)
13–24 months	21.7 (19.7–23.8)	20.1 (18.6–21.8)	21.7 (19.8–23.8)
25–36 months	18.2 (16.4–20.1)	19.2 (17.7–20.9)	19.2 (17.4–21.1)
37–48 months	21.6 (19.8–23.4)	20.4 (18.9–21.9)	20.2 (18.5–22.1)
49–59 months	15.2 (13.5–17.1)	15.2 (13.8–16.8)	14.4 (12.8–16.1)
	NS	NS	0.126
Birthweight			
LBW	2.8 (1.9–4.1)	0.9 (0.5–1.4)	7.2 (5.0–10.3)
NBW	97.2 (95.9–98.1)	99.1 (98.6–99.5)	92.8 (89.7–95.0)
	NS	<0.0001	<0.0001
Stunted			
No	34.8 (32.6–37.0)	30.8 (28.8–32.9)	25.7 (23.5–28.1)
Yes	65.2 (63.0–67.4)	69.2 (67.1–71.2)	74.3 (71.9–76.5)
p	<0.0001	0.0007	0.007
Type of place of residence			
Urban	31.7 (28.2–35.4)	33.7 (30.3–37.2)	40.5 (36.7–44.4)
Rural	68.3 (64.6–71.8)	66.3 (62.8–69.7)	59.5 (55.6–63.3)
p	0.013	<0.0001	0.003
Mother's education			
No education	56.0 (52.5–59.4)	48.2 (45.0–51.5)	43.4 (40.2–46.8)
Primary	18.4 (16.4–20.6)	19.3 (17.4–21.5)	35.0 (31.8–38.3)
Secondary/Higher	25.6 (22.9–28.5)	32.4 (29.6–35.4)	21.6 (19.3–24.0)
p	<0.0001	NS	<0.0001
Father's education			
No education	45.0 (41.3–48.8)	40.0 (36.5–43.5)	51.5 (48.3–54.7)
Primary	18.9 (16.8–21.1)	19.6 (17.7–21.7)	28.9 (25.7–32.2)
Secondary/Higher	36.1 (33.0–39.4)	40.4 (37.5–43.4)	19.6 (17.6–21.9)
p	<0.0001	NS	<0.0001
Wealth status			
Poor	53.9 (49.8–57.9)	51.7 (47.9–55.4)	60.8 (57.0–64.5)
Non-Poor	46.1 (42.1–50.2)	48.3 (44.6–52.1)	39.2 (35.5–43.0)
p	<0.0001	0.071	<0.0001
Number of children 5 and under in household			
≤2	5.8 (4.5–7.4)	4.8 (3.4–6.6)	3.4 (2.3–4.9)
3–4	30.8 (28.7–32.9)	27.6 (25.4–29.8)	25.9 (23.4–28.4)
>4	63.4 (60.8–66.0)	67.6 (65.0–70.2)	70.7 (67.9–73.4)
p	0.039	NS	<0.0001

NDHS = Nigeria Demographic and Health Survey. The 95%CI are presented between brackets.

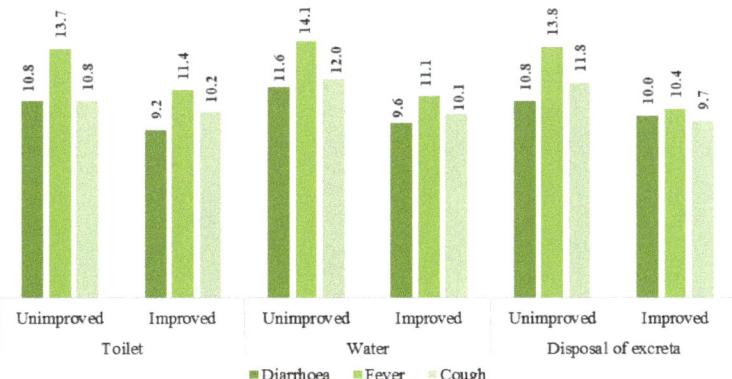

Figure 1. Prevalence of diarrhoea, fever and cough among under-5 children stratified by type of toilet, water, and child's excreta disposal facilities.

Figure 2 showed the regional disparities in the prevalence of diarrhoea, fever and cough. It reveals that the individual and combines prevalence of all these three diseases tended to be highest in the Northeast region and lowest in the South West.

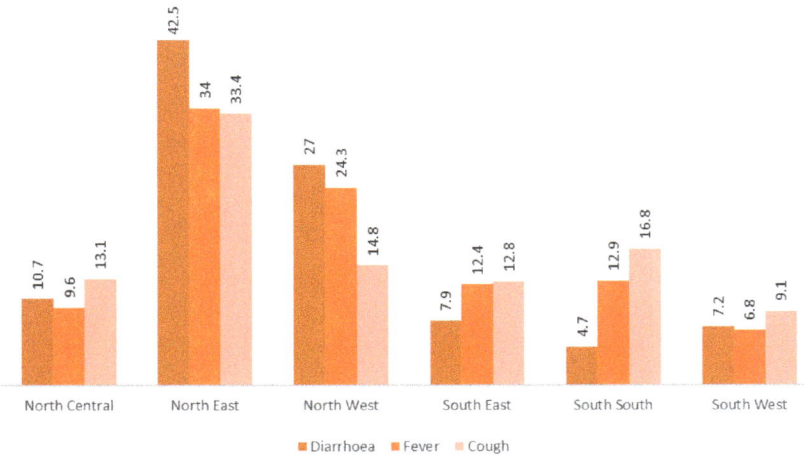

Figure 2. Prevalence of diarrhoea, fever and cough among under-5 children by region.

Figure 3 illustrates the regional disparities in the accessibility to improved toilet, water and child's excreta disposal facilities. It appears that the situation is worst in the North East and Northwest region, with South East and South West regions having comparatively better scenarios.

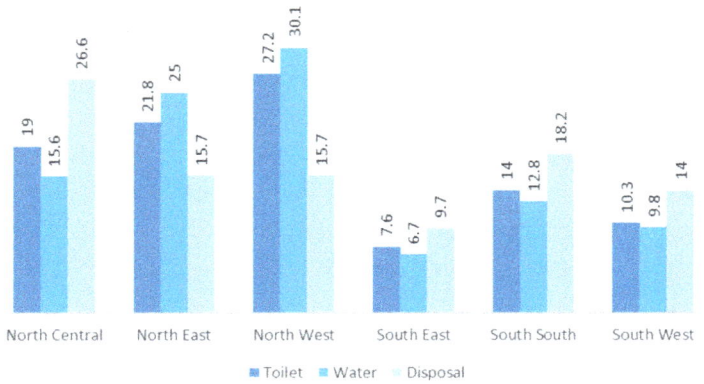

Figure 3. Percentage of households lacking access to improved toilet, water and child's excreta disposal facilities by region.

3.2. Regression Analysis

The results of multivariable regression measuring the associations between the three types of illnesses with household's access to sanitation, clean water and child's excreta disposal facilities were presented in Table 4. Access to sanitary toilet did not appear to be a significant predictor of any of the three diseases. The odds of suffering from diarrhoea were 1.6 [AOR = 1.602, 95% CI = 1.217–2.343, $p < 0.001$] and that of suffering from fever was 2.2 times [AOR = 2.193, 95% CI = 1.544–4.618, $p < 0.001$] as high among those with lack of access to clean water. Insanitary disposal of child's excreta also showed 1.17 time [AOR = 1.172, 95% CI = 1.022–1.344, $p < 0.001$] higher odds of suffering from diarrhoea and 1.39 times [AOR = 1.393, 95% CI = 1.041–3.028] higher odds of suffering from fever. Finally, household that lacked all three types of facilities had respectively 1.33 [AOR = 1.329, 95% CI = 1.046–1.947, $p < 0.001$], 1.24 [AOR = 1.242, 95% CI = 1.050–1.468, $p < 0.001$] and 1.43 times [AOR = 1.432, 95% CI = 1.113–2.902, $p < 0.001$] higher odds of suffering from diarrhoea, fever and cough.

Table 4. Regression analysis on the association between lack of access to toilet, water and child excreta disposal facilities with the three types of diseases.

Variables	Diarrhoea		Fever		Cough	
	COR	AOR	COR	AOR	COR	AOR
Toilet facilities (yes)						
No	1.104 (0.950–1.283)	0.972 (0.841–1.124)	1.054 (0.456–2.438)	1.029 (0.480–2.203)	1.240 (0.629–2.443)	1.149 (0.627–2.107)
Water facilities (yes)						
No	**1.179 (1.010–1.376)**	**1.602 (1.217–2.343)**	1.428 (0.616–3.311)	**2.193 (1.544–4.618)**	1.310 (0.721–2.379)	1.059 (0.924–1.214)
Child's excreta Disposal facilities (yes)						
No	0.927 (0.804–1.069)	**1.172 (1.022–1.344)**	1.013 (0.442–2.325)	**1.393 (1.041–3.028)**	1.388 (0.771–2.498)	1.245 (0.673–2.303)
Toilet + water + disposal facilities (yes)						
No	1.137 (0.968–1.336)	**1.329 (1.046–1.947)**	1.180 (0.568–2.449)	**1.242 (1.050–1.468)**	**1.220 (1.050–1.418)**	**1.432 (1.113–2.902)**

N.B. AOR/COR = Adjusted/Crude odds ratio. (yes) = Reference category. Bold numbers indicate significant associations ($p < 0.05$). The 95%CI are presented between brackets.

4. Discussion

In this study, attempts were made to provide an updated scenario of water and sanitation situation in Nigeria. Prevalence rates of three common childhood diseases namely diarrhea, fever and cough were also measured and was checked for their independent association with household's access to improved water and sanitation facilities. Results indicate that fever was the most prevalent of the three diseases followed by diarrhoea and cough. In line with previous reports, the prevalence rates were higher among households that lacked access to improved WASH facilities [21]. In the bivariate analysis; stunting, parents' educational achievement and household wealth status also appeared to be significantly associated especially with diarrhoea and cough. These observations are quite as expected because less educated parents are more likely to be unaware of the health risks associated with substandard water and sanitation quality and show poor hygiene behavior [22,23]. Higher socioeconomic status can act as a strong enabling factor for the utilization of WASH technologies, as well as a determinant of better self-efficacy for proper hygiene practices. Bivariate analysis also indicated a significant relationship between access to improved water and sanitation and the prevalence of the three types of diseases. The negative impact of poor WASH conditions on child growth and development have been shown to result from sustained exposure to enteric pathogens as well as various social and economic mechanisms [14,24].

Important regional variations were also noted in the prevalence of all three diseases, and of household's access to improved WASH facilities. It appeared that household in the North East and Northwest regions share the highest burden of the diseases and have the lowest rate of access to WASH facilities. These findings are hard to explain in light of the current analysis, however can be implicated to the socioeconomic disparities across the six regions. There has been a marked North/South polarity in the country in terms of infrastructure, sociopolitical prosperity and human development indicators since the colonial times [25]. Hence, it is very likely that the relatively deeper impoverishment is the North partly accounts for the poorer health indicators. This finding therefore embodies an important message for the ongoing WASH projects in the country as conflicting geopolitical interests can significantly hamper the success of all development efforts.

The results also revealed statistically significant associations between the lack of WASH facilities with the occurrence of diarrhoea, fever and cough. These findings are similar with those from an Ethiopian study conducted among children (aged 0–50 months) in the slum areas of Addis Ababa. The study reported a diarrheal prevalence of 11.9% which is close to that in Nigeria. However, the rate of access to improved sanitation facilities was remarkably low (5.4%), perhaps because of study areas being slums, and was found to be a strong risk factor for diarrhoea [26]. In a nationally representative study in Uganda (Uganda Demographic and Health Survey 2011), a quarter of the infants were reported to have suffered from diarrhea during the past two weeks, a significant proportions of which were living in poorest WASH conditions [27,28]. Another Nigerian study showed evidences of infant mortality risks of from both unimproved water and sanitation [4]. Thus, the findings of the present study add further evidence to the current literature, and calls for heightened stress on WASH.

It is evident that as one of the fastest growing economy in the world, Nigeria is undergoing rapid demographic and epidemiological transitions in terms of the emergence of diseases and risk factors, changing trends in morbidity and mortality from certain disease groups. These altogether translate to mounting challenges for the healthcare sector due mainly to financial and infrastructure constraints to address the rising healthcare needs of the population. From this perspective, promoting WASH facilities and their proper utilization offer a key opportunity to minimize healthcare related constraints and promote population health in resource-poor settings [12]. This is particularly the case with respect to children's health who are usually the most at-risk group for infectious disease and malnutrition related morbidities [29]. There are also documented evidences that poor WASH is associated with increased vulnerabilities to epidemics as widespread as HIV/AIDS [30] and tuberculosis [31]. It is therefore an urgent public health imperative to scale up WASH initiatives by ensuring multi-sectoral collaboration, especially by establishing closer cooperation between WASH and childcare stakeholders [6]. It is hoped that the current study provides important insights for researchers and interest groups involved in policy making in the areas of child health and sanitation issues. As a general recommendation for program managers and policy makers, special emphasis needs to be given on the underlying sociopolitical factors that engender inequality and barrier progress to the health promotion programs in the country since lack of organizational accountability and transparency is known to be rife among both public and private sectors [32].

As far as we are concerned, this is the first study to report on the relationship between WASH and diarrhea and selected ARIs. The data were cross-sectional, however large enough to help make meaningful conclusions, and more so since the samples were selected nationwide. One particular strength is that that analysis was adjusted for several important confounders including stunting and birth weight which have been found to be strong predictors of diarrhoea. Apart from that, we also considered three different types of communicable diseases instead of diarrhoea alone which can serve as a good reference for future researches in this area. Among the limitations were the self-reported nature of the variables that incurs the risks of recall and reporting biases, and lack of information on medication and presence of other disease conditions that could have influenced the strength of the association to certain degrees. Also, only a small of range of indicators were available for WASH as few others e.g., handwashing was not possible to include due to very limited amount of observations. As the data were secondary, we were unable to account for several important determinants of WASH such as gender equity, cultural and behavioural practices which need to explored through in-depth qualitative investigations. Further studies should be performed by considering a wider range of infectious diseases and using more proximate indicators of WASH to develop a deeper understanding of the causal relationships.

5. Conclusions

Based on secondary analysis of nationally representative data from Nigeria Demographic and Health Survey, the study drew several important conclusions which might of high interest for child health and WASH related stakeholders in the country. The magnitude of the burden of diarrhoea, fever and cough were alarming, as was the prevalence of households living without improved WASH facilities. Of particular concern was the presence of marked regional (North/South) disparities in WASH condition and morbidity of the diseases. Not having access to WASH facilities also appeared to be an important predictor of the disease conditions under study. In light of the current scenario, it is perceivable that special efforts will be required to ensure optimum WASH coverage for huge proportion of the population to produce observable benefits on child health outcomes. Qualitative studies are required to investigate the gender, cultural and behavioural aspects of WASH with respect to common infectious diseases among under-5 children.

Author Contributions: Z.H., G.B. and D.Z. conceptualized the study and data collection. Z.H., G.B., D.Z. and S.Y. were responsible for data management and analysis. Z.H. and G.B. contributed to initial drafting and interpretation of the results. G.B., Y.Z., Z.H., Z.C. were responsible of the linguistic. All authors read the final manuscript and gave approval for publication.

Funding: This research was funded by National Social Science Foundation of China (No. 2013-GM-048).

Acknowledgments: We are appreciate the authors of Ottawa University, who contributed a lot in data collection and analysis. Meanwhile, we are appreciate the authors of Southwest University of Political Science and Law, who contributed to initial drafting and writing. Finally, we thanks to the National Social Science Foundation of China, which provides the funding support.

Conflicts of Interest: The authors declare no conflict of interest.

Abbreviations

ARIs	Acute Respiratory Infections
DHS	Demographic and Health Survey
SDGs	Sustainable Development Goals
WASH	Water, Sanitation, and Hygiene
WHO	World Health Organization.
LBW	Low Birthweight
NBW	Normal Birthweight

References

1. Ijaiya, H.; Joseph, O.T. Rethinking Environmental Law Enforcement in Nigeria. *Beijing Law Rev.* **2014**, *5*, 306. [CrossRef]
2. Ishaku, H.T.; Majid, M.R.; Ajayi, A.A.; Haruna, A. Water Supply Dilemma in Nigerian Rural Communities: Looking Towards the Sky for an Answer. *J. Water Resour. Prot.* **2011**, *3*, 598. [CrossRef]
3. Umezulike, C. Challenges in The Nigerian Water Sector—If the Problem Is Not Lack of Comprehensive Regimes, Then What Is It? 2017. Available online: http://www.connecteddevelopment.org/1963-2/ (accessed on 27 October 2017).
4. Ezeh, O.K.; Agho, K.E.; Dibley, M.J.; Hall, J.; Page, A.N. The Impact of Water and Sanitation on Childhood Mortality in Nigeria: Evidence from Demographic and Health Surveys, 2003–2013. *Int. J. Environ. Res. Public Health* **2014**, *11*, 9256–9272. [CrossRef] [PubMed]
5. Roche, R.; Bain, R.; Cumming, O. A long way to go—Estimates of combined water, sanitation and hygiene coverage for 25 sub-Saharan African countries. *PLoS ONE* **2017**, *12*, e0171783. [CrossRef]
6. Progress on Drinking Water, Sanitation and Hygiene: 2017 Update and SDG Baselines. UNICEF. Available online: https://www.unicef.org/publications/index_96611.html (accessed on 25 May 2018).
7. Wardlaw, T.; Salama, P.; Brocklehurst, C.; Chopra, M.; Mason, E. Diarrhoea: Why children are still dying and what can be done. *Lancet* **2010**, *375*, 870–872. [CrossRef]
8. Velleman, Y.; Mason, E.; Graham, W.; Benova, L.; Chopra, M.; Campbell, O.M.; Gordon, B.; Wijesekera, S.; Hounton, S.; Mills, J.E.; et al. From Joint Thinking to Joint Action: A Call to Action on Improving Water, Sanitation, and Hygiene for Maternal and Newborn Health. *PLoS Med.* **2014**, *11*, e1001771. [CrossRef] [PubMed]
9. Mascarini-Serra, L. Prevention of Soil-transmitted Helminth Infection. *J. Glob. Infect. Dis.* **2011**, *3*, 175–182. [CrossRef] [PubMed]
10. WHO | Controlling Infectious Diseases in the Environment. WHO. Available online: https://www.ncbi.nlm.nih.gov/books/NBK310829/ (accessed on 27 October 2017).
11. WHO | Water, Sanitation and Hygiene Interventions and the Prevention of Diarrhoea. WHO. Available online: http://www.who.int/elena/titles/bbc/wsh_diarrhoea/en/ (accessed on 25 May 2018).
12. Bartram, J.; Cairncross, S. Hygiene, Sanitation, and Water: Forgotten Foundations of Health. *PLoS Med.* **2010**, *7*, e1000367. [CrossRef] [PubMed]
13. WHO | Safer Water, Better Health. WHO. Available online: http://www.who.int/quantifying_ehimpacts/publications/saferwater/en/ (accessed on 27 October 2017).
14. Cumming, O.; Cairncross, S. Can water, sanitation and hygiene help eliminate stunting? Current evidence and policy implications. *Matern. Child Nutr.* **2016**, *12* (Suppl. 1), 91–105. [CrossRef] [PubMed]
15. Tony. Nigeria Faces Disease Epidemics as 63 m Lack Access to Safe Water. Vanguard News. 2017. Available online: https://www.vanguardngr.com/2017/06/nigeria-faces-disease-epidemics-63m-lack-access-safe-water/ (accessed on 27 October 2017).
16. UNICEF Nigeria—Media Centre—Launch of Hand Washing Campaign in Abuja. Available online: https://www.unicef.org/nigeria/media_2364.html (accessed on 27 October 2017).
17. USAID Launches New Water and Sanitation Project in Nigeria. Available online: https://www.usaid.gov/nigeria/news-information/press-releases/usaid-launches-new-water-and-sanitation-project-nigeria (accessed on 28 October 2017).

18. NPC/Nigeria NPC-, International ICF. Nigeria Demographic and Health Survey 2013. Published Online First: 2014. Available online: http://dhsprogram.com/publications/publication-fr293-dhs-final-reports.cfm (accessed on 30 November 2017).

19. Stotzer, P.-O.; Abrahamsson, H.; Bajor, A.; Kilander, A.; Sadik, R.; Sjövall, H.; Simrén, M. Are the definitions for chronic diarrhoea adequate? Evaluation of two different definitions in patients with chronic diarrhoea. *United Eur. Gastroenterol. J.* **2015**, *3*, 381–386. [CrossRef] [PubMed]

20. Ghose, B.; Feng, D.; Tang, S.; Yaya, S.; He, Z.; Udenigwe, O.; Ghosh, S.; Feng, Z. Women's decision-making autonomy and utilisation of maternal healthcare services: Results from the Bangladesh Demographic and Health Survey. *BMJ Open* **2017**, *7*, e017142. [CrossRef] [PubMed]

21. Anthonj, C.; Rechenburg, A.; Kistemann, T. Water, sanitation and hygiene in wetlands. A case study from the Ewaso Narok Swamp, Kenya. *Int. J. Hyg. Environ. Health* **2016**, *219*, 606–616. [CrossRef] [PubMed]

22. Dreibelbis, R.; Winch, P.J.; Leontsini, E.; Hulland, K.R.; Ram, P.K.; Unicomb, L.; Luby, S.P. The Integrated Behavioural Model for Water, Sanitation, and Hygiene: A systematic review of behavioural models and a framework for designing and evaluating behaviour change interventions in infrastructure-restricted settings. *BMC Public Health* **2013**, *13*, 1015. [CrossRef] [PubMed]

23. Curtis, V.; Kanki, B.; Cousens, S.; Diallo, I.; Kpozehouen, A.; Sangaré, M.; Nikiema, M. Evidence of behaviour change following a hygiene promotion programme in Burkina Faso. *Bull. World Health Organ.* **2001**, *79*, 518–527. [PubMed]

24. Cairncross, S.; Bartram, J.; Cumming, O.; Brocklehurst, C. Hygiene, sanitation, and water: What needs to be done? *PLoS Med.* **2010**, *7*, e1000365. [CrossRef] [PubMed]

25. Why Nigeria's North South Distinction Is Important| HuffPost. Available online: https://www.huffingtonpost.com/amb-john-campbell/why-nigerias-north-south-_b_817734.html (accessed on 30 October 2017).

26. Adane, M.; Mengistie, B.; Kloos, H.; Medhin, G.; Mulat, W. Sanitation facilities, hygienic conditions, and prevalence of acute diarrhea among under-five children in slums of Addis Ababa, Ethiopia: Baseline survey of a longitudinal study. *PLoS ONE* **2017**, *12*, e0182783. [CrossRef] [PubMed]

27. Hirai, M.; Roess, A.; Huang, C.; Graham, J. Exploring geographic distributions of high-risk water, sanitation, and hygiene practices and their association with child diarrhea in Uganda. *Glob. Health Action* **2016**, *9*, 32833. [CrossRef] [PubMed]

28. Fuller, J.A.; Clasen, T.; Heijnen, M.; Eisenberg, J.N. Shared Sanitation and the Prevalence of Diarrhea in Young Children: Evidence from 51 Countries, 2001–2011. *Am. J. Trop. Med. Hyg.* **2014**, *91*, 173–180. [CrossRef] [PubMed]

29. Cordell, R.; Pickering, L.; Henderson, F.W.; Murph, J. Infectious Diseases in Childcare Settings1. *Emerg. Infect. Dis.* **2004**, *10*, e9. [CrossRef]

30. Wegelin-Schuringa, M.; Kamminga, E. Water and sanitation in the context of HIV/AIDS: The right of access in resource-poor countries. *Health Hum. Rights* **2006**, *9*, 152–172. [CrossRef] [PubMed]

31. Bishwajit, G.; Ide, S.; Ghosh, S. Social Determinants of Infectious Diseases in South Asia. *Int. Sch. Res. Notices* **2014**, *2014*, 135243. [CrossRef] [PubMed]

32. Smith, D.J. AIDS NGOS and corruption in Nigeria. *Health Place* **2012**, *18*, 475–480. [CrossRef] [PubMed]

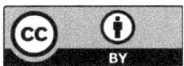

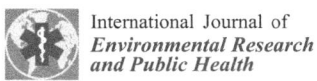

Article

Dramatic Reduction in Diarrhoeal Diseases through Implementation of Cost-Effective Household Drinking Water Treatment Systems in Makwane Village, Limpopo Province, South Africa

Resoketswe Charlotte Moropeng *, Phumudzo Budeli, Lizzy Mpenyana-Monyatsi and Maggy Ndombo Benteke Momba *

Department of Environmental, Water and Earth Sciences, Arcadia Campus, Tshwane University of Technology, P/B X 680, Pretoria 0001, South Africa; Bphumu@gmail.com (P.B.); monyatsil@tut.ac.za (L.M.-M.)
* Correspondence: moropengrc@tut.ac.za (R.C.M.); mombamnb@tut.ac.za (M.N.B.M.);
   Tel.: +27-12-382-6365 (M.N.B.M.); Fax: +27-12-382-6233 (M.N.B.M.)

Received: 16 January 2018; Accepted: 20 February 2018; Published: 27 February 2018

Abstract: The main purpose of this study was to implement cost-effective household water treatment systems in every household of Makwane Village for the reduction of diarrhoeal diseases. These household water treatment systems were constructed with locally available materials and consisted of the biosand zeolite-silver impregnated granular clay filters and the silver-impregnated porous pot filters. During the study period (April 2015 to September 2015), the entire village had 88 households with a population size of 480. Prior to the implementation, a survey was conducted and results revealed that 75% (360/480) of the Makwane residents suffered from diarrhoeal disease and the majority of the cases were reported in children that were less than five years of age. Out of the 480 participants, 372 (77.5%) from 70 households accepted the installation of the systems (intervention group) and 108 (25.5%) from 18 households were reluctant to use the systems (the control group). To date, in the intervention group, only 3.8% (14/372) of participants reported cases of diarrhoea. In the control group, 57.4% (62/108) participants reported cases of diarrhoea and most of the episodes of diarrhoea were reported in children of less than five years old (85%), followed by the group aged ≥56 years (75%). The findings of the current study unequivocally demonstrated that the BSZ-SICG and SIPP filters were able to reduce the incidence of diarrhoea by 96.2%. These findings further demonstrate the importance of household water treatment systems (HWTS) interventions in rural areas to bring about meaningful reductions in diarrhoeal diseases by providing safe potable water.

Keywords: diarrhoeal disease; HWTS implementation; water and sanitation

1. Introduction

Target 7.C of Goal 7 of the Millennium Development Goals (MDGs) for water is to reduce by half the proportion of people without sustainable access to safe drinking water by 2015 [1]. While the MDG target of 88% coverage for access to improved drinking water was met in 2010, the report by WHO/UNICEF Joint Monitoring Programme (JMP) [2], highlighted that 748 million people still depend on unsafe drinking water sources and approximately half of them live in sub-Saharan Africa.

Lack of basic services such as safe drinking has a great impact on individuals, households, communities, and the country as a whole. It has been reported that nearly 2 million people suffer devastating waterborne diseases on an annual basis, and these even result in high mortality for certain cases [3], among which an estimated 6000 children under the age of five years are the first victims [4] and the majority of deaths occurring in developing countries. Approximately 88% of these diseases have been reported to be attributable to unsafe drinking water supply, inadequate sanitation, and poor hygiene [5]. It has been estimated that waterborne diseases are the second most common cause of death in children under the age of five years and the majority of deaths occur in sub-Saharan Africa and Southern Asia [6–8].

Access to safe drinking water supply is currently one of the most complex challenges facing a number of rural communities of South Africa, especially for those living in scattered rural areas. A report issued by the Statistics South Africa in 2013 [9] pointed out that access to safe drinking water for poor households has increased to 71.6% in 2011 [10]. This report also revealed a decrease in the incidence of diarrhoea per 1000 children less than five years of age, down from 121.4 per 1000 children in 2004 to 102.1 per thousand children in 2011. In spite of this decrease, a recent report shows that diarrhoea still remains one of the leading causes of morbidity and mortality in under-five children in South Africa; however, the true burden of childhood diarrhoea is not accurately known [11].

Due to an increase in the number of deaths that are caused by diarrhoea reported every year as a result of contaminated drinking water, point-of-use (POU) water treatment systems are encouraged in rural areas. A home-made water treatment system can produce safe drinking water using any easily reached water sources, such as rivers, streams, ponds, and canals, regardless of their quality and allows for people to adapt to any seasonal disparity. Implementation of household water treatment systems (HWTS) in rural areas without access to safe drinking water sources allows the treatment of drinking water at POU and also improves the quality of the water. This household drinking-water supply intervention can be considered as a quick and sustainable solution to address the burden of disease caused by lack of access to safe drinking water in scattered rural communities of South Africa.

As part of a Water Research Commission project undertaken between 2010 and 2012 by the Tshwane University of Technology Water Research Group (TUT WRG) a range of homemade water purification devices were trialled under laboratory conditions and were then found to be cost-effective [12,13]. The five types of low-cost filters that seemed to hold the greatest potential for South African conditions included: the silver-impregnated porous pot (SIPP) filter (a TUT Product), the ceramic candle filter (CCF), the biosand filter (BSF), a modified biosand filter with zeolite (BSF-Z—a TUT product), and a bucket filter (BF). With the exception of the CCF, these low-cost filters were designed and built by the TUT WRG. Among these HWTS devices, two filters were found to have higher performance in terms of pollutant removals. The SIPP filter was found to be efficient in achieving complete removal of waterborne pathogens from a variety of water sources; however, it could not deliver sufficient volume of water as its flow rates ranged from 0.05 to 2.49 L/h. In contrast, the BSF-Z filter, which had a higher flow rate up to 19.2 L/h showed waterborne pathogen removal rates ranging between 1 and 4.8 log (90–99.99%) and required a disinfection step to render the filtered water safe for drinking [12,14]. These two HWTS devices therefore required some modifications prior to their implementation in rural communities. The BSF-Z and SIPP filters could play a vital role in providing safe drinking water to rural communities without access to improved drinking water sources

The aim of the present study was threefold: firstly, to enhance the performance of the BSF-Z and SIPP filters in terms of pathogen removal and flow rate; secondly, to deploy these devices in every household of the Makwane Village and investigate their performance while they are in use in homes; and, thirdly, to ascertain their performance in eradicating or reducing the burden of diarrhoeal diseases.

2. Methodology

2.1. Modification of BSF-Z and SIPP Filters

The project team worked closely with Cermalab cc (Materials Testing Laboratory, CSIR, Pretoria, South Africa) for manufacturing of the biosand zeolite-silver impregnated granular clay (BSZ-SICG) and silver-impregnated porous pot (SIPP) filters to enhance their performance. The SIPP filter was modified in terms of the flow rate, which increased from 2.49 L/h to 27.5 L/h. The BSZ-SICGs were modified from the biosand filters with zeolite (BSF-Z) that were previously constructed by [12]. A layer of silver-impregnated granular clay, which was prepared by mixing ball clay, sawdust, paper fibre, and silver nitrate ($AgNO_3$), and moulded into small granulates prior to firing was added to the BSF-Z filter to form a BSZ-SICG filter. The size of these filters was scaled down to 25 L in order to ensure that the filter would not take up too much space in homes of rural communities. Moreover, the spigot was elevated to allow for the filters to maintain a 5 cm of biological layer above the surface of fine sand to prevent it from drying out. The flow rate of this filter was increased from 19.2 L/h to 38.6 L/h. With these improved flow rates, both HWTS devices achieved the required volume of 25 L/person/d. Fifty-five (55) SIPP filters and thirty-five (35) BSZ-SICG filters were thereafter manufactured between December 2014 and March 2015. All of these HWTS devices were tested in the laboratory in terms of pathogen removal and the leaching of silver into the treated drinking water. They were found to produce safe drinking water that complied with SANS 241-1:2011 [15] and also with the WHO [16] guideline values of 0.1 mg/L silver in final drinking water that is meant for human consumption. Figure 1 provides a schematic representation of the modifications made to the BSF-Z filter to produce the BSZ-SICG filter and Figure 2 shows a schematic representation of a SIPP filter.

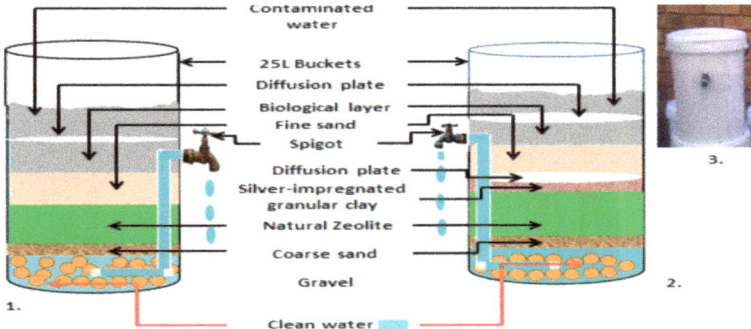

Figure 1. Schematic representation of biosand filters: 1. BSF-Z; and 2. modified BSF with zeolite and silver-impregnated granular clay; 3. BSZ-SICG filter (7 mm gravel; 0.95 mm coarse sand; 3 mm natural zeolite; silver-impregnated granular clay; 0.15 mm fine sand).

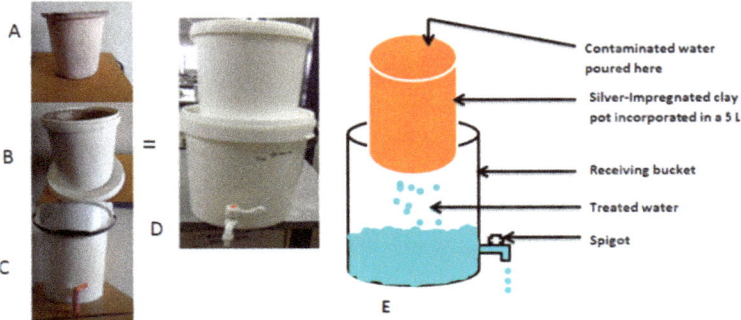

Figure 2. (**A**) Silver-impregnated porous pot (SIPP) filter; and (**B**) 5 L bucket with silver impregnated clay pot inside; (**C**) 10 L receiving bucket; (**D**) Complete SIPP filter; and, (**E**) Schematic representation of SIPP filter.

2.2. Deployment of the Filters in Makwane Village

2.2.1. Description of the Study Area

Makwane Village was the target rural community without access to improved drinking water sources; the village is situated in the Elias Motsoaledi Local Municipality of the Limpopo Province. This Village comprises four sections: Nkakaboleng, New Stands, Lepururu and Ditakaneng which are surrounded by streams (Figure 3). The village had 88 households and a population of 480 with one primary school during the study period. Residents of this village have limited infrastructure and live in close proximity to domestic animals (goats, cows, sheep, dogs, etc.), which drink from and defecate in the same primary water sources that are used by the community for drinking and domestic purposes.

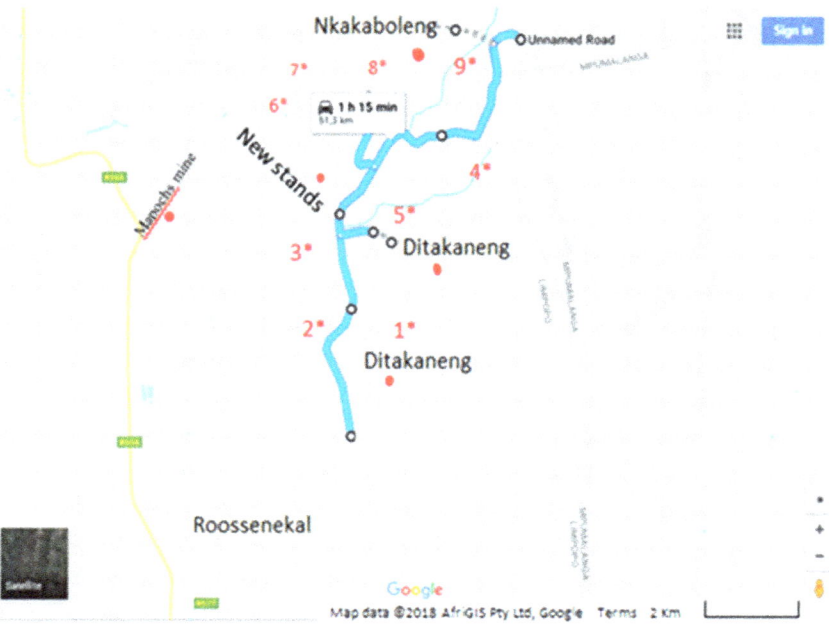

Figure 3. Map of Makwane Village showing all the sections and the surrounding streams/rivers where some of the samples were collected in addition to water collected from households. Source: [17].

2.2.2. Ethical Approval

The study was conducted in accordance with the Declaration of Helsinki, and approved by the Faculty of Science Research Ethics Committee (FCRE) at the Tshwane University of Technology (TUT), where the study was registered (Ref: FCRE 2015/03/040 (2) (SCI)). Access to Makwane Village was obtained through the local pastor and community leaders. Furthermore, authorisation to conduct the study was also obtained from the municipal manager, the municipal councillor, and the local municipal committee. All of the households that were selected for participation were given informed consent forms to sign (Supplementary File 1) at the beginning of the project. The project expectations and respective obligations by both the participants and investigators were explained and any questions were answered. The participants were not subjected to risks of any kind as a result of the project. The investigators provided feedback and information to the participants at regular intervals, conducting the project in the most open manner possible.

2.2.3. Deployment of the Filters in Households of Makwane Village

A total of 90 HWTS devices (35 BSZ-SICG and 55 SIPP) were transported to Makwane Village subsequent to modification for implementation. Two systems were deployed at a local school in Makwane village, while 88 systems were implemented in every household of the Makwane community. Out of 88 households, 18 households were later used as controls in the study because these householders were reluctant to use the systems. All of the households equipped with HWTS devices were also provided with a 25 L improved storage container with a tap installed 5 cm from the base of the bucket. The intervention phase of the study included weekly household observations from April 2015 to September 2015. Householders were advised to use only treated water from HWTS for cooking and drinking purposes. All of the households that participated in the intervention and the control groups continued to provide detailed information on a weekly basis of diarrhoeal disease incidents. In each household, water quality parameters, such as turbidity and bacterial (pathogenic *E. coli*) counts were measured every week during the first three months and thereafter every second week of the last three months. Figure 4 below illustrates how the research team worked hand-in-hand with the Makwane community during deployment of the HWTS devices.

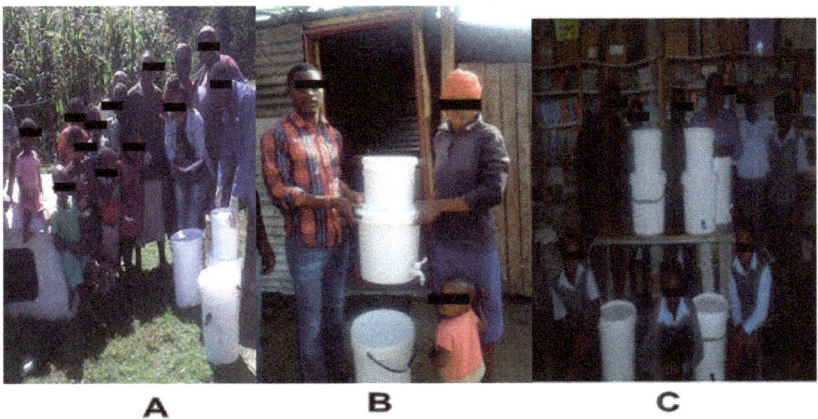

Figure 4. Deployment of the household water treatment systems (HWTS) devices in Makwane Village: (**A**,**B**) deployment in some of the households of Makwane community; (**C**) Deployment at a local primary school in Makwane Village.

2.3. Water Quality Assessment

Samples of drinking water were collected during household visits from both control households and households with HWTS (intervention households). Control households provided a sample of untreated water used for drinking from their storage containers, while intervention households provided drinking water samples from the storage containers (untreated water), directly from BSZ-SICG and SIPP filter outlet tubes and treated water that had been stored in improved storage containers for drinking. Turbidity was tested using a Hach 2100P Portable turbidity Meter (Eutech Instrument Turbidimeter TN-100, Thermo Scientific, Johannesburg, South Africa) during sampling.

2.3.1. Cuture-Based Methods for the Isolation of Presemptive Pathogenic *E. coli*

In order to determine the presence of presumptive pathogenic *E. coli*, water samples were collected in a 250 mL sterile bottle and transported on ice to the in-field laboratory and analyses were performed within two hours using culture-based techniques. Briefly, MacConkey agar with sorbitol (Merck, Johannesburg, South Africa) was used for the detection of *E. coli* O157H:7 (enterohaemorrhagic

E. coli—EHEC) and MacConkey agar without sorbitol (Merck, Johannesburg, South Africa) was used for the detection of other pathogenic *E. coli* (enteropathogenic *E. coli*—EPEC; enterotoxigenic *E. coli*–ETEC; enteroaggregative *E. coli*—EAEC and enteroinvasive *E. coli*—EIEC). Individual colonies were randomly selected based on their sizes, shape, and colour, and inoculated in 2 mL Brain Heart Infusion Broth (BHIB). The samples were then incubated overnight at 37 °C upon which they were archived by 20% glycerol and transported on ice packs to the TUT laboratory for further analysis.

The archived isolates were streaked onto nutrient agar plate (Merck, Johannesburg, South Africa) and incubated at 37 °C for 24 h. The colonies were further purified at least three times employing the same methods and medium before Gram-staining. Subsequently, oxidase tests were conducted on those colonies that were Gram-negative. Thereafter, the oxidase-negative colonies were inoculated into a 2 mL Eppendorf tube containing nutrient broth and incubated at 37 °C for 24 h. The preservation of these colonies was done with 20% glycerol and kept at 20 °C until they were used for molecular studies.

2.3.2. Molecular Identification of Pathogenic *E. coli*

A total of 250 oxidase-negative isolates were used for the molecular study. Each individual isolate was streaked onto nutrient agar and incubated at 37 °C for 24 h. The total genomic DNA from the bacterial isolates was subsequently extracted by boiling method described by Theron et al. (2000) with some modifications. Briefly, a loopful of colonies was transferred into 1.5 mL of nuclease-free water containing 7 μL of Triton X-100. The samples were then vortexed and boiled at 99 °C for 30 min. The DNA was collected through centrifugation at 12,000 rpm for 15 min. The genomic DNA was quantified using the NanoDrop^{TM} 2000 spectrophotometer (Thermo Scientific, Johannesburg, South Africa).

The DNA templates were subjected to multiplex PCR with specific primers (Table 1), as previously described by [18], for the detection of the following virulence genes of *E. coli*: *stx1* (Shiga-toxin 1 of EHEC), *bfpA* (structural gene for the bundle-forming pilus of EPEC), *estA* (ST) (heat-stable toxin of ETEC), *aaiC* (chromosomal secreted protein of EAEC), and *ipaH* (invasion plasmid antigen H of EIEC). The PCR assay was performed with a 25 μL reaction mixture containing 2.5 μL of template DNA, 12.5 μL of DreamTaq Green PCR Master Mix (2X), which is a ready-to-use solution containing DreamTaq DNA polymerase (2X DreamTaq Green Buffer, dATP, dCTP, dGTP, and dTTP, 0.4 mM each, and 4 mM MgCl$_2$) and 0.2 μL of each primer. Nuclease-free water was added to a final volume of 25 μL. The amplification cycles consisted of an initial DNA denaturation at 94 °C for 7 min, followed by 39 cycles of denaturation at 94 °C for 30 s, primer annealing at 57 °C for 30 s, extension at 72 °C for 1 min, and a final extension at 72 °C for 10 min. Negative controls, substituting DNA template with nuclease-free water (Inqaba, Pretoria, South Africa), were included in all PCR runs. The DNA extracted from *E. coli* ATCC 25922 (Quantum Biotechnologies, Johannesburg, South Africa) was used as a positive control. The PCR products (8 μL) were evaluated with a 1.5% (wt/vol) agarose gel (Life Technologies, Johannesburg, South Africa) at 120 mV for 60 min. A molecular marker (100 bp DNA ladder; Inqaba, Pretoria, South Africa) was run concurrently. All of the results were captured using a gel documentation system (Syngene, Cambridge, UK).

Table 1. Oligonucleotides used in this study for the amplification of several genes representing *E. coli* pathotypes.

Primer Name	Sequences 5′→3′	Target Genes	Size	Reference
EHEC-423	F-TGGAAAAACTCAGTGCCTCT- R-CCAGTCCGTAAATTCATTCT-	*stx1*	423 bp	[18]
EPEC-300	R-GGAATCAGACGCAGACTGGTAGT- F-GGAAGTCAAATTCATGGGGGTAT-	*bfpA*	300 bp	[18]
ETEC-187	F-GCTAAACCAGTAGAGGTCTTCAAAA- R-CCCGGTACAGAGCAGGATTACAACA-	*estA* (ST)	187 bp	[18]
EIEC-508	R-CACACGGAGCTCCTCAGTC- F-CCCCCAGCCTAGCTTAGTTT-	*ipaH*	508 bp	[18]
EAEC-215	R-ACGACACCCCTGATAAACAA- F-ATTGTCCTCAGGCATTTCAC-	*aaiC*	215 bp	[18]

2.4. Surveillance of Episodes of Diarrhoea before and after Implementation

One elderly person in each household was identified as the primary respondent during the recruitment period. A structured 10-min interview was conducted weekly in Sepedi (a local language of the Makwane community) in collecting information on the respondents' personal and domestic hygiene practices, sanitation systems, and the episodes of diarrhoea for all the members of the household during the previous seven days. Diarrhoea was defined as three or more loose or watery stools containing blood or mucus during a period of 24 h and also the frequency of visits to the toilet by a person with diarrhoea within a 24-h period. The diarrhoea reduction percentage (% DR) after HWTS implementation was calculated as follows:

$$\% \, DR = \frac{(number \, of \, households \, with \, or \, without \, HWTS - diarrhoeal \, cases)}{(number \, of \, households \, with \, or \, without \, HWTS \,)} \times 100 \qquad (1)$$

2.5. Turbidity Removal Efficiency

The level of turbidity in water samples before and after filtration was determined using a portable turbidity meter (2100P Hach, Process Instrument (Pi), Burnley, UK). Turbidity reduction percentage achieved by all of the HWTS devices was calculated according to [19], as follows

$$\% \, turbidity \, reduction = \frac{(\text{turbidity unfiltered} - \text{turbidity filtered})}{(turbidity \, unfiltered)} \times 100 \qquad (2)$$

2.6. Monitoring of Silver Leached from BSZ-SICG and SIPP Filters

The concentration of silver in water treated by BSZ-SICG SIPP filters was monitored on a monthly basis throughout the study period. Samples were sent to the Department of Chemistry (Tshwane University of Technology, Pretoria, South Africa) for analysis of leached silver. The SPECTRO ARCOS ICP spectrometer (SPECTRO ANALYTICAL INSTRUMENTS (PTY) LDT, Kempton Park, Johannesburg, South Africa) was used to detect and determine the concentration of silver in treated water samples.

2.7. Efficiency of the HWTS Devices in Removing Pathogenic E. coli Strains from Makwane Water Sources

The efficiency of the HWTS devices in removing pathogenic *E. coli* was determined by comparing the concentrations of all the target pathogenic strains before and after treatment. Enumeration of presumptive *E. coli* before and after treatment was done by standard methods. The log reductions were calculated using the equation below and were converted to the percentage *E. coli* removed [19]:

$$\% \, E.coli \, \text{removal} = 100 - \frac{(\text{survival counts})}{(initial \, counts \,)} \times 100 \qquad (3)$$

2.8. Statistical Analysis of Data

Paired and independent *t*-tests were run on Excel using the XLSTAT statistical software (XLSTAT 2017: Data Analysis and Statistical Solution for Microsoft Excel) to determine any significant differences between control and intervention groups. Pearson's correlation coefficient (r) was used to determine the correlation between *E. coli* removal efficiency and leaching silver from SIPP and BSZ-SICG filters. The effect of using the BSZ-SICG and SIPP filters on diarrhoeal disease was determined by comparing the prevalence of diarrhoeal disease for all the households in each group. In this study, the classification of diarrhoeal diseases was carried out according to the WHO (2006) definition of three or more loose or watery stools in any 24-h period. Unpaired *t*-tests were used to compare geometric mean *E. coli* concentrations and turbidity between groups.

3. Results

3.1. Demographic Information of the Study Area

During the study period (April 2015 to September 2015), the entire village had 88 households with a population size of 480. Among this population, the most dominant groups were between 22 and 55 years (35.8%) and children less than five years old (20.6%). The demographic information of the Makwane Village community during the study period is provided in Figure 5.

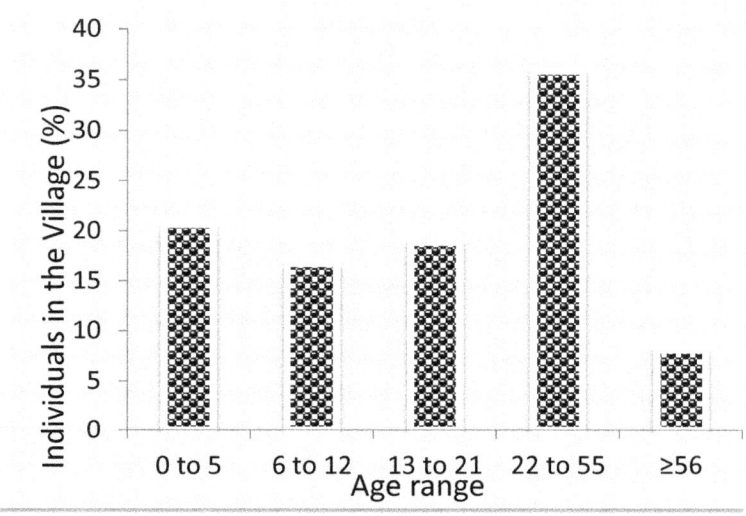

Figure 5. Population distribution of Makwane Village by major age groups.

3.2. Characteristics of Study Population Based on Episodes of Diarrhoea, and Water and Sanitation Facility Per Household

Prior to HWTS implementation in Makwane Village, a higher incidence of diarrhoeal diseases was reported (Table 2). The statistical analysis showed a significant difference between households that never experienced diarrhoea (25%) and those that had experienced diarrhoea (75%) with a p-value of 0.000176115. Moreover, all of the households in Makwane Village use water directly from the available sources without prior treatment. The majority of households (70.5%) use water obtained directly from the streams (surface water), while 13.6% use water obtained from springs/wells. About 9.1% of the households have boreholes in their yards and they use water from the boreholes without any treatment. In addition, during rainy seasons 6.8% of the households use roof-harvested rain water. Out of 88 households, 52 (59.1%) households have access to proper sanitation facilities, while 36 (40.9%) had no access to sanitation facilities and the difference was not statistically significant (p = 0.369174254). Table 2 shows the characteristics of the study population based on episodes of diarrhoea prior to HWTS implementation, as well as water and sanitation per household.

Table 2. Episodes of diarrhoea prior to HWTS implementation and water and sanitation per household in Makwane Village.

Characteristics		Frequency (*n* = 88)	Percentage (%)	*p*-Value
Episodes of diarrhoea	No	22	25	*p* = 0.000176115
	Yes	66	75	
Diarrhoeal episodes based on water source	Roof water harvesting	06	6.8	
	River/stream water	62	70.5	
	Open spring	12	13.6	
	Borehole	8	9.1	
	Municipal treated tap water	NA	NA	
Access to proper sanitation *	With access	52	59.1	*p* = 0.369174254
	No access	36	40.9	

* Proper sanitation was characterised by any type of latrine; NA: there were no municipal tap water in the village.

3.3. Water Quality Analysis

3.3.1. Average Mean *E. coli* Reduction, Turbidity Reduction, Temperature and pH of Untreated Water from Control Households and Treated Water from Intervention Households in Makwane Village

The average Log10 *E. coli* and percentage removal efficiency together with turbidity reduction, temperature, and pH, are summarised in Table 3 below. Much higher average *E. coli* counts (4.3830 Log10 CFU/100 mL) were observed in the control households, than those observed in the intervention households (0.4770 Log10 CFU/100 mL) that were using BSZ-SICG filters. The difference was statistically significant with a *p*-value of 0.000004201. Although *E. coli* counts were detected in the drinking water of the intervention households that were using the BSZ-SICG filters, none of the pathogenic strains were detected. The water that is produced by the SIPP filter (% *E. coli* reduction = 100%) and the BSZ-SICG filter (% *E. coli* reduction = 89.1%) was consistently free of the target bacteria regardless of the quality of the water source. The average turbidity of the untreated water in the control households was found to be 168 nephelometric units (NTU), which exceeded the WHO guideline limits. All of the households equipped with HWTS devices showed a significant reduction in turbidity when compared to the control households (*p* = 0.000025949). The SIPP filters produced drinking water that had the lowest turbidity (0.85 NTU) and was within the recommended limits (SANS 241: <1 NTU; EPA: ≤1; WHO: 5 NTU), while the BSZ-SICG filters produced water with a turbidity of 2.34 NTU, which was within the WHO guideline limits. Untreated water was found to have the highest temperature (25.1 °C), while the treated water had lower temperatures, namely 19.8 °C and 22.5 °C for BSZ-SICG and SIPP filters, respectively. All of the temperature values were within the limits set by both SANS 241 and WHO. The pH values of both untreated and treated water were also within the EPA guideline limits (6.5–8.5). Untreated water had a mean pH value of 8.2, whereas the treated water had a mean pH value of 7.8 and 7.5 for BSZ-SICG and SIPP filters, respectively.

Table 3. Mean *E. coli* reduction, turbidity reduction, temperature, and pH of untreated and treated water from control and intervention households.

Water Quality Parameters	Control Households	Intervention Households		*p*-Value
	Untreated Water	BSZ-SICG	SIPP	
E. coli	4.3830 Log10 * CFU/100 mL	0.4770 Log10 CFU/100 mL	** NG	0.000004201
% *E. coli* reduction	-	89.1%	100%	
Turbidity (*** NTU)	168	2.34	0.85	0.000025949
% Turbidity reduction	-	98.6%	99.5%	
Temperature (°C)	25.0	19.8	22.5	
pH	8.2	7.8	7.5	

* CFU—colony-forming unit per 100 mL of the water sample; ** NG—no growth noted from water filtered by SIPP; *** NTU—nephelometric turbidity unit.

3.3.2. The Leaching of Silver Ions into Water Treated by SIPP and BSZ-SICG Filters over the Study Period (April 2015–September 2015) versus *E. coli* Removal Efficiency

After manufacturing and prior to deployment of the HWTS in Makwane village, the leaching silver was above the WHO recommended limit. In an attempt to reduce the concentration of the silver in HWTS, the SIPP filters were soaked in containers containing municipal treated tap water, while for the BSZ-SIGC, this water passed through the filters until the recommended silver concentration limit was reached. The HWTS devices were subsequently deployed in Makwane village and evaluated for silver leaching in the treated water for 12 weeks between April and September 2015. Figure 6 shows the concentration of silver leached from SIPP and BSZ-SICG filters into treated water throughout the study period. Slower depletion of the silver concentration was observed in the SIPP filters than in the BSZ-SICG filters with the concentration of 0.100 mg/L to 0.045 mg/L and 0.100 mg/L to 0.016 mg/L for SIPP and BSZ-SICG filters, respectively. Moreover, the silver leached from both SIPP and BSZ-SICG filters into the treated water was within the guideline limits set by the EPA (2012), which is 0.10 mg/L. It was observed that the presumptive *E. coli* removal efficiency decreased with a decrease in the concentration of silver that leached into the treated water.

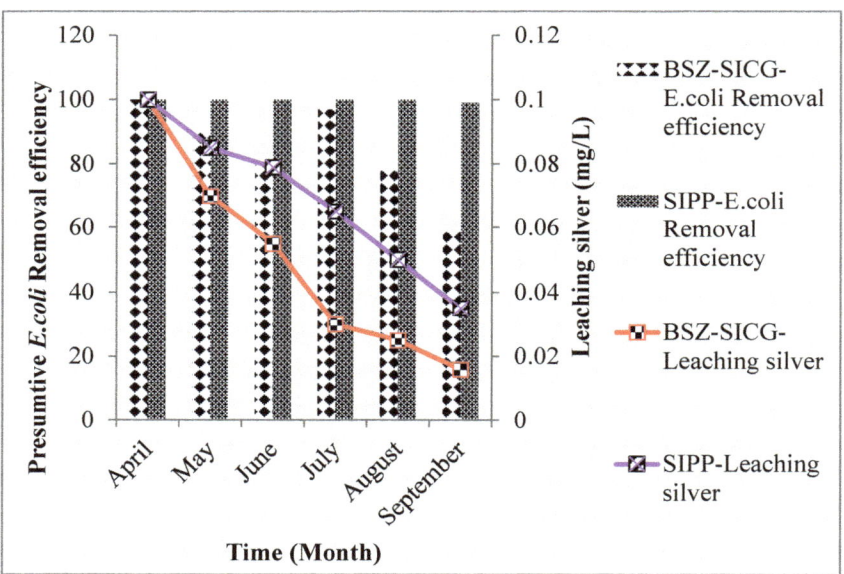

Figure 6. The concentration of silver leached from SIPP and BSZ-SICG filters into treated water versus *E. coli* removal efficiency.

3.3.3. Pearson's Correlation between Presumtive *E. coli* Removal Efficiency and Silver Leached into Water Treated by BSZ-SIGC and SIPP Filters at POU

The results revealed a strong positive correlation between *E. coli* and silver leached into the water treated by the BSZ-SIGC filter ($r = 0.678627405$) and the SIPP filter ($r = 0.705154424$). However, the relationship between silver leached and *E. coli* concentration in the water treated by BSZ-SIGC and SIPP filters was not statistically significant ($p = 4.59594 \times 10^{-13}$ and $p = 7.48692 \times 10^{-6}$, respectively).

3.3.4. Amplification of Pathogenic *E. coli* Strains of by Multiplex PCR

All of the water samples that were presumptively positive for five targeted pathogenic *E. coli* strains were randomly selected for molecular characterisation. However, none of the five pathogenic strains of *E. coli* were detected in water samples after using the BSZ-SICG and SIPP filters (Figure 7A). The *stx1* gene coding for EHEC was the most frequently detected gene in surface water, borehole water, and storage containers with a prevalence of 36.7%, 30.9%, and 33.6%, respectively. The *ipaH* gene coding for EIEC was the least isolated with a prevalence of 8.3% (surface water), 1.2% (spring water), 6.7% (borehole water), and 8.3% (storage containers). All of the results are presented in Figure 7A below. A typical result after agarose gel electrophoresis of PCR products showing several genes representing *E. coli* pathotypes isolated from water sources of Makwane Village is given in Figure 7B.

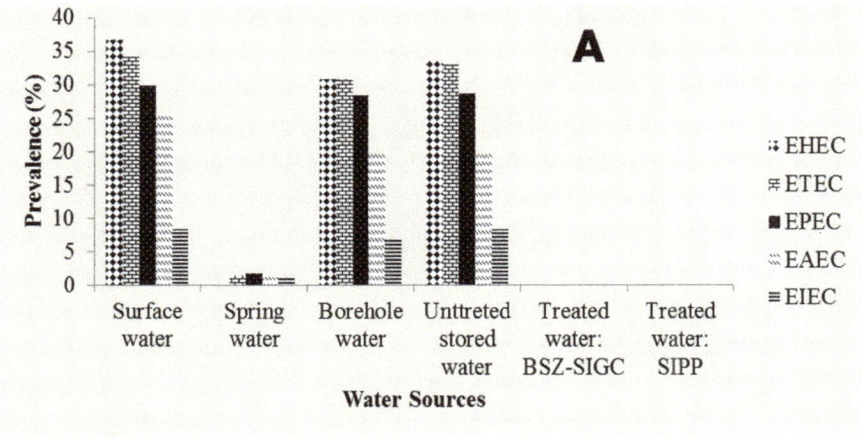

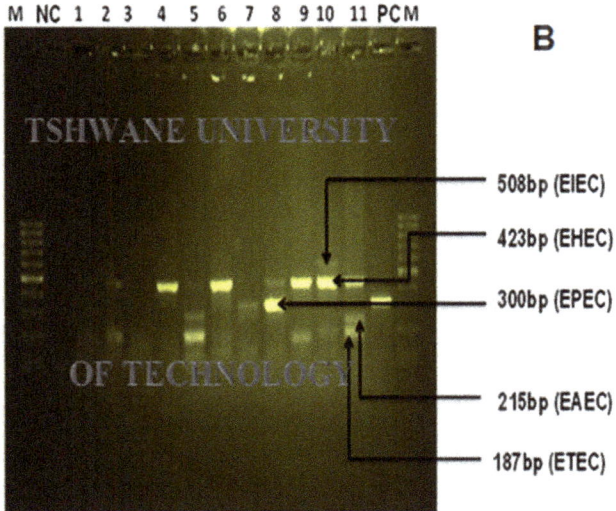

Figure 7. (**A**) Prevalence of pathogenic stains of *E. coli* from different water sources over the study period; and (**B**) agarose gel electrophoresis of PCR products showing several genes representing *E. coli* pathotypes using published primer (M—molecular marker (100 bp); NC—negative control; PC—positive control; and, 1 to 11—samples from different sources).

3.4. Diarrhoeal Disease Incidence per Age Group and Stool Consistency Subsequent to HWTS Implementation in Makwane Village

Subsequent to HWTS implementation in Makwane Village, episodes of diarrhoea were found to be more prevalent in control households than in intervention households. The majority of the diarrhoea episodes were reported in children that were less than five years old from both the control and intervention households with a prevalence of 85% and 5.1%, respectively. The difference was statistically significant with a *p*-value of 0.000000105. The second highest incidence of diarrhoeal disease was observed in the elderly group of ≥56 years with a prevalence of 75% (control households) and 11.11% (intervention households). The statistical analysis showed a significant difference with a *p*-value of 0.0005018. Conclusively, 57.4% of the respondents in control households reported episodes of diarrhoea, while only 3.8% of the respondents in the intervention households reported episodes of diarrhoea. The incidence of diarrhoea was thus reduced by 96.2% in the intervention households. In general, watery diarrhoea was the main type of diarrhoea reported by Makwane Village residents. In control households, 62 cases of diarrhoea were reported (57.4%), most of which were watery diarrhoea (69.3%), followed by mucus diarrhoea (21%) and bloody diarrhoea (9.7%), while 14 cases of diarrhoea were reported in intervention households (3.8%), all of which (14/14) were watery diarrhoea. All of the results are summarised in Table 4.

Table 4. Episodes of diarrhoea per age group and stool consistency subsequent to HWTS implementation in Makwane Village.

Characteristics		Control Households (n = 108)		Intervention Households (n = 372)		*p*-Value
Age Groups	Episodes of Diarrhoea	Frequency	Percent (%)	Frequency	Percent (%)	
0–5	Yes	17	85	4	5.1	0.0000105
	No	3	15	75	94.9	
6–12	Yes	9	60	3	4.6	0.0000959
	No	6	40	62	95.4	
13–21	Yes	7	36.8	1	1.4	0.0001004
	No	12	63.2	70	98.6	
22–55	Yes	20	47.6	3	2.3	0.0000096
	No	22	52.4	127	97.7	
≥56	Yes	9	75	3	11.1	0.0005018
	No	3	25	24	88.9	
Stool consistency	Watery	43/62	69.3	14/14	100.0	
	Bloody	6/62	9.7	0/14	0	
	Mucus	13/62	21	0/14	0	
Overall episodes of diarrhoea in control households			Overall episodes of diarrhoea in intervention households			
62/108 (57.4%)			14/372 (3.8%)			

4. Discussion

According to [2], most of the rural communities in sub-Saharan Africa still face significant challenges in gaining access to improved drinking water and are struggling to meet the MDG targets for water and sanitation. It has been estimated that about 16 million people in South Africa have no access to adequate water and sanitation [20], and the lack of such services significantly contribute to diarrhoeal diseases worldwide. To address these issues, a study on the effect of HWTS implementation was undertaken in one of the rural villages in South Africa; these HWTS devices were deployed in every household of the village that was willing to participate and their performance was assessed in terms of their ability to reduce the burden of diarrhoeal diseases in the community. Prior to HWTS implementation in Makwane Village, 75% of the householders had reported episodes of diarrhoea and it was also found that the majority of the households (70.5%) in Makwane use water obtained directly from the river/surface without prior treatment (Table 2). The episodes of diarrhoea that were reported in the study area could be due to a lack of improved water sources and proper sanitation (Table 2), as it has been previously reported that a lack of such facilities contributes significantly to diarrhoeal diseases with higher cases reported in children aged five years and less [5–8,11]. Therefore, the high number of children under the age of five years old in this study indicates the potential vulnerability of this community. Successful HWTS implementation will therefore be a solution to reduce the burden of diarrhoeal diseases in the study area, as improved household water management and storage ensures that the drinking water is microbiologically safe at the point of use.

Water Quality

Surface water is an important supply of drinking water for many populations worldwide, principally in rural areas. Therefore, it is imperative that it must be judiciously managed and protected. Safe drinking water must have an acceptable quality that complies with physical, chemical, and bacteriological parameters that are set by [21–23]. The surface water used by the Makwane community was shown to have mean pH and temperature values that are within the limits set by EPA (2012) for drinking and domestic purposes, which is 7.0–8.12 for pH and $\leq 25\ ^\circ$C for temperature (Table 3). The cause of a decrease in temperature can be attributed to the second law of thermodynamic, which state "in a closed system, the potential energy of the system will always be less than that of the initial state" [24]. The HWTS implemented in Makwane were closed systems and there is a possibility that they can exchange heat with the surroundings, so when untreated water is filtered it will exchange temperature with the content of the systems as a result the temperature of the final product will be less than the initial temperature. Even though the pH and the temperature of the Makwane water sources cannot cause any health risk to the community, their surface water sources were found to have high average turbidity levels of up to 268 NTU, which by far exceeded the limit (5 NTU) that is set by the [23] guidelines. Turbidity in drinking water is caused by particulate matter that may be present in the water source such as clay, silt, organic matter, inorganic matter, plankton, and other microscopic organisms [25]. Moreover, high levels of turbidity in the water are associated with poor water quality and promote the survival of microorganisms [25]. The turbidity reduction in intervention households (households using BSZ-SICG and SIPP systems) was statistically significant as compared to untreated water in the control households (Table 3), suggesting that HWTS implementation in Makwane Village households had improved the turbidity of the water. The average percentage reduction in turbidity obtained during the period of the study was 98.6% (2.34 NTU) and 99.5% (0.84 NTU) for BSZ-SICG and SIPP filters, respectively. The average turbidity level achieved complies with the turbidity limits set by [21,23], and they also compare well to previous findings in which the percentage reduction in turbidity ranged from 88% to 99% for ceramic candle filters [26]. The results of this study in terms of percentage reduction in turbidity levels are also similar to the results reported by [27], with average turbidity reduction levels of between 83% and 99% being achieved for ceramic silver-coated water filters. Another similar study conducted in South Africa by [12,14] reported that a range of locally produced point-of-use water filters, including BSF and SIPP, consistently reduced the turbidity of surface water in the laboratory with an average turbidity of up to 98%.

In order to determine whether the leached out silver from the BSZ-SICG and SIPP filters complies with EPA 2012, guidelines (0.1 mg/L), the silver concentration was measured in the filtered water prior to and after HWTS implementation over the study period (six months). The mean silver concentration leached in filtered water from both HWTS devices was found to be within the limits recommended by [6,22]. Results for both silver leached and the *E. coli* removal efficiency are clearly shown in Figure 6. The findings of this study revealed that the silver level in the BSZ-SICG filter was depleted much faster compared to SIPP filters. However, the difference is not clearly understood as in both cases silver is incorporated within the clay.

This study also assessed the efficiency of the BSZ-SICG and SIPP filters in removing pathogenic *E. coli* strains from various water sources of Makwane Village. A significant improvement in household water quality was documented in this study for pathogenic *E. coli* strains (EHEC, ETEC, EPEC, EIEC, and EAEC) during the six-month assessment period (Figure 7). Since the proportion of the population in this village without access to improved drinking water is high (Table 2) and the water that was assessed was found to have high levels of microbial contamination (4.3830 Log10 CFU/100 mL of *E. coli*) and often very turbid (Table 3), this study further provides important evidence regarding HWTS implementation in sites where access to safe water is inadequate.

During the study period, the BSZ-SICG filter demonstrated an average reduction of 89.1% for *E. coli* (Table 4) in Makwane water sources. Moreover, none of the pathogenic strains of *E. coli* was detected in water treated by the BSZ-SICG filter (Figure 7). These results were found to be in line with the results of other studies in some countries, which reported 60% to 100% *E. coli* removal efficiencies of the BSF filters both in the field and laboratory [28,29]. A laboratory-scale study conducted by [14] showed a reduction in indicator bacteria of between 60% and 100% and 90% and 100%, respectively, in the biosand filter with zeolite (BSZ-SICG) and the SIPP filter. The findings of this study also compare well to those of previous studies reported by different researchers that showed that the BSF could achieve 90% to 99.99% *E. coli* removal [30,31]. A higher reduction of the target bacteria by the BSZ-SICG filter may be due to the presence of silver-impregnated clay granules in the system, which is reported to have bactericidal properties [32,33]. However, it was also observed that even though the silver concentration in the BSZ-SICG filter system was low, the systems continued to remove pathogenic *E. coli* from water. This could be attributed to the unknown pore size of the BSZ-SICG systems. In addition, it was reported that the removal of bacteria by biosand filters at the initial stage occurs by sedimentation and straining, and that with frequent use of these filters, the removal efficiencies increased, sometimes up to 99.99% [31]. However, this was not found to be the case in this study, as the pathogen removal efficiency of the BSZ-SICG filter was found to decrease with frequent use (down to 78.9%). This might have been due to the fine sand that managed to penetrate the diffusion plate with some bacteria attached and moved to the bottom layer of the BSZ-SICG filter system. Silver ions did not have any effect on the bacteria attached to the fine sand as it was also shown to deteriorate with frequent use of the systems; hence, at low concentration, Ag^+ does not have an antibacterial effect. As a result, the quality of treated water deteriorated. However, an increase in the efficiency to remove pathogenic *E. coli* of up to 96.9% was observed in the BSZ-SICG filters after they had been washed during the third month of being used. Therefore, the maintenance of these systems is important and, depending on the volume of water filtered, they need to be washed every third month of use to ensure good quality drinking water.

The SIPP filter also demonstrated a total reduction of pathogenic *E. coli* (Table 4 and Figure 7). These findings are similar to the results of a study done by [34], where the author attempted to determine the highest possible reduction of target pathogenic bacteria by a silver-impregnated clay-pot filter which resulted in 99.99% reduction. Other similar studies conducted both in the laboratory and in the field for BSF, SIPP, and other filtration technologies showed the pathogen reduction ranging between 90% and 100% [12,14,31,35–38]. Greater removal efficiency (100%) of target pathogenic bacteria by the SIPP filter in this study might have been achieved by silver (Ag) nanoparticles, which were embedded within the clay during manufacturing [39]. A study by [40] also revealed that the Ag-impregnated pot was significantly more effective in removing *E. coli*, when compared to the control pot without silver.

In this study, an overall and significant reduction (96.2%) in the incidence of diarrhoeal disease was documented in households that were using BSZ-SICG and SIPP filters as compared to the control households. These results suggest greater or comparable reduction in diarrhoeal disease in comparison to randomised control trials of ceramic water filters in SA and Zimbabwe, which demonstrated an 80% reduction in diarrhoeal diseases [36]. These results also compare well to studies of other HWTS devices such as the concrete BSF in Cambodia, the Dominican Republic, and Kenya which demonstrated a 47% reduction in diarrhoeal disease (both Cambodia and Dominican Republic), and a 54% reduction in Kenya, in children under the age of five years [35,41,42]. A related study conducted in Ghana also showed a 60% reduction in diarrhoeal diseases in households that were requested to use the plastic

BSF as compared to control households [43]. In general, the results for diarrhoeal disease reduction in intervention households as compared to control households (Table 4) observed in this study suggest greater reductions compared to those obtained during trials of concrete BSF and ceramic filters in other regions of the world.

In addition, as children under the age of five years were a subgroup of interest in this study, data on diarrhoeal disease were also analysed by age groups (Table 4). The results showed a major reduction (90.5%) in diarrhoeal disease in children less than five years old in the BSZ-SICG and SIPP intervention as compared to the control households and the difference was statistically significant ($p < 0.01$). These results suggest a greater reduction in diarrhoeal disease when compared to the 44% reduction in diarrhoeal disease in children under the age of five years reported in Cambodia [41]. Therefore, in rural areas were people still mainly rely on untreated water for drinking and domestic purposes, the implementation of BSZ-SICG and SIPP filters is substantiated by the results of this study.

5. Conclusions

This study investigated the performance of two cost-effective household water treatment systems in reducing the burden of diarrhoeal diseases, while they were in use in homes of the Makwane village. Prior to their deployment, they were subjected to some modifications to enhance their performance. Both the BSZ-SICG and SIPP filters were found to be effective in removing pathogenic *E. coli* from water sources used by the community of the Makwane Village. Furthermore, they have demonstrated their capability to reduce the incidence of diarrhoeal diseases by 96% in the Makwane Village community of the Limpopo Province, South Africa. These cost-effective technologies can be recommended in rural areas without access to improved drinking water supply. In addition, research on HWTS technologies shall attempt to measure health impacts in more objective ways that can assist in eliminating bias. These may include incorporating diagnostic procedures to detect intestinal infections in children in order to compare the organisms found in water with those found in stool samples.

Supplementary Materials: The following are available online at www.mdpi.com/1660-4601/15/3/410/s1, Supplementary File 1: Informed consent form.

Acknowledgments: The authors would like to extend their gratitude to the National Research Foundation and the SARChI (South African Research Chair Initiative) Chair for Water Quality and Wastewater Management for funding this project. Lastly we would like thank all of the study participants from Makwane Village community, Limpopo Province, South Africa, for their time and support during this study.

Author Contributions: Resoketswe Charlotte Moropeng, Lizzy Mpenyana-Monyatsi and Maggy Ndombo Benteke Momba conceived and designed the experiments; Resoketswe Charlotte Moropeng and Phumudzo Budeli performed the experiments; Resoketswe Charlotte Moropeng and Maggy Ndombo Benteke Momba analyzed the data; Resoketswe Charlotte Moropeng wrote the paper.

Conflicts of Interest: The authors declare that there are no conflicts of interest.

References

1. United Nations (UN) General Assembly. United Nations Millennium Declaration, Resolution Adopted by the General Assembly. A/RES/55/2. 18 September 2000. Available online: http://www.refworld.org/docid/3b00f4ea3.html (accessed on 21 February 2018).
2. WHO/UNICEF Joint Monitoring Programme (JMP). *Progress on Sanitation and Drinking Water—2014 Update*; WHO Press: Geneva, Switzerland, 2014.
3. Hardberger, A. Life, Liberty and the pursuit of water: Evaluating water as human right and the duties and obligations it creates. *Northwest. Univ. J. Int. Hum. Rights* **2005**, *4*, 331–362. [CrossRef]
4. Fitzmaurice, M. The human rights to water. *Fordham Environ. Law Rev.* **2007**, *18*, 537–585.
5. Prüss, A.; Kay, D.; Fewtrell, L.; Bartram, J. Estimating the burden of disease from water, sanitation, and hygiene at a global level. *Environ. Health Perspect.* **2002**, *110*, 537–542. [CrossRef] [PubMed]
6. Black, R.E.; Cousens, S.; Johnson, H.L.; Lawn, J.E.; Rudan, I.; Bassani, D.G.; Jha, P.; Campbell, H.; Walker, C.F.; Cibulskis, R.; et al. Child Health Epidemiology Reference Group of WHO and UNICEF. *Lancet* **2010**, *375*, 1969–1987. [CrossRef]

7. Santosham, M.; Chandran, A.; Fitzwater, S.; Fischer-Walker, C.; Baqui, A.H.; Black, R. Progress and barriers for the control of diarrhoeal disease. *Lancet* **2010**, *376*, 63–67. [CrossRef]
8. Liu, L.; Johnson, H.L.; Cousens, S.; Perin, J.; Scott, S.; Lawn, J.E.; Rudan, I.; Campbell, H.; Cibulskis, R.; Li, M.; et al. Global, regional, and national causes of child mortality: An updated systematic analysis for 2010 with time trends since 2000. *Lancet* **2012**, *379*, 2151–2161. [CrossRef]
9. Statistics South Africa (Stats SA). *Millennium Development Goals, Country Report 2013*; Stats SA: Pretoria, South Africa, 2013.
10. Statistics South Africa (Stats SA). *Census 2011: Statistical Release*; Statistics South Africa: Pretoria, South Africa, 2012; pp. 52–53.
11. Chola, L.; Michalow, J.; Tugendhaft, A.; Hofman, K. Reducing diarrhoea deaths in South Africa: Costs and effects of scaling up essential interventions to prevent and treat diarrhoea in under five children. *BMC Public Health* **2015**, *15*, 394. [CrossRef] [PubMed]
12. Mwabi, J.K.; Adeyemo, F.E.; Mahlangu, T.O.; Mamba, B.B.; Brouckaert, B.M.; Swartz, C.D.; Offringa, G.; Mpenyana-Monyatsi, L.; Momba, M.N.B. Household water treatment systems: A solution to the production of safe drinking water by the low-income communities of Southern Africa. *J. Phys. Chem. Earth.* **2011**, *36*, 1120–1128. [CrossRef]
13. Mahlangu, T.O.; Mamba, B.B.; Momba, M.N.B. A comparative assessment of chemical contaminant removal by three household water treatment filters. *Water SA.* **2012**, *38*, 39–47. [CrossRef]
14. Mwabi, J.K.; Mamba, B.B.; Momba, M.N.B. Removal of waterborne bacteria from surface water and groundwater by cost-effective household water treatment systems (HWTS): A sustainable solution for improving water quality in rural communities of Africa. *Water S. Afr.* **2012**, *39*, 445–447. [CrossRef]
15. South African Bureau of Standards (SABS). *SANS 241-1: 2011, South African National Standard (SANS), Drinking Water. Part 1: Microbiological, Physical, Aesthetic and Chemical Determinands*; South African Bureau of Standards (SABS): Pretoria, South Africa, 2011.
16. World Health Organization. *The World Health Report 2006—Working Together for Health*; World Health Organization: Geneva, Switzerland, 2006.
17. Map of Makwane Village Showing All the Sections and the Surrounding Streams/Rivers Where Some of the Samples Were Collected in Addition to Water Collected from Households. Available online: https://www.google.com/maps/dir/-25.1631288,29.9473028/-25.0873681,29.9861423/@-25.142823, 29.9184398,12.2z/data=!4m2!4m1!3e0?hl=en (accessed on 27 February 2018).
18. Nguyen, T.V.; Le Van, P.; Le Huy, C.; Gia, K.N.; Weintraub, A. Detection and characterization of diarrheagenic Escherichia coli from young children in Hanoi, Vietnam. *J. Clin. Microbio.* **2005**, *43*, 755–760. [CrossRef] [PubMed]
19. Broezel, V.S.; Cloete, T.E. Effect of storage time and temperature on the aerobic plate count and on the community structure of two water samples. *Water S. Afr.* **1991**, *17*, 289–300.
20. Heleba, S. Access to sufficient water in South Africa: How far have we come? *Law Democr. Dev.* **2012**, *15*, 1–35. [CrossRef]
21. South African Bureau of Standards (SABS). *SANS 241-1: 2015, South African National Standard (SANS), Drinking Water. Part 1: Microbiological, Physical, Aesthetic and Chemical Determinands*; South African Bureau of Standards (SABS): Pretoria, South Africa, 2015.
22. Environmental Protection Agency. *Water Quality in Small Community Distribution Systems*; EPA: Sacramento, CA, USA, 2012.
23. WHO (World Health Organization). *Guidelines for Drinking-Water Quality*, 4th ed.; World Health Organization: Geneva, Switzerland, 2011.
24. Carnot, N.L.S. *Reflections on the Motive Power of Heat, Accompanied by Kelvin W. T. "An Account of Carnot's Theory"*, 2nd ed.; Thurston, R.H., Ed.; John Willey & Sons: New York, NY, USA, 1897.
25. Department of Water Affairs and Forestry. *South African Water Quality Guidelines, Volume 1: Domestic Use*, 2nd ed.; Department of Water Affairs and Forestry: Pretoria, South Africa, 1996; p. 1.
26. Franz, A. A Performance Study of Ceramic Candle Filters in Kenya, Including Tests for Coliphage Removal. Master's Thesis, Department of Civil and Environmental Engineering, Massachusetts Institute of Technology, Cambridge, MA, USA, 2004.

27. Low, J. Appropriate Microbiological Indicator Tests for Drinking Water in Developing Countries and Assessment of Ceramic Water Filters. Master's Thesis, Department of Civil and Environmental Engineering, Massachusetts Institute of Technology, Cambridge, MA, USA, 2002.

28. Ngai, T.K.K.; Shrestha, R.R.; Dangol, B.; Maharjan, M.; Murcott, S.E. Design for sustainable development—Household drinking water filter for arsenic and pathogen treatment in Nepal. *J. Environ. Sci. Health Part A* **2007**, *42*, 1879–1888. [CrossRef] [PubMed]

29. Devi, R.; Alemayehu, E.; Singh, V.; Kumar, A.; Mengistie, E. Removal of fluoride, arsenic and coliform bacteria by modified homemade filter media from drinking water. *Bioresour. Technol.* **2008**, *99*, 2269–2274. [CrossRef] [PubMed]

30. Murphy, H.M.; McBean, E.A.; Farahbakhsh, K. Nitrification, denitrification and ammonification in point-of-use biosand filters in rural Cambodia. *J. Water Health* **2010**, *8*, 804–817. [CrossRef] [PubMed]

31. Elliott, M.A.; Stauber, C.E.; Koksal, F.; DiGiano, F.A.; Sobsey, M. Reductions of *E. coli*, echovirus type 12 and bacteriophages in an intermittently operated household-scale slow sand filter. *Water Res.* **2008**, *42*, 2662–2670. [CrossRef] [PubMed]

32. Nangmenyi, G.; Xao, W.; Mehrabi, S.; Mintz, E.; Economy, J. Bactericidal activity of Ag nanoparticle-impregnated fibreglass for water disinfection. *J. Water Health*, **2009**, *7*, 657–663. [CrossRef] [PubMed]

33. Michen, B.; Meder, F.; Rust, A.; Fritsch, J.; Aneziris, C.; Graule, T. Virus removal in ceramic depth filters based on diatomaceous earth. *Environ. Sci. Technol.* **2012**, *46*, 1170–1177. [CrossRef] [PubMed]

34. Van Halem, D. Ceramic Silver-Impregnated Pot Filters for Household Drinking Water Treatment in Developing Countries. Master's Thesis, Delft University of Technology, Delft, The Netherlands, 2006.

35. Tiwari, S.; Schmidt, W.P.; Darby, J.; Kariuki, Z.G.; Jenkins, M.W. Intermittent slow sand filtration for preventing diarrhoea among children in households using unimproved water sources: A randomized controlled trial. *Trop. Med. Int. Health* **2009**, *14*, 1374–1382. [CrossRef] [PubMed]

36. Du Preez, M.; Conroy, R.M.; Wright, J.A.; Moyo, S.; Potgieter, N.; Gundry, S.W. Use of ceramic water filtration in the prevention of diarrheal disease: A randomized controlled trial in rural South Africa and Zimbabwe. *Am. J. Trop. Med. Hyg.* **2008**, *79*, 696–701. [PubMed]

37. Duke, W.F.; Nordin, R.N.; Baker, D.; Mazumder, A. The use and performance of BioSand filters in the Artibonite Valley of Haiti: A field study of 107 households. *Rural Remote Health* **2006**, *6*, 570. [PubMed]

38. Clasen, T.F.; Brown, J.; Collin, S.M. Preventing diarrhoea with household ceramic water filters: Assessment of a pilot project in Bolivia. *Int. J. Environ. Health Res.* **2006**, *16*, 231–239. [CrossRef] [PubMed]

39. Michen, B.; Diatta, A.; Fritsch, J.; Aneziris, C.G.; Graule, T. Removal of colloidal particles in ceramic depth filters based on diatomaceous earth. *Sep. Purif. Technol.* **2011**, *81*, 77–87.

40. Momba, M.N.B.; Offringa, G.; Nameni, G.; Brouckaert, B. *Development of a Prototype Nanotechnology-Based Clay Filter Pot to Purify Water for Drinking and Cooking in Rural Homes*; WRC Report No. KV 244/10; Water Research Commission: Pretoria, South Africa, 2010; pp. 27–32.

41. Stauber, C.E.; Ortiz, G.M.; Loomis, D.P.; Sobsey, M.D. A randomized controlled trial of the concrete biosand filter and its impact on diarrheal disease in Bonao, Dominican Republic. *Am. J. Trop. Med. Hyg.* **2009**, *80*, 286–293. [PubMed]

42. Liang, K.; Sobsey, M.; Stauber, C. *Field Note: Improving Household Water Quality—Use of Biosand Filters in Cambodia*; Water and Sanitation Program: Hagar, Cambodia, 2010.

43. Stauber, C.E.; Printy, E.R.; McCarty, F.A.; Liang, K.R.; Sobsey, M.D. Cluster randomized trial of the plastic biosand water filter in Cambodia. *Environ. Sci. Technol.* **2012**, *46*, 722–728. [CrossRef] [PubMed]

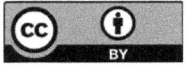

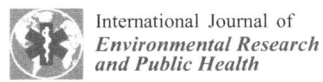

International Journal of
*Environmental Research
and Public Health*

Article

Assessing the Impact of a Risk-Based Intervention on Piped Water Quality in Rural Communities: The Case of Mid-Western Nepal

Dorian Tosi Robinson [1], Ariane Schertenleib [1], Bal Mukunda Kunwar [2], Rubika Shrestha [2], Madan Bhatta [2] and Sara J. Marks [1,*]

[1] Eawag, Swiss Federal Institute of Aquatic Science and Technology, Überlandstrasse 133, 8600 Dübendorf, Switzerland; dorian.tosirobinson@gmail.com (D.T.R.); ariane.schertenleib@eawag.ch (A.S.)

[2] Helvetas Swiss Intercooperation Nepal, Jhamshikhel Dhobi Ghat, Lalitpur, GPO Box 688 Kathmandu, Nepal; Bal.Kunwar@helvetas.org (B.M.K.); Rubika.Shrestha@helvetas.org (R.S.); Madan.Bhatta@helvetas.org (M.B.)

[*] Correspondence: sara.marks@eawag.ch; Tel.: +41-58-765-56-31

Received: 30 June 2018; Accepted: 27 July 2018; Published: 31 July 2018

Abstract: Ensuring universal access to safe drinking water is a global challenge, especially in rural areas. This research aimed to assess the effectiveness of a risk-based strategy to improve drinking water safety for five gravity-fed piped schemes in rural communities of the Mid-Western Region of Nepal. The strategy was based on establishing community-led monitoring of the microbial water quality and the sanitary status of the schemes. The interventions examined included field-robust laboratories, centralized data management, targeted infrastructure improvements, household hygiene and filter promotion, and community training. The results indicate a statistically significant improvement in the microbial water quality eight months after intervention implementation, with the share of taps and household stored water containers meeting the international guidelines increasing from 7% to 50% and from 17% to 53%, respectively. At the study endline, all taps had a concentration of <10 CFU *Escherichia coli*/100 mL. These water quality improvements were driven by scheme-level chlorination, improved hygiene behavior, and the universal uptake of household water treatment. Sanitary inspection tools did not predict microbial water quality and, alone, are not sufficient for decision making. Implementation of this risk-based water safety strategy in remote rural communities can support efforts towards achieving universal water safety.

Keywords: *E. coli*; monitoring; drinking water; water safety plan; sanitary inspection; gravity-fed piped water scheme; risk management

1. Introduction

In recent years, water sector professionals have made considerable progress improving access to drinking water worldwide. The Millennium Development Goal (MDG) for drinking water was met in 2015, with 2.6 billion people gaining access to an improved drinking water source since 1990 [1]. However, the additional sanitary protection offered by an improved drinking water source does not ensure that the water is safe to drink, because it is not guaranteed to be free from fecal contamination [2,3]. Half a million people worldwide died in 2012 due to consumption of unsafe water [4]. The MDGs thus underscored an urgent need to prioritize interventions designed to limit the hazards to human health by meeting the international guidelines for drinking water safety [5].

To address this issue, the water sector adopted Sustainable Development Goal (SDG) 6, which now includes measures of availability, accessibility, and quality as core standards in its definition of safely managed drinking water [6]. With these considerations, over a quarter of the global population currently lacks access to safely managed drinking water [7]. Water sector practitioners, therefore, face the challenging objective to deliver "universal and equitable access to safe and affordable drinking water for all by 2030" (SDG 6.1).

In Nepal, only a quarter of the rural population was estimated to have access to safely managed drinking water in 2015 [7], with access rates being lowest in the most remote areas where treatment is virtually non-existent and microbial contamination of water supplies is well documented. For example, Shrestha et al. (2017) reported inadequate water, sanitation, and hygiene (WASH) conditions in rural Nepal [8]. In the hilly areas of Mid-Western Nepal, a previous study reported a high health risk associated with the consumption of water from public taps, with 69% of samples collected testing positive for *Escherichia coli (E. coli)*. One in ten samples contained more than 100 colony forming units (CFU) of *E. coli*/100 mL [9], considered at very high risk per World Health Organization (WHO) classifications [5]. Another study in this region reported high daily variability and peak concentrations of fecal contamination [10].

These studies indicate a need for a comprehensive risk management strategy in place of end-of-pipe testing. Shrestha et al. (2017) recommended regular monitoring of water quality to generate missing information regarding seasonal variations [8]. The authors additionally suggested several mitigation actions, such as source protection, regular inspections, and targeted upgrades, with an emphasis on community engagement and water treatment measures. Such activities align with the World Health Organization (WHO)'s Water Safety Plan (WSP) approach that has been (and continues to be) widely promoted for improving drinking water safety from the source to the consumer. This approach is based on the identification of hazards and the mitigation of risks to achieve multibarrier protections for public health safety [5]. WSPs can be adapted to the needs of any drinking water project, including small communities' water supplies [11,12]. One tool used in small community WSPs is the sanitary inspection form to systematically assess vulnerabilities throughout the water scheme. These assessment forms proactively identify hazards at critical locations, thereby informing the management team regarding the potential sources of contamination to the water system and the mitigation efforts required.

While the WSP approach supports operational management processes for drinking water supplies, String and Lantagne point to a need for "evidence-based, documented impacts to both water supply and health after WSP implementation" [13]. Evidence regarding the implementation and impacts of WSPs on water quality is especially lacking in remote rural settings, where monitoring activities are hindered by low access to laboratory resources and technical expertise. Additionally, the suitability of sanitary inspection tools for assessing water safety is questioned, with previous studies showing contradictory conclusions regarding the predictability of fecal pollution levels based on sanitary risk scores alone [14–16]. It is therefore argued that effective risk management for water supplies should combine sanitary protection indicators with regular water quality testing [3,16]. In addition, the WHO has developed a revised set of forms that better suit the reality of small water supplies in rural contexts [17].

The objective of this research was to describe and evaluate a risk-based water safety strategy within five rural communities served by gravity-fed piped water supply schemes in the Dullu municipality in Mid-Western Nepal. Using a controlled before-and-after study design, we assessed the impact of a suite of interventions on the microbial water quality at different points throughout the system over an eight-month period. The interventions included the reinforcement of a pre-existing household water treatment and safe storage (HWTS) promotion campaign and targeted infrastructural and management improvements to the water schemes. Regular water quality monitoring was established using two solar-powered field laboratories equipped for microbial testing, and adapted sanitary inspections tools were used to systematically assess risks to the water systems. Intensive community participation and training were core features throughout the project's implementation.

In addition to the main objective of evaluating intervention impacts on the microbial water quality, other research questions of interest were as follows: (1) How did community members engage with the risk management process for their water system? (2) To what extent were the water safety interventions taken up by the communities by the study endline? (3) Did sanitary inspection scores align with water quality testing results? The project was implemented by Helvetas Swiss Intercooperation Nepal's (hereafter referred to as Helvetas-Nepal) Integrated Water Resources Management (IWRM) program, in collaboration the Swiss Federal Institute of Aquatic Science and Technology (hereafter referred to as Eawag) and REACH: Improving Water Security for the Poor (a program led by Oxford University and funded by the United Kingdom (UK) Government). The study commenced with baseline data collection from 120 households across five intervention communities and three control communities. To assess outcomes, an endline assessment was performed eight months after the baseline to capture changes in the microbial water quality and in households' perceptions and behavior regarding their drinking water.

The water safety strategy showed promising results towards achieving SDG 6.1 in rural communities dependent on gravity-fed piped schemes. Within intervention communities, we observed water quality improvements at taps and within households, improved hygiene behavior, and increased community capacity to proactively identify and mitigate the risks identified through regular monitoring. However, the microbial water quality did not meet the international guidelines by the study's endline for 100% of the water points assessed, indicating that further efforts are needed to ensure universal access to safe drinking water in this setting. This study also revealed the limitations of sanitary inspection scores and concluded that such tools should be combined with regular water quality testing for a complete risk management approach.

2. Materials and Methods

2.1. Study Site

Nepal is a landlocked country in Southern Asia that is situated in the Himalayas and shares borders with India and China. Three main regions compose the country's landscape and climate: a flat tropical area called the Terai, an intermediate hilly region, and the Himalayan mountains [18]. In 2017, the population was estimated to be 29 million people [19], 81% of whom were living in rural areas in 2015 [20]. Nepal ranked at the poorest end of the United Nations Development Programme Human Development Index in 2016, in the 144th position out of 188 countries [21]. Water scarcity is a common issue in the country [22,23] that is exacerbated by ongoing climate change impacts [24]. Developmental efforts in the past years have mainly focused on meeting the water supply demand and increasing freshwater accessibility. In addition, recent national development initiatives have focused on eliminating open defecation and achieving universal improved drinking water access, especially in rural areas [25]. The Nepal Water Supply, Sanitation, and Hygiene Sector Development Plan for 2016–2030 [26] highlights poor drinking water quality and the lack of an effective monitoring and surveillance system as a barrier to the implementation of the National Drinking Water Quality Standards [27].

The study was conducted in the Dullu municipality in the Dailekh district of the Mid-Western Development Region (Figure 1). This intermediate hilly region was selected as the study location because it is representative of the rural, hilly settings of Nepal, with the additional advantages of close proximity to sufficient projects within the Helvetas-Nepal IWRM service area and relatively convenient road access. In total, eight communities with gravity-fed piped drinking water schemes were selected for this study: five schemes where risk-based water safety intervention took place (hereafter called intervention schemes) and three control schemes where no risk-based water safety interventions were implemented.

Before the study, all eight communities had received a new piped water system with private or public taps constructed by Helvetas-Nepal between 2012 and 2016. Alongside system installation in each community, the program additionally established a water and sanitation users' committee, promoted improved household hygiene practices, distributed ceramic filters for household water treatment, and trained a female community health volunteer and a village maintenance worker responsible for repairing the water supply system. These pre-baseline activities, which defined the starting scenario of all the study communities, are summarized in Table 1.

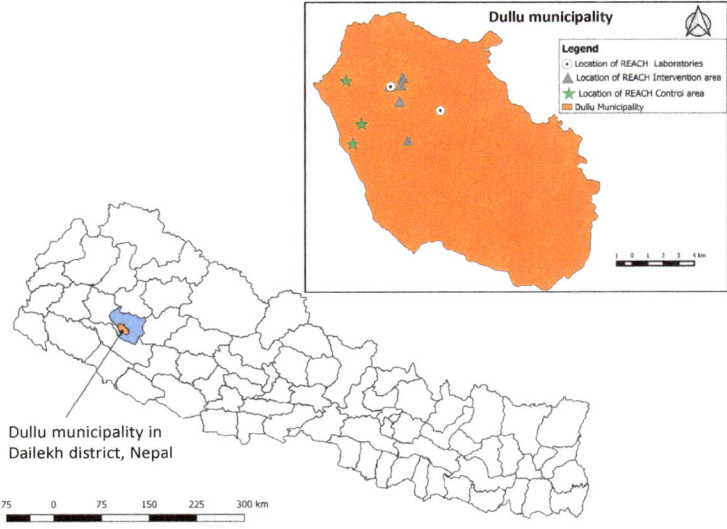

Figure 1. Map of Nepal with the district borders highlighting Dailekh district in blue and the intervention area, Dullu municipality, in orange. The map inset expands on the intervention area, showing the locations of the intervention and control schemes in relation to the field laboratories.

Table 1. Activities carried out before and during the study period within intervention and control communities.

Activity	Intervention Communities	Control Communities
Helvetas-Nepal program activities established before the study	Constructed piped water scheme Established water users' committee Conducted household hygiene campaign Installed ceramic water filters Trained community health volunteer and village maintenance worker	Same as intervention schemes
Data collection at study baseline and endline	Household survey Water quality sampling System sanitary inspection	Same as intervention schemes
Physical upgrades to water schemes	Source protection Intake improvement Scheme level chlorination [1] Small repairs 3R measures (Recharge, Retention, Reuse)	None
Management interventions	Creation of the Water Safety Plan task force Regular monitoring of sanitary state and water quality Laboratory coverage Improved maintenance	None
Behavior change interventions	Promotion of good handling practices for ceramic candle filter Household sanitary inspections	None

[1] Two of the five intervention schemes received chlorination.

2.2. Description of Drinking Water Schemes

The selected water schemes were constructed between 2012 and 2016; all were completed at least one year prior to this research. All are simple gravity-fed piped networks with spring sources, except one that includes a solar-powered lifting pump to deliver water from a downhill reservoir to the uphill distribution tanks. All the schemes provide intermittent water services with variable opening times and service durations throughout the year, as is common in the hilly region. They are all similar in their layout with a spring source that is connected to a reservoir tank by a distribution line, with water then flowing to the taps (Figure 2). All the selected schemes deliver water to public taps except one that has private taps only.

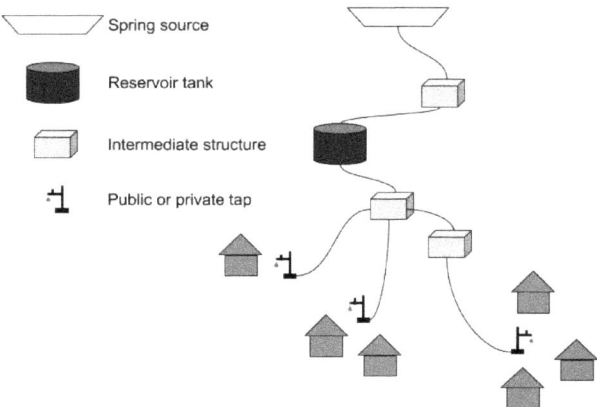

Figure 2. Sketch of a typical gravity-fed piped water scheme (or sub-scheme). Each scheme is composed of 1–4 sub-schemes. Sub-schemes comprise one water project for the same community but make use of independent water sources. Within a sub-scheme, one water source can feed several reservoir tanks that distribute water to different areas of the village. The intermediate structures can be distribution and collection chambers, purge valve chambers, break pressure tanks or interruption chambers, and air valve chambers.

2.3. Study Design and Sample Strategy

Two distinct research strategies were used: one for the baseline and endline surveys and the other for regular monitoring. The baseline and endline surveys aimed to assess community members' perceptions and behaviors regarding their drinking water. The sanitary state of the water schemes and the microbial water quality were also assessed at the baseline and the endline to measure changes before and after the water safety intervention. By contrast, regular monthly monitoring activities served as less intensive "spot checks" to capture temporal variations in water quality and sanitary indicators. In this way, regular monitoring data informed the ongoing implementation of interventions within each scheme by gauging their effectiveness and identifying any unaddressed system vulnerabilities.

2.3.1. Baseline and Endline Surveys

The baseline data collection took place in June 2017 and the endline data collection in January 2018. The field teams were composed of staff members of Eawag, Helvetas-Nepal, and the local non-governmental organization (NGO) Social Services Center. All the questionnaires were translated and conducted in Nepali. Only households using the water scheme were eligible for enrollment. Eligible households were selected randomly from the water project beneficiaries list and enrolled following informed consent about the project's purpose and anonymity of the questionnaire. At the study baseline, if the household declined to participate in the study or if no adult was available at the time of the visit, another household was selected randomly as a replacement. A total of 15 households were enrolled at each water scheme for a total of 120 surveys. During the endline period, the same households from the baseline were interviewed. The survey questions probed the households' drinking water supply characteristics, sanitation and hygiene practices, and socio-economic statuses. A drinking water sample was taken at each household by collecting 100 mL of water in the same manner as if getting a cup of water to drink. At each of the 8 study schemes, water samples were also taken at the inlet of all reservoir tanks and from three randomly selected taps during the baseline and endline visits.

2.3.2. Regular Monitoring

At each of the five intervention schemes, one source, one reservoir tank, one tap, and one household were regularly monitored every three–six weeks between August and December 2017 for both drinking water quality and sanitary status (Table 2). Sanitary inspection forms for sources, reservoir tanks, taps, and stored water were developed based on the updated forms provided by the WHO [17], with modifications made to suit the field context. Each form was composed of 10 yes/no questions from which a risk score out of 10 points was calculated, with a higher risk score indicating a greater health risk posed at the specific point (see Table A1 for the content of each sanitary inspection form). A trained person from each WSP task force was responsible for selecting monitoring points, taking the water samples, and performing the sanitary inspections. Monitoring points were rotated each month and were all water-connected: the household used water from the corresponding tap that was connected to the reservoir tank and the source that was being monitored. Care was taken to ensure that households were not aware of monitoring visits in advance. Regular monitoring is planned to be continued after the study's end as an integral part of the water safety framework. Further details on the regular monitoring strategy are provided in Supplementary Materials Section S1.

Table 2. Quantity of water samples at each phase of sampling.

Sampling Phase	Household	Tank	Tap
Baseline	120	21	23
Regular monitoring	23	23	23
Endline	115	25	23

2.4. Water Safety Plan, Interventions, and Laboratories

A WSP approach was adopted within the intervention communities. A WSP task force was formed as a subgroup of the pre-existing water users' committee. The task force members' main responsibilities were to evaluate and identify risks to their water scheme and to support efforts towards improved water security management practices. Based on the full sanitary inspection performed at the baseline, the WSP task force and Helvetas-Nepal's technical team collaboratively decided on one or more scheme upgrades to improve the water quality and devised a participatory approach for implementation.

The five intervention schemes received the system upgrade measures shown in Table 1 during November and December 2017. Additional details on the water scheme upgrades are provided in the Supplementary Materials Section S2. The upgrading process was based on a participatory approach that emphasized community members' involvement in the decision making to increase their sense of ownership over the project [28]. The communities also contributed to the system upgrade efforts by providing unskilled labor and local materials for construction.

In addition, two water quality laboratories were installed at a village health post and a secondary school close to the five interventions schemes. These laboratories consisted of a simple field incubator connected to a solar photovoltaic setup and all the materials required to perform the microbial water quality analysis (*E. coli* and total coliforms). The laboratory technicians received targeted group training followed by supervised field work. All the data gathered during the regular monitoring was collected by the trained WSP task force members and lab technicians under the supervision of a local NGO staff member who had also previously received intensive training.

2.5. Data Collection Tools and Water Quality Analysis

2.5.1. Mobile Data Collection

All the data, including the baseline and endline household surveys and regular sanitary inspections, were collected using tablets (Samsung Galaxy Tab A, Seoul, Korea) equipped with the Akvo Flow application (Akvo Foundation, Amsterdam, The Netherlands). The data were uploaded to the cloud and made available to project team members to be analyzed remotely.

2.5.2. Water Sampling and Microbial Water Quality Testing Protocol

Water samples collected at the reservoir tanks were taken directly from the inlet, which is the closest point to the water source that was available to sample; therefore, the sample collected is representative of the water entering but not the water being stored at the reservoir tank. At the taps, water was run for 30 s before sampling to wash out any deposited residue and ensure a representative sample from the piped system. The household water samples were collected at the point of consumption (i.e., 100 mL of water was collected in the same way a glass of water for drinking would be prepared). All the water samples from a single scheme were collected on the same day. The water samples were collected in sterile 100 mL Whirl-Pak sampling bags (Nasco, Fort Atkinson, USA). For chlorinated schemes, Whirl-Pak Thio-bags (Nasco, Fort Atkinson, USA) containing sodium thiosulfate were used to inactivate any residual chlorine. Because the electricity required to support a cold chain was not available, the samples were transported to the field laboratories in cooler boxes without ice. The samples were processed by membrane filtration using Nissui Compact Dry EC plates (Nissui Pharmaceuticals, Tokyo, Japan) and a modified filtration device (DelAgua, UK), followed by incubation at $35 \pm 2\,^{\circ}\text{C}$ for 24 h. All the samples were transported and processed within two hours of collection. If transportation to laboratories within two hours was impossible, the samples were processed on site and incubated later. A detailed protocol for the membrane filtration method and further information on the construction of the field incubators are available in the Supplementary Materials Sections S3 and S4, respectively.

2.5.3. Bacteria Enumeration and Quality Control

After incubation, *E. coli* and total coliform were enumerated on Compact Dry EC according to the manufacturer's instructions. Counts higher than 300 colonies per plate were reported as too numerous to count (TNTC). The results are reported as colony forming units (CFU) of total coliforms or *E. coli* per 100 mL (CFU/100 mL). To assess the replicability of the method, a duplicate was performed every tenth sample during the baseline and endline data collection. In addition, a random duplicate was taken from one of the sampled sites (tank, tap, or household) during each round of a scheme's regular monitoring. Negative controls (blanks) were processed daily. The statistical analyses of all control measures are found in the Supplementary Materials Section S5.

2.6. Data Analysis

Water quality and survey data were initially compiled and cleaned using Excel 10 (Microsoft, Redmond, WA, USA). Coding and statistical tests of intervention effects were performed using IBM SPSS (IBM, New York, NY, USA). The microbial concentrations were observed to be exponentially distributed; therefore, bivariate comparisons made use of non-parametric tests (e.g., Mann–Whitney U test and central tendency reported as median CFU/100 mL) or parametric tests (e.g., Student's *t*-test for independent samples following Log_{10} transformation of *E. coli* data and central tendency reported as mean CFU/100 mL). For all Log_{10} transformations, zero counts were set to 0.5 CFU/100 mL and TNTC values were set to the upper limit of detection (300 CFU/100 mL).

2.7. Ethics Statement

All participating households gave their informed consent before being interviewed. The research was conducted in accordance with the Declaration of Helsinki, and the protocol was approved by the Eawag ethics committee (protocol 16_09_072017). The study received government approval in Nepal as part of the Helvetas-Nepal IWRM research program.

3. Results

3.1. Household and Drinking Water Scheme Characteristics

3.1.1. Generalities

The average household had 6.5 (SD = 2.3) family members, with 0.8 children who were 5 years old or younger. Virtually all of the interviewed households (99%) were active in agricultural and farming activities. The monthly expenses per household ranged from 1550 to 50,000 Nepalese Rupees (NPR, M = 10,610, SD = 7800), corresponding to 15.5–500 United States Dollars (USD, M = 106, SD = 78) using a rounded average currency exchange rate of 2017 (Exchange rate calculator, http://www.x-rates.com/average/?from=USD&to=NPR&amount=1&year=2017). When asked about their main concern within their community in the baseline survey, households most frequently mentioned water supply services (31% of intervention and 53% of control households). Most of the households interviewed had walls made of wood or mud (>73%), a floor made of mud, sand, or dirt (>87%), and a roof made of metal (>36%) or thatch (>14%). Concerning sanitation, most of the households reported using an improved private latrine (>89%). There was no electrical grid in the project area, but most households had installed small private solar systems to power lighting and mobile phones (>89%). A further description of the household characteristics is available in the Supplementary Materials Section S6.

3.1.2. Hygiene Practices and Reported Illness

At the baseline visit, most households reported washing their hands after going to the toilet (>91%), before eating (>93%), and before cooking (>67%). The frequency of soap use during handwashing increased from 43% to 63% between the baseline and endline among the households using the intervention schemes, whereas the frequency decreased from 80% to 60% among the control schemes over the same period. The availability of dedicated handwashing stations with a faucet increased at the intervention schemes from 65% to 83% and stayed constant at the control schemes at 82%. The Supplementary Materials Section S6 contains detailed results of the households' handwashing practices.

Most households (96%) did not report having experienced any diarrhea or respiratory illness cases among their family members in the week prior to the survey. A total of six people at the baseline and four people at the endline had experienced a case of diarrhea or respiratory illness, with about half of these cases being children under the age of five. All the households reporting illness during the baseline were using the interventions schemes, whereas at the endline most of the households reporting illnesses (three of the four) were using a control scheme.

3.1.3. Perception of Drinking Water Quality and Water Treatment Practices

At the baseline visit, most households perceived their drinking water taste and smell as good (>98%), color as clear/good (>92%), and as generally safe to drink (>85%). By the endline visit, the share of households reporting their drinking water was safe had increased slightly in the intervention schemes (99%) and decreased in the control schemes (79%) (Figure 3). However, households using the interventions schemes that received chlorination as part of the WSP intervention reported greater dissatisfaction with the taste of the water by the endline visit; among the two schemes where chlorination was introduced, chlorine taste and "bad or funny smelling water" was reported by

15% and 14%, respectively, of the 29 households interviewed. Further details on the perceptions of the drinking water quality are available in the Supplementary Materials Section S6.

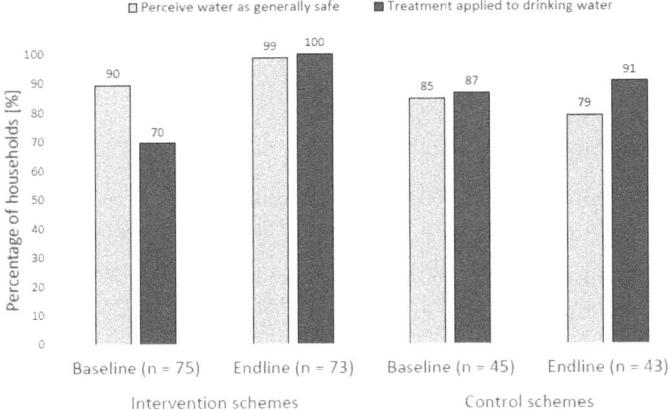

Figure 3. Drinking water safety perception and treatment coverage among the households served by the intervention and the control schemes from the baseline to the endline period.

Regarding water treatment practices, at the baseline visit, fewer households in the intervention schemes reported treating their drinking water (70%) compared with the households in the control schemes (85%). The share of the households adopting the treatment practices increased among all households from the baseline to endline visits (Figure 3). However, the observed difference in the treatment coverage was only statistically significant among the intervention schemes (c^2 (1, $n = 147) = 26.18$, $p = 0.00$), with all the households reporting that they practiced some form of household water treatment by the endline.

At the baseline, the households that said their drinking water was not generally safe indicated the main reasons as being an unprotected source (36%) or animal waste (29%). However, more than a quarter (29%) of the households did not know why they thought the water was unsafe. At the endline, half of the households that did not consider their water to be safe reported toilet waste as the major reason. The other major concerns mentioned at the endline included animal waste (38%), an unprotected source (25%), and chemicals (13%).

3.1.4. Water Supply Characteristics

In Nepal, efforts have been made in recent decades to provide access to an improved drinking water supply for all rural households. In the study area, the designs of the gravity-fed schemes are all similar, with source water directed to one or several reservoir tanks, which are then opened daily for distribution. The study schemes served from 29 to 108 households or 177–683 people (see the additional scheme characteristics in Table 3). The water services were intermittent, meaning that reservoir tanks were manually opened once or twice per day at a defined hour. The opening times and durations varied throughout the year depending on the source water availability and the time required to fill the reservoir. Usually, the opening duration ranged from one to two hours, with shorter times during the dry season.

All the water points within the study communities were functional at the time of the research team's baseline and endline visits. Most households (>80%) reported that their water supply scheme functioned well in general, and most (>85%) reported that they were confident that their water system would still be functional in a year. Most of the interviewed households (>82%) had access to a public tap, and among these households, nearly all (>95%) reported it as their main drinking water source.

The average reported time taken for a round trip to the drinking water source, including queuing time, was 10 min (SD = 9). A trained local maintenance worker was responsible for regular maintenance and repairs for each scheme. Most interviewed households (>87%) reported that they could get help from their local maintenance worker for necessary repairs and that repairs could be completed within a week (>71%). A water tariff system had been implemented prior to the start of this study, with most households (>85%) reporting that user fees were collected to pay for repairs on an as-needed basis. Detailed water supply characteristics are available in the Supplementary Materials Section S6.

Table 3. Description of water supply schemes characteristics: mean (standard deviation), [range].

Characteristics	Intervention Schemes	Control Schemes
Households served	66.8 (32.2), [29 to 108]	84.3 (30.4), [50 to 108]
Population served	411.8 (209.5), [177 to 683]	511.7 (194.9), [292 to 664]
Spring sources	2.6 (1.1), [1 to 4]	3.3 (1.2), [2 to 4]
Reservoir tanks	3.2 (1.5), [1 to 5]	3.7 (0.6), [3 to 4]
Taps	19.4 (3.6), [15 to 24]	26.7 (14.2), [18 to 43]

3.1.5. Water Supply Management

The household survey probed the community members involved in the management, operation, and maintenance of their water supply scheme. A total of 44% of the households interviewed at the endline indicated having a family member who was either a member of the water and sanitation users' committee or the WSP task force or had served as a maintenance worker, community health volunteer, or tap stand care taker. The water users' committee met together regularly (most often monthly) to discuss issues related to the water supply scheme. During the construction of the scheme, the water users' committee also met with community members monthly to discuss the project, establish a fund for operation and maintenance, assign maintenance workers, collect contributions toward construction, and eventually, conduct public reviews of the committee's income and expenditures. After construction was completed, the water users' committee generally met with community members only once every year or every second year to perform the aforementioned duties, as well as reform the water users' committee as needed. During the baseline, 60% and 40% of households using the intervention and control schemes, respectively, indicated that they were aware of the water users' committee meetings within their community. At the endline, these percentages increased to 79% and 67% for the intervention and control schemes, respectively, suggesting that the study served to raise awareness regarding the water users' committee activities. More detailed results are available in the Supplementary Materials Section S6.

3.1.6. Activities within Intervention Schemes

Among the households served by the intervention schemes only, additional questions were asked at the endline visit to assess the activities taking place during the WSP implementation. Nearly all (88%) the households served by the intervention schemes were aware of the WSP strategy, and among these households, about half (54%) had participated in its development and implementation through their membership in the WSP task force, involvement in the regular scheme chlorination, or the installation of the intake filter. A total of 93% of households had heard about the laboratories that had been installed for monthly water quality testing, and 71% said that the results of the microbial analysis had been reported back to them by local NGO staff members or members of the water users' committee. Among the 51 households that had received their test results, 37% indicated that their water quality was contaminated. In response, all of these households had begun to treat their water using a ceramic candle filter (100%) and boiling (16%). When asked about their desire for future water quality testing, 96% of interviewees responded positively and said they would pay up to 500 NPR (or 4.78 USD) per test, with a median value of 50 NRP (or 0.48 USD) per test (Exchange rate calculator, http://www.x-rates.com/average/?from=USD&to=NPR&amount=1&year=2017).

Among the nine households served by intervention schemes that had a family member in the water users' committee, all had been informed about the results of the monthly water quality monitoring. All but one of the households had then discussed these results with the water users' committee, and in about half of the instances (44%), actions to improve the water scheme had been undertaken. Further details on the activities within the intervention schemes are provided in the Supplementary Materials Section S6.

3.2. Water Quality Analysis

3.2.1. Household Stored Water Sample Characteristics

Among all the households, most of the water samples collected from the stored water containers were clear at both the baseline (>96%) and the endline (>81%) visits. The share of stored water samples treated by household ceramic filters or boiling among the intervention schemes increased from 63% at the baseline to 100% at the endline (Table 4). By the endline visit, three-quarters of these samples had also received some form of scheme-level treatment, such as chlorination; however, no monitoring of chlorine residual in the stored water was conducted as confirmation. By contrast, the share of stored water samples that had been treated at the household level within control schemes remained relatively constant, from 76% at the baseline to 86% at the endline (see the Supplementary Materials Section S6 for additional details).

Table 4. Characteristics of stored water samples collected from households.

Sample Characteristic	Intervention Schemes		Control Schemes	
	BL (%)	EL (%)	BL (%)	EL (%)
Sample collected from:				
Ceramic candle filter outlet	57	99	78	81
Gagri/jerrycan/bucket	43	1	22	19
Visual quality:				
Clear	100	97	96	81
Somewhat turbid	0	3%	4	19
Very turbid	0	0	0	0
Received treatment at:				
Household level only	59	25	76	86
Scheme level only	0	0	0	0
Both household and scheme level	3	75	6	0
No treatment	37	0	18	14

BL: Baseline; EL: Endline.

3.2.2. Baseline Water Quality and Qualitative Sanitary Observations

At the study baseline, the microbial water quality was assessed at each of the surveyed households, as well as at the all the reservoir tanks and three taps per scheme. All the data were analyzed based on *E. coli* concentrations unless otherwise stated. Table 5 shows the median and the mean Log_{10} *E. coli* contamination at the intervention and control schemes. The Mann–Whitney U tests showed no statistical differences in the *E. coli* concentrations between sampling points at the intervention and controls schemes at the baseline ($p \geq 0.05$).

Table 5. *Escherichia coli* concentrations at each sample location for the intervention and control schemes, with bivariate comparisons of the mean *E. coli* contamination at the baseline and endline measurements.

Location	Sampling Phase	Intervention Schemes				Control Schemes			
		n	Median [CFU/100 mL]	Mean (SD), [Range] [Log_{10}(CFU/100 mL)]	Student's t-test	n	Median [CFU/100 mL]	Mean (SD), [Range] [Log_{10}(CFU/100 mL)]	Student's t-Test
Household	Baseline	75	24	1.25 (1.00), [−0.30 to 2.48]	$t = -5.645$, df = 145, $p < 0.001$	45	8	1.01 (0.97), [−0.30 to 2.48]	$t = -1.026$, df = 86, $p = 0.308$
	Endline	72	0	0.36 (0.92), [−0.30 to 2.48]		43	4	0.80 (0.98), [−0.30 to 2.48]	
Tank	Baseline	11	12	1.00 (0.80), [−0.30 to 2.04]	$t = -1.120$, df = 24, $p = 0.274$	10	50	1.52 (0.86), [0.00 to 2.48]	$t = -1.381$, df = 18, $p = 0.184$
	Endline	15	4	0.63 (0.87), [−0.30 to 2.08]		10	9	0.98 (0.89), [−0.30 to 2.48]	
Tap	Baseline	14	11	1.14 (0.79), [−0.30 to 2.18]	$t = -4.086$, df = 26, $p < 0.000$	9	38	1.54 (1.01), [0.00 to 2.48]	$t = -2.040$, df = 16, $p = 0.058$
	Endline	14	1	0.13 (0.49), [−0.30 to 0.85]		9	3	0.65 (0.82), [−0.30 to 2.48]	

The sanitary inspections of the water schemes at the baseline visit indicated high risk scores at all the spring sources due to inadequate protection measures. The infiltration of contaminated runoff water and open intakes were the main hazards identified. Additionally, for most of the spring sources, the inspections revealed that intake maintenance was not possible without compromising the integrity of the intake covering and the protective gravel and sand layers. Any blockage at the intake would require the removal of these covering layers, thereby risking that the intake would not be properly covered afterwards. Generally, the other structures, such as the reservoir tanks and the distribution pipes, were in good condition. Nevertheless, the tank covers were pinpointed as vulnerabilities, because contamination could enter during rain events or when the covers were opened. Occasional pipe leaks were observed, and the taps were found to be damaged or leaking in some of the schemes.

3.2.3. Monthly Monitoring of Intervention Schemes

Regular monitoring of the intervention schemes included water quality testing and structured sanitary inspections that provided a calculated risk score. Figure 4 shows the mean risk scores and mean *E. coli* concentrations at the source, reservoir tank, tap, and household. The microbial water quality was not measured at the sources because no samples could be collected without damaging the integrity of their protective structures.

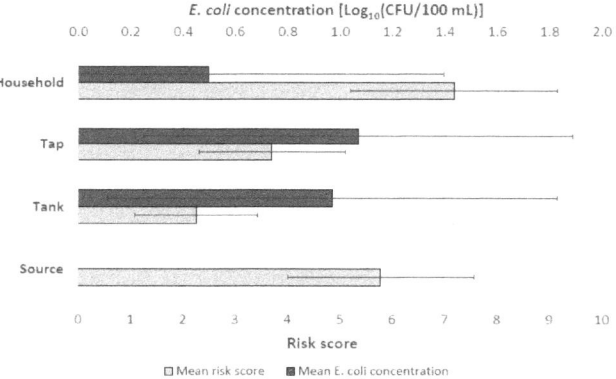

Figure 4. Mean risk scores from monthly sanitary inspections and mean *Escherichia coli* concentrations from monthly sampling (*n* = 23, standard deviation bars shown). The maximum risk score is 10.

The average risk score was higher at the sources (due to poor protective measures) and the households (due to recontamination vulnerabilities) than at the taps and reservoir tanks. However, the microbial water quality of household stored water was on average better than at the taps and reservoir tanks. With these results, the sanitary inspections did not accurately predict the water quality test results at each given point. The household water treatment practices appeared to improve the stored water quality, even if the overall sanitary state of the household was poor according to the inspection forms. Rain events during the monitoring day and the preceding day were recorded in the sanitary inspection forms and examined as a potential factor explaining variations in the microbial water quality. However, the results did not reveal any meaningful impact of rain on the observed microbial concentrations.

3.2.4. Endline Water Quality and Qualitative Sanitary Observations

Water quality at the endline was assessed at the same points as during the baseline (Table 5). The Mann–Whitney U tests showed a small but significant difference in the *E. coli* contamination levels of the household stored water samples between the intervention (median = 0 CFU/mL) and control schemes (median = 4 CFU/100 mL), U = 1073, p = 0.004. No significant differences in the *E. coli* contamination of the intervention and control scheme reservoir tanks or taps were observed ($p \geq 0.05$).

The sanitary inspections during the endline visit showed that all the source intakes of the intervention schemes had been structurally improved. Each had a new intake filter made of fine sand and gravel layered and packed in a net. The intake was also topped with a plastic cover to avoid surface water infiltration. Rain water diversion ditches were constructed around the source intakes to prevent rainwater runoff from entering the intake area. In some cases, additional shields against landslides were installed as added protection. Protection and regeneration of the micro-catchment through the 3R (Recharge, Retention, Reuse) intervention (see Table 1) were observed but only at their early stages. It is expected that this plantation work will deliver its full potential as a conservation measure several years after its completion. The intervention schemes were also improved through the replacement or repair of leaking pipes throughout the network and improved maintenance of the public taps.

3.3. Comparisons of Fecal Contamination at the Baseline and Endline Measurement

3.3.1. Average Contamination by Scheme and Sampling Point

The mean *E. coli* contamination of household stored water is shown in Figure 5a. These results showed that the contamination during the baseline was on average greater in the intervention schemes than in the control schemes. By the endline visit, the opposite situation was observed, with most intervention schemes having lower contamination levels within the stored water on average, as compared with the control schemes. At most reservoir tanks and taps at the intervention and control schemes, the water quality at the baseline had improved by the endline visit (Figure 5b,c). A particularly high level of fecal contamination was observed in the reservoir tanks and taps of the control scheme number six during the baseline visit.

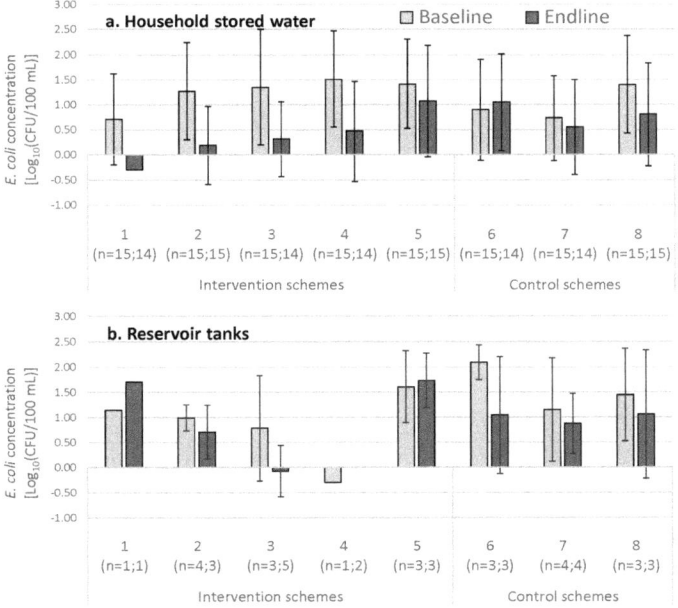

Figure 5. *Cont.*

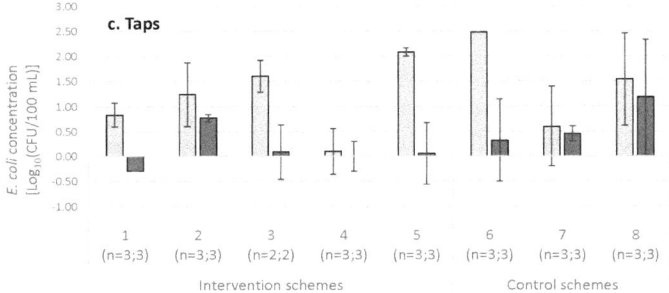

Figure 5. Mean *E. coli* concentrations of the (**a**) household stored water containers, (**b**) reservoir tanks, and (**c**) taps at the baseline and endline for each of the eight schemes. The standard deviation bars are shown.

Figure 6 shows the mean *E. coli* concentrations for the intervention and control schemes at each sampling location. The greatest reductions in the contamination between the baseline and endline measurements are seen at the households and taps among the interventions schemes (see the Supplementary Materials for additional microbial analyses across the sampling points (Section S7); within the chlorinated schemes specifically (Section S8); among the households using and not using ceramic water filters (Section S9); and other detailed microbial results (Section S10)).

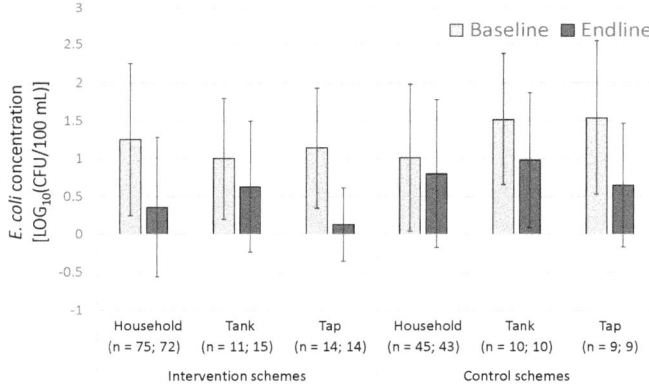

Figure 6. Mean *E. coli* contamination at each sampling point at the baseline and endline measurements for the intervention and control schemes. The standard deviation bars are shown.

3.3.2. Statistical Comparisons of Fecal Contamination at the Baseline and Endline Measurements for Intervention and Control Schemes

A Student's *t*-test was used to compare the *E. coli* contamination levels at the baseline to the endline measurements within the intervention and control schemes (Table 5). The results show a statistically significant difference in mean contamination levels at the households and the taps within the intervention schemes only. The mean Log_{10} *E. coli* concentration at the households served by the intervention schemes was 1.25 CFU/100 mL at the baseline and 0.36 CFU/100 mL at the endline. At the intervention scheme taps, a reduction in the mean Log_{10} *E. coli* concentration from 1.14 CFU/100 mL to 0.13 CFU/100 mL was observed. No significant difference in the average contamination levels between the baseline and the endline was observed at the intervention reservoir tanks or at any of the sampling points in the control schemes (see the Supplementary Materials Section S10 for further discussion and statistical analysis).

When examining whether the samples met the WHO guidelines for drinking water safety (<1 CFU *E. coli*/100 mL), the results show that the share of the household stored water samples from the intervention schemes with no detectable *E. coli* increased significantly from 17% at the baseline to 53% at the endline (c^2 (1, $n = 147$) = 24.01, $p = 0.00$). Also significant was the increase in the tap samples from the intervention schemes that met the WHO guidelines, from 7% at the baseline to 50% at the endline (c^2 (1, $n = 28$) = 6.30, $p = 0.03$), with all the tap samples at the endline having less than 10 CFU *E. coli*/100 mL. Other sampling points did not yield meaningful changes in the share of samples meeting the WHO criteria (see Table A2 for detailed results and the Supplementary Materials Section S11 for temporal representations of the baseline, endline, and regular monitoring data).

3.3.3. Difference-in-Differences Analysis

A difference-in-differences analysis was used to compare the household water quality data from the intervention and control schemes at the baseline and the endline. Estimating the natural change at the control sites and subtracting it from the intervention sites indicated that the effect of the interventions on the household water quality caused a decrease of the mean Log_{10} concentration of *E. coli* of 0.681 CFU/100 mL (SE = 0.26, $n = 235$, $t = -2.614$, $p = 0.01$) among the intervention schemes.

The difference-in-differences analysis for the water quality at the reservoir tanks was +0.168 Log_{10} CFU/100 mL and at the taps was −0.13 Log_{10} CFU/100 mL. This is interpreted as meaning that the interventions were responsible for an increase in the contamination at the reservoir tanks and a decrease at the taps (reservoir tanks: DD = 0.168, SE = 0.512, $t = 0.329$, $p = 0.744$, $n = 46$; taps: DD = −0.13, SE = 0.464, $t = -0.281$, $p = 0.78$, $n = 46$). This unexpected finding could be explained by the fact that the control scheme number six showed exceptionally high contamination at the baseline as compared with all the other schemes (Figure 5b), resulting in a large improvement of the mean water quality at the control schemes' reservoir tanks. The difference-in-differences analysis at the taps is aligned with the results presented above and indicates a statistically significant improvement in the water quality due to the interventions.

4. Discussion

4.1. Study Novelty and Insights

While past studies have investigated water safety interventions in rural areas of Nepal, to the authors' knowledge, no study to date has reported outcomes based on comparison to a set of control communities. The aims of this research were to describe an approach for improving the drinking water safety that is adapted to this unique setting, as well as to rigorously evaluate whether this strategy was capable of achieving measurable improvements in the water quality. The findings reported here will be of interest to government agencies, water program managers, system operators, and program managers throughout Nepal and are applicable to other remote rural areas dependent on gravity-fed piped supplies.

This study revealed several insights relevant to the rural water sector. First, we observed universal uptake of the household water treatment (ceramic water filters and/or boiling) within the intervention communities. This finding suggests that the suite of water safety interventions delivered through the WSP, including the intensive WASH promotion activities, were very effective in motivating behavior change over an eight-month period. The WASH promotion activities included the communication of the stored water quality results to most households following testing. The survey data revealed that all the households who received the results indicating contamination of their stored water subsequently adopted treatment practices. Moreover, nearly all the survey respondents said that they would be interested in further water quality testing at an average price of 0.70 USD per test.

Int. J. Environ. Res. Public Health **2018**, *15*, 1616

The high uptake of the household water treatment and increased demand for water quality testing among the households could also be attributed to a generally high level of awareness and involvement among the community members. For example, 88% of survey respondents said they knew about the WSP activities within their community. Over half of these households had served as an official member of the WSP task force or participated in infrastructural improvements, such as the installation of intake filters or the implementation of chlorine dosing. Taken together, these results suggest the broad level of engagement by the households in the planning and implementation of their water safety interventions contributed to the successful outcome observed over an eight-month period. More generally, the study findings suggest a dynamic interaction between the community members' participation in the water supply stewardship, the delivery of targeted water quality information, and the demand for safe drinking water.

A second insight from this research is that the sanitary inspection risk scores did not accurately predict the microbial water quality at different points across the system. According to the sanitary inspection metric used, the risks were on average greatest at the sources and households and lowest at the reservoir tanks and taps. These findings were driven by the poor physical protection of the sources and factors indicating the recontamination potential of the stored drinking water at the household level. Surprisingly, however, the water quality measurements revealed the opposite trend; the fecal contamination of the household stored water was on average lower than at the collection taps and reservoir tanks (it was not possible to measure the microbial water quality at the source). These findings may be explained by the uptake and consistent use of ceramic water filters by the households following enrollment in the study, thereby improving the water quality even if other measures of the household's sanitary state remained poor according to the inspection form.

Finally, statistical comparisons of the microbial water quality revealed improvements at all points monitored for both the intervention and control schemes. However, the improvements observed in the average *E. coli* concentrations from the baseline to the endline were only statistically significant for the taps and the household stored water containers in the intervention group (and not so in the control group). Examining the microbial data at the scheme level, we found that the household stored water quality consistently improved from the baseline to the endline for all the intervention schemes, whereas an inconsistent trend was observed for the three control schemes. In addition, the intervention communities showed universal adoption of household water treatments by the endline, resulting in over half of the households having stored water meeting the WHO guidelines for water safety (0 CFU *E. coli*/100 mL). The reduction in the fecal contamination among the intervention taps is notable as well, with half of the taps meeting the WHO guidelines (up from only 7% at the baseline) and all the taps delivering water with less than 10 CFU *E. coli*/100 mL. These results, while promising, do not indicate perfect compliance with international water safety guidelines for all the intervention schemes. Thus, the water safety interventions applied may be considered as an effective and viable interim solution in efforts to eventually achieve universal access to safely managed drinking water in rural settings.

4.2. Study Limitations

Some features of this study design limit our ability to generalize the findings beyond the sampled population. Most notable is the generally high level of water service experienced within both the intervention and control schemes. Nine out of every 10 survey respondents reported at the baseline that their main water source tasted and smelled good and was generally safe to drink. Moreover, all the water points were functioning at the time of the research team's visit, and most survey respondents believed it would likely continue to function well over the coming year. This generally high level of satisfaction and confidence among water users may be unique to the program setting and is likely a driving factor in the households' willingness to pay for water services and engage in stewardship of the infrastructure over time.

Another issue is the enrollment of only three control schemes as compared with the five intervention schemes. This research design limitation was driven by both resource constraints and

Int. J. Environ. Res. Public Health **2018**, *15*, 1616

ethical considerations; within a set budget, there was the need to ensure the potential benefits of the study (water supply upgrades) outweighed the potential costs (lost time due to participation). As a result, the sample sizes in the control group were roughly three-fifths the size of those in the intervention group, which underpowered comparisons of small effective sizes. Finally, the follow-up period for this study was eight months, which only allows for preliminary conclusions to be made regarding the sustainability of the interventions examined. Future research should ideally monitor the outcomes reported here over a longer period (at least one year and ideally up to five years). This is especially critical for understanding the sustainability of behavioral measures known to decline over time, such as household ceramic filter use.

4.3. Recommendations for Water Sector Policy and Practice

There are several recommendations for water sector practitioners arising from this research. First, these study results indicate that over the short term (eight months), the applied water safety interventions were highly effective in motivating uptake and use of household water treatments. Such promotional activities were tailored to the needs of the households in rural Nepal and were integrated into a broader WSP framework. To replicate this success, program managers should strive for a comprehensive approach that merges household-centered WASH promotional activities with system-scale water safety efforts. Second, sanitary inspection scores did not reliably predict the microbial concentrations at various sampling points and are therefore insufficient for assessing actual health risks due to drinking water consumption. Based on these findings, standardized sanitary inspection packages should be combined with regular water quality testing for a comprehensive risk management approach. Finally, the applied interventions, while effectively improving water quality at the taps and in the household stored water containers, did not achieve perfect compliance with the international guidelines over the eight-month study period, in part, because interventions such as micro-catchment restoration required more time to deliver their intended benefits. Future research should therefore explore additional treatment options, for example, disinfection by automated chlorine dosing or ultraviolet treatment devices.

5. Conclusions

This study characterized and assessed a risk-based strategy for improving the drinking water quality of gravity-fed piped schemes in the hilly regions of Mid-Western Nepal. This research was motivated by the need to accelerate progress towards achieving universal access to safely managed drinking water in similar contexts, where effective treatment and regular monitoring of piped supplies is often challenged by geography, limited resources, and unreliable supply chains. The results showed that simplified field laboratories equipped for microbial testing can inform ongoing decision-making regarding targeted system upgrades and mitigation measures. These interventions led to positive changes in the drinking water quality at the taps and within the households over eight months of implementation. Of particular note was the achievement of 100% coverage of household water treatments with ceramic filters and boiling across all intervention schemes. In addition, the results showed high levels of involvement by the households in planning and implementing the WSP within their community, especially through regular engagement with the local water and sanitation users' committee.

The study also revealed the inconsistent predictability of microbial contamination using standard sanitary inspection forms alone. This finding suggests that such forms, while useful for identifying potential hazards, should be combined with regular water quality testing for a comprehensive risk management approach for piped schemes. By the study endline visit, half of the samples collected from households' stored water containers and taps were free of fecal contamination—a significant improvement from the baseline visit when only 17% and 7% of the households and the taps, respectively, met the international guidelines for microbial safety. Despite all the water points sampled not meeting the stated guidelines, the applied strategy nevertheless proved promising as an intermediate step towards achieving universal access to safe drinking water in rural areas.

Supplementary Materials: The following are available online at http://www.mdpi.com/1660-4601/15/8/1616/s1. Section S1: The Regular Monitoring Strategy; Section S2: Water Scheme Upgrades; Section S3: Membrane Filtration Protocol; Section S4: Construction of Field Incubators; Section S5: Water Quality Tests Validity Measurements; Section S6: Detailed Household Survey Results; Section S7: Comparison of Individual Sampling Points; Section S8: Details of Chlorinated Schemes; Section S9: Comparison between Use and Non-Use of Ceramic Candle Filters; Section S10: Detailed Microbial Results; and Section S11: Temporal View of Baseline, Regular Monitoring, and Endline Microbial Data. Scheme-level water quality data are also provided as a supplementary file.

Author Contributions: Conceptualization, M.B. and S.J.M.; Methodology, D.T.R., A.S., B.M.K., M.B., and S.J.M.; Validation, R.S.; Formal Analysis, D.T.R. and S.J.M.; Resources, M.B.; Data Curation, D.T.R., A.S., and R.S.; Original Draft Preparation, D.T.R.; Review and Editing of Manuscript, D.T.R., A.S., B.M.K., R.S., M.B., and S.J.M.; Visualization, R.S.; Supervision, A.S., B.M.K., M.B., and S.J.M.; Project Administration, B.M.K., M.B., and S.J.M.; Funding Acquisition, M.B. and S.J.M. All authors read and approved the final manuscript.

Funding: This research was supported by the Swiss Agency for Development Cooperation and the REACH programme funded by UK Aid from the UK Department for International Development (DFID) for the benefit of developing countries (Aries Code 201880). The views expressed and information contained in this manuscript are not necessarily those of or endorsed by these agencies, which can accept no responsibility for such views or information or for any reliance placed upon them.

Acknowledgments: The authors thank the community members in the study area who served as laboratory technicians, water samplers, WSP task force members, and household survey participants. Jiban Singh, Manuel Holzer, the Helvetas staff, and the local enumerator teams provided excellent field support during the training and data collection. Many thanks to Arnt Diener for contributing to the REACH grant submission and Tim Julian for constructive comments on the results section of the manuscript.

Conflicts of Interest: The authors declare no conflict of interest.

Abbreviations

CFU	colony forming units
HWTS	household water treatment and safe storage
IWRM	integrated water resources management
MDGs	Millennium Development Goals
NGO	non-governmental organization
NPR	Nepalese Rupee
3R	recharge, retention, and reuse
SDGs	Sustainable Development Goals
Eawag	Swiss Federal Institute of Aquatic Science and Technology
WASH	water, sanitation and hygiene
WSP	water safety plan
WHO	World Health Organization
USD	United States Dollar

Appendix A

Table A1. Sanitary inspection forms for the household water storage containers, piped water taps, reservoir tanks, and sources. Each "yes" answer is scored as 1, and each "no" answer is scored as 0. The risk score equation is given, with the maximum risk score possible being 10.

	Question	Score (yes = 1, no = 0)
	HOUSEHOLD STORED WATER CONTAINER	
1	Are the drinking water storage containers used only for storing drinking and cooking water?	
2	Are the drinking water storage containers kept above ground level?	
3	Are the drinking water storage containers' lids or covers present and in place?	
4	Are the drinking water storage containers sanitary and free from cracks?	
5	Is the area around the drinking water storage containers sanitary?	
6	Are animals prevented from accessing the area around the drinking water storage containers?	
7	Are the taps or utensils used to draw water from the drinking water storage containers sanitary?	
8	Is the water treated in any way before drinking?	
9	Has the water supply been continuous over the past 10 days?	
10	Is the water obtained from only one source?	
	RISK SCORE = (10 − total # yes answers) =	
	PIPED WATER TAP	
1	Does the tap stand leak?	
2	Is any part of the tap stand cracked or broken?	
3	Is there standing water around the tap stand?	
4	Are there any visible pipe leaks between the tank and the tap stand?	
5	Is the area uphill from the tap stand visibly eroded? (roughly 30m)	
6	Are pipes visibly exposed nearby the tap stand? (roughly 10m)	
7	Is excreta or garbage found within 10 m of the tap stand?	
8	Are there any animals within 10 m of the tap stand?	
9	Is there a sewer or latrine within 10 m of the tap stand?	
10	Has there been discontinuity within the past 10 days at the sample site?	
	RISK SCORE = (total # yes answers) =	
	RESERVOIR TANK	
1	Are there any visible pipe leaks between the source and the tank?	
2	Is there standing water around the tank?	
3	Is the area uphill from the tank visibly eroded? (roughly 30m)	
4	Are pipes visibly exposed close to the tank? (roughly 10m)	
5	Are excreta, garbage, or animals found within 10 m of the tank?	
6	Is there a sewer or latrine within 10m of the tank?	
7	Has there been discontinuity within last 10 days at the sample site?	
8	Are there signs of leaks around the tank?	
9	Is the tank cracked or damaged?	
10	Are the air vents or inspection covers unsanitary, damaged, or open?	
	RISK SCORE = (total # yes answers) =	
	SOURCE	
1	Is the water protected from surface contamination (masonry, concrete wall, or spring box)?	
2	Is the structure protecting the source in good condition?	
3	Is there a locked sanitary inspection cover?	
4	Is there a sanitary air vent in the structure?	
5	Is there a sanitary overflow pipe in the structure?	
6	Is there a functional surface water diversion ditch above the source?	
7	Is the source free from contaminating silt or animal excreta?	
8	Is the area around the source properly fenced?	
9	Are animals prevented from entering within 10 m of the source?	
10	Is the area within 10 m of the source free from the presence of latrines?	
	RISK SCORE = (total # yes answers) =	

Table A2. Baseline and endline water quality at the intervention and control schemes for the households, reservoir tanks, and taps: percentages at guidelines, low risk, and high risk.

Description	Baseline						Endline					
	Households		Tanks		Taps		Households		Tanks		Taps	
	I (n = 75)	C (n = 45)	I (n = 11)	C (n = 10)	I (n = 14)	C (n = 9)	I (n = 72)	C (n = 43)	I (n = 15)	C (n = 10)	I (n = 14)	C (n = 9)
Median [CFU/100 mL]	24	8	12	49.5	10.5	38	0	4	4	8.5	0.5	3
% of samples at the WHO guidelines [0 CFU/100 mL]	17.3	20.0	18.2	0	7.2	0	52.8	23.3	26.7	10.0	50.0	11.1
% of samples at low risk [1–10 CFU/100 mL]	25.3	31.1	27.3	30.0	42.8	33.3	22.2	32.6	40.0	40.0	50.0	66.7
% of samples at higher risk [11-TNTC CFU/100 mL]	57.3	48.9	54.5	70.0	50.0	66.7	25.1	44.2	33.3	50.0	0	22.2

I = Intervention, C = Control.

References

1. WHO/UNICEF Joint Monitoring Programme. *Progress on Drinking Water, Sanitation and Hygiene: Update and MDG Assessment*; WHO Press: Geneva, Switzerland; New York, NY, USA, 2015; ISBN 9789241509145.
2. Onda, K.; Lobuglio, J.; Bartram, J. Global access to safe water: Accounting for water quality and the resulting impact on MDG progress. *Int. J. Environ. Res. Public Health* **2012**, *9*, 880–894. [CrossRef] [PubMed]
3. Bain, R.; Cronk, R.; Wright, J.; Yang, H.; Slaymaker, T.; Bartram, J. Fecal contamination of drinking-water in low- and middle-income countries: A systematic review and meta-analysis. *PLoS Med.* **2014**, *11*, e1001644. [CrossRef] [PubMed]
4. Prüss-Ustün, A.; Bartram, J.; Clasen, T.; Colford, J.M.; Cumming, O.; Curtis, V.; Bonjour, S.; Dangour, A.D.; De France, J.; Fewtrell, L.; et al. Burden of disease from inadequate water, sanitation and hygiene in low- and middle-income settings: A retrospective analysis of data from 145 countries. *Trop. Med. Int. Health* **2014**, *19*, 894–905. [CrossRef]
5. World Health Organization (WHO). *Guidelines for Drinking Water Quality*, 4th ed.; WHO Press: Geneva, Switzerland, 2011; ISBN 9789241548151.
6. World Health Organization (WHO). *Safely Managed Drinking Water—Thematic Report on Drinking Water*; WHO Press: Geneva, Switzerland, 2017; ISBN 9789241565424.
7. WHO/UNICEF Joint Monitoring Programme. *Progress on Drinking Water, Sanitation and Hygiene: 2017 Update and SDG Baselines*; WHO Press: Geneva, Switzerland; New York, NY, USA, 2017; ISBN 9789241512893.
8. Shrestha, A.; Sharma, S.; Gerold, J.; Erismann, S.; Sagar, S.; Koju, R.; Schindler, C.; Odermatt, P.; Utzinger, J.; Cissé, G. Water quality, sanitation, and hygiene conditions in schools and households in Dolakha and Ramechhap Districts, Nepal: Results from a cross-sectional survey. *Int. J. Environ. Res. Public Health* **2017**, *14*, 89. [CrossRef] [PubMed]
9. Marks, S.J.; Diener, A.; Bhatta, M.; Sihombing, D.; Meierhofer, R. Researching Water Quality, Consumer Preferences and Treatment Behaviour. Available online: https://www.eawag.ch/fileadmin/Domain1/Abteilungen/sandec/schwerpunkte/WST/researching_water_quality.pdf (accessed on 27 July 2018).
10. Diener, A.; Kenea, M.A.; Pratama, I.Y.; Bhatta, M.; Bhatta, M.; Marks, S.J. Safer Water for Remote Nepal—Novel Pathways Towards SDG 6.1. Available online: https://www.eawag.ch/fileadmin/Domain1/Abteilungen/sandec/schwerpunkte/WST/safer_water_remote_nepal.pdf (accessed on 27 July 2018).
11. World Health Organization (WHO). *Water Safety Planning for Small Community Water Supplies: Step-By-Step Risk Management Guidance for Drinking-Water Supplies in Small Communites*; WHO Press: Geneva, Switzerland, 2012; ISBN 9789241548427.
12. Rickert, B.; Schmoll, O.; Rinehold, A.; Barrenberg, E. *Water Safety Plan: A Field Guide to Improving Drinking-Water Safety in Small Communities*; WHO Regional Office for Europe: Copenhagen, Denmark, 2014; ISBN 9789289050074.
13. String, G.; Lantagne, D. A systematic review of outcomes and lessons learned from general, rural, and country-specific Water Safety Plan implementations. *Water Sci. Technol. Water Supply* **2016**, *16*, ws2016073. [CrossRef]
14. Ercumen, A.; Naser, A.M.; Arnold, B.F.; Unicomb, L.; Colford, J.M.; Luby, S.P. Can sanitary inspection surveys predict risk of microbiological contamination of groundwater sources? Evidence from shallow tubewells in rural Bangladesh. *Am. J. Trop. Med. Hyg.* **2017**, *96*, 561–568. [CrossRef] [PubMed]
15. Mushi, D.; Byamukama, D.; Kirschner, A.K.T.; Mach, R.L.; Brunner, K.; Farnleitner, A.H. Sanitary inspection of wells using risk-of-contamination scoring indicates a high predictive ability for bacterial faecal pollution in the peri-urban tropical lowlands of Dar es Salaam, Tanzania. *J. Water Health* **2012**, *10*, 236–243. [CrossRef] [PubMed]
16. Misati, A.G.; Ogendi, G.; Peletz, R.; Khush, R.; Kumpel, E. Can sanitary surveys replace water quality testing? Evidence from Kisii, Kenya. *Int. J. Environ. Res. Public Health* **2017**, *14*, 152. [CrossRef] [PubMed]
17. World Health Organization (WHO). Sanitary Inspection Package Update. In *WHO Meeting on the Guidelines for Drinking-Water Quality: Small Water Supplies and Small Drinking-Water Supplies: A Guide to Field Work*; WHO Regional Office for Europe: Chisinau, Moldova, 2017.
18. Shrestha, N.R. *In the Name of Development: A Reflection on Nepal*; University Press of America: Lanham, MD, USA; Oxford, UK, 1997; ISBN 0761807594.

19. United Nations Department of Economic and Social Affairs/Population Division. *Volume I: Comprehensive Tables (ST/ESA/SER.A/399)*; United Nations: New York, NY, USA, 2017.

20. World Bank. The World Bank Open Data Portal. Available online: http://data.worldbank.org/ (accessed on 1 April 2018).

21. United Nations Development Programme (UNDP). *Human Development Report*; United Nations: New York, NY, USA, 2016; ISBN 9789211264135.

22. Udmale, P.; Ishidaira, H.; Thapa, B.; Shakya, N. The status of domestic water demand: Supply deficit in the Kathmandu Valley, Nepal. *Water* **2016**, *8*, 196. [CrossRef]

23. Merz, J.; Nakarmi, G.; Shrestha, S.K.; Dahal, B.M.; Dangol, P.M.; Dhakal, M.P.; Dongol, B.S.; Sharma, S.; Shah, P.B.; Weingartner, R. Water: A scarce resource in rural watersheds of Nepal's middle mountains. *Mt. Res. Dev.* **2003**, *23*, 41–49. [CrossRef]

24. Xu, J.; Grumbine, R.E.; Shrestha, A.; Eriksson, M.; Yang, X.; Wang, Y.; Wilkes, A. The melting Himalayas: Cascading effects of climate change on water, biodiversity, and livelihoods. *Conserv. Biol.* **2009**, *23*, 520–530. [CrossRef] [PubMed]

25. Government of Nepal. *Nepal Drinking Water Quality Surveillance Guideline*; Ministry of Health and Population: Kathmandu, Nepal, 2010.

26. Government of Nepal. *Nepal Water Supply, Sanitation and Hygiene Sector Development Plan (2016–2030) 2016*; Ministry of Water Supply and Sanitation: Kathmandu, Nepal, 2016.

27. Government of Nepal. *National Drinking Water Quality Standards*; Ministry of Water Supply and Sanitation: Kathmandu, Nepal, 2005.

28. Marks, S.J.; Davis, J. Does user participation lead to sense of ownership for rural water systems? Evidence from Kenya. *World Dev.* **2012**, *40*, 1569–1576. [CrossRef]

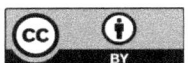

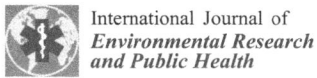

International Journal of
Environmental Research and Public Health

MDPI

Review

A Systematic Review of the Time Series Studies Addressing the Endemic Risk of Acute Gastroenteritis According to Drinking Water Operation Conditions in Urban Areas of Developed Countries

Pascal Beaudeau

Santé Publique France, 14 rue du Val-d'Osne, 94415 Saint-Maurice CEDEX, France;
pascal.beaudeau@santepubliquefrance.fr; Tel.: +33-179-416-822

Received: 28 February 2018; Accepted: 24 April 2018; Published: 26 April 2018

Abstract: Time series studies (TSS) can be viewed as an inexpensive way to tackle the non-epidemic health risk from fecal pathogens in tap water in urban areas. Following the PRISMA recommendations, I reviewed TSS addressing the endemic risk of acute gastroenteritis risk according to drinking water operation conditions in urban areas of developed countries. Eighteen studies were included, covering 17 urban sites (seven in North-America and 10 in Europe) with study populations ranging from 50,000 to 9 million people. Most studies used general practitioner consultations or visits to hospitals for acute gastroenteritis (AGE) as health outcomes. In 11 of the 17 sites, a significant and plausible association was found between turbidity (or particle count) in finished water and the AGE indicator. When provided and significant, the interquartile excess of relative risk estimates ranged from 3–13%. When examined, water temperature, river flow, and produced flow were strongly associated with the AGE indicator. The potential of TSS for the study of the health risk from fecal pathogens in tap water is limited by the lack of specificity of turbidity and its site-sensitive value as an exposure proxy. Nevertheless, at the DWS level, TSS could help water operators to identify operational conditions most at risk, almost if considering other water operation indicators, in addition to turbidity, as possible relevant proxies for exposure.

Keywords: acute gastroenteritis; risk; tap water; time series study; turbidity; urban area; water operation data

1. Introduction

In 1992, the Milwaukee Cryptosporidiosis outbreak revealed that sophisticated urban drinking water treatment plants (DWTP) did not always fully prevent fecal contamination of finished water, resulting in disease outbreaks. This event also raised the issue of the endemic share of waterborne infections (sporadic cases of disease) in urban facilities [1]. To date, results from the few randomized trials [2–4] and case-control intervention studies [5,6] investigating this issue have provided inconsistent risk estimates, leading to controversy about the possible presence of methodological flaws resulting in an inherent bias in risk estimates [7,8]. These studies may also have been too short to prevent the evaluation of risk estimates being overly weighted by specific one-off situations [9]. Insufficient study duration and sampling frequency are primarily due to the cost of water microbial analyses.

In the 1990s, the development of healthcare databases provided new resources for public health surveillance. Concurrently, continuous monitoring of water turbidity and chlorine became more widespread, making large datasets available which could be used to build proxies for exposure. The availability of both health and water records encouraged the use of time series studies (TSS) [10].

Since data were continuously available and free, TSS could last long enough to meet the study requirements in terms of adequate statistical power and representativeness for the most common combinations of epidemiological and hydrological contexts, and yield a robust estimate of the risk.

Turbidity measures the light diffraction capacity of suspended particles in water to estimate the particle load. By analogy with a study of the adverse effect of air pollution on health [11], where the measurement of fine particle concentration in air was extensively used as an exposure surrogate, epidemiologists believed finished water turbidity could act as a possible generic proxy for the pathogen load in water.

In this paper I reviewed published and unpublished water TSS. A quite similar review, carried out by Mann et al. in 2007 [12], covered nine studies. A second one, released in 2017 by De Roos et al. [13], incorporated 14 studies, but it did not include the reports of the multicentric study of the French public health agency [14–18]. Furthermore, the authors of both reviews focused on water turbidity, while water monitoring offers additional daily recorded indicators worthy to be considered as possible complementary proxies for the remaining contamination of finished water by fecal pathogens. In the discussion, I propose a renewed interpretation of operational risk factors and highlight the scientific strengths and limits of the TSS approach from a public health perspective.

2. Materials and Methods

My review process complied with the "Preferred reporting items for Systematic Reviews and Meta-Analysis" (PRISMA) recommendations [19].

I first collected all published TSS addressing the association between water turbidity or precipitation and acute gastroenteritis (AGE). My search of the Medline database (the last search was in November 2017) was based on the occurrence of ("Time series*" AND ("Drinking water" OR Waterborne) AND (Gastrointestinal* OR gastroenteritis OR Diarrhea OR Infection) AND (Turbidity OR Precipitation) NOT Review) in the tittle, abstract or keyword list. All terms were MeSH terms, apart from "Time series", "Turbidity", and "Precipitation". No constraint on the publication date was imposed. I completed the search by examining the reference lists in the primary set of articles. I also considered reports available on university and public health agency websites.

I excluded reviews and original studies according to the following criteria:

- Studies focusing on an outbreak;
- Studies which design prevents the marginal risk estimate;
- Prospective studies which used self-reported health outcome were excluded to prevent reporting biases due to individuals' perception of exposure. Only health care-related databases were used, including on-line remote diagnosis data from calls for medical advice;
- Studies showing inadequate mathematical control of potential confounding factors (i.e., resulting in bias);
- Studies where the number of AGE cases included was under 1000, (excluded to prevent insufficient statistical power);
- Studies with a duration of two years or less (excluded to achieve minimal representativeness of the hydro-epidemiological conditions diversity); and
- Studies mapping complex distribution zones (DZ) resulting in major exposure misclassification.

From the selected articles and reports, I first characterized the studied population and the health outcomes. I then characterized the type of water resources, treatment, fecal contamination of raw water (fecal bacteria indicators were under the limits of detection in all sites' finished water), and the turbidity or particle load in raw and finished water. When the authors did not specify the treatment or the quality of the raw water, I recovered further information from the internet.

I then focused on the risk associated with turbidity in finished water (Tu_FW), in raw water (Tu_RW) or precipitation. I considered associations which met the following conditions:

- Minimal significance ($p < 0.1$) of the turbidity-risk function (TRF);

- Sufficient plausibility of the shape of the TRF: an increasing TRF was required for the shape to be considered plausible; and
- Good fit between (1) the turbidity-AGE latency observed in the model and (2) the delay for both water transit through the distribution network and infection incubation in sick people.

I also evaluated the robustness of the TRF through documenting (i) the consistency of the TRF over several consecutive lags; (ii) its reproducibility in different age classes, in different health indicators, and in mono- and multi-exposure models (i.e., where several exposure proxies were included together in the risk model); and (iii) when extreme values of exposure were excluded from the dataset.

When possible, I homogenized the exposure scenarios used by the authors to express risks, in order to enable comparisons of the risk levels between the studies. To that end, I expressed the excess of relative risk as both a conventional increase in turbidity of finished water (e.g., 0.01 Nephelometric Turbidity Units (NTU)) and an inter-percentile increase (e.g., inter-quartile (IQ) change). The latter method enabled me to compare inter-site risks irrespective of turbidity levels. When the TRF levelled off at high turbidity values, the P10–P50 scenario (turbidity change from 10% percentile to median) was used instead of the IQ scenario.

Finally, I synthesized the exploratory approach performed in some studies (covering nine French sites), which consist in drawing additional exposure proxies from water operation data to complement turbidity.

3. Results

3.1. Selected Studies

I defined a drinking water system (DWS) as a distribution network and the resources and the drinking water treatment plants (DWTP) which feed that distribution network. "Site" refers to the urban area serviced by one or several DWS.

From the reference search request, I identified nine articles (Figure 1). Including other articles and reports quoted in these nine articles, and reports posted on the French National Public Health agency's website, I finally gathered 24 documents (17 articles and seven reports) concerning 22 different sites (20 urban, two rural). One report included three different sites studied separately [17] and, therefore, considered separate studies here. I did not distinguish between different DWS which were fed by similar resources and subject to pooled analyses.

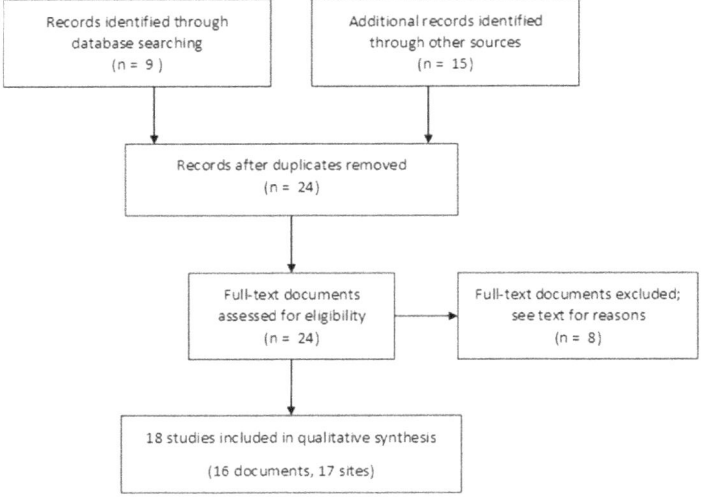

Figure 1. Preferred reporting items for Systematic Reviews and Meta-Analysis (PRISMA) flow diagram of the selection of the studies included in the review.

From these 26 studies (24 documents) I excluded:

- The Milwaukee studies [1,20,21] which specifically addressed the Milwaukee outbreak and the period preceding the outbreak where other possible contamination episodes by *Cryptospodidium* oocysts may have occurred;
- The Egorov et al. study [22] because of its short duration, the small population size, and the use of self-reported health outcomes;
- The Drayna et al. study [23] because it focused on the relationship between precipitation and AGE in Wisconsin (USA), irrespective of distribution zone (DZ) locations and organization;
- The Harper et al. [24] and Uejio et al. [25] studies focusing on rural areas; and
- The first study carried out in Le Havre [26] that used a moving average model yielding conditional risk estimates.

Among selected sites, several DWS shew complex production-distribution patterns with DZ fed by several DWTP (Le Havre, Paris, New York) and including sectors with time-varying water origin; but no exposure misclassification remained at the population level, since adequate operation data (e.g., daily records of turbidity and produced flow) were available for all DWTP involved, thus allowing to calculate unbiased exposure estimates (e.g., mean turbidity weighed by produced flows).

Eighteen studies, therefore, met selection criteria (Table 1), and concerned 17 different sites corresponding to nine articles and seven reports. Seven sites were located in North America, nine in France, and one in Sweden. Among the American sites, three covered several DWS, but with DWTP servicing separated DZ (no risk of misclassification): Philadelphia, Vancouver, and Atlanta.

Table 1. Description of the selected sites and associated risks.

Site	Period	Serviced Population	AGE Indicator	Age Classes (Years)	Number of Resources, DWTP and DZ Covered by the Study	Type of Resource	Turbidity in Raw Water: Mean (Max) (NTU)	[E.coli] in Raw Water: Mean (Max.) (CFU/100 mL)	Treatment Facilities [a]	Turbidity in Finished Water: Mean (Max) (NTU)	Number of AGE Cases Included	Exposure Scenario	ERR Related to Exposure Scenario	Significant Lags (Days) [b]	Proxies Tested as Exposure with Significance and Reproducibility [c]	Study
Philadelphia (USA)	1989–1993	1.2 M	Visits and admissions to hospital	<16	2-3-3	Rivers	9–19 (100–150) [d]	20–40 (1000)	PCh, CFD, RFi, pChm	0.17–0.20	3282	Tu_FW IQ change (lag 4): 0.16–0.20 NTU	all cases: 7% [3; 12]	1, 4, 6–7 [†], 7–9 [†], 8, 10, 13	Tu_FW **[]◊	Schwartz et al., 1997 [10]
Philadelphia (USA)	1992–1993	1.2 M	Admissions to hospital	>64	2-3-3	Rivers	9–19 (100–150) [d]	20–40 (1000)	PCh, CFD, RFi, pChm	0.17–0.20	6021	Tu_FW IQ change (lag 9–11): 0.16–0.21 NTU	all cases: 9% [5; 13]	4–6 [†], 9, 10, 11	Tu_FW **	S2: Schwartz et al., 2000 [27]
Edmonton (Canada)	1993–1998	845,000	Admissions to hospital, visits to emergency department, visits to GP	All, 2–18, 19–65, >65	1-2-3	River	35 (1500)	400 (15,000)	CFD, RFi, Ch, pChm	0.04 (0.38)	62,060				Precipitation, Tu_RW, coliforms in raw water, Tu_FW, particle count, air temperature, change in the location of water abstraction point (0/1)	Lim et al., 2003 [28]
Québec (Canada)	2000–2002	240,000	Calls for medical advice	All	1-1-1	River	1.7–3.2	62 (340)	PCh, CFD, RFi, Oz, pCh	0.27 (0.75)	3555	Tu_FW daily change from min. to max.: 0.11–0.75 NTU	33–76% depending on the lag	11, 15, 17	Tu_FW **, precipitation	Gilbert et al., 2006 [29]
Atlanta (USA)	1993–2004	3.0 M	Visits to emergency department	All	3-9-8	Rivers	Hourly max: 1.5–55 (1984)	100 (1000) [e]	CFD, RFi, Ch (UV for 3 DWTPs), pCh	0.03–0.17	240,925	IQ change in Tu_FW: 0.04–0.09 NTU (lags 4–6)10 NTU change in Tu_RW over three weeks	0.5% [−0.2; 1.2] (NS except for 1/8 distribution zones: 6% [4; 8])	4–11	Tu_RW ***	Tinker et al., 2010 [30]
Nantes (France)	2002–2007	410,000	Consultations of GP	<16, >15	1-1-1	River	20 (124)	120 (7000)	CFD, RFi, Oz, pCh	0.05 (0.35)	103,149	Tu_FW IQ change (lags 7–9): 0.04–0.06 NTU	4.2% [1.5; 6.9] (child.), 2.9 [0.5; 5.4] (ad.)	7–15	Precipitation, Tu_RW, Tu_FW **◊, air temperature ***◊, river flow ***◊, produced flow **◊, free chlorine, interventions for broken pipe *, hydrant flushes	Boudeau et al., 2014 [31]

Table 1. *Cont.*

Site	Period	Serviced Population	AGE Indicator	Age Classes (Years)	Number of Resources, DWTP and DZ Covered by the Study	Type of Resource	Turbidity in Raw Water: Mean (Max) (NTU)	[E.coli] in Raw Water: Mean (Max.) (CFU/100 mL)	Treatment Facilities [a]	Turbidity in Finished Water: Mean (Max) (NTU)	Number of AGE Cases Included	Exposure Scenario	ERR Related to Exposure Scenario	Significant Lags (Days) [b]	Proxies Tested as Exposure with Significance and Reproducibility [c]	Study
Gothenburg (Sweden)	2008–2011	500,000	Calls for medical advice	All	2-1-1	River and lake	5 (40)	36 (6500)	CFD, Rfi, Ch	<0.05	25,659	40 mm precipitation in 24 h (lag 5)	17% [7; 27]	4–7	Precipitation **, number of consecutive dry days, number of consecutive wet days **	Tornevi et al., 2013 [32]
Paris-Est (France)	2002–2007	379,000	Consultations of GP	<16, >15	2-2-1	Rivers	15–16 (124–149)	6200–6700 (125,000–240,000)	[CFD], RFi or Flot, Sti, Oz, pCh (syst. 1); Coag,RFi, Sti, Oz, pCh (syst. 2)	0.03–0.05 (0.14–0.19)	99,315	Tu_FW P10-P50 change (lags 6–8): 0.03–0.04 NTU	13% [4; 18] (child.), 14% [4; 16] (ad.)	6–8 [†]	Precipitation, Tu_RW **, Tu_FW **◊, water temperature **◊, river flow **◊, produced flow *, free chlorine	Rambaud et al., 2014 [16]
Paris area—Nord (France)	2002–2007	673,000	Consultations of GP	<16, >15	1-2-1	River	20 (147)	1600 (40,000)	CFD, RFi, Oz, NanoFi, UV, pCh (DWTP 1); CFD, RFi, Oz, Ch (DWTP 2)	0.04 (0.05)	246,165	IQ change of particle count in filtered water (lags 6–8): 147–333 units/mL (0.03–0.05 NTU)	ERR = 12.1% [7.5; 17.0] (child.), 8.5% [4.3; 12.9] (ad.)	6–8 [†], 5–13	Tu_RW, turbidity in filtered water *, particle count in filtered water ***◊, TOC in raw water ***◊, water temperature ***◊, river flow ◊, proportion of nanofiltered water, produced flow ***◊	Rambaud et al., 2015 [17]
Paris area—Est (France)	2002–2007	874,000	Consultations of GP	<16, >15	1-1-1	River	30 (320)	3100 (48,000)	CFD, RFi, Oz, Ch	0.04 (0.05)	322,773	IQ change in particle count in filtered water (lags 6–8): 52–150 units/mL (0.04–0.04 NTU)	NS		Tu_RW, turbidity in filtered water **, Tu_FW, particle count in filtered water, TOC in raw water **◊, TOC in filtered water, water temperature ***◊, river flow ***◊, produced flow ***	Rambaud et al., 2015 [17]
Paris area—Sud (France)	2002–2007	1.4 M	Consultations of GP	<16, >15	1-1-1	River	16 (220)	1600 (43,000)	CFD, RFi, Oz, Ch	0.03 (0.14)	375,613	IQ change in particle count in filtered water (lags 6–8): 25–65 units/mL (0.03–0.03 NTU)	ERR = 3.8% [1.0; 6.7] (child.), 2.7% [-0.3; 5.7] (ad.)	6–10	Tu_RW *, turbidity in filtered water **, Tu_FW, particle count in filtered water ***◊, TOC in raw water **◊, TOC in filtered water *, water temperature ***◊, river flow *◊, produced flow ***	Rambaud et al., 2015 [17]

Table 1. Cont.

Site	Period	Serviced Population	AGE Indicator	Age Classes (Years)	Number of Resources, DWTP and DZ Covered by the Study	Type of Resource	Turbidity in Raw Water: Mean (Max) (NTU)	[E.coli] in Raw Water: Mean (Max.) (CFU/100 mL)	Treatment Facilities [a]	Turbidity in Finished Water: Mean (Max) (NTU)	Number of AGE Cases Included	Exposure Scenario	ERR Related to Exposure Scenario	Significant Lags (Days) [b]	Proxies Tested as Exposure with Significance and Reproducibility [c]	Study
Nancy (France)	2002–2007	247,000	Consultations of GP	<16, >15	1-2-1	River	8 (290)	2,000 (16,000)	PCh, CFD, Oz, pCh	0.07 (0.23)	87,007	Tu_FW IQ change (lags 5–7): 0.06–0.08 NTU	NS		Tu_RW, Tu_FW, water temperature ***◊, river flow, produced flow **, water cuts, interventions for broken pipe	Rambaud et al., 2016 [18]
Vancouver (Canada)	1992–1998	2.1 M	Visits to GP; admissions to hospital	All, <16, >64	3-3-3	Reservoirs	0.5–1.3 (8–19)	1–2 (38–51)	Ch	0.5–1.3 (8–19)	14,571 H admission; 1,102 M visits to GP	Turbidity > 1 NTU	Attributable Risk: 0.8–2.1 visits to GP; 0.2–1.3% H visits	3–6 †, 6–9 †, 12–16 †, 21–29 †	Turbidity ***◊, precipitation, fecal coliform	Aramini et al., 2000 [33]
Boston (USA)	1998–2008	1.5 M	Visits to hospital	>64	1-1-1	Reservoirs	0.34 (0.68)	1.5 (43)	Ch/Oz, pChm	0.34 (0.68)	36,456	Turbidity IQ change (lags 8–12): 0.28–0.39 NTU	ERR = 3.7% [1.2; 6.3]	8–12 †, 13–17 †, 18–22 †, 23–27 †, 28–32 †, 33–37 †	Precipitation, turbidity corrected from algae **, water temperature **, fecal coliforms *, cyanobacteria *, ozone *, abs.UV350, CT	Beaudeau et al., 2014 [34]
New York (USA)	2002–1999	9.2 M	Visits to emergency department	All, 1–4, 5–17	3-3-1	Reservoirs	0.98–1.0 (2.80–2.85)	1–2 (14–57) †	Ch	0.97 (2.38)	438,000	Turbidity IQ change (lag 6): NA	5% [36] in spring, NS in other seasons	3–11	Turbidity ***◊ (only in spring)	Hsieh et al., 2015 [35]
Le Havre (France)	1994–1996; 1997–2000	80,000	Drug sales	All	2-2-1	Karstic springs	4 (>200) (syst. 1); 0.1 (1) (syst. 2)	80 (1000) (syst. 1); 8 (50) (syst. 2)	[CFD], Rfi, Ch (syst. 1); Ch (syst. 2)	0.3 (>1.5) (syst. 1); 0.1 (1.0) (syst. 2)	14,600 drug boxes (2500 cases)	IQ change in Tu_FW over lags 6–8:0.13–0.27 NTU (syst. 1); 0.08–0.11 NTU (syst. 2)	2.8 [−1.06;7.2] (syst. 1); 9.4 [5.2; 13.7] (syst. 2)	6–8 †, 9–10 (syst. 1); 13–15 (syst. 1)	Precipitation, turbidity ** (syst. 2), Tu_RW (syst. 1), Tu_FW* (syst. 1); produced flow, free chlorine (hourly min.) ** (syst. 2), decantation * (syst. 1)	Beaudeau et al. 2012 [36]
Angoulême (France)	2002–2007	50,000	Consultations of GP	<16, >15	1-1-1	Karstic spring	4 (27)	31 (1700)	CoagRFi, Ch	0.14 (2)	21,336	P10-P50 change in Tu_RW over lags 7–9: 1.1–2.9 NTU	30% [0; 60] (child.), 15% [−15; 45] (ad.)	7–9 †, 13–15 †	Precipitation, Tu_RW *, Tu_FW, air temperature *◊, produced flow *◊, interventions for broken pipe *◊	Rambaud et al., 2013a [14]
Paris-Centre (France)	2002–2007	160,000	Consultations of GP	<16, >15	3-1-1	Karstic springs	0.08–0.23 (0.50–0.73)	1–8 (14–150)	Ch	0.17 (0.66)	26,526	IQ change in Tu_FW over lags 7–9: 0.11–0.22 NTU	11.8% [1.2; 22.5] (child.), 4.1% [−0.2; 8.8] (ad.)	7–9 †, 10–11	Precipitation, turbidity **◊, air temperature *** free chlorine, produced flow *◊, contribution of the most fecally contaminated resource in the produced flow *	Rambaud et al., 2013b [15]

[a] Treatment facilities: PCh: Pre-chlorination; CFD: Coagulation-flocculation-decantation; [CFD]: CFD operated if high turbidity; RFi: Rapid filtration; CoagRFi: Coagulation and RFi; SFi: Slow filtration; NanoFi: Nanofiltration; Oz: Ozone disinfection; Ch: Chlorine disinfection; UV: UV-disinfection; pCh: Post-chlorination; pChm: Post-chloramination; Syst.: System; couple (resource + DWTP). [b] Significant lags: $p < 0.05$; †: Combined lags. [c] Significance and robustness of the exposure-AGE risk functions: * $p < 0.1$; ** $p < 0.01$; *** $p < 0.001$; ◊ Association reproduced in different populations, age classes, or with different health indicators. Consulted websites for raw water quality: [d] [37]; [e] [38]; [f] [39].

With respect to the statistical power of the selected TSS and the robustness of the risk estimates (Figure 2), four studies included fewer than 10,000 AGE cases: the study performed in Le Havre, the two in Philadelphia, and the study in Québec. The second Philadelphia study lasted only two years and its study periods was embedded within the period of the previous study, while the Québec study lasted three years. In contrast, I counted 10 studies each with a study period of at least six years and each with approximately 100,000 AGE cases: Atlanta (with the longest study period of 12 years); New York; Nantes; Paris-Est; and the three sites in the Paris area (PA), defined as follows: PA-Nord, PA-Est (N.B.: not to be confused with Paris-Est), PA-Sud, Nancy, Vancouver (with the largest dataset of 1.1 million included cases), and Boston.

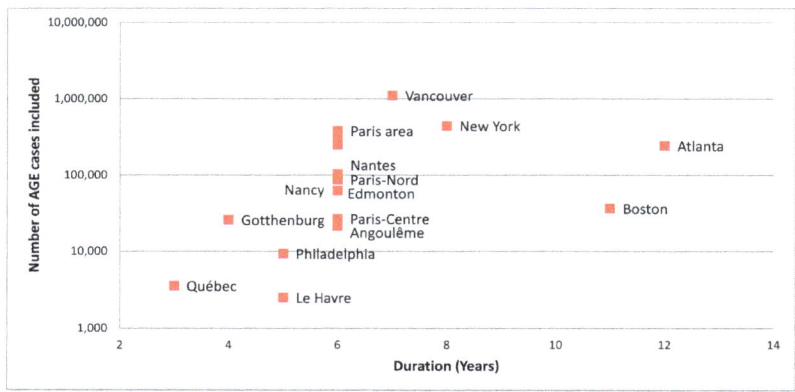

Figure 2. Duration of the selected studies and number of acute gastroenteritis (AGE) cases included.

3.2. Serviced Populations and Water Systems

Table 1 summarizes all the characteristics of the selected studies and sites and provides references. The size of the studied populations was greater in North America than in other countries: five of the seven sites there provided over one million people with tap water (maximum, New York: 9.2 M; minimum, Québec: 240,000). In contrast, only one of the 10 European sites included supplied over one million people (maximum, PA-Sud: 1.4 M; minimum, Angoulême: 50,000).

I distinguished three types of DWS according to the type of resource: (1) "river DWS" fed by rivers with moderate to high fecal pollution and which had treatment systems incorporating full clarification facilities, i.e., at least coagulation-flocculation-decantation and rapid sand filtration facilities; (2) "reservoir DWS" served by protected reservoirs and treatment facilities limited to disinfection; and (3) "karst DWS" fed by karstic springs and involving diversified treatment processes including clarification or not.

Eleven river sites were fed exclusively by river DWS. This category was relatively homogenous in terms of both resources and treatments. Eight were fed by a single DWS: Nantes, Québec, Paris-Est, Gothenburg, PA-Nord, PA-Est and PA-Sud, and Nancy. The remaining three were fed by several DWS: Philadelphia, Edmonton, and Atlanta. Atlanta exhibited the more complex scheme with three resources, nine DWTP, and eight DZ. The potential heterogeneity in exposure in the serviced populations in these three sites was limited by the sharing of common resources and treatments. Mean turbidity and *E.coli* concentrations in resources ranged from moderate (<5 NTU and <100 FCU/100 mL) in Gothenburg and Québec, to high in the Paris-Est and the three PA sites (>15 NTU and >1000 FCU/100 mL). Both particulate and fecal contaminations were higher following heavy rain episodes, in proportion to each site's baseline contamination level (40–100 NTU and 500–50,000 FCU/100 mL). All 11 river DWS had full clarification treatments, including, at least, coagulation-flocculation-decantation (CFD) facilities. Paris-Est additionally operated slow sand filtration downstream of CFD. The PA-Nord site used membrane ultra-filtration in one of the two plants servicing the DZ. DWTP operated ozonation in seven of the river sites. In the other four sites, chlorination (Philadelphia, Edmonton) or UV irradiation (in some DWTP feeding Atlanta and PA-Nord) were operated, followed by post-chlorination. Given the high efficiency of clarification facilities, Tu_FW was kept very low (mean <0.07 NTU), except in two American sites: Philadelphia (0.17 NTU), Québec (0.27 NTU). *E. coli* was not detected in any of the 11 river DWS.

The "reservoir sites" category comprised only three North American sites: Vancouver, divided in three reservoir DWS, Boston, and New York, which were fed by a single DSW. This category was also relatively homogenous in both resources and treatments, being limited to disinfection, and consequently finished water qualities were also similar. Due to wildlife protection policies in the USA and Canada, mean *E. coli* concentrations were low (1–2 FCU/100 mL) but could rise slightly following heavy rain episodes or when geese were present on the water surface; *E. coli* maxima ranged from 14 to 57 FCU/100 mL depending on the resource. In addition, baseline turbidity levels were low to moderate (0.3 NTU in Boston and 1.3 NTU in New York and Vancouver) and rose when algal blooms or muddy runoffs occurred, with daily maxima staying below 1 NTU in Boston and 3 NTU in New York, but reaching 19 NTU in Vancouver reservoirs. In the absence of clarification facilities, turbidity did not significantly change from reservoir to taps. Again, *E. coli* was not detected at any time in finished water thanks to heavy chlorination (Vancouver, New-York) or ozonation (Boston).

Karst water may be viewed as groundwater episodically mixed with surface water from a flooding river or surface runoff. Baseline microbial contamination and particle load vary substantially between these two hydrological stages (recession in dry weather vs. turbid high water following heavy rain episodes), as well as between springs. The "karst sites" category comprised three French sites, each corresponding to one DWS: Le Havre, which was fed by two different springs and DWTP, referred to as systems 1 and 2, Angoulême and Paris-Centre. The hydrology of the Paris-Centre and Le Havre (syst. 2) aquifers showed discrete karstic patterns, with turbidity varying from 0.1 NTU in dry weather conditions to 0.5–1 NTU in wet weather conditions and fecal contamination from 1 to 14 FCU/100 mL. On the contrary, Le Havre springs (syst. 1) had higher baseline contamination (4 NTU and 80 FCU/100 mL) and were hit by frequent and intense periods of high turbidity (>100 NTU and >1000 FCU/100 mL). Tu_FW depended on both Tu_RW and the clarification process: in sites with no clarification facilities, i.e., Paris-Centre and Le Havre (syst. 2), turbidity did not change from the springs to the tap, while in Angoulême, coagulation and rapid sand filtration achieved the local target of <0.2 NTU in finished water. In the Le Havre DWTP (syst. 1), water was only filtered in dry weather and decantation was implemented when turbidity in the spring water exceeded 3 NTU. Consequently, consumers experienced lower Tu_FW in wet weather conditions (0.1 NTU) and higher Tu_FW in dry weather (0.4 NTU). *E. coli* was not detectable at any time in finished water from karst DWS.

3.3. Health Outcomes

AGE is used in epidemiology as a generic indicator for infections arising from fecal pathogens, as the syndrome is very common [40,41]. This provides potential sensitivity, and as AGE has a short incubation period, it also provides good reactivity to environmental triggers. AGE indicators used in TSS depend on the availability of syndromic data, i.e., on the local health care system. Indicators should, however, meet sensitivity and specificity if referring to a symptomatic definition of a case to achieve an accurate risk assessment, and remain stable over time.

In the US, the availability constraint led epidemiologists to examine visits and admissions to hospital emergency departments from different data providers. Both diagnosis by medical staff and the use the International Classification of Diseases (AGE related codes in ICD9: 001 to 009.9; 276; 558.9; 787) for coding, guarantee a high and stable specificity of the health indicator. Furthermore, sensitivity towards the symptomatic definition of AGE cases is low as the cases admitted to, or visiting, the hospital are the most serious. In the USA, with all routes of infection and causal pathogens being taken into account, the incidence rate of visits to emergency hospital departments was five visits a year per 1000 people in the Atlanta study, whereas 17 visits a year per 1000 people >65 years old was measured in hospitals in Boston, resulting in two elderly patient visits per 1000 people a year in the general population. The sensitivity may vary across time according to the capacity of the patients to pay their health care bills. That is one of the reasons why some authors [27,34] restricted their recruitment to elderly people supported by the Medicare program.

In France, epidemiologists used prescriptions of General Practitioners (GP) from a health insurance database [42]. The indicator results from the application of an algorithm based on the test of the nature and quantity of prescribed drugs, which enables true cases of AGE to be discriminated from others. The evaluation of this algorithm [42] concluded that sensitivity was acceptable (approximately ten percent of true medicalized cases were wrongly rejected) and specificity (approximately ten percent of included cases were not cases of AGE). The indicator was also calibrated with the consensus symptom-based definition of AGE cases [43]: MG consultations accounted for 33% of total cases, according to Majovicz's definition [41]. Thus, the French health insurance database provided enough sensitivity to perform separate analyses in children and adults in cities with over 50,000 people. According to a case definition based on drug prescription analysis with all routes of infection being taken into account [42], the mean incidence rate of GP consultations for AGE in France was approximately 47 a year per 1000 people in Nantes and 90 in children under 16 years of age, resulting in 14 pediatric cases a year per 1000 people, when taking the whole community as the denominator. Incidence rates of AGE prescription were quite similar in other French cities. Again, the prescription-based indicator was moderately insensitive to the variations of patient's income, because health expenditures are largely covered by the French social security system. Furthermore, the reduced turnover of drugs dedicated to AGE care, and the yearly adaptation of the discriminating algorithm to changes in medication, made it possible to maintain a relatively constant specificity of the indicator over time.

Other data sources were used to perform TSS. Prescribed and over-the-counter drug sales were used in the Le Havre study, and phone calls for medical advice in the Québec study (with a yearly incidence rate of 19 per 1000 people). In France, drug sales are a very sensitive and relatively stable indicator of AGE case, but specificity is poor [42]. I did not find in the literature a systematic evaluation of the phone call data for epidemiological use.

3.4. Model Designs

In all the TSS included in the review, authors basically used Poisson regression most often adapted to over-dispersed counts (e.g., by using quasi-Poisson regression) to model daily counts of AGE cases and implemented the generalized additive model (GAM). When specified, the criterion for fitting the model was the absence of autocorrelation in residuals, which provides optimal risk estimates when health outcomes follow marked seasonal variations [44,45]. Control covariates were mostly similar: trends and seasonal patterns were modelled with a spline or Loess function of time, day of the week, and school vacation periods.

The main differences between the studies reviewed stem from the different sets of exposure variables included in the models used (Table 2), from the shape of the risk functions, and from the width and position of the time window used to average exposure variables included in the GAM. Some authors forced the linearity of the TRF, whereas others considered non-linear risk functions modelled by spline or Loess functions. I also observed a large diversity in the width of the time window used for exposure assessment. The earliest studies used single day windows over 0–15 or 0–40 day lags [33], whereas later studies calculated means over several consecutive lags (e.g., 5–7 up to 0–21). All French studies systematically assigned a three-day width to the time window to take into account the spread of response and a six- or seven-day delay for the start of the window, in order to exclude the latency period. One study [32] used a distributed lag non-linear model over a 0–21 day lag to optimize the time window shape instead of forcing it to be rectangular.

Table 2. Indicators tested as exposure proxies in the selected time series studies (TSS).

Indicator	Shape of the Risk Function	Commentary	Frequency of Positive Tests [a]	Sites
Concentration of fecal coliform or *Escherichia coli* in raw water	Increasing, linear	Lack of sensitivity to viral or protozoan contamination.	1/3	Edmonton, Boston *, Vancouver
Cyanobacteria	Increasing, linear	Possibly relevant for reservoir waters in the absence of clarification facilities.	1/1	Boston *
Turbidity in finished water (in the presence of clarification facilities)	Increasing	Suspended particles may carry pathogens. May indicate resource contamination and/or treatment transient weaknesses. May interact with river flow.	5/12	Philadelphia *, Edmonton, Québec *, Atlanta, Nantes *, Paris-Est *, PA-Nord, PA-Est, PA-Sud, Nancy, Le Havre * (syst. 1), Angoulême
Particle count in filtered/finished water (in the presence of clarification facilities)	Increasing	Alternative to turbidity in finished water. More precise when turbidity is very low.	2/4	Edmonton, PA-Nord *, PA-Est, PA-Sud *
Turbidity in raw/finished water (in the absence of clarification facilities)	Increasing	The availability of algae data makes possible to correct turbidity from algae influence (Boston). May interact with water temperature or season.	5/5	Vancouver *, Boston *, New York *, Le Havre (sys. 2) *, Paris-Centre *
Turbidity in raw water (in the presence of clarification facilities)	Increasing	May better correlate to AGE than turbidity in finished water.	5/10	Atlanta *, Edmonton, Nantes, Paris-Est *, PA-Nord, PA-Est, Paris-Sud *, Nancy, Le Havre (sys. 1) *, Angoulême *
Precipitation	Increasing with threshold	Alternative to turbidity in raw water.	1/10	Edmonton, Québec, Nantes, Paris-Est, Gothenburg *, Vancouver, Boston, Le Havre, Angoulême, Paris-Centre
Numbers of consecutive days of wet weather	Increasing	Derived from precipitation. Surrogate for wetness of soils (facilitating surface runoff).	1/1	Gothenburg *
Numbers of consecutive days of dry weather	No expectation	Derived from precipitation. Unclear.	1/1	Gothenburg
total organic carbon (TOC) in raw water	No expectation	Unclear. May interact with river flow.	3/3	PA-Nord *, PA-Est *, PA-Sud *
total organic carbon (TOC) in filtered water	No expectation	Unclear.	1/2	PA-Est, PA-Sud *
River flow	U-shaped	High or low flows may be associated to fecal pollution. Heavy precipitations bring about both high river flows and river contaminations. Low flows result in less dilution of urban effluents. May modify the turbidity risk function.	5/6	Nantes *, Paris-Est *, PA-Nord *, PA-Est *, PA-Sud *, Nancy
Water temperature	U-shaped	High or low temperature may enhance the AGE risk (via waterborne or other route exposure), possibly depending on climate. May modify the turbidity or TOC.-AGE association.	6/6	Paris-Est *, PA-Nord *, PA-Est *, PA-Sud *, Nancy *, Boston *
Air temperature	U-shaped	Beside a possible direct and synchronous effect on health care pursue (Boston and New York), may also serve as a surrogate to water temperature (exposure).	3/4	Edmonton, Nantes *, Angoulême *, Paris-Centre *
Produced flow	U-shaped or increasing	Sub optimal operation conditions at low or high produced flow.	8/9	Nantes *, Paris-Est *, PA-Nord *, PA-Est *, PA-Sud *, Nancy *, Le Havre, Angoulême *, Paris-Centre *
CT (disinfectant concentration × time of contact)	Decreasing	Measure of the disinfection power; available in the USA.	0/1	Boston
Free chlorine concentration at the outlet of the treatment plant	Decreasing with threshold	Hourly minimum may be relevant to highlight a risk associated to transient breakdowns, if direct distribution (i.e., no buffer effect of storage).	1/4	Nantes, Le Havre *, Paris-Est, Paris-Centre

Table 2. *Cont.*

Indicator	Shape of the Risk Function	Commentary	Frequency of Positive Tests [a]	Sites
Permanent change in abstraction or treatment facilities (Boolean)	Improvement	E.g., change in abstraction point, implementation of ozonation instead of chlorination.	1/2	Edmonton, Boston * (respectively)
Episodic change in treatment (Boolean)	Improvement	Decantation implementation interacts with turbidity on AGE incidence.	1/1	Le Havre *
Daily number of water cuts	Increasing, linear	Adverse impact limited to the inhabitants next downstream of the intervention point. TSS are poorly adequate to address this risk.		Nancy
Daily number of interventions for broken pipe	Increasing, linear	Idem.	2/3	Nantes *, Nancy, Angoulême *
Daily number of hydrant flushings	Increasing, linear	Idem.	0/1	Nantes
Daily number of consumers' complaints	Increasing	Idem. Additional limitation: few complaints are specific to fecal contamination.	0/1	Nantes

[a] Number of sites with positive test/number of sites testing the indicator. *: Site with positive test (i.e., meeting significance (p-value < 0.10) and plausibility criteria).

3.5. Turbidity-Related Risk

Significant, robust and plausible associations between Tu_FW and AGE incidence were found in 9 of the 16 sites where Tu_FW was tested as a proxy of exposure (9 positive/16 total sites tested, since Gothenburg did not test turbidity, but only precipitation, as a candidate exposure variable). Moreover, in Atlanta, the risk associated with Tu_FW and estimated using pooled data from all DWS was noticeable, but not significant, and the risk latency was consistent with the expected latency (see Discussion: Standardizing the Time Window for Exposure Assessment). The insufficient resolution of the turbidimeters at very low turbidity levels (Tu_FW < 0.05 NTU) may have prevented the authors from observing a possible risk associated with the presence of suspended particles in finished water in the Paris area sites, but the availability of particle count data (particle size detection range 1.5–15 μm) for PA-Nord and PA-Sud enabled them to do so. Considering both turbidity and particle counts, a significant association between the particle load of finished water and AGE was observed in 11 of these 16 sites (11/16). I did not observe significant differences in the frequencies of positive results between the three DWS categories, but all DWTP servicing people with unfiltered water exhibited a significant and plausible turbidity related risk (5/5). Tu_RW was also correlated to AGE (five positive in 10 sites equipped with clarification facilities). In two of these four positive sites (Atlanta, Angoulême) Tu_FW was not significantly correlated to AGE. Precipitation, which can be viewed as the primary driver of turbidity, was rarely correlated to AGE in the reviewed studies (1/10). Daily measurements of *E. coli* in resource water were rarely available and, consequently *E. coli* was rarely tested as a possible indicator of exposure. It did not closely correlate to AGE incidence (1/3).

As health risk was modelled as a function of the turbidity, in order to express the size of the risk using only one number, an exposure scenario needs to be chosen. Two types of scenarios were used: an absolute increase in turbidity and an interquartile variation in turbidity. The first leads to an expression of the risk which is dependent on turbidity, whereas the second leads an expression of the risk which is site-dependent. I was able to calculate both expressions for six DWS corresponding to seven DWTP (Figure 3). The average interquartile (IQ) excess of relative risk (ERR) ranged from 3–13%, whereas the averaged ERR per +0.01 NTU was between 0.2% and 13%. ERR were generally higher in children [14,15,17,31] and in the elderly [27,33] than in adults. In Philadelphia, elderly people >75 years old were at a higher risk than those aged 65–74 [27]. In the five French studies where medical prescriptions were used as health outcome, the children-adult ERR ratio was between one and three. In the New York study, authors found similar ERR levels in both children and the population as a whole, and did not notice any turbidity-AGE association in the elderly.

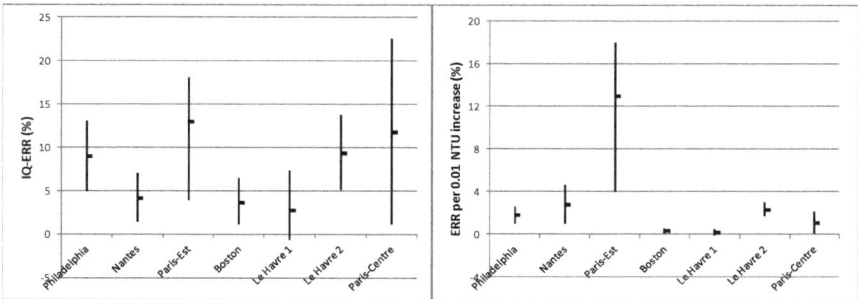

Figure 3. Excess of relative risk (ERR) associated to turbidity increase in finished water in six urban areas.

In the Vancouver study, authors systematically tested both hospital admission and visits to GPs and found that hospital admission data yielded a risk attributable to tap water turbidity which was approximately half that from visits to GPs (0.6% vs. 1.6%).

The shapes of the risk function were not always linear or quasi-linear. On the contrary, the use of spline functions showed that non-linearity was a common feature. In four sites (Nantes, Boston, Paris-Centre, and Paris-Sud), non-linear TRF leveled off and became inaccurate at high turbidity values. This suggests that an additional variable was needed in the model to correctly characterize the risk at high turbidity.

3.6. In Search for Additional Exposure Proxies from Water Operation Data

In all of the French studies, water operation and weather data were systematically explored to identify alternative or complementary proxies of exposure to waterborne pathogens. Fourteen variables were tested in total, or 22 when distinguishing the different measurement points inside the treatment chain (e.g., Tu_RW and Tu_FW) and derived variables (e.g., the number of consecutive dry days derived from the precipitation time series) (Table 2). Some variables were tested only once and others repeatedly, according to the availability of data. This exploration stage highlighted four variables as major contributors to the risk model: qualitative change in treatment (2/2), river flow for river DWS (5/6; Figure 4), supply water temperature (6/6; Figure 5) and produced flow (8/9; Figure 6). The levels of risk associated with these alternative exposure proxies were higher and more significant than the risk associated with turbidity. Since no strong collinearity was observed within the exposure set or between exposure levels and control covariates, risk estimates did not change with the removal of other exposure variables from the model. In addition, variations in the dataset used to adjust the model, e.g., adult instead of children health data, did not affect the set of significant exposures or the shape of the risk functions.

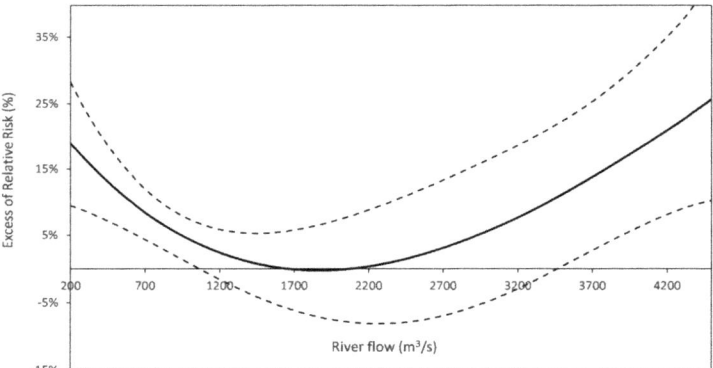

Figure 4. AGE risk function for the river flow (Nantes). The right branch may miss (e.g., PA sites). The delay considered for the health response to the river flow is homogenous with that used for turbidity.

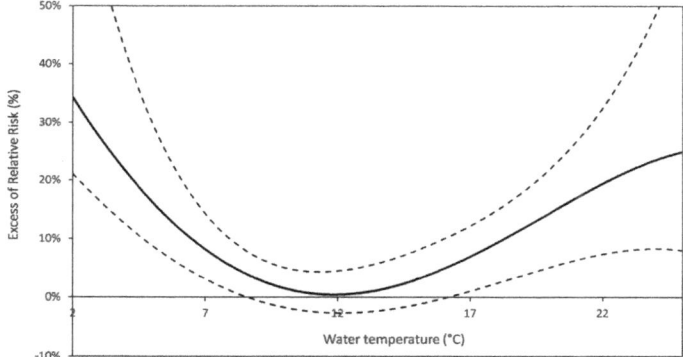

Figure 5. AGE risk function for the water temperature (PA-Nord). The right branch may miss (e.g., Boston). The delay considered for the health response to the river flow is homogenous with that used for turbidity.

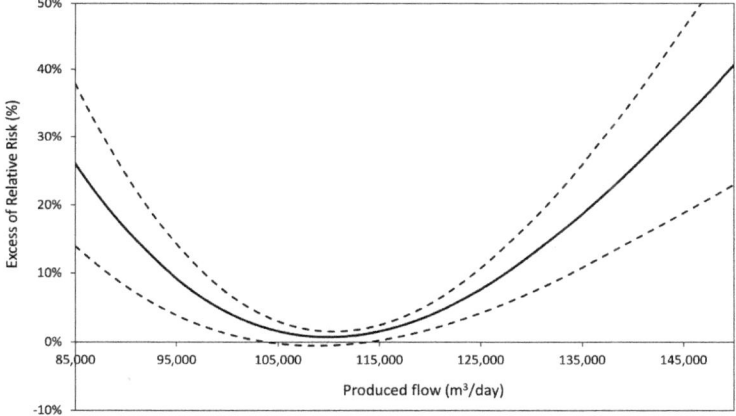

Figure 6. AGE risk function for the produced flow (Nantes). The left branch may miss (e.g., PA and Paris sites). The delay considered for the health response to the river flow is homogenous with that used for turbidity.

The Le Havre study showed that decantation—triggered when Tu_RW exceeded 3 NTU (syst. 1)—strongly modified the TRF associated with Tu_FW, with a shift from a high risk (IQ-ERR = 18% (14; 22)) in the absence of decantation, to a low and non-significant risk (IQ-ERR = 3% (0; 7)) with decantation. As well, the Boston study highlighted a possible decrease in risk due to the change from chlorination to ozonation. However, the disinfection-related proxies were generally not correlated to AGE incidence, except in one case (1/4).

River flow was a consistent factor in exposure (5/6). Basically, the U-shaped relationship between river flow and AGE indicated an increased risk at extreme flows (Figure 4). Both branches of the U could co-exist (e.g., in Nantes), whereas only the falling left branch remained in Paris-Est and the three sites in the Paris area, exhibiting a risk at lowest flow. Water temperature (6/6) or air temperature, as surrogates of water temperature (3/4), were also factors in exposure (6/6), with an associated risk exceeding by far (Boston) the turbidity related risk. As with the river flow, the temperature-risk functions decreased (Boston, Paris-Sud) or were U-shaped (other French DWSs), indicating that the risk was concentrated at extreme temperatures.

River flow also modified the TRF in Nantes and Paris-Est, and the water temperature in Boston and PA-Sud. These interactions (i.e., river flow—turbidity and water temperature—turbidity) were modelled as a tensor product smooth (TPS) which provided better estimations of risk than the cubic splines of each variable, taken together. The examination of the bivariate relative risk TPS (Tu_FW, river flow) and TPS (Tu_FW, water temperature) provides some clues to help explain the common lack of accuracy of the TRF at the high-level domain of turbidity (e.g., Nantes, Paris-Est, and Boston). Higher risks resulted from a combination of high Tu FW and extreme river flow (Nantes) or only low river flow (Paris-Est). In Boston, low temperature combined with turbidity, increased the risk whereas, in Paris-Est and PA-Sud, high temperature combined with Tu_FW or particle counts, respectively, increased the risk. Season may also modify the TRF, as was the case in New York, where AGE incidence was only related to drinking water turbidity after the spring snowmelt.

Produced flow was correlated to AGE incidence (8/9). The risk function varied from linearly increasing to U-shaped (Figure 5). The authors did not observe any interaction between the produced flow and other exposure proxies. IQ-ERR (when the risk function was increasing) or P50-P90 ERR (U-shaped risk function) often exceeded the corresponding turbidity related risk estimates.

No proxy related to distribution incidents (e.g., leaking pipes, cuts in the water supply) or repair interventions was strongly associated with the AGE incidence (overall: 2/5, details in Table 2).

Considering the subset of multi-exposure models, I calculated, when available, the difference in risk between all the exposure variables (Tu_FW or particle count, water temperature, produced flow, and river flow for river DWS) at the 75th percentile (in the direction of increasing risk) and at the 25th percentile. I observed, in most cases (4/6), that the contribution of Tu_FW in the IQ-ERR sum was lower than that of two or three other variables (max = 33 %).

4. Discussion

4.1. An Underestimated Established Risk

"It is likely that an association between turbidity and gastro-intestinal illness exists in some settings or over a certain range of turbidity", concluded Mann et al. in their review [12]. The findings of the updated review by De Roos et al. (12 sites studied vs. five in Mann's review) confirm that conclusion, as well as this review, which has kept nine sites in common with the De roos' review and incorporated seven additional sites. With 11 sites exhibiting an association between particle content of finished water and AGE incidence, the results from TSS clearly favor the existence of a residual risk of AGE from tap-water intake in the cities of developed countries. Risk could be higher with unfiltered water drawn from reservoirs and karst aquifers. On the other hand, TSS also show that even enhanced treatment (i.e., slow sand filtration instead of rapid filtration in Paris-Est) cannot fully cope with river water of poor microbial quality, and that joint watershed protection and water disinfection measures do not lead to an undetectable risk in people serviced by reservoir DWS.

The design of TSS is suitable for studying risks which vary from day to day. TSS are, however, unable to capture the full risk arising from fecal contamination of tap water. Specifically, TSS cannot capture an (improbable) time-steady risk, nor the risk acquired during the distribution stage, e.g., backflows of contaminated waters into the distribution network which cause a significant proportion of waterborne outbreaks [46,47] and possibly sporadic cases [48]. Furthermore, French TSS, which add other exposure proxies to the risk model, show that turbidity does not cover the full risk generated upstream of the DWTP outlet.

4.2. How to Improve Inter-Site Comparison of Turbidity-Related Risks

Despite the statistical modelling framework and options being quite similar in almost all the studies included, the diversity of the indicators used in the studies for both health and exposure hindered me from generating a comparison of the risks.

4.2.1. About Health Outcomes

The AGE indicators used in studies depended on their availability, i.e., on the organization of each country's health care system. Visits and admissions to hospital in North America and GP prescriptions in France are the two main sources of AGE indicators used in published TSS. They demonstrate adequate specificity and stability over time to target symptomatic cases of AGE, thanks to standardized coding (ICD) and regular revision of the discrimination algorithm, respectively. The diversity of AGE indicators corresponded to different degrees of symptom seriousness and to different age groups. Accordingly, the sensitivity of the available AGE indicators dictated the minimum population size needed to obtain sufficient statistical power to establish the presence of a risk. Indicators based on GP activity data were almost 10 times more sensitive than those based on hospital activity, this resulting in different ranges of population sizes between the North American and French sites. Irrespective of the sensitivity level, the stability, (i.e., the limited change in sensitivity and specificity over time) of most AGE indicators used for TSS meets the conditions to carry out TSS.

Children and elderly people were often targeted in the studies reviewed, because (i) they are at higher risk of infection than adults [40,41], and (ii) they are less subject to misclassification of exposure [31]. Indeed, compared with the whole community, these two subpopulations include fewer people who commute daily for work reasons, and so who drink tap water from different DSW. As such, a misclassification is a priori independent of health outcomes, the resulting bias is not differential, and only brings the risk estimate to zero. In the French studies, where models developed in children were systematically tested in adults, risk levels in adults were approximately half those in children. Both higher susceptibility to infections and lower misclassification rates could have participated in generating differences in estimated risk levels. The choice to study one particular population (i.e., children or the elderly), as opposed to studying the population as a whole, results in a trade-off between the loss of statistical power due to population restrictions and underestimation of the risk attributable to misclassification bias, arising from people commuting to areas with different DWS.

4.2.2. Need to Standardize the Time Window for Exposure Assessment

One practical condition needed to make an accurate inter-site comparison of the risks of gastroenteritis in tap water is that the formulation of the turbidity-based exposure variables must be similar between studies. In this review, the diversity of the time windows used for exposure assessment—from the earlier studies which used daily mean turbidity as exposure to the Atlanta study where a 0–21 day window was considered for statistical testing—advocates for future standardization. Exposure time windows should exclude the latency period accounting for water transit to consumers' taps (e.g., 1–2 days), incubation of AGE causing pathogens (e.g., 1–10 days and 4–6 days for the modal delay) and search for medical help (e.g., one day). The width of the window should also match the distribution of the incubation durations of all pathogens potentially involved in the risk, and the variability in the times of water transit from the drinking water treatment plant (DWTP) outlet to taps. Restricting the time windows (e.g., 6–10 days) to exclude inconstant, if not implausible, early and late responses would facilitate the comparison of risks between studies.

4.2.3. Need for Long Duration Studies

In addition to providing increased statistical power, a longer study duration would most probably have a crucial effect on the robustness of the risk estimates, because the contamination of finished water results from highly diversified combinations of pathogen shedding, resource contamination and treatment options to be covered by the study period.

Basically, hydrological conditions drive the fecal contamination of surface resources and of aquifers influenced by surface waters. In dry weather, fecal contamination is minimal, with a baseline level depending mainly on human pressure, i.e., the discharge of upstream waste water treatment plants (WWTP) located upstream of the DWTP intake. In the case of urban rivers, at the lowest flows, discharges from WWTP are less diluted and may cause a dramatic increase in the fecal contamination of river water, e.g., in the Paris area sites. Rain downpours first result in urban runoff and sewage overflow [49] causing the release of raw urban waste water (i.e., fecal pollution of human origin) into the rivers. Stronger or extended episodes of rain may further trigger rural runoffs contaminated by cattle and wildlife or manure spread on fields. In addition, sudden rises in river flows cause the re-suspension of the contaminated mud previously settled on river beds. Accordingly, high flows most often correspond to high fecal contaminations (e.g., 2 log-units or more above baseline) of surface water and of influenced groundwater bodies.

Fecal pollution in raw water does not necessarily mean a high pathogen content. The shedding of a given pathogen may vary yearly, seasonally, and in much shorter timescales, depending on the pathogen carriage level in humans and animals. Consequently, at a given time, fecal indicators may be correlated to the presence of one dominant pathogen (e.g., norovirus in January), several pathogens (as some outbreak investigations have shown), but may also occur in the quasi-absence of pathogens in resources, as shown by the fact that fecal accidental contaminations of drinking water outnumber outbreaks.

Finally, in addition to resource contamination by pathogens as a necessary condition, the contamination of finished water also necessitates that pathogens break through barriers provided by treatment. For sophisticated DWTP, permanently maintaining the barrier effect of treatment challenges the capacity of timely treatment adaptation to short-term changes in raw water quality, especially peaks in turbidity and organic matter.

To summarize, finished water contamination involves three time-varying conditions (shedding of pathogens, transport, and inadequate treatment) combining in a large variety of events. Thus, robust risk assessment not only requires the inclusion of a sufficient number of AGE cases but also long duration study periods, e.g., 5–10 years (Figure 2). Accordingly, the findings of long-duration studies (Atlanta, Boston) are more reliable than short duration studies (Québec, Gothenburg) where the risk functions may be attached to one-off situational conditions.

4.3. Microbiological vs. Operational Interpretations of Turbidity

"Microorganisms are only a tiny portion of the total number of suspended particles in water and pathogenic microbes are likely to be only a tiny fraction of the total microbial population" [27]. Given this, turbidity cannot be simply considered an indicator of pathogen content, but only a surrogate, the relevance of which relies on the statistical association between turbidity and pathogen load, i.e., the rain-driven concurrent presence in water resources of particles from soil erosion and pathogens from sewage overflow and manure entrainment.

The association between organo-mineral particles and pathogens is not only statistical, but also physical: bacteria may form biofilms on particles [50]. Furthermore, other viral and protozoan pathogens may also bind to particles [51,52]. Some experiments have shown that most bacteria, viruses, and protozoa in treated waste waters, as well as surface runoffs [52] and natural waters [53–55], are attached to, or embedded in, organo-mineral particles suspended within the water body. Accordingly, organo-mineral particles may act as Trojan horses, permitting the entry of infectious pathogens into distribution networks.

Chemical disinfection is expected to ensure that particle-free fecal bacteria are totally inactivated, and free viruses are totally or partially inactivated, depending on the disinfectant and dose used. However, it may fail to inactivate protozoan parasites, especially *Cryptosporidium* [56], although the World Health Organization stated that high rates of ozonation can bring about *Cryptosporidium* inactivation [57]. Studies performed in real conditions show that pathogen inactivation rates vary substantially in time and may be episodically low [56]. Some factors of ineffective disinfection have been well described, for example low temperatures or dead zones in disinfection reactors. However, the key factor when focusing on turbidity as a proxy for exposure is that suspended particles in water greatly hinder disinfection by harboring pathogens [57,58]. This is an especially important issue for waters from reservoirs and karsts which are distributed without clarification. However, information in the literature on the particles-pathogen association and the harboring effect which protects against disinfection is scarce.

Additionally, little is known about the relationship between particles and pathogens in clarified waters [59]. The key condition to efficient rapid sand filtration, i.e., which significantly retains pathogens, is upstream well-operated coagulation [57]. Hijnen and Medema recommend conservative values for real-condition removal rates of coagulation-filtration: 0–4 log for viruses, 1–3 log for bacteria and 1–5 log for *Cryptosporidium* oocysts [56]. Discrepancies between operational and theoretical removal rates, the latter corresponding to the upper boundaries of the aforementioned ranges, reflect difficulties in maintaining the efficiency of treatments all of the time when faced with changes in raw water quality.

Although some biological elements of plausibility advocate for the use of turbidity as an indicator for exposure to pathogens, the findings from this review of TSS do not entirely support this. The expression of ERR by 0.01 NTU led to over-dispersed estimates of risks (0.2–13%) among the six different DWS sites where ERR was calculable (Figure 3), whereas the range of estimated IQ-ERR values was tighter (3–13%). Moreover, ERR, whatever their expression, were independent of Tu_FW baseline levels. These observations question the biological interpretation of Tu_FW as a universal proxy for the pathogen content of finished water. On the contrary, they suggest that Tu_FW could be considered a site-specific proxy for the general functioning of a DWTP and that only relative changes in Tu_FW matter in risk assessment. This latter interpretation also rejects the impossibility of observing a significant risk below 0.2 NTU, which was argued in the earliest TSS [7].

In conclusion, there are two possible and, in a certain extent, compatible interpretations of turbidity as a proxy for pathogen exposure: the biological interpretation and the operational interpretation. The operational interpretation may be more suitable for river DWS, as Tu_FW mainly reflects the accuracy and timeliness of on-line treatment adaptation to changes in raw water quality, whereas turbidity in unfiltered reservoir water can be more directly interpreted in terms of environmental conditions.

4.4. Public Health Issues

4.4.1. TSS Do Not Support the Quantitative Health Impact Assessment

In a former review [60], authors stated that the set of published TSS is still inadequate to draw a meta-risk estimate representative of the risk in cities of developed countries. The insufficiency of the dataset not only results from the small number of available studies and from the recruitment provisions leading to an overrepresentation of "good performers", but mainly from the intrinsic heterogeneity of turbidity that makes pooled analyses irrelevant.

The quantitative health impact assessment [61] aims to predict the possible effect of prevention actions on risk. It is based on the existence of a robust causal risk function. TSS do not offer an interesting perspective for the building of a generic meta-TRF. Even when considering a single site, the specific TRF (if any) does not enable operators to forecast the effect on risk of a reduction in turbidity. For instance, the implementation of enhanced treatment facilities (e.g., clarification) probably lowers the turbidity baseline in finished water, but also changes its composition by differential selection of particles, according to their size, shape, density, and electric properties. The relationship between Tu_FW and the pathogen presence would also probably change under new treatment conditions, as some real-world experiences of decantation implementation have suggested [36], making the TRF irrelevant for such inference.

4.4.2. TSS Do Not Help Identify Causative Pathogens

The description of the DWS provides some clues about the pathogens which may survive in finished water. In the case of reservoir DWS, the exclusion of human activities and livestock from the reservoir watershed makes wildlife the main (theoretically, the only) source of pathogens: the pathogens at the inlet of DWTP should, therefore, encompass bacteria and protozoa and exclude viruses. Infective protozoa may only possibly remain at the outlet of DWTP, considering the strength of the disinfection implemented. On the contrary, the finished water from river DWS should mainly contain viruses since humans are probably the main source of pathogen discharge into the river in urbanized watersheds. Protozoa may also be present in the case of inefficient clarification [1]. For all studied DWS, the presence of infective fecal bacteria is improbable because of the disinfection provisions.

To date, results from TSS have added little information about the causative agents involved in water-related AGE cases. Long latency in the health effects associated with the reservoir DWS turbidity, i.e., more than two weeks, could suggest the presence of protozoa in finished water [1,33,34], whereas the early response suggests pathogens with short incubation durations, e.g., viruses. Alternative interpretations of late responses may, however, be put forward: (i) long distribution time in remote parts of the distribution network; (ii) secondary cases infected by contact with primary water-related cases [20]; or (iii) increased incubation times due to lower pathogen doses ingested by consumers than referenced infective doses observed in outbreak investigations or experimented in controlled trials [62].

4.4.3. But TSS Can Teach Water Operators about High Risk Conditions

Risk functions formulated as operation conditions may directly help water operators in developing prevention measures without having to go through a formal pathogen identification step. To improve water microbial quality, multi-exposure models provide more useful information to achieve prevention measures than models where exposure is limited to turbidity. Indeed, this review highlighted three variables worthy of examination as exposure indicators in addition to turbidity: produced flow, river flow (for river DWS), and water temperature.

TSS results consistently (8/9) showed the adverse health effects of the high production of drinking water, irrespective of the effect of turbidity, possibly due to the shortening of transit time of water across treatment facilities and the consequent lowering of retention and inactivation rates. For other DWS, the U-shaped produced flow-AGE functions suggest the existence of optimal flow conditions (Figure 6).

French studies also suggested an adverse effect of extreme river flow on the risk of AGE observed in five of the six sites where river flow was tested. The J- or U-shape of the risk function (Figure 4) is in line with prior knowledge about the drivers of contamination (see § Need for long-duration studies). Furthermore, the modifying effect of river flow on the TRF, highlighted in Nantes and Paris-Est, suggests that, in extreme flow conditions, a similar amount of particles in finished water may shelter (or be associated with) significantly more pathogens than in intermediate flows.

Temperature heavily influences the risk of AGE both as control and exposure (Figure 5). High temperatures enhance the dehydration risk in patients with AGE symptoms and encourage people to seek medical help earlier. The absence of latency in the health effect supports this interpretation. In addition to the likely direct effect of air temperature on symptom seriousness, present in the Boston and New York studies, water temperature (or air temperature as a surrogate) also factors in exposure (9/10), whatever the route (tap water, food, or contact), as suggested by the delayed response of the risk of AGE to temperature, consistently with the incubation duration of the AGE-related infections. Moreover, the presence of interactions between water temperature and Tu_FW on the risk in Boston and PA-Sud advocates for a waterborne effect. Considering the delayed influence, extreme temperatures result in higher and plausible risks. Low temperatures mean greater survival of pathogens in the environment [63–65] and slower disinfection [56] and coagulation dynamics [66]. At high temperatures, dissolved organic matter may rise in the surface water and cause an unexpected chlorine demand, thus temporarily compromising disinfection power. In addition to its waterborne effect, water temperature may also be influential in other routes of infection. For instance, cold weather favors indoor confinement and consequent cross-infection from contact between people and fomites. Accordingly, temperature should be involved in waterborne exposure, but only partially.

Some of the identified risk factors are environmental constraints for water operation (river flow, water temperature), while others may only be marginally controlled (produced flow). Turbidity remains the only risk factor that may be lowered by improved operational provisions. However, since decreased turbidity may mean a change in the nature of the particles, cutting the risk by decreasing turbidity could be a false solution when seeking to improve the microbial quality of finished water. Prevention actions could target other factors than turbidity, for instance, increased disinfection during episodes deemed to be at higher risk. Authors should discuss the results and how they can be interpreted in the perspective of previous studies and of the working hypotheses. The findings and their implications should be discussed in the broadest context possible. Future research directions may also be highlighted.

5. Conclusions

In the history of the epidemiology of waterborne infections, priority has been given to microbiology to specify both the health effects and the exposure level. When opportunities for an alternative approach appeared, based on syndromic and water operation data, TSS seemed to be a cost-reasonable solution to study waterborne risks in cities.

Despite this advantage, TSS have not caught on in this field for several reasons. Scientifically, the lack of specificity of turbidity as a proxy for exposure appears to be the main limitation to obtaining accurate estimates of the risk at the site level. Furthermore, inter-site heterogeneity of turbidity prevents further meta-risk assessment and limits the review to a qualitative approach. TSS could help provide safer finished water, provided that models increase the set of relevant exposure variables drawn from operational data.

Acknowledgments: This study was fully funded by Santé Publique France (Public Health France). My thanks to Jude Sweeney for the English revision and editing of my manuscript.

Conflicts of Interest: The author declares no conflict of interest.

Abbreviations

AGE	Acute gastroenteritis
CFD	Coagulation-flocculation-decantation
DWS	Drinking water system
DWTP	Drinking water treatment plant
DZ	Distribution zone
ERR	Excess of relative risk
GAM	Generalized additive model
GP	General Practitioner
ICD	International classification of diseases
IQ	Interquartile
NTU	Nephelometric turbidity unit
P10	10th Percentile
PA	Paris area
PRISMA	Preferred reporting items for Systematic Reviews and Meta-Analysis
TRF	Turbidity risk function
TSS	Time series study
Tu_FW	Turbidity of finished water
Tu_RW	Turbidity of raw water
USA	United States of America
UV	Ultraviolet

References

1. Morris, R.D.; Naumova, E.N.; Griffiths, J.K. Did Milwaukee experience waterborne cryptosporidiosis before the large documented outbreak in 1993? *Epidemiology* **1998**, *9*, 264–270. [CrossRef] [PubMed]
2. Payment, P.; Richardson, L.; Siemiatycki, J.; Dewar, R.; Edwardes, M.; Franco, E. A randomized trial to evaluate the risk of gastrointestinal disease due to consumption of drinking water meeting current microbiological standards. *Am. J. Public Health* **1991**, *81*, 703–708. [CrossRef] [PubMed]
3. Payment, P.; Siemiatycki, J.; Richardson, L.; Renaud, G.; Franco, E.; Prevost, M. A prospective epidemiological study of gastrointestinal health effects due to the consumption of drinking water. *Int. J. Environ. Health Res.* **1997**, *7*, 5–31. [CrossRef]
4. Hellard, M.E.; Sinclair, M.I.; Forbes, A.B.; Fairley, C.K. A randomized, blinded, controlled trial investigating the gastrointestinal health effects of drinking water quality. *Environ. Health Perspect.* **2001**, *109*, 773–778. [CrossRef] [PubMed]
5. Goh, S.; Reacher, M.; Casemore, D.P.; Verlander, N.Q.; Charlett, A.; Chalmers, R.M.; Knowles, M.; Pennington, A.; Williams, J.; Osborn, K.; et al. Sporadic cryptosporidiosis decline after membrane filtration of public water supplies, england, 1996–2002. *Emerg. Infect. Dis.* **2005**, *11*, 251–259. [CrossRef] [PubMed]
6. Lake, I.R.; Harrison, F.C.; Chalmers, R.M.; Bentham, G.; Nichols, G.; Hunter, P.R.; Kovats, R.S.; Grundy, C. Case-control study of environmental and social factors influencing cryptosporidiosis. *Eur. J. Epidemiol.* **2007**, *22*, 805–811. [CrossRef] [PubMed]
7. Sinclair, M.I.; Fairley, C.K. Drinking water and endemic gastrointestinal illness. *J. Epidemiol. Community Health* **2000**, *54*, 728. [CrossRef] [PubMed]
8. Schwartz, J.; Levin, R. Drinking water turbidity and health. *Epidemiology* **1999**, *10*, 86–90. [CrossRef] [PubMed]
9. Beaudeau, P. Surveillance Syndromique Des Gastroentérites Aigües: Une Opportunité Pour la Prévention du Risque Infectieux Attribuable à L'ingestion D'eau du Robinet. [Syndromic Surveillance of Acute Gastroenteritis: An Opportunity for the Prevention of the Infectious Risk Attributable to Tap Water]. Ph.D. Thesis, Université de Rennes, Rennes, France, 2012. Available online: https://tel.archives-ouvertes.fr/tel-00795215/document (accessed on 1 November 2017).
10. Schwartz, J.; Levin, R.; Hodge, K. Drinking water turbidity and pediatric hospital use for gastrointestinal illness in Philadelphia. *Epidemiology* **1997**, *8*, 615–620. [CrossRef] [PubMed]
11. Schwartz, J.; Dockery, D.W. Particulate air pollution and daily mortality in Steubenville, Ohio. *Am. J. Epidemiol.* **1992**, *135*, 12–19. [CrossRef] [PubMed]
12. Mann, A.G.; Tam, C.C.; Higgins, C.D.; Rodrigues, L.C. The association between drinking water turbidity and gastrointestinal illness: A systematic review. *BMC Public Health* **2007**, *7*, 256–262. [CrossRef] [PubMed]
13. De Roos, A.J.; Gurian, P.L.; Robinson, L.F.; Rai, A.; Zakeri, I.; Kondo, M.C. Review of epidemiological studies of drinking-water turbidity in relation to acute gastrointestinal illness. *Environ. Health Perspect.* **2017**, *125*, 086003. [CrossRef] [PubMed]
14. Beaudeau, P.; Rambaud, L.; Zeghnoun, A.; Corso, M. *Qualité de L'eau Distribuée à Angoulême et Incidence Des Gastro-Entérites Aiguës, 2002–2007 [Quality of Water Distributed in Angoulême (France) and Incidence of Acute Gastroenteritis, 2002-7]*; Institut de Veille Sanitaire: Saint-Maurice, France, 2013; p. 36. ISBN 978-2-11-131096-4. Available online: http://invs.santepubliquefrance.fr (accessed on 1 November 2017).
15. Rambaud, L.; Zeghnoun, A.; Corso, M.; Beaudeau, P. *Qualité de L'eau Distribuée à Paris-Centre et Incidence Des Gastro-Entérites Aiguës, 2002–2007 [Quality of Water Distributed in Paris (France) and Incidence of Acute Gastroenteritis, 2002-7]*; Institut de Veille Sanitaire: Saint-Maurice, France, 2013; p. 43, ISBN 978-2-11-138332-6. Available online: http://invs.santepubliquefrance.fr (accessed on 1 November 2017).
16. Rambaud, L.; Zeghnoun, A.; Corso, M.; Beaudeau, P. *Qualité de L'eau Distribuée à Paris-Est et Incidence Des Gastroentérites aiguës, 2002–2007 [Quality of Water Distributed in East of Paris (France) and Incidence of Acute Gastroenteritis, 2002-7]*; Institut de Veille Sanitaire: Saint-Maurice, France, 2014; p. 46, ISBN 979-10-289-0071-4. Available online: http://invs.santepubliquefrance.fr (accessed on 1 November 2017).
17. Rambaud, L.; Zeghnoun, A.; Corso, M.; Beaudeau, P. *Qualité de L'eau Distribuée en Banlieue Parisienne et Incidence Des Gastro-Entérites aiguës, 2002–2007 [Quality of Water Distributed in Paris Suburbs (France) and Incidence of Acute Gastroenteritis, 2002-7]*; Institut de Veille Sanitaire: Saint-Maurice, France, 2015; p. 83, ISBN 979-10-289-0170-7. Available online: http://invs.santepubliquefrance.fr (accessed on 1 November 2017).

18. Rambaud, L.; Zeghnoun, A.; Corso, M.; Beaudeau, P. *Qualité de L'eau Distribuée à Nancy et Incidence Des Gastro-Entérites Aiguës, 2002–2007 [Quality of Water Distributed in Nancy (France) and Incidence of Acute Gastroenteritis, 2002-7]*; Institut de Veille Sanitaire: Saint-Maurice, France, 2016; p. 41, ISBN 979-10-289-0195-0. Available online: http://invs.santepubliquefrance.fr (accessed on 1 November 2017).

19. Moher, D.; Liberati, A.; Tetzlaff, J.; Altman, D.G. Preferred reporting items for systematic reviews and meta-analyses: The prisma statement. *J. Clin. Epidemiol.* **2009**, *62*, 1006–1012. [CrossRef] [PubMed]

20. Morris, R.D.; Naumova, E.N.; Levin, R.; Munasinghe, R.L. Temporal variation in drinking water turbidity and diagnosed gastroenteritis in Milwaukee. *Am. J. Public Health* **1996**, *86*, 237–239. [CrossRef] [PubMed]

21. Naumova, E.N.; Egorov, A.I.; Morris, R.D.; Griffiths, J.K. The elderly and waterborne *Cryptosporidium* infection: Gastroenteritis hospitalizations before and during the 1993 Milwaukee outbreak. *Emerg. Infect. Dis.* **2003**, *9*, 418–425. [CrossRef] [PubMed]

22. Egorov, A.I.; Naumova, E.N.; Tereschenko, A.A.; Kislitsin, V.A.; Ford, T.E. Daily variations in effluent water turbidity and diarrhoeal illness in a Russian city. *Int. J. Environ. Health Res.* **2003**, *13*, 81–94. [CrossRef] [PubMed]

23. Drayna, P.; McLellan, S.L.; Simpson, P.; Li, S.H.; Gorelick, M.H. Association between rainfall and pediatric emergency department visits for acute gastrointestinal illness. *Environ. Health Perspect.* **2010**, *118*, 1439–1443. [CrossRef] [PubMed]

24. Harper, S.L.; Edge, V.L.; Schuster-Wallace, C.J.; Berke, O.; McEwen, S.A. Weather, water quality and infectious gastrointestinal illness in two Inuit communities in Nunatsiavut, Canada: Potential implications for climate change. *Ecohealth* **2011**, *8*, 93–108. [CrossRef] [PubMed]

25. Uejio, C.K.; Yale, S.H.; Malecki, K.; Borchardt, M.A.; Anderson, H.A.; Patz, J.A. Drinking water systems, hydrology, and childhood gastrointestinal illness in central and Northern Wisconsin. *Am. J. Public Health* **2014**, *104*, 639–646. [CrossRef] [PubMed]

26. Beaudeau, P.; Payment, P.; Bourderont, D.; Mansotte, F.; Boudhabay, O.; Laubiès, B.; Verdière, J. A time series study of anti-diarrheal drug sales and tap-water quality. *Int. J. Environ. Health Res.* **1999**, *9*, 293–311. [CrossRef]

27. Schwartz, J.; Levin, R.; Goldstein, R. Drinking water turbidity and gastrointestinal illness in the elderly of Philadelphia. *J. Epidemiol. Community Health* **2000**, *54*, 45–51. [CrossRef] [PubMed]

28. Investigating the Relationship Between Drinking Water and Gastroenteritis in Edmonton: 1993–1998. Available online: https://www.canada.ca/en/health-canada/services/environmental-workplace-health/reports-publications/water-quality/investigating-relationship-between-drinking-water-gastroenteritis-edmonton-1993-1998.html?wbdisable=true (accessed on 1 November 2017).

29. Gilbert, M.L.; Levallois, P.; Rodriguez, M.J. Use of a health information telephone line, info-sante clsc, for the surveillance of waterborne gastroenteritis. *J. Water Health* **2006**, *4*, 225–232. [PubMed]

30. Tinker, S.C.; Moe, C.L.; Klein, M.; Flanders, W.D.; Uber, J.; Amirtharajah, A.; Singer, P.; Tolbert, P.E. Drinking water turbidity and emergency department visits for gastrointestinal illness in atlanta, 1993–2004. *J. Expo. Sci. Environ. Epidemiol.* **2010**, *20*, 19–28. [CrossRef] [PubMed]

31. Beaudeau, P.; Zeghnoun, A.; Corso, M.; Lefranc, A.; Rambaud, L. A time series study of gastroenteritis and tap water quality in the Nantes area, France, 2002–2007. *J. Expo. Sci. Environ. Epidemiol.* **2014**, *24*, 192–199. [CrossRef] [PubMed]

32. Tornevi, A.; Axelsson, G.; Forsberg, B. Association between precipitation upstream of a drinking water utility and nurse advice calls relating to acute gastrointestinal illnesses. *PLoS ONE* **2013**, *8*, e69918. [CrossRef] [PubMed]

33. Aramini, J.; Allen, B.; Copes, R.; Holt, J.; Mc Lean, M.; Sears, W.; Wilson, J. *Drinking Water Quality and Health Care Utilization for Gastrointestinal Illness in Greater Vancouver*; University of Guelph and Vancouver Richmond Health Board, Guelf: Guelph, ON, Canada, 2000; p. 78.

34. Beaudeau, P.; Schwartz, J.; Levin, R. Drinking water quality and hospital admissions of elderly people for gastrointestinal illness in Eastern Massachusetts, 1998–2008. *Water Res.* **2014**, *52*, 188–198. [CrossRef] [PubMed]

35. Hsieh, J.L.; Nguyen, T.Q.; Matte, T.; Ito, K. Drinking water turbidity and emergency department visits for gastrointestinal illness in new york city, 2002–2009. *PLoS ONE* **2015**, *10*, e0125071. [CrossRef] [PubMed]

36. Beaudeau, P.; Le, T.A.; Zeghnoun, A.; Zanobetti, A.; Schwartz, J. A time series study of drug sales and turbidity of tap water in Le Havre, France. *J. Water Health* **2012**, *10*, 221–235. [CrossRef] [PubMed]

37. U.S. Department of the Interior, U.S. Geological Survey. USGS Water-Quality Data for USA. Available online: https://waterdata.usgs.gov/nwis/qw (accessed on 1 November 2016).

38. Gregory, M.B.; Frick, E.A. Fecal-coliform bacteria concentrations in streams of the Chattahoochee River National Recreation Area, Metropolitan Atlanta, Georgia, May–October 1994 and 1995. U.S. Geological Survey Water-Resources Investigations Report 00-4139; 2000; p. 8. Available online: https://pubs.usgs.gov/wri/wri004139/pdf/wrir00-4139.pdf (accessed on 1 November 2016).

39. NYC Environmental Protection. New York City 2009 Drinking Water Supply and Quality Report. 2010; p. 16. Available online: http://www.nyc.gov/html/dep/pdf/wsstate09.pdf (accessed on 1 November 2016).

40. Jones, T.F.; McMillian, M.B.; Scallan, E.; Frenzen, P.D.; Cronquist, A.B.; Thomas, S.; Angulo, F.J. A population-based estimate of the substantial burden of diarrhoeal disease in the United States; FoodNet, 1996–2003. *Epidemiol. Infect.* **2007**, *135*, 293–301. [CrossRef] [PubMed]

41. Van Cauteren, D.; de Valk, H.; Vaux, S.; Le, S.Y.; Vaillant, V. Burden of acute gastroenteritis and healthcare-seeking behaviour in France: A population-based study. *Epidemiol. Infect.* **2012**, *140*, 697–705. [CrossRef] [PubMed]

42. Bounoure, F.; Beaudeau, P.; Mouly, D.; Skiba, M.; Lahiani-Skiba, M. Syndromic surveillance of acute gastroenteritis based on drug consumption. *Epidemiol. Infect.* **2010**, *139*, 1388–1395. [CrossRef] [PubMed]

43. Majowicz, S.E.; Hall, G.; Scallan, E.; Adak, G.K.; Gauci, C.; Jones, T.F.; Sockett, P.N. A common, symptom-based case definition for gastroenteritis. *Epidemiol. Infect.* **2008**, *136*, 886–894. [CrossRef] [PubMed]

44. Peng, R.D.; Dominici, F.; Louis, T.A. Model choice in time series studies of air pollution and mortality. *J. R. Stat. Soc. A* **2006**, *169*, 179–203. [CrossRef]

45. Perrakis, K.; Gryparis, A.; Schwartz, J.; Tertre, A.L.; Katsouyanni, K.; Forastiere, F.; Stafoggia, M.; Samoli, E. Controlling for seasonal patterns and time varying confounders in time-series epidemiological models: A simulation study. *Stat. Med* **2014**, *33*, 4904–4918. [CrossRef] [PubMed]

46. Kramer, M.H.; Quade, G.; Hartemann, P.; Exner, M. Waterborne diseaeses in Europe: 1986–1996. *Am. Water Work. Assoc.* **2001**, *93*, 48–53. [CrossRef]

47. Craun, G.F.; Calderon, R.L.; Nwachuku, N. Causes of waterborne outbreaks reported in the United States, 1991–1998. In *Drinking Water and Infectious Disease: Estblishing the Links*; Hunter, P.R., Waite, M., Ronchi, E., Eds.; CRC Press: Boca Raton, FL, USA, 2003; pp. 119–126.

48. Ercumen, A.; Gruber, J.S.; Colford, J.M., Jr. Water distribution system deficiencies and gastrointestinal illness: A systematic review and meta-analysis. *Environ. Health Perspect.* **2014**, *122*, 651–660. [CrossRef] [PubMed]

49. Jagai, J.S.; Li, Q.; Wang, S.; Messier, K.P.; Wade, T.J.; Hilborn, E.D. Extreme precipitation and emergency room visits for gastrointestinal illness in areas with and without combined sewer systems: An analysis of Massachusetts data, 2003–2007. *Environ. Health Perspect.* **2015**, *123*, 873–879. [CrossRef] [PubMed]

50. Liu, G.; Ling, F.Q.; van der Mark, E.J.; Zhang, X.D.; Knezev, A.; Verberk, J.Q.; van der Meer, W.G.; Medema, G.J.; Liu, W.T.; van Dijk, J.C. Comparison of particle-associated bacteria from a drinking water treatment plant and distribution reservoirs with different water sources. *Sci. Rep.* **2016**, *6*, 20367. [CrossRef] [PubMed]

51. Medema, G.J.; Schets, F.M.; Teunis, P.F.; Havelaar, A.H. Sedimentation of free and attached *Cryptosporidium* oocysts and *Giardia* cysts in water. *Appl. Environ. Microbiol.* **1998**, *64*, 4460–4466. [PubMed]

52. Krometis, L.A.; Characklis, G.W.; Simmons, O.D., III; Dilts, M.J.; Likirdopulos, C.A.; Sobsey, M.D. Intra-storm variability in microbial partitioning and microbial loading rates. *Water Res.* **2007**, *41*, 506–516. [CrossRef] [PubMed]

53. Mahler, B.J.; Personné, J.-C.; Lods, G.F.; Drogue, C. Transport of free and particulate-associated bacteria in karst. *J. Hydrol.* **2000**, *238*, 179–193. [CrossRef]

54. Jamieson, R.; Joy, D.M.; Lee, H.; Kostaschuk, R.; Gordon, R. Transport and deposition of sediment-associated escherichia coli in natural streams. *Water Res.* **2005**, *39*, 2665–2675. [CrossRef] [PubMed]

55. Servais, P.; Garcia-Armisen, T. Partitioning and fate of particle-associated *E. coli* in river waters. *Water Environ. Res.* **2009**, *81*, 21–28.

56. Hijnen, W.A.M.; Medema, G.J. *Elimination of Micro-Organisms by Water Treatment Processes*; IWA Publishing: London, UK, 2010; ISBN 9781843393733.

57. LeChevallier, M.W.; Au, K. *Water Treatment and Pathogen Control: Process Efficiency in Achieving Safe Drinking-Water*; World Health Organization and IWA Publishing: London, UK, 2004; ISBN 1-84339-069-8.

58. LeChevallier, M.W.; Evans, T.M.; Seidler, R.J. Effect of turbidity on chlorination efficiency and bacterial persistence in drinking water. *Appl. Environ. Microbiol.* **1981**, *42*, 159–167. [PubMed]

59. Kaegi, R.; Wagner, T.; Hetzer, B.; Sinnet, B.; Tzvetkov, G.; Boller, M. Size, number and chemical composition of nanosized particles in drinking water determined by analytical microscopy and libd. *Water Res.* **2008**, *42*, 2778–2786. [CrossRef] [PubMed]

60. Craun, G.F.; Calderon, R.L. Observational epidemiologic studies of endemic waterborne risks: Cohort, case-control, time-series, and ecologic studies. *J. Water Health* **2006**, *4* (Suppl. S2), 101–119. [CrossRef] [PubMed]

61. Medina, S.; Ballester, F.; Chanel, O.; Declercq, C.; Pascal, M. Quantifying the health impacts of outdoor air pollution: Useful estimations for public health action. *J. Epidemiol. Community Health* **2013**. [CrossRef] [PubMed]

62. Haas, C.N.; Rose, J.B.; Gerba, C.P. *Quantitative Microbial Risk Assessment*; John Wiley & Sons: New York, NY, USA, 1999; p. 449. ISBN 9781118145296.

63. Beaudeau, P.; Tousset, N.; Bruchon, F.; Lefevre, A.; Taylor, H.D. In situ measurement and statistical modelling of Escherichia coli decay in small rivers. *Water Res.* **2001**, *35*, 3168–3178. [CrossRef]

64. Menon, P.; Billen, G.; Servais, P. Mortality rates of autochthonous and fecal bacteria in natural aquatic ecosystems. *Water Res.* **2003**, *37*, 4151–4158. [CrossRef]

65. Gerba, C.P. Chapter 5 Virus occurrence and survival in the environmental waters. In *Perspectives in Medical Virology*; Bosch, A., Ed.; Elsevier: New York, NY, USA, 2007; Volume 17, pp. 91–108. ISBN 0168-7069.

66. Gregory, J. *Particles in Water, Properties and Processes*; CRC Press and IWA Publishing: Boca Raton, FL, USA, 2006; p. 180. ISBN 9781587160851.

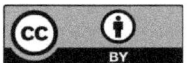

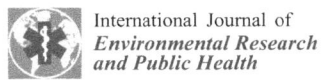

International Journal of
*Environmental Research
and Public Health*

Article

Waterborne Disease Outbreak Detection: A Simulation-Based Study

Damien Mouly [1,*], Sarah Goria [1], Michael Mounié [2], Pascal Beaudeau [1], Catherine Galey [1], Anne Gallay [1], Christian Ducrot [3] and Yann Le Strat [1]

[1] Santé Publique France, the French National Public Health Agency, 94 410 Saint-Maurice, France; sarah.goria@santepubliquefrance.fr (S.G.); pascal.beaudeau@santepubliquefrance.fr (P.B.); catherine.galey@santepubliquefrance.fr (C.G.); anne.gallay@santepubliquefrance.fr (A.G.); yann.lestrat@santepubliquefrance.fr (Y.L.S.)

[2] Unité D'évaluation Médico-Economique, Université Paul Sabatier, CHU 31059 Toulouse, France; mounie.michael.12@gmail.com

[3] Institut National de la Recherche Agronomique, UR346-Unité d'Épidémiologie Animale, 63 122 Saint Genès Champanelle, France; christian.ducrot@inra.fr

* Correspondence: damien.mouly@santepubliquefrance.fr

Received: 24 June 2018; Accepted: 10 July 2018; Published: 17 July 2018

Abstract: Waterborne disease outbreaks (WBDOs) remain a public health issue in developed countries, but to date the surveillance of WBDOs in France, mainly based on the voluntary reporting of clusters of acute gastrointestinal infections (AGIs) by general practitioners to health authorities, is characterized by low sensitivity. In this context, a detection algorithm using health insurance data and based on a space–time method was developed to improve WBDO detection. The objective of the present simulation-based study was to evaluate the performance of this algorithm for WBDO detection using health insurance data. The daily baseline counts of acute gastrointestinal infections were simulated. Two thousand simulated WBDO signals were then superimposed on the baseline data. Sensitivity (Se) and positive predictive value (PPV) were both used to evaluate the detection algorithm. Multivariate regression was also performed to identify the factors associated with WBDO detection. Almost three-quarters of the simulated WBDOs were detected (Se = 73.0%). More than 9 out of 10 detected signals corresponded to a WBDO (PPV = 90.5%). The probability of detecting a WBDO increased with the outbreak size. These results underline the value of using the detection algorithm for the implementation of a national surveillance system for WBDOs in France.

Keywords: waterborne disease outbreak; simulation study; health insurance data; space–time detection

1. Introduction

Outbreaks of infectious waterborne diseases are still a public health concern in developed countries [1,2]. Most of the time, acute gastrointestinal infections (AGIs) are the syndrome involved. In most of the waterborne disease outbreaks (WBDOs) reported in the last decade in Europe, the United States of America, and Canada, several hundred to several thousand people became ill after drinking water contaminated by infectious pathogenic agents. In rare cases, tens of thousands of people were affected. This occurred for example in two waterborne cryptosporidiosis outbreaks which occurred in 2010 and 2011 in Sweden, infecting 27,000 and 20,000 people, respectively [3,4], and in the 1993 disaster in Milwaukee, which affected 400,000 people [5]. There is also concern in France with respect to WBDOs [6], but to date, in the absence of a specific nationwide surveillance system, the detection of these events is mainly based on the voluntary reporting of clusters of AGIs by general practitioners to health authorities. The mean outbreak size of reported WBDOs (ranging from several hundred to thousands of AGI cases) suggests that only the most important events are reported. Despite the need for the development of a specific nationwide surveillance system to improve the detection of outbreaks caused by contaminated drinking water in France, and accordingly help health authorities with the microbial risk management of drinking water, the creation of such a specific surveillance system is a challenge for French authorities.

For several years, *Santé publique France* (the French Public Health Agency) has been using the French Health Insurance Administrative Database (*Système national d'information inter régimes de l'Assurance maladie*, SNIIRAM) for the syndromic surveillance of the medicalized AGI cases by employing a specifically developed algorithm [7]. Medicalized AGI cases are aggregated by day and by zip code. Although not all medicalized AGI cases can be specifically attributed to drinking water contamination, the correspondence between AGI cases and water distribution zones (DZs) at a local level provides the opportunity to study the ecological relationship between tap water and infectious gastrointestinal diseases. Medicalized AGI data have already proven relevant for studying the relationship between tap water quality parameters (e.g., turbidity) and the incidence of AGIs [8,9], and also for retrospectively identifying and describing outbreaks of AGIs notified by general practitioners [8,10]. Consequently, using these data to develop a specific automated nationwide system for local WBDO detection offers a promising way forward.

By so doing, an integrated approach to detect and localize WBDOs using medicalized AGI cases from SNIIRAM data was published in 2017 by Coly et al. [11]. The authors' approach relied on a space–time statistical method developed by Kulldorff [12] used to detect local outbreaks of AGIs. Their approach integrates the DZ as the ecological unit of exposure to tap water. A detected outbreak of AGIs localized in a DZ (compared with no outbreak in the surrounding DZs) is considered as a potential WBDO and is characterized by epidemiological criteria (day one of detected signal, duration, number of expected cases, and number of observed cases, DZ identity code). Each outbreak is retrospectively investigated in terms of various environmental criteria during the days before the onset of the outbreak: weather (e.g., heavy rain) and technical incidents in drinking water treatment (e.g., chlorination breakdown, alarm malfunction) or in the distribution system (e.g., water pipe breaks). However, the performance of this integrated approach in the implementation of nationwide retrospective automated WBDO detection has not been evaluated to date. Another detection method, inspired by field investigator practices in France and based on the comparison of the incidence ratio mean between the zip code and specific French administrative districts (called *départements*) was published in 2016 [13]. However we did not decide to select this method for evaluation as its theoretical foundations were considered insufficient [14].

A simulation-based study was performed to evaluate Coly et al.'s detection algorithm in order to implement a nationwide surveillance system. Simulation studies were performed to evaluate surveillance methods and disease control measures [15,16]. To our knowledge, to date, no simulation-based study has been specifically developed to evaluate an automated WBDO detection system. One of the major challenges regarding outbreak detection systems of contaminated water is to identify the largest number of clusters corresponding to real WBDO (i.e., maximizing the sensitivity) while avoiding clusters that are inconsistent with WBDO assumption (i.e., minimizing the number of false positives).

The objective of our study was therefore to evaluate, through simulations, the performance of the integrated approach developed by Coly et al. for WBDO detection [11] and to highlight the DZ and outbreak features which most influence WBDO detection.

2. Materials and Methods

2.1. Study Area and Period

Two French *départements*, Puy-de-Dôme and Isère, with 655,498 and 1,253,410 inhabitants, respectively [17], were selected. Puy-de-Dôme was included in the previous study by Coly et al.

for the construction of the WBDO detection algorithm. Isère is known for chronic microbiological pollution of DZ. The period studied extended from 1 January 2010 to 31 December 2013.

2.2. Reference Health Data

Health data represented medicalized AGI cases from the French National Health Insurance Information System (*Système national d'information inter régimes de l'Assurance maladie*, SNIIRAM). SNIIRAM aims to evaluate beneficiaries' healthcare consumption and associated expenditures. It covers more than 98% of the French population and records all patient reimbursements for out-of-pocket medical procedures, medications, and payments to professionals for consultations [18]. Almost all medicalized AGI cases in France, irrespective of the route of infection (contaminated drinking water, person-to-person transmission, food poisoning), can be identified from SNIIRAM using a specifically developed algorithm detailed elsewhere [7]. Using the algorithm, medicalized AGI cases were selected from people who consulted a general practitioner and went to a pharmacy to buy medications prescribed to treat AGI. To be included, the individual had also to meet a set of conditions regarding the delay of purchase after the visit to doctor, and the combination of drugs prescribed. A national survey study showed that 33% of individuals with symptomatic AGI consulted a doctor in France [19]. Cases were aggregated by day and residence zip code at the municipality level (note: *départements* are comprised of smaller municipal areas).

2.3. Simulation Study

Several steps were implemented to simulate WBDOs (Figure 1).

We simulated the daily baseline counts of AGI at the zip code level using the SNIIRAM data. A variety of simulated WBDO signals were then superimposed on the baseline data. The simulation study was based on a methodology developed to evaluate the performance of an algorithm for outbreak detection of infectious diseases, which met the objectives of our study [15].

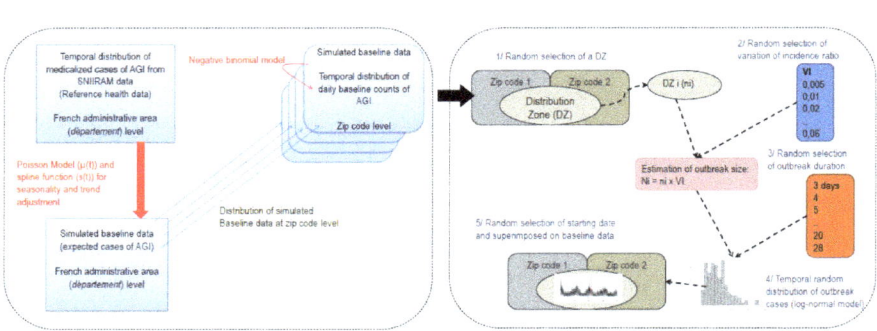

DZ: distribution zone, WBDO: waterborne disease outbreak, VI: variation of incidence ratio; ni: population serviced by DZi; Ni: outbreak size

Figure 1. Algorithm of the overall process for simulation of baseline data and WBDOs. SNIRAM: *Système national d'information inter régimes de l'Assurance maladie* (the French Health Insurance Administrative Database); AGI: acute gastrointestinal infection.

2.4. Simulation of Baseline Data

Baseline counts of AGI were first generated at the *département* level (1) and then at the zip code level (2).

(1) A Poisson regression was used to model the daily observed counts of AGI at the *département* level (SNIIRAM data). A thin-plate regression spline [20] was used to model trend and seasonality

in order to account for the seasonality of the AGI, in particular the variability of winter viral pandemic of AGI. Adjustments were made for days of the week and holidays [21].

(2) The estimated expected values obtained from the regression model at (1) were then distributed at the zip code level in proportion to the number of cases observed in the SNIIRAM data. Finally, to introduce stochasticity, daily counts of AGI cases were simulated using a negative binomial distribution [15,21] (Figure 2).

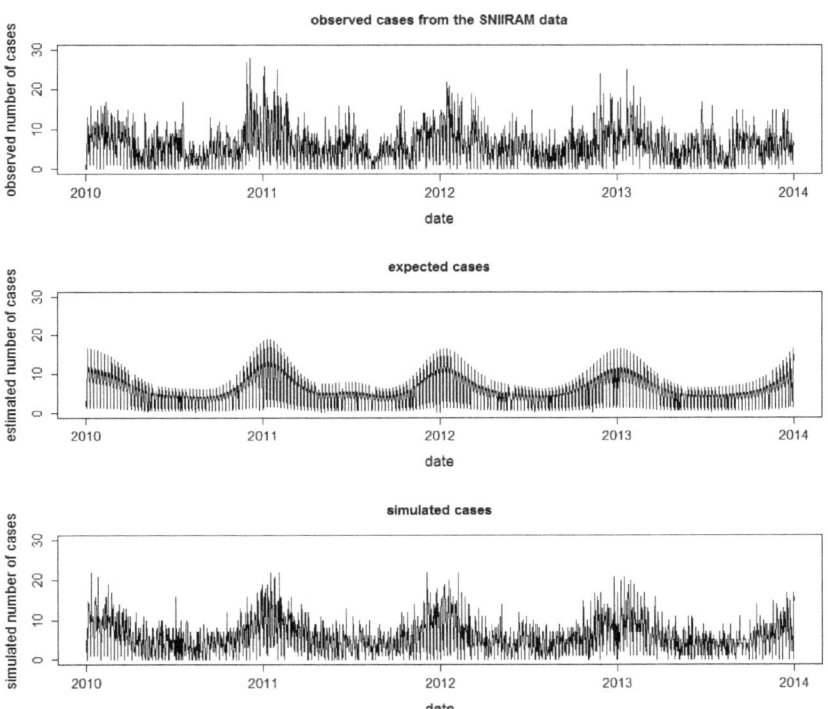

Figure 2. Simulation of time series of incident AGI cases before the inclusion of the simulated WBDO: daily number of observed AGI cases from the French Health Insurance Administrative Database (SNIIRAM) between 1 January 2010 and 31 December 2013 (*n* = 8677) (**top**), number of estimated expected cases (**middle**), and number of simulated cases (**bottom**) for a zip code with 18,541 inhabitants.

2.5. The Simulation Process of Waterborne Disease Outbreaks

The spatial unit of interest for the WBDO simulation in our study was the DZ. By definition, a DZ delivers water of homogenous quality to consumers, meaning that all people serviced by the same DZ are exposed to the same risk in terms of water quality apart from situations of backflows, and where contamination directly enters the network. There are 25,000 DZs and 35,000 zip codes in France. As the health outcome (i.e., AGI cases) was simulated at the zip code level, when the selected DZ serviced more than one zip code, AGI outbreak daily cases were distributed according to the proportion of inhabitants serviced by the DZ in each zip code [22].

1. DZs were randomly selected. DZs servicing fewer than 200 inhabitants were excluded from the simulation study to ensure statistical power of detection and because of their reduced impact on public health.

2. For each simulation, the variation of incidence ratio (VI), defined as the proportion between the number of outbreak AGI cases and the number of expected cases of AGI (baseline data) during the outbreak period, was randomly selected between 0.5% and 6%. These values were chosen according to what we observed in previous WBDOs [10].

3. The outbreak duration was randomly selected between 3 and 28 days in accordance with the observed values in reported WBDOs [6].

4. The outbreak size, that is, the number of AGI cases in the outbreak, was generated by multiplying the VI by the number of inhabitants serviced by the DZ.

5. Finally, outbreak cases were distributed over time according to a log-normal distribution [15,21] (Figure 3). The parameters of the log-normal distribution used to shape the time distribution of the outbreak AGI cases were randomly chosen between 0.33 and 0.5 for the median, and fixed at 0.5 for the standard deviation [10,21]. When the selected DZ serviced more than one zip code, daily cases in the AGI outbreak were then distributed according to the proportion of inhabitants serviced by the DZ in each zip code.

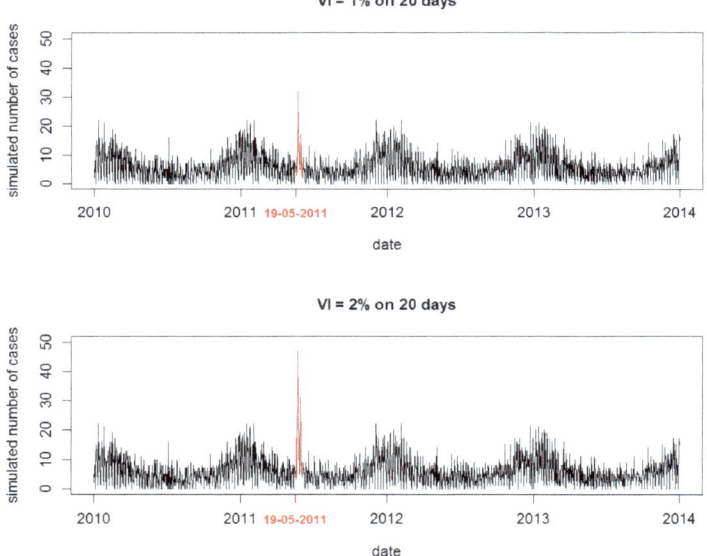

Figure 3. Illustration of two simulated outbreaks starting on 22 September 2011 in a zip code of 18,541 inhabitants serviced by only one DZ, with a variation of incidence ratio (VI) of 1% (**top**) and 2% (**bottom**), and with a 20-day duration.

A total of 2000 simulations were run (1000 for each of the two French *départements* studied). Each simulated set included the simulation of the baseline data and a WBDO.

The simulation study was performed using the R software version 3.3.0 (R foundation for Statistical Computing, Vienna, Austria).

2.6. Detection of Simulated Waterborne Disease Outbreaks

The WBDO detection method used is detailed elsewhere [11]. First, an algorithm was used for grouping zip codes (and corresponding AGI cases) which share the same DZ so that tap water exposure could be taken into account in the detection process. Then the space–time permutation scan statistic developed by Kulldorff et al. [12] was applied to grouped zip codes. The scan statistic was based on overlapping cylinders to define a scanning window. In our study, the scanning window is represented by grouping zip codes sharing the same DZ and defined by the algorithm.

With a space–time permutation scan statistic, expected cases are calculated using observed cases. A generalized likelihood ratio is then used as a measure of the evidence that a tested cylinder contains an outbreak (i.e., number of observed cases exceeds the number you would typically expect to see in a comparable period of time). The cylinder with the maximum generalized likelihood ratio constitutes the space–time cluster of cases least likely to occur by chance, and consequently it is the primary candidate for a true outbreak. Within the space–time permutation model, adjustments were made for days of the week and holidays.

This detection study was performed using SaTScan version 9.3 [23] and R version 3.3.0.

2.7. Data Analysis

2.7.1. Evaluation Method

The running of the scan on the simulated dataset generated a set of clusters. All clusters associated with a statistical threshold (*p*-value) of 0.05 were considered, whether they revealed a true alarm (i.e., WBDO detected) or not. A true alarm was declared if at least one detected day and one detected zip code corresponded to the days and zip codes involved in the simulated WBDOs [15]. The other clusters were considered as false alarms.

To evaluate the performance of the WBDO detection method we considered the sensitivity (Se) and the positive predictive value (PPV). Sensitivity was estimated as the ratio between the true alarm and the number of simulated WBDOs (i.e., 1000 WBDOs generated per administrative area). The PPV was defined as the ratio between the number of true alarm and the number of all the clusters detected associated with a statistical threshold of 0.05. The Se and VPP were described by administrative area, by DZ size (inhabitants served), by outbreak size, and by season.

2.7.2. Factors Associated with WBDO Detection

A multivariate Poisson regression was performed on true alarms to identify the factors associated with WBDO detection and to estimate the strength of these associations [21]. Five dependent variables were considered: outbreak duration, size of the DZ population, outbreak incidence ratio, outbreak size, and season ("winter" for December, January, February and March/"other seasons" for April to November). We tested for potential interactions among these factors. Incidence rate ratios (IRRs) and their 95% confidence intervals (CIs) were computed. The IRR is the ratio between the incidence rate in a considered group and the incidence rate in the reference group. All analyses were performed using Stata 12.0 (StataCorp LP, College Station, TX, USA).

3. Results

3.1. Description of Simulated WBDO

Simulated WBDOs involved between 1 and 7392 AGI outbreak cases (median = 22; mean = 96). Most (90%) included 200 AGI cases or fewer (Table 1). The mean outbreak duration was 15 days (3 to 28 days). All DZ sizes were represented: 35.8% of the randomly selected DZs serviced 200 to 500 people, 21.9% between 500 and 1000 people, 15.5% between 1000 and 2000 people, 21.1% between 2000 and 10,000, and 5.9% more than 10,000 people. Among all the simulated WBDOs, 26.7% (*n* = 534/2000) involved a DZ which serviced more than one zip code: 162 WBDOs generated for Isere with 2 to 13 zip codes were serviced by the same DZ, and 372 WBDOs for Puy-de-Dôme with 2 to 53 zip codes were serviced by the same DZ.

Table 1. Description of simulated WBDOs by *département*.

Variables	n	Both *départments*					Puy-de-Dôme					Isère				
		Total	Detected	%	Undetected	%	Total	Detected	%	Undetected	%	Total	Detected	%	Undetected	%
		2000	1460		540		1000	726		274		1000	734		266	
DZ size (number of inhabitants served by DZ)																
	200–500	715	353	49.4	362	50.6	385	201	52.2	184	47.8	330	152	46.1	178	53.9
	501–1000	437	330	75.5	107	24.5	204	153	75.0	51	25.0	233	177	76.0	56	24.0
	1001–2000	309	264	85.4	45	14.6	128	107	83.6	21	16.4	181	157	86.7	24	13.3
	200–10,000	421	396	94.1	25	5.9	188	171	91.0	17	9.0	233	225	96.6	8	3.4
	>10,000	118	117	99.2	1	0.8	95	94	98.9	1	1.1	23	23	100.0	0	0.0
Outbreak size (number of simulated cases of AGI)																
	Min	1	5		1		2	6		2		1	5		1	
	p10	5	11		2		5	11		2		5	12		2	
	Median	22	38		6		22	35		6		23	39		6	
	Mean	96.2	128.8		8.1		122.5	165.3		8.9		69.9	92.6		7.3	
	p90	199	271		14		255	412		15		140	187		14	
	Max	7392	7392		133		5551	5551		133		7392	7392		33	
Duration (days)																
	Min	3	3		3		3	3		3		3	3		3	
	Median	16	15		17		15	14		16		16	15		18	
	Mean	15.4	15.0		16.4		15.2	14.8		16.3		15.6	15.2		16.5	
	Max	28	28		28		28	28		28		28	28		28	
DZ area (number of municipalities served)																
	1	1466	1042	71.1	424	28.9	628	445	70.9	183	29.1	838	597	71.2	241	28.8
	>1	534	418	78.3	116	21.7	372	281	75.5	91	24.5	162	137	84.6	25	15.4
Season																
	Winter	605	414	68.4	191	31.6	298	199	66.8	99	33.2	307	215	70.0	92	30.0
	Other seasons	1395	1046	75.0	349	25.0	702	527	75.1	175	24.9	693	519	74.9	174	25.1

3.2. Sensitivity and Positive Predictive Value of the Detection Method

Almost three-quarters of the 2000 simulated WBDOs were detected (sensitivity = 73.0%). More than 9 out of 10 detected signals corresponded to a simulated WBDO (PPV = 90.5%). Sensitivity increased with DZ size and with outbreak size (Table 2). Moreover, WBDOs in non-winter seasons (hereafter "other seasons") were better detected than WBDO simulated during the winter season. Indeed, to reach the same sensitivity value of 75%, WBDO size had to be greater in the winter season than in other seasons (at least 15 cases versus 10 cases) (Figure 4).

Table 2. Sensitivity and predictive positive value of the detection method according to outbreak size, distribution zone (DZ) size, season, and DZ area.

Variables	Total Se %	Total Se N1	Total PPV %	Total PPV N2	Isère Se %	Isère Se N1	Isère PPV %	Isère PPV N2	Puy-de-Dôme Se %	Puy-de-Dôme Se N1	Puy-de-Dôme PPV %	Puy-de-Dôme PPV N2
	73.0	2000	90.5	1614	73.4	1000	89.0	825	72.6	1000	92.0	789
DZ size (number of inhabitants served by DZ)												
200–500	49.3	715	88.0	401	46.0	330	82.1	185	52.2	385	93.0	216
501–1000	75.5	437	91.4	361	75.9	233	92.6	191	75.0	204	90.0	170
1001–2000	85.4	309	92.9	284	86.7	181	91.2	172	83.5	128	95.5	112
2001–10,000	94.0	421	91.4	433	96.5	233	89.2	252	90.9	188	94.4	181
>10,000	99.1	118	86.6	135	100.0	23	92.0	25	98.9	95	85.4	110
Outbreak size (number of simulated cases)												
1–10	15.2	466	77.1	92	13.8	224	77.5	40	16.5	242	76.9	52
11–15	68.5	312	91.4	234	64.6	150	85.8	113	72.2	162	96.6	121
16–20	86.4	170	91.8	160	83.3	90	90.3	83	90.0	80	93.5	77
21–50	95.3	449	90.8	471	97.9	240	89.0	264	92.3	209	93.2	207
>50	99.5	603	91.3	657	100.0	296	91.0	325	99.0	307	91.5	332
Season												
Winter *	68.4	605	87.7	472	70.0	307	84.3	255	66.7	298	91.7	217
Other season	74.9	1395	91.5	1142	74.8	693	91.0	570	75.0	702	92.1	572
DZ area (number of municipalities served)												
1	71.0	1466	90.2	1155	71.2	838	88.7	673	70.8	628	92.3	482
>1	78.2	534	91.0	459	84.5	162	90.1	152	75.5	372	91.5	307

Se: sensitivity; PPV: positive predictive value; N1: number of WBDO simulated; N2: number of clusters detected with *p*-value $\leq$ 0.05; DZ: distribution zone; * Winter: December, January, February, March.

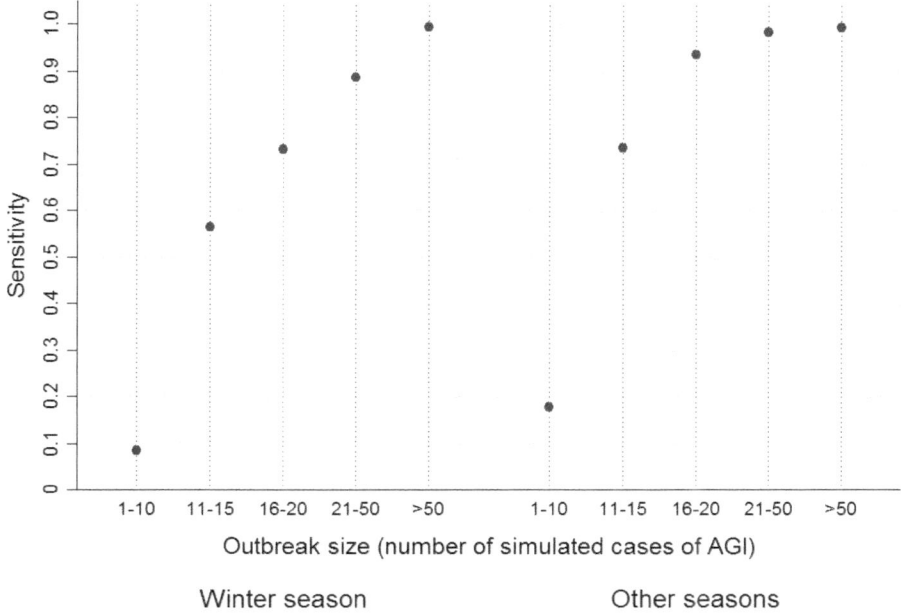

Figure 4. Sensitivity of detection method according to outbreak size (number of simulated AGI cases) and season (winter: December, January, February, March).

For WBDOs occurring in more than one zip code (a total of 534 for both departments studied), the sensitivity of detection was higher than for WBDO associated with a DZ servicing only one zip code (78.3% and 71.1%, respectively), while the PPV was stable (90.2% versus 91.1%, respectively). For half of the WBDOs associated with a DZ servicing several zip codes, 80% of these zip codes were included in the detected signal for Isere and 50% for Puy-de-Dôme.

The undetected WBDOs involved mostly small DZ (200–500 inhabitants) and few outbreak cases (Table 1).

3.3. Factors Associated with WBDO Detection

In the multivariate Poisson regression, the outbreak size, the VI, and the duration and the season of WBDOs were all significantly associated with detection (Table 3). The interaction of VI and the outbreak size was significant. WBDOs involving at least 10 AGI cases, with a 14-day duration or less, and occurring between April and November, had a higher probability of being detected. The variable "outbreak size" had the strongest association with detection.

Table 3. Final multivariate regression model with factors significantly associated with WBDO detection, stratified by variation of the incidence ratio.

Variables	VI: 0.5%–2.0%			VI: 2.0%–4.0%			VI: 4.0%–6.0%		
	n = 642	IRR	[95% CI]	n = 659	IRR	[95% CI]	n = 699	IRR	[95% CI]
Outbreak size (number of simulated cases)									
1–10	331	ref		129	ref		6	ref	
11–15	79	7.70	[5.03–11.74]	130	2.01	[1.55–2.61]	103	1.59	[0.71–3.58]
16–20	40	10.30	[6.79–15.60]	51	2.62	[2.02–3.39]	79	1.91	[0.86–4.28]
21–50	96	12.80	[8.71–18.82]	151	2.85	[2.24–3.62]	202	1.96	[0.88–4.37]
>50	96	13.70	[9.29–20.07]	198	2.92	[2.30–3.70]	309	2.03	[0.91–4.53]
Season									
Winter *	193	ref		193	ref		219	ref	
Other seasons	449	1.37	[1.20–1.56]	466	1.11	[1.03–1.19]	480	1.05	[1.01–1.10]
Outbreak duration (days)									
3–7	131	ref		136	ref		133	ref	
8–14	173	0.84	[0.73–0.97]	180	1.00	[0.92–1.09]	184	0.97	[0.94–1.01]
15–21	178	0.77	[0.66–0.90]	170	0.89	[0.81–0.97]	178	0.94	[0.90–0.99]
22–28	160	0.64	[0.54–0.76]	173	0.89	[0.81–0.98]	204	0.93	[0.89–0.97]

VI: variation of the incidence ratio; IRR: incidence rate ratio; CI: confidence Interval; WBDO: waterborne disease outbreak; * winter: December, January, February, March.

4. Discussion

4.1. Simulation Process

The first step of this simulation-based study was to generate the baseline incidence of the disease. This step employed a published method [15] adapted for AGI epidemiology by adding a flexible adjustment function (spline) to account for high winter incidence of AGIs due to the enteric virus outbreak. Days of the week and holidays were adjusted for to reflect the closure of pharmacies during weekends and holidays. This ensured an acceptable representativeness of seasonality and of AGI incidence (Figure 1).

Simulated WBDOs were generated using a log-normal distribution model [15]. The parameters used to build these epidemic signals were inspired by past outbreaks of waterborne AGIs. Accordingly, the chosen epidemic duration ranging (from 3 to 28 days) and the chosen VI (between 0.5% and 6%) are realistic. When compared with the health impact of WBDOs assessed in cohort studies in which the attack rate varied between 30% and 50%, the AGI outbreak cases observed in SNIIRAM data are less frequent. This difference is probably due to several factors, including healthcare-seeking behaviors: in France, the mean consultation rate for AGI is quite low at 32% [19] and depends on age and pathogen agent. The true distribution of cases during outbreaks is described in a previous article which compared, for two WBDOs, the true distribution of cases identified in cohort studies among the impacted population and the true distribution of medicalized cases identified in the SNIIRAM database [10]. Results highlighted a good temporal correlation between both data sources. Moreover, a descriptive study of 11 WBDOs reported in France between 1998 and 2006 gives the main parameters of outbreak distributions [6].

One limitation of this study was the choice not to perform WBDO simulations for DZ servicing fewer than 200 inhabitants. This prevented us from being able to evaluate the algorithm for these DZs. However the public health concern is less important for these small zip codes.

Another limitation regards the use of the SNIIRAM database. Disease severity associated with an epidemic may be a criterion that influences control measures. Nevertheless, medicalized AGI cases (i.e., those who consulted a doctor and subsequently went to the pharmacy with a prescription) identified from the health insurance database cannot be distinguished in terms of illness severity in the absence of a specific association between severity and the drugs prescribed. This said, medicalized AGI cases represented almost 32% of AGI cases in one French national survey [19]. In that study, less than 1% of all individuals with an AGI went to a hospital for consultation. The main reported reasons for consulting were: prolonged symptoms (49%), vomiting (31%), diarrhea (28%), and unusual symptoms (27%). The main reasons for not consulting were: quick recovery/no serious symptoms (64%) and feeling that a consultation was not necessary (47%). After multivariate analysis, gender, age, duration of illness, and symptoms (headache) were associated with consultation for AGIs. Given these results, AGI medicalized cases can be considered as the most severe cases.

4.2. Algorithm Performance for WBDO Detection

Globally, the algorithm has a high sensitivity (detecting 73% of simulated WBDOs) and a high positive predictive value among the detected signals (90.5% corresponded to simulated WBDOs). These indicators reached, respectively, 99.2% and 86.7%, for DZs servicing more than 10,000 people (Table 2). The performance (sensitivity and positive predictive value) of the algorithm mainly depended on the serviced population size and the outbreak size. The influence of the season and the number of zip codes served by the same DZ were less important (Tables 2 and 3). If we focus on the influence of the serviced population size, a threshold of 500 inhabitants resulted in increased sensitivity, from 50% (fewer than 500 people served) to more than 75% (more than 500 people served) of detected WBDO. Likewise, when the outbreak size exceeded 10 AGI cases, the sensitivity was four times greater than with smaller outbreaks (10 cases or fewer). For these two parameters, the most significant variations in sensitivity were observed when between 200 and 2000 people were serviced (from 49.4% to 94.1%,

Int. J. Environ. Res. Public Health **2018**, *15*, 1505

respectively) and between fewer than 10 AGI cases to over 50 (17.2% and 99.3%). Nevertheless, the 10-case sensitivity threshold should be treated with caution and is not the main consideration for the implementation of surveillance system of WBDO. With respect to the positive predictive value, there is no outbreak size threshold which could influence detection. Therefore, the criterion for considering large epidemics or large DZ is a criterion of public health efficiency (avoided cost from an avoided case).

4.3. Factors Influencing Detection

In addition to the evaluation of the performance of the detection algorithm, the simulation study also allowed us to identify and quantify the three factors which most influence the performance of WBDO detection as follows: outbreak size, duration and season ("winter" or "other seasons"). The existence of a significant interaction between the outbreak size and the variation of incidence led us to consider the results according to three classifications of the incidence ratio (0.5% to 2%; 2% to 4%; 4% to 6%) (Table 3).

From the results of our analysis, outbreak size had the strongest association with detection sensitivity, especially for a variation of incidence value below 4%. Above this value, outbreak size was no longer associated with detection. For variation of incidence rate between 0.5% and 2%, the outbreak size has a dominant effect (vis-à-vis duration and season), with a detection capacity 13 times greater for an outbreak of 20 AGI cases or more than for an outbreak of 10 or fewer cases (the incidence rate ratio is 7.7 when going from fewer than 10 cases to 15 cases). For a variation of incidence between 2% and 6%, the detection ratio (IRR) did not exceed 3 between the most extreme values (more than 50 cases versus fewer than 10 cases). These results suggest a strong improvement in detection ability for WBDOs with more than 10 AGI cases and a variation of incidence greater than 2%. These values are consistent with the previous study's results which described the detection algorithm and its application to real health data [11]. Of the 11 clusters detected in this study, the values of the medication rate in the population (indicator close to the variation of incidence) ranged from 0.7% to 4.8%, and the cluster size from 21 to 67 AGI cases.

As mentioned above, "duration" and "season" also affected detection but much less substantially than outbreak size. WBDOs with a lower variation of incidence (0.5–2%) were primarily affected by these three factors. Accordingly, the number of detected WBDO was 1.3 times higher in non-winter season outbreaks of AGI. Similarly, outbreaks which lasted less than 14 days were better detected than longer outbreaks.

4.4. International Comparison

To our knowledge, few previously published simulation studies on WBDO detection exist. Different Canadian research studies have presented an agent-based simulation model for generating realistic multivariable outbreak signals [24]. This model was used to simulate a WBDO caused by *Cryptosporidium*, taking into account parameters for population, water consumption, and disease progression. To verify whether the simulation model produced credible results, the authors attempted to replicate the largest documented WBDO of cryptosporidiosis, which occurred in Milwaukee in 1993. During that outbreak, over 400,000 people were estimated to have diarrhea attributable to acute *Cryptosporidium* infection [5]. The results showed that the simulated curve was slightly more positively skewed and peaked one to two days earlier than the historically observed curves. These simulated data were then used to improve early outbreak detection using a hidden Markov model [25].

Although French health insurance data constitute an adequate source for the retrospective surveillance of WBDO, they do not allow—at least for the moment—the possibility of implementing a prospective approach within the context of a public health alert system.

5. Conclusions

Our study presents a global approach for simulating AGI baseline data using reference health data and superimposing simulated WBDOs. The algorithm for WBDO detection was evaluated as being able to detect almost 90% of WBDOs, with few false positive alarms. We also estimated the factors which most influence WBDO detection. The results of our study underline the value of using the detection algorithm for the implementation of a national surveillance system for WBDOs in France upon which to base public health action.

Author Contributions: Conceptualization, D.M., S.G., M.M., P.B., C.G., A.G., C.D. and Y.L.S.; Data curation, S.G. and M.M.; Formal analysis, D.M. and S.G.; Methodology, S.G., P.B., C.G., A.G., C.D. and Y.L.S.; Project administration, D.M., A.G. and C.D.; Software, M.M.; Supervision, D.M.; Validation, Y.L.S.; Writing—original draft, D.M.; Writing—review & editing, D.M., S.G., P.B., A.G., C.D. and Y.L.S.

Funding: This research received no external funding.

Acknowledgments: The authors wish to express their appreciation and gratitude to the National Health Insurance for access to data from SNIIRAM, to Magali Corso of the French national public health agency for the preparation of case data of acute gastroenteritis using this data, to Loïc Rambaud of the French national public health agency for his contribution to the conceptualization of the study, to the Health Ministry and Henri Davezac for water data drawn from the Sise-Eaux database, and to Farida Mihoub and Jude Sweeney for their help in translating and revising the English version of the manuscript.

Conflicts of Interest: The authors declare no conflicts of interest.

References

1. Craun, G.F.; Brunkard, J.M.; Yoder, J.S.; Roberts, V.A.; Carpenter, J.; Wade, T.; Calderon, R.L.; Roberts, J.M.; Beach, M.J.; Roy, S.L. Causes of outbreaks associated with drinking water in the United States from 1971 to 2006. *Clin. Microbiol. Rev.* **2010**, *23*, 507–528. [CrossRef] [PubMed]

2. Hrudey, S.E.; Hrudey, E.J. *Safe Drinking Water: Lessons from Recent Outbreaks in Affluent Nations*; IWA Publishing: London, UK, 2004.

3. Widerstrom, M.; Schonning, C.; Lilja, M.; Lebbad, M.; Ljung, T.; Allestam, G.; Ferm, M.; Bjorkholm, B.; Hansen, A.; Hiltula, J.; et al. Large outbreak of Cryptosporidium hominis infection transmitted through the public water supply, Sweden. *Emerg. Infect. Dis.* **2014**, *20*, 581–589. [CrossRef] [PubMed]

4. Rehn, M.; Wallensten, A.; Widerstrom, M.; Lilja, M.; Grunewald, M.; Stenmark, S.; Kark, M.; Lindh, J. Post-infection symptoms following two large waterborne outbreaks of Cryptosporidium hominis in Northern Sweden, 2010–2011. *BMC Public Health* **2015**, *15*, 529. [CrossRef] [PubMed]

5. MacKenzie, W.R.; Schell, W.L.; Blair, K.A.; Addiss, D.G.; Peterson, D.E.; Hoxie, N.J.; Kazmierczak, J.J.; Davis, J.P. Massive outbreak of waterborne cryptosporidium infection in Milwaukee, Wisconsin: Recurrence of illness and risk of secondary transmission. *Clin. Infect. Dis.* **1995**, *21*, 57–62. [CrossRef] [PubMed]

6. Beaudeau, P.; De Valk, H.; Vaillant, V.; Mannschott, C.; Tillier, C.; Mouly, D.; Ledrans, M. Lessons learned from ten investigations of waterborne gastroenteritis outbreaks, France, 1998–2006. *J. Water Health* **2008**, *6*, 491–503. [CrossRef] [PubMed]

7. Bounoure, F.; Beaudeau, P.; Mouly, D.; Skiba, M.; Lahiani-Skiba, M. Syndromic surveillance of acute gastroenteritis based on drug consumption. *Epidemiol. Infect.* **2011**, *139*, 1388–1395. [CrossRef] [PubMed]

8. Beaudeau, P. Syndromic Surveillance of Acute Gastroenteritis: An Opportunity for the Prevention of the Infectious Risk Attributable to Tap Water. Ph.D. Thesis, Université de Rennes, Rennes, France, 2012.

9. Beaudeau, P.; Le Tertre, A.; Zeghnoun, A.; Zanobetti, A.; Schwartz, J. A time series study of drug sales and turbidity of tap water in Le Havre, France. *J. Water Health* **2012**, *10*, 221–235. [CrossRef] [PubMed]

10. Mouly, D.; Van Cauteren, D.; Vincent, N.; Vaissiere, E.; Beaudeau, P.; Ducrot, C.; Gallay, A. Description of two waterborne disease outbreaks in France: A comparative study with data from cohort studies and from health administrative databases. *Epidemiol. Infect.* **2016**, *144*, 591–601. [CrossRef] [PubMed]

11. Coly, S.; Vincent, N.; Vaissiere, E.; Charras-Garridol, M.; Gallay, A.; Ducrot, C.; Mouly, D. Waterborne disease outbreaks detection: An integrated approach using health administrative databases. *J. Water Health* **2017**. [CrossRef] [PubMed]

12. Kulldorff, M.; Heffernan, R.; Hartman, J.; Assuncao, R.; Mostashari, F. A space-time permutation scan statistic for disease outbreak detection. *PLoS Med.* **2005**, *2*, e59. [CrossRef] [PubMed]

13. Rambaud, L.; Galey, C.; Beaudeau, P. Automated detection of case clusters of waterborne acute gastroenteritis from health insurance data—Pilot study in three French districts. *J. Water Health* **2016**, *14*, 306–316. [CrossRef] [PubMed]

14. Goria, S.; Mouly, D.; Rambaud, L.; Guillet, A.; Beaudeau, P.; Galey, C. *Evaluation of Different Methods of Detection of Aggregates of Cases of Medicalized Acute Waterborne Gastroenteritis*; Santé Publique France: Saint Maurice, France, 2017.
15. Noufaily, A.; Enki, D.G.; Farrington, P.; Garthwaite, P.; Andrews, N.; Charlett, A. An improved algorithm for outbreak detection in multiple surveillance systems. *Stat. Med.* **2013**, *32*, 1206–1222. [CrossRef] [PubMed]
16. Buckeridge, D.L.; Jauvin, C.; Okhmatovskaia, A.; Verma, A.D. Simulation Analysis Platform (SnAP): A tool for evaluation of public health surveillance and disease control strategies. *Annu. Symp. Proc.* **2011**, *2011*, 161–170.
17. Insee. Available online: https://www.insee.fr (accessed on 8 December 2015).
18. Tuppin, P.; Rudant, J.; Constantinou, P.; Gastaldi-Ménager, C.; Rachas, A.; De Roquefeuil, L.; Maura, G.; Caillol, H.; Tajahmady, A.; Coste, J.; et al. Value of a national administrative database to guide public decisions: From the système national d'information interrégimes de l'Assurance Maladie (SNIIRAM) to the système national des donneés de santé (SNDS) in France. *J. Epidemiol. Community Health* **2017**, *65S*, 149–167. [CrossRef] [PubMed]
19. Van Cauteren, D.; De Valk, H.; Vaux, S.; Le Strat, Y.; Vaillant, V. Burden of acute gastroenteritis and healthcare-seeking behaviour in France: A population-based study. *Epidemiol. Infect.* **2012**, *140*, 697–705. [CrossRef] [PubMed]
20. Wood, S.N. *Generalized Additive Models: An Introduction with R*; Chapman and Hall: Boca Raton, FL, USA, 2006.
21. Buckeridge, D.L.; Okhmatovskaia, A.; Tu, S.; O'Connor, M.; Nyulas, C.; Musen, M.A. Predicting outbreak detection in public health surveillance: Quantitative analysis to enable evidence-based method selection. *Annu. Symp. Proc.* **2008**, *15*, 76–80.
22. French Ministry of Health. *French Database on Public Drinking Water Quality*; French Ministry of Health: Paris, France, 2011.
23. Kulldorff, M. *SaTScanTM v8.0: Software for the Spatial and Space-Time Scan Statistics*; Information Management Services, Inc.: Calverton, MD, USA, 2006.
24. Okhmatovskaia, A.; Verma, A.D.; Barbeau, B.; Carriere, A.; Pasquet, R.; Buckeridge, D.L. A simulation model of waterborne gastro-intestinal disease outbreaks: Description and initial evaluation. *Annu. Symp. Proc.* **2010**, *2010*, 557–561.
25. Morrison, K.; Charland, K.; Okhmatovskaia, A.; Buckeridge, D. A Framework for Detecting and Classifying Outbreaks of Gastrointestinal Disease. *Online J. Public Health Inform.* **2013**, *5*. [CrossRef]

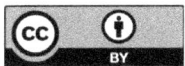

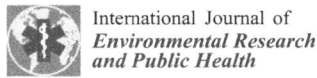

Article

The Seasonality of Nitrite Concentrations in a Chloraminated Drinking Water Distribution System

Pirjo-Liisa Rantanen [1,*], Ilkka Mellin [2], Minna M. Keinänen-Toivola [3], Merja Ahonen [3] and Riku Vahala [1]

[1] Department of Built Environment, School of Engineering, Aalto University, 02150 Espoo, Finland; riku.vahala@aalto.fi
[2] Department of Mathematics and Systems Analysis, Aalto University, School of Science, 02150 Espoo, Finland; ilkka.mellin@aalto.fi
[3] Faculty of Technology, Satakunta University of Applied Sciences, 26101 Rauma, Finland; minna.keinanen-toivola@samk.fi (M.M.K.-T.); merja.ahonen@samk.fi (M.A.)
* Correspondence: pirjo.rantanen@aalto.fi

Received: 28 June 2018; Accepted: 10 August 2018; Published: 15 August 2018

Abstract: We studied the seasonal variation of nitrite exposure in a drinking water distribution system (DWDS) with monochloramine disinfection in the Helsinki Metropolitan Area. In Finland, tap water is the main source of drinking water, and thus the nitrite in tap water increases nitrite exposure. Our data included both the obligatory monitoring and a sampling campaign data from a sampling campaign. Seasonality was evaluated by comparing a nitrite time series to temperature and by calculating the seasonal indices of the nitrite time series. The main drivers of nitrite seasonality were the temperature and the water age. We observed that with low water ages (median: 6.7 h) the highest nitrite exposure occurred during the summer months, and with higher water ages (median: 31 h) during the winter months. With the highest water age (190 h), nitrite concentrations were the lowest. At a low temperature, the high nitrite concentrations in the winter were caused by the decelerated ammonium oxidation. The dominant reaction at low water ages was ammonium oxidation into nitrite and, at high water ages, it was nitrite oxidation into nitrate. These results help to direct monitoring appropriately to gain exact knowledge of nitrite exposure. Also, possible future process changes and additional disinfection measures can be designed appropriately to minimize extra nitrite exposure.

Keywords: nitrite; disinfection by-product; drinking water distribution systems; seasonality

1. Introduction

Disinfection of drinking water is necessary to maintain hygienically good water quality in large drinking water distribution systems (DWDSs). When monochloramine (NH_2Cl) is used for secondary disinfection in DWDSs, nitrite is quite often formed as a disinfection by-product (DBP). Nitrite is a potentially harmful compound when ingested by humans. In humans, nitrite can cause methemoglobinemia, which is a specific type of anemia. Infants younger than one year are more susceptible to methemoglobinemia than older children and adults. In methemoglobinemia, nitrite reacts with the hemoglobin of blood and disrupts oxygen transfer [1]. Furthermore, nitrite has been observed to cause several types of cancer in animals and may potentially do so in humans. Moreover, nitrite has been found to be potentially cancerous in animal tests, when ingested together with amines and amides or in conditions where the formation of organic nitroso compounds is possible [2].

Monochloramine is often favored in secondary disinfection because it significantly reduces the formation of trihalomethanes and other chlorination by-products compared to other forms of chlorine [3]. Nevertheless, when monochloramine decomposes in disinfection or during other reactions, ammonium is formed. Frequently, ammonium reacts to form nitrite in a biochemical oxidation reaction, called nitrification, in the biofilms on the inner surface of the pipes and reservoirs of the DWDS. In such cases, typical nitrite concentrations are 0.05–0.5 mgN l^{-1}, but concentrations above 1 mgN l^{-1} have been observed in the stagnant parts of some DWDSs [4,5]. Furthermore, nitrite concentrations in drinking water can originate from polluted groundwater [6]. Due to the potential toxicity of nitrite, its concentrations are regulated in drinking water. In Finland, the statutory limit for nitrite in drinking water is 0.5 mg l^{-1} (0.15 mgN l^{-1}) [7], following EU legislation [8]. The statutory limits require constant monitoring of the nitrite concentrations in distributed drinking water.

This article discusses the seasonal patterns of nitrite concentrations in drinking water. A term often connected to monochloramine use in DWDSs is a nitrification episode, which in itself implies that nitrification and nitrite occur in relation to time and location. Nevertheless, very few actual studies of nitrite seasonality in DWDSs exist. Wilczak et al. [4] studied the seasonality of nitrite concentrations in summer and winter conditions and observed that the majority of the water samples with increased nitrite in the DWDS were collected in the summer. However, elevated nitrite concentrations occurred during the winter conditions also. Schullehner et al. [6] conducted a large and systematic research of nitrite in Danish distributed groundwater that contained nitrite pollution, but did not find any seasonality. The number of ammonia oxidizing bacteria (AOB) in DWDSs has been found to be higher in summer than in winter [9–11]. In a 15-month study, Pinto et al. [12] found distinct seasonality in the bacterial dynamics of a DWDS using monochloramine. Stanish et al. [13] noted that in DWDSs with seasonal monochloramine use, the monochloramine increased the abundances of nitrifiers and *Nitrospira*-like organisms. In connection to nitrification episodes in DWDSs, *N*-nitrosodimethylamine (NDMA) and other DBPs have also been found to increase [14]. Woods et al. found NDMA to occur in higher concentrations at a lower temperature in a large urban DWDS [15].

In Finland, the main source of drinking water is tap water. The consumption of bottled water in 2016 was 14 l cap^{-1}, which was only 13% of the European average [16]. Thus, the nitrite formed from the added monochloramine in the DWDSs is ingested with the drinking water and increases the nitrite exposure. Consequently, the production of drinking water is compelled to keep a balance between preserving the good microbiological quality of the distributed water and the nitrite formation in the DWDS. For this purpose, precise knowledge of the nitrite formation is required. In this research, we studied the nitrite concentrations of the distributed drinking water in the Helsinki Metropolitan Area, Finland. The aim of the study was to evaluate how the nitrite exposure originating from the added chloramine is distributed seasonally and what the main drivers leading to seasonality are.

2. Materials and Methods

2.1. Water Quality Monitoring Data

In the Helsinki Metropolitan Area, the monitoring of the quality of distributed drinking water is organized by the local water company, the Helsinki Region Environmental Services Authority (HSY). The company has two main drinking water treatment plants (WTPs), located at Pitkäkoski and Vanhakaupunki. The annual drinking water production of HSY was 89.7 Mm^3 in 2015 [17]. Monochloramine is used in both WTPs for secondary disinfection, and nitrite concentrations have been observed to increase in the DWDSs [18,19]. The target ratio of chlorine and ammonia when feeding the chemicals is 4 mg Cl$_2$ l^{-1} per 1 mgN l^{-1}, and the target concentration of total chlorine in the freshly produced potable water is 0.35–0.4 mg Cl$_2$ l^{-1}. The general quality of the produced drinking water is displayed in Table 1.

Table 1. The quality of the drinking water at the Pitkäkoski water treatment plant (WTP) from 2010 to 2015. The analyses are from the analytically extensive monitoring which was organized 4–6 times a year by Helsinki Region Environmental Services Authority (HSY) [20].

Analysis	Units	Median	Minimum	Maximum	N
Dissolved oxygen	$mgO_2\,l^{-1}$	15.0	12.2	16.1	24
Total chlorine	$mgCl_2\,l^{-1}$	0.39	0.33	0.48	25
Ammonium	$mgN\,l^{-1}$	0.13	0.10	0.19	23
Temperature	°C	7.5	3.3	11.8	24
pH		8.5	8.0	8.7	25
Hardness	$Mmol\,l^{-1}$	0.53	0.46	0.62	23
Turbidity	FTU	0.08	0.06	0.12	25
Conductivity	$mS\,m^{-1}$	15.1	14.2	16.5	24
Total organic carbon	$Mg\,l^{-1}$	1.6	1.4	2.0	25
Total microbes (R2A)	$cfu\,ml^{-1}$	<10	<10	45	19
Trihalomethanes	$\mu g\,l^{-1}$	<2	<2	<2	23

The obligatory monitoring of the quality of the distributed drinking water was organized by HSY, and the sampling and analysis were conducted by an accredited laboratory, Metropolilab [21]. In total, the obligatory monitoring data for the cities of Helsinki and Vantaa for the years 2010–2013 included water samples from approximately 900 drinking water taps. However, the data only included 16 locations with a long time series of water quality (lengths: 12–47 months). All these sampling sites were located in the city of Vantaa, inside the DWDS of Pitkäkoski WTP (Figure 1). Nitrite was analyzed from most of the drinking water samples. Thus, the formed nitrite concentration time series consisted of 10–35 analysis results each.

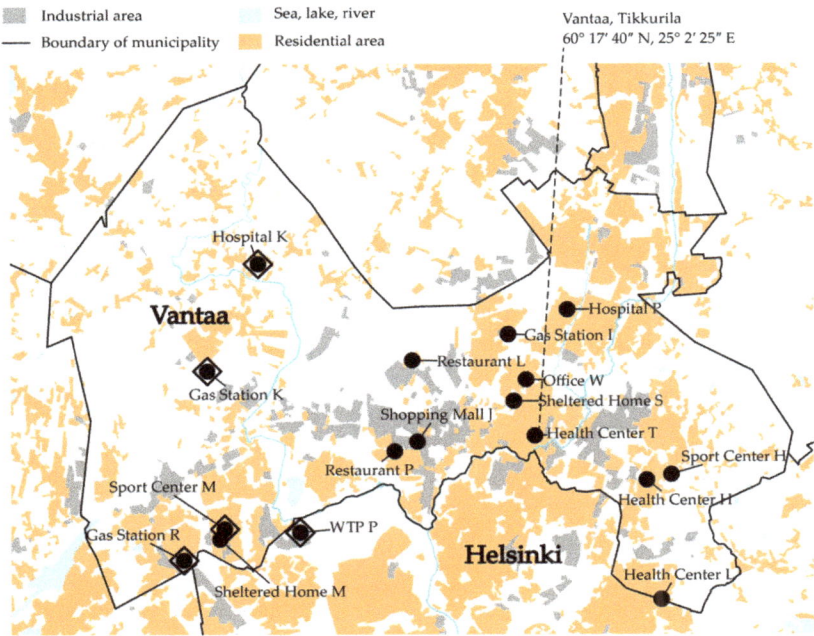

Figure 1. A map of the study area. The black circles are obligatory monitoring locations and the large open diamonds are sampling campaign locations.

2.2. Sampling Campaign

To gather more information on nitrite and other nitrogen compounds in distributed drinking water, a one-year sampling campaign was organized in a section of a DWDS between 1 July 2014 and 2 June 2015 (Figure 1). The section is isolated from the rest of the DWDS in the east, south and north. The Pitkäkoski WTP is situated in the southeastern corner of the section. In the west there are two connections to the rest of the DWDS, one of which is closed.

We chose four sampling locations that were included in the obligatory monitoring (Sport Center M, Gas Station R, Gas Station K and Hospital K; Figure 1). The drinking water at the Pitkäkoski WTP was sampled from a pipe leading to the laboratory, located at the site of the WTP. Additionally, water at the end of Process Line 1 in the WTP was sampled between 9 December 2014 and 2 June 2015. Sampling tours were organized approximately once a month, with 3–7-week intervals, on Tuesdays starting at 08:00 and ending at 13:00. All the samples were stored in cool boxes with freezer blocks during the sampling tour. The temperatures inside the cool boxes were between 4 °C and 15 °C, depending on the initial temperature of the samples. The samples were analyzed the same day they were collected. If the analysis took more than one day, the samples were stored at a temperature of 4 °C, without preservation.

The sampling procedure included discharging water from the tap before taking the samples. At first, the samples were taken after a 5-min discharge of water from the tap. The water quality change during the discharge was evaluated on 9 September 2014. The results indicated that a discharge of 150–200 l was sufficient to stabilize the water quality according to the ammonium and total chlorine analyses. Thus, the sampling procedure was to discharge at least for 15 min or 200 l of water, depending on the flow of the tap. This sampling procedure was adopted into use from 30 September 2014 to 2 June 2015. Roeselers et al. [22] have also used 15 min extra flushing when sampling drinking water in their study.

The drinking water samples for nitrite, oxidized nitrogen (nitrite + nitrate) and total nitrogen analyses were collected in amber glass bottles with ground-glass stoppers. The samples above were analyzed in the laboratory of the Water and Environmental Engineering Group of Aalto University with standard methods (see Section S1 in the Supplementary Materials). Ammonium concentrations were analyzed in the laboratory of HSY, at the Pitkäkoski WTP. These samples were collected in plastic bottles that were completely filled. The samples were analyzed with the standard method (see Section S1 in the Supplementary Materials). All samples were analyzed as duplicates, and the mean values of the analyses were reported as the analysis results. The ammonium analysis included ammonia, ammonium and chloramines. The limits of quantification (LoQs) of the ammonium and nitrite analyses are provided in the Section S1 in the Supplementary Materials.

2.3. Data Collection, Statistical Methods and Calculations

The statistical analyses were executed in MathWorks Matlab and IBM SPSS Statistics. Seasonal indices (SI; see Equation (1)) were utilized to inspect the seasonal properties of nitrite time series. The nitrite concentrations were calculated as two-month or three-month averages, because there were gaps in the monthly data. It was not possible to fill all the gaps with this method and the remaining gaps of one concentration were filled with the averages of adjacent two-month concentrations. The gaps of two or more concentrations were not filled. The seasonal indices were calculated from the two-month and three-month averages of nitrite concentrations according to Equation (1):

$$SI = \frac{x_i}{\hat{x}} \tag{1}$$

where SI = seasonal index, based on one-year data, x_i = the mean nitrite concentration in a two-month season i, $\hat{x}$ = the annual mean nitrite concentration, and i = the numbers of the two-month ($i = 1$–6) or three-month ($i = 1$–4) periods in a year.

The data was depicted as time series and boxplots. The nitrite data in the obligatory monitoring and the sampling campaign were not normally distributed (as assessed by the Anderson-Darling test), and thus we used non-parametric tests. Spearman's rank-order correlation coefficients were used to define the correlation between two variables, with the limit of significance being $p < 0.05$. The water age was a maximum water age (Table 2), estimated with a model of the DWDS [19,23]. The calculations with the analysis results lower than the LoQ were done with the numerical value of the half of the LoQ.

Table 2. The modeled maximum water ages in the sampling locations [19,23].

Location	Water Age (h)	Location	Water Age (h)
Sheltered Home M	5.0	Sheltered Home S	27.3
Sport Center M	5.0	Restaurant L	26.7
Gas Station R	6.7	Hospital P	28.7
Shopping Mall J	63.6	Health Center T	12.9
Gas Station I	31.2	Sport Center H	47.1
Health Center H	53.9	Restaurant P	5.8
Health Center L	29.7	Office W	30.4
Gas Station K	33.0	Hospital K	190

3. Results and Discussion

3.1. Obligatory Monitoring Data

3.1.1. Seasonality of the Nitrite Time Series

The seasonality of nitrite concentrations in the distributed drinking water was first studied in the obligatory monitoring data. Quite a few of the nitrite time series showed distinct seasonality with annual crests and troughs (Figure 2). Nitrification is strongly dependent on temperature; thus, the time series were first inspected visually by comparing them to the time series of the water temperature at the WTP. According to this inspection, the data included time series with a seasonality similar to the seasonality of the temperature (Figure 2a–d), a seasonality reversed to the temperature (Figure 2e–h), time series with variation, but no clear seasonality (Figure 2i–l), short time series (Figure 2m–o) and a time series with no variation (Figure 2p). The first group had crests during the warm period of the year and the second group during the cold period.

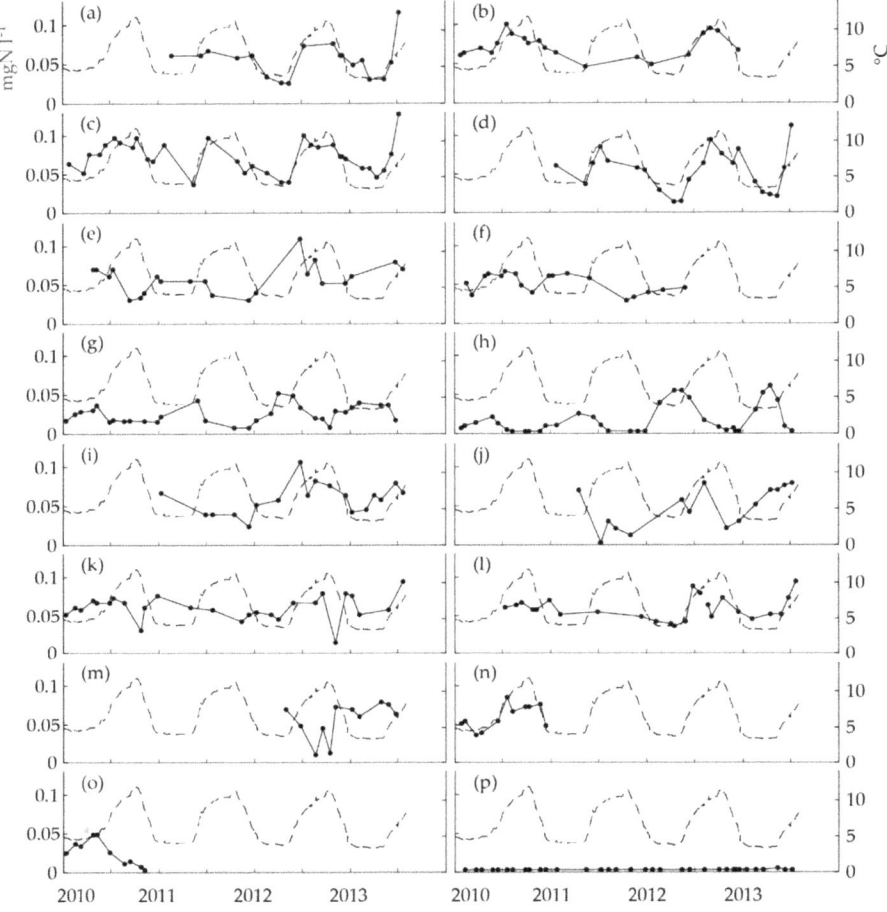

Figure 2. The time series of nitrite concentrations in the drinking water distribution system (DWDS) in the obligatory monitoring data collected between January 2010 and July 2013 (the unbroken line with dots, the left *y*-axis: one dot represents one analysis) and temperature at the WTP (the dashed line, the right *y*-axis) for (**a**) Sheltered Home M, (**b**) Sport Center M, (**c**) Gas Station R, (**d**) Shopping Mall J, (**e**) Gas Station I, (**f**) Health Center H, (**g**) Health Center L, (**h**) Gas Station K, (**i**) Sheltered Home S, (**j**) Restaurant L, (**k**) Hospital P, (**l**) Health Center T, (**m**) Sport Center H, (**n**) Restaurant P, (**o**) Office W and (**p**) Hospital K. The number of nitrite analyses for each time series = 10–35.

3.1.2. Seasonal Index of a Nitrite Time Series

To conduct a more systematic inspection, we calculated the two-month seasonal indices (Equation (1)) for the single time series. The seasonal indices included 1–3 nitrite values each. We have drawn boxplots of the single-year seasonal indices to depict the inter-year variation of the values. In nine of the time series, the seasonal variation was largely substantial (Figure 3a,c,d,g,h,j,m–o), while in four it was clear but less eminent (Figure 3b,e,f,l). The seasonal index revealed that no clear seasonality existed in two time series, even though there was variation in the values (Figure 3i,k). No seasonal index was calculated for the time series of Hospital K (Figure 2p), because the values did not vary. The evaluation of the seasonal patterns of the time series was decided according to both the time series and the seasonal indices. In equivocal cases, the seasonal index was given more weight.

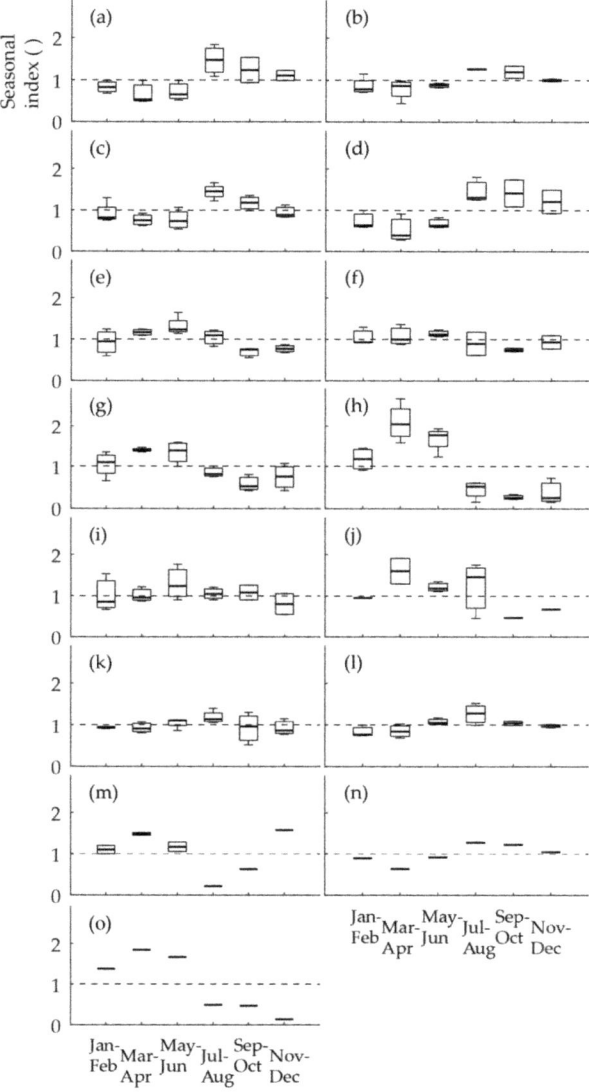

Figure 3. The two-month seasonal indices of the nitrite time series recorded in obligatory monitoring data between January 2010 and July 2013 for (**a**) Sheltered Home M, (**b**) Sport Center M, (**c**) Gas Station R, (**d**) Shopping Mall J, (**e**) Gas Station I, (**f**) Health Center H, (**g**) Health Center L, (**h**) Gas Station K, (**i**) Sheltered Home S, (**j**) Restaurant L, (**k**) Hospital P, (**l**) Health Center T, (**m**) Sport Center H, (**n**) Restaurant P and (**o**) Office W. In the boxplots, the middle values are medians, the boxes are the upper and lower quartiles, and are the whiskers the minima and the maxima.

The time series were found to be of four types. Firstly, the annual maximum occurred during the warm period of the year (months 7–12) and the minimum during the cold period (months 1–6). This type of series was called a summer maximum and included the time series of Sheltered Home M, Sport Center M, Gas Station R, Shopping Mall J, Health Center T, and Restaurant P. Secondly, the nitrite maximum concentrations occurred during the cold period and the minimum concentrations occurred during the warm period. This type was called a winter maximum and included the time series of Gas Station I, Health Center H, Health Center L, Gas Station K, Restaurant L, Sport Center H and Office W. The third type indicated no clear seasonality, though the concentrations varied over time. This type was called mixed seasonality and included the time series of Sheltered Home S and Hospital P. Finally, one time series, that of Hospital K, with no variation and values below the LoQ, formed the fourth type, was called no seasonality.

We included the short one-year time series to the relevant seasonality groups, because the seasonality of distributed drinking water quality is quite often studied in time series with only one year of data [4,15,24]. Additionally, the seasonal patterns in the time series (Figure 2m–o) and in the seasonal indices (Figure 3m–o) were quite clear in all three cases.

3.1.3. Nitrification in the Sampling Line Running to the on-Site Laboratory

Unexpectedly, the nitrite concentrations at the Pitkäkoski WTP followed a seasonal pattern (Figure 4a). The pattern had a crest in the warm period and a trough in the cold period. The nitrite concentrations varied between 0.005 mgN l^{-1} and 0.039 mgN l^{-1} (median 0.019 mgN l^{-1}). The seasonal indices confirmed the seasonality (Figure 4b). However, nitrite could not have been formed in the treatment process, because monochloramine was added to the drinking water as the last step. According to the theoretical calculations by Fleming et al. [25] the monochloramine dose (Table 1) was not high enough to prevent nitrite formation in the biofilm [19]. The tap from which samples were taken had a constant uninterrupted flow of 1.9 l min^{-1}. The retention time of the sampling line is not known, but most probably it amounts to minutes or tens of minutes at maximum. Supposedly, chloramine was decomposed and ammonium was nitrified into nitrite in the biofilm formed inside the sampling line. This supposition was confirmed during the sampling campaign. However, the total microbes (Table 1) were below 10 cfu ml^{-1}, with one exception of 45 cfu ml^{-1}, which indicated that the formation of the possible biofilm was not extensive. In the middle of the sampling campaign, the WTP personnel noticed that the nitrite and ammonium concentrations were different at the end of the process line compared to the sampling tap. The maximum concentration after the final step of the process line was 0.0057 mgN l^{-1} and at the tap in the laboratory it was seven-fold: 0.041 mgN l^{-1} (Figure 5a,b). Thus, most probably the nitrite concentrations in the water entering the DWDS were close to or below the LoQ.

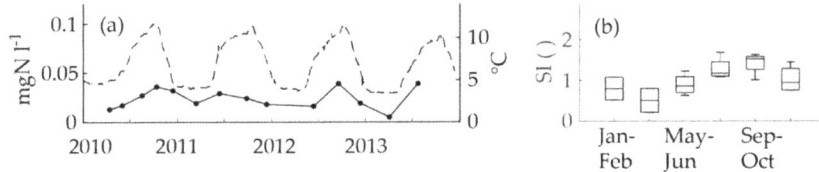

Figure 4. The parts of the figure: (**a**) The nitrite concentrations time series (black dots and an unbroken line; the left *y*-axis; one dot represents one analysis) and the temperature at the WTP (the dashed line; the right *y*-axis) and (**b**) a boxplot of the seasonal indices of the nitrite (each seasonal index included 1–2 nitrite analyses) in the distributed water from the laboratory tap at the Pitkäkoski WTP in the in-house control data recorded between 2010 and 2013. In the boxplot, the middle line is the median, the boxes are the lower and upper quartiles and the whiskers are the minima and maxima.

3.2. Sampling Campaign

The nitrite concentrations at the locations of Pitkäkoski WTP, Sport Center M, Gas Station R, Gas Station K and Hospital K, were analyzed in a separate sampling campaign to complement the findings based on the obligatory monitoring data. The same methods as above were utilized to inspect the seasonality of the obligatory monitoring data (Figure 5). The nitrite concentration time series were compared to the temperature at the Pitkäkoski WTP (Figure 5a–f). Seasonality occurred in two time series: the taps at Pitkäkoski laboratory and Gas Station K. On the contrary, the time series of Sport Center M and Gas Station R had variation, but no clear seasonality. The seasonal indices confirmed these observations (Figure 5g–j). The time series of Hospital K was flat with no variation (Figure 5f). As a summary, three out of five time series behaved similarly seasonally as in the obligatory monitoring and in-house control data of the WTP (WTP P, Gas Station K, and Hospital K) and two behaved differently (Sport Center M and Gas Station R).

At Sport Center M and Gas Station R, seasonality was not observed in the data of the sampling campaign, which, however, did not necessarily mean that there was no seasonal behavior of nitrite concentrations. The longer time series of obligatory monitoring had already proved that seasonality featured in the nitrite concentrations of these sampling locations, and the one-year data of the sampling campaign did not override this notion. Furthermore, the median values of the nitrite concentrations of Sport Center M and Gas Station R in the sampling campaign and obligatory monitoring were almost equal (Sport Center M: 0.067 mgN l^{-1} and 0.068 mgN l^{-1}; Gas Station R: 0.070 mgN l^{-1} and 0.072 mgN l^{-1} respectively) and the ranges overlapped (Sport Center M: 0.054–0.093 mgN l^{-1} and 0.028–0.10 mgN l^{-1}; Gas Station R: 0.038–0.118 mgN l^{-1} and 0.037–0.128 mgN l^{-1} respectively). The explanation for the mixed seasonal behavior in these locations is not known; however, a possible explanation is variations in the water consumption in the premises.

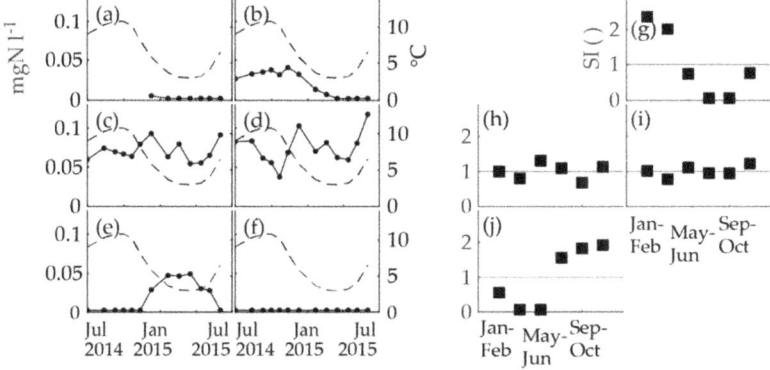

Figure 5. The nitrite concentrations (the black dots and an unbroken line; the left *y*-axis) compared to the temperature (the dashed line; the right *y*-axis) at the WTP and the two-month seasonal indices of nitrite concentrations (the black squares, *N* of nitrite analyses for each box = 2–3) of the sampling campaign. The parts of the figure are as follows: (**a**) nitrite at Pitkäkoski WTP (Process Line 1), (**b**) nitrite at Pitkäkoski WTP (a tap in the on-site laboratory), (**c**) nitrite at Sport Center M, (**d**) nitrite at Gas Station R, (**e**) nitrite at Gas Station K, (**f**) nitrite at Hospital K, (**g**) seasonal indices of nitrite at Pitkäkoski WTP (a tap in the on-site laboratory), (**h**) seasonal indices of nitrite at Sport Center M, (**i**) seasonal indices of nitrite at Gas Station R, and (**j**) seasonal indices of nitrite at Gas Station K.

3.3. Evaluation of the Methods

The seasonal index is routinely used in detecting the seasonal patterns of time series, especially in economic analysis [26,27]. Biochemical reactions in DWDSs follow intra-year changes, pre-eminently of temperature, and thus it is reasonable to study nitrite formation with methods designed to understand seasonal properties. A seasonal index is a simple method to evaluate seasonality. More advanced methods, for example an ARIMA time series analysis, could not be used, because the sampling intervals were not equidistant.

Visual inspection was an even more simple method than the seasonal index. In addition, the visual categorization of some of the nitrite time series was debatable (e.g., Sheltered Home S in Figure 2i and Restaurant L in Figure 2j). However, the seasonal index helped in this categorization problem.

To test our method of determining the seasonal index, we calculated another set of seasonal indices of the nitrite time series in the obligatory monitoring data with a different division of the seasons, starting from December and not January. This division of seasons would have fitted better with the seasonality pattern of the temperature, and we wanted to observe whether this division would have altered the seasonality types of nitrite. Most of the time series were classified similarly, compared to the method of starting the division from January (Figure 3). Nevertheless, the method of starting the division from December did not improve the classification of the nitrite seasonality types. On the contrary, the location of Gas Station I was classified as a mixed seasonality, even though it expressed an evident winter maximum according to the nitrite time series (Figure 2e). Nevertheless, this did not affect the final decisions of the seasonality types of the nitrite time series. In addition, we tested a method of three-month division starting from January, which flattened the seasonal features slightly, though it gave a similar classification as the method of the two-month averages starting from January (Figure 3). These additional analyses of the method are provided in Supplementary Materials Section S2.

During the calculation of the seasonal indices, we experimented with filling the gaps in the data. It was found that all the choices of not filling the gaps, filling only one-season gaps with interpolation, or filling all the gaps gave the same final results for the seasonality types. Thus, without additional restrictions, we chose a conservative filling strategy: only one-season gaps were interpolated.

The nitrite time series of Hospital P (Figure 2k), in the obligatory monitoring data, was scrutinized more closely to decide whether it showed seasonality or not. The time series had two sharp peaks, which were considered as possible outliers. When these were removed, the seasonal indices of the six seasons had less variation. It was concluded that nitrite concentrations analyzed from the water at Hospital P did not have annual seasonality according to the available data. Nitrification in the premises' plumbing system [28] can increase the nitrite concentrations in drinking water. Obviously, the sharp changes downwards in nitrite concentration in Figure 2k were not a result of this phenomenon. It was noted that the low concentrations were both observed on Mondays. We suspected that water may have been stagnating during the weekend, thus possibly causing lower nitrite concentrations. However, it was discovered that most of the samples were taken on Mondays (84% of all samples). Thus, Monday sampling did not implicitly cause decreased nitrite concentrations, but the high percentage of Monday sampling may have caused some other, unknown bias to the nitrite data.

3.4. Nitrite Concentrations in Seasonality Groups

When all the nitrite concentrations of obligatory monitoring were combined (excluding monitoring for Hospital K) and depicted as a monthly boxplot (Figure 6a), seasonality was only observable to a lesser extent. The highest monthly median and maximum nitrite concentrations both occurred in July. On the other hand, distinct seasonality can be observed in the nitrite concentrations of the conjoined data of summer maxima (Figure 6b) and winter maxima (Figure 6c). In the summer maximum group (Figure 6b), the highest median nitrite concentrations occurred during July. This is interesting, because it coincided with the sharp rise in temperature, but not the highest temperature. We investigated whether the sampling schedule caused bias and possible higher concentrations, but this was not the case; all the locations included in the group were sampled during July. The winter maximum group was more heterogeneous than the summer maximum group (Figure 6c). The highest monthly median occurred in April. Nevertheless, the highest maximum occurred during June, which again coincided with the sharply rising temperature. In all the months from July to December, the lowest values were below the LoQ. The mixed seasonality group revealed the maximum nitrite in June, but interestingly lacked the lowest nitrite concentrations (below or close to the LoQ; Figure 6d). This was possibly because the low concentrations were masked by the high concentrations, when waters were mixed in the junctions of the DWDS.

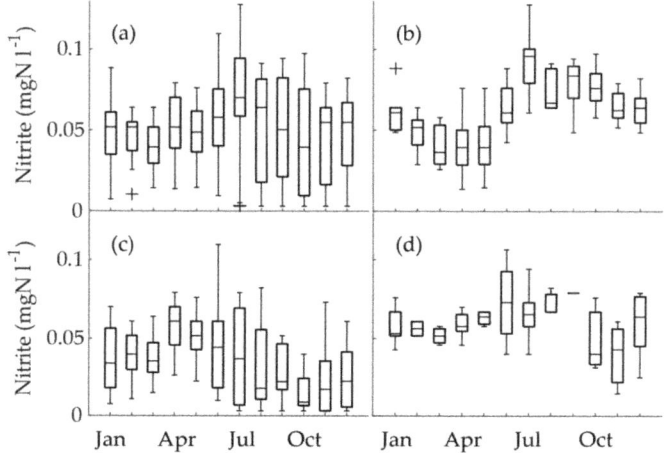

Figure 6. The monthly boxplots of nitrite seasonality in obligatory monitoring data for (**a**) all of the time series (excluding Hospital K, $N = 317$), (**b**) the time series with the summer maximum ($N = 129$), (**c**) the time series with the winter maximum ($N = 143$), and (**d**) the time series with mixed seasonality ($N = 45$).

In the Helsinki Metropolitan Area, nitrite levels had been observed to increase in the DWDS in succession to the commissioning of a granular activated carbon (GAC) filtration unit at the Vanhakaupunki WTP to reduce organic matter in the drinking water [18,29]. A similar process is currently in use at the Pitkäkoski WTP. Nevertheless, the nitrite concentrations were somewhat lower in the Vanhakaupunki DWDS (0.005–0.05 mgN l^{-1}) compared to our study.

In a recent study, Schullehner et al. [6] examined nitrite and other nitrogen species at WTPs and DWDSs in a research that included the whole of Denmark. However, they did not find seasonal variation in nitrite concentrations. Their method of evaluating seasonality in their vast data resembled Figure 6a in our research. As we have seen in our research, when large data is inspected as a whole, opposing seasonalities can override each other. These, among other factors, may have hidden the seasonality of nitrite in the Danish study. However, we have to note that the drinking water in Denmark is abstracted from groundwater, which is polluted by nitrite and nitrate. Thus, the nitrite did not originate from monochloramine addition.

3.5. Nitrite Seasonality in Relation to Temperature and Water Age

We studied the relation of the temperature at the WTP and the nitrite concentrations in the obligatory monitoring data with a correlation analysis. The Spearman rank-ordered correlation coefficient of temperature and nitrite in the summer maximum group was 0.69 ($p < 0.001$), in the winter maximum group it was -0.50 ($p < 0.001$), and in the whole nitrite time series data it was merely 0.07 ($p = 0.23$). Thus, the winter maximum group had ostensibly reversed temperature dependence and the whole data did not have any dependence. The kinetic parameters of nitrification depend on temperature following the Arrhenius equation [30], and the maximum growth rate of nitrification bacteria roughly doubles between 12 and 26 °C [31]. Moreover, the number of AOB has been found to be 100–1000 times higher in DWDSs in the summer compared to the winter [9–11]. Thus, the reversed correlation requires an explanation.

When the seasonality types of nitrite concentrations were inspected against water age, it was found that in the summer maximum group the water age was shorter (median: 6.7 h; range: 5–64 h) than in the winter maximum group (median: 31 h; range: 27–54 h). In the summer maximum group, the nitrite crests were observed at the median temperature of 9.1 °C (range: 7.7–9.6 °C), and in the winter maximum group they were observed at the median temperature of 5.0 °C (3.7–7.7 °C). Thus, at a low temperature, a longer reaction time for nitrite formation was required, and the contradictory observation of maximum nitrite concentrations in cold temperature resulted from the decelerated ammonium oxidation.

Possibly, in complicated DWDSs, nitrite seasonality can be distorted by mixing the waters from different directions. As we noticed, water age impacts the nitrite concentrations, and if in a junction of DWDS two or more waters with different water ages and nitrite concentrations were mixed, the result was probably no clear seasonality, or alternating seasonalities, depending on the changing shares of flows from the different directions. This could explain the time series with mixed seasonality.

We observed that there were two types of low nitrite concentrations. Firstly, at low water age, low nitrite concentrations occurred because nitrite had not yet been formed. However, we have to add that nitrite started to form very rapidly when the conditions were favorable, i.e., when the water was in contact with a nitrifying biofilm. As we observed in the sampling line at the WTP, this happened in minutes. Secondly, low nitrite concentrations occurred when nitrite had been oxidized into nitrate. The time series without variation (Hospital K, with a water age of 190 h) was a result of nitrite oxidation occurring completely, with the final nitrogen compound being fully oxidized nitrate. Generally, nitrite occurs in stagnating water, meaning at a high water age [32], which disagrees with our observations. The general observation is probably a result of a higher monochloramine dose (1–3 $mgCl_2 \ l^{-1}$ [4]), which prevents nitrification initially, but further in the DWDS the lowered concentration is not capable of inhibiting the AOB inside the biofilm. Our results were received from a DWDS with a low initial monochloramine dose (median: 0.39 $mgCl_2 \ l^{-1}$).

Wilczak et al. [4] noted that a higher share of high nitrite occurred during the summer season, but nitrite occurred also during the winter season. This corroborates our findings that nitrification is not totally inhibited during cold temperature, but is slowed down significantly. Moreover, AOB and NOB have been observed in DWDSs elsewhere in Finland, in spite of the low temperatures of water [33]. Unfortunately, this study did not include an evaluation of the seasonality.

Woods et al. [15] studied the seasonality of NDMA in DWDSs with monochloramine disinfection and utilized the temperature of water as a reference of seasonal behavior of the NDMA concentrations. They noted that the NDMA concentrations increased in temperatures lower than 10 °C. Their approach to evaluating seasonality was somewhat similar to our first method (Figure 2) and strengthens the notion that temperature is a very important background variable in the seasonality of water constituents in DWDSs.

3.6. Nitrite's Correlation to Other Nitrogen Forms in Relation to Seasonality

Generally, when nitrite concentrations increase in the DWDS, ammonium concentrations should decrease accordingly [4]. However, nitrite concentrations of the sampling campaign data (excluding Hospital K) did not correlate negatively or even significantly with ammonium concentrations (Spearman's rho = 0.04, *p* = 0.79). Nevertheless, ammonium correlated negatively with oxidized nitrogen (nitrite + nitrate) (Spearman's rho = -0.94, *p* = 1.3×10^{-24}). Usually, both nitrite and nitrate concentrations increase together in the DWDSs [4,6], but in our data nitrate correlated negatively with nitrite (Spearman's rho = -0.27, *p* = 0.053).

Next, we inspected the correlation separately in the locations with a summer maximum (Pitkäkoski WTP, Sport Center M, and Gas Station R; water ages up to 6.7 h) and the location with a winter maximum (Gas Station K, water age 33 h) in the sampling campaign data. Furthermore, we noticed that the ammonium and nitrite scatterplot suggested a curvilinear dependence (Figure 7a), which could have resulted from two subgroups with different types of correlations. This appeared to be accurate: the correlation of ammonium and nitrite was clearly negative and significant in the locations with a summer maximum (Spearman's rho = −0.69, p =1.4 × 10^{-6}). On the other hand, in the data with a winter maximum, a positive correlation appeared (Spearman's rho = 0.80, p = 0.001). Both of these correlations were more significant than the correlation in the combined data. Furthermore, the correlations indicated that, at low water ages, ammonium decreased while nitrite increased, but at a higher water age, both nitrite and ammonium decreased. The latter interpretation was corroborated by the fact that both nitrite and ammonium were below the LoQ at the farthest point examined (Hospital K) with the water age of 190 h.

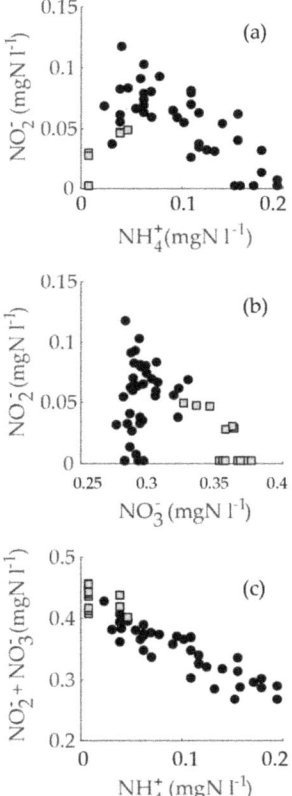

Figure 7. A scatterplot of inorganic nitrogen species in the sampling campaign. Groups are divided by the seasonality type of the sampling location; black dots indicate a summer maximum (in the locations of Pitkäkoski WTP, Sport Center M, and Gas Station R); grey squares indicate a winter maximum (Gas Station K). The graphs show (**a**) ammonium vs. nitrite, (**b**) nitrate vs. nitrite, and (**c**) ammonium vs. nitrite + nitrate.

A similar inspection was conducted for the correlations of nitrite and nitrate (summer maximum, Spearman's rho = 0.25, p = 0.12; winter maximum, Spearman's rho = −0.63, p = 0.02). Thus, at lower water ages, nitrite and nitrate both increased, but at a higher water age nitrite decreased while nitrate increased (Figure 7b). Additionally, when we inspected the correlation of ammonium to oxidized nitrogen, the correlations inside subgroups were of the same sign (summer maximum, Spearman's rho = -0.90, $p = 2.7 \times 10^{-15}$; winter maximum, Spearman's rho = -0.43, $p = 0.15$). On a scatterplot, the correlation was evidently linear, and the subgroups did not stand out from the whole of the data (Figure 7c).

Thus, according to the correlation analysis of the nitrogen species, ammonium oxidation into nitrite was the dominant reaction in the summer maximum group with lower water ages, and nitrite oxidation into nitrate was the dominant reaction in the winter maximum group with a higher water age.

3.7. Denitrification

Denitrification organisms have been observed in DWDSs [34]. Denitrification can decrease the nitrite and nitrate concentrations if the conditions in the biofilm are anoxic. This could have impacted our interpretation of the decreasing nitrite concentrations. To investigate whether denitrification played a significant role, the total nitrogen data of the sampling campaign at different water ages was plotted as a boxplot (Figure 8). A slight decline in total nitrogen, especially at the water age of 190 h, can be observed. On the other hand, the non-significant Spearman correlation of the data (Spearman's rho = -0.13, $p = 0.29$) did not corroborate the observation. However, the possibility of denitrification was not completely excluded, even though the extent of denitrification was evidently small. When the sum of nitrogen species (ammonium, nitrite, and nitrate) was investigated, it was noted that the concentrations did not decline with increasing water age and the Spearman correlation with water age was insignificant (Spearman's rho = 0.08, $p = 0.53$). This implies that the decline in total nitrogen was not inorganic nitrogen, but organic nitrogen, which is included in the analysis of total nitrogen. Furthermore, it is probable that the loss of nitrogen at water ages of 33 and 190 h was due to assimilation into the growth of microorganisms. The loss of total nitrogen at the water age of 190 h was 2.7% from the mean total nitrogen of the rest of the data of the sampling campaign. This percentage is close to those observed in wastewater treatment, for example, in a sequencing batch reactor the assimilation percentage has been recorded to be 3.7% [35] and in a granular sludge process it has been recorded to be less than 5% of all nitrogen in wastewater sludge [36].

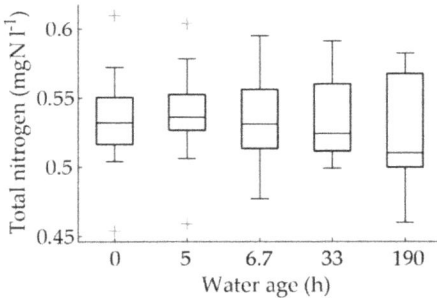

Figure 8. The variation of the total nitrogen concentrations by water age.

3.8. Nitrite Exposure

Nitrite in drinking water increased in the DWDS in the Helsinki Metropolitan Area compared to the water at the WTP. According to our results, the dense population consuming drinking water with water ages below 50–60 h received drinking water with elevated nitrite concentrations due to monochloramine addition. This observation applied even to the lowest studied water ages. The nitrite exposure was unevenly distributed during the year, depending on the water age: lower water ages (median: 6.7 h) implied a maximum nitrite exposure during summer and higher water ages (median:

31 h) during winter. Interestingly, the scattered population consuming drinking water with the highest water age was least exposed to nitrite. In a previous study of this region, it was noted that the area of elevated nitrite was slightly larger at a temperature below 9 °C than above 9 °C, suggesting that a larger population was exposed to nitrite at the lower temperature [19]. Our findings of seasonality in winter months, due to delayed nitrite formation, corroborate this observation.

In another earlier study in the Helsinki Metropolitan Area, the increase of nitrite in the Vanhakaupunki DWDS due to the commissioning of a GAC filtration to remove organic matter, in 1998, was totally unexpected [18,29]. It was speculated that AOB increased in the DWDS because of the lessened competition from heterotrophic microorganisms, though definite reasons were not detected [29]. Recently, HSY has been considering introducing membrane filtration at the WTPs to alter the process of organic matter removal [37]. While it is unknown, whether this will influence nitrification or nitrite concentrations in any way, a proper analysis of the nitrite concentrations in the DWDS and the reasons leading to it is advisable before commissioning any process modifications. The altered process may require various other measures in the treatment process to balance good water quality, including extra disinfection. Our results help to design these measures appropriately, taking into account the nitrite exposure of consumers and minimizing it. Also, our results help to notice possible seasonal changes in the concentrations and to direct the monitoring appropriately, taking into account the unexpectedly high winter concentrations.

In our study, the nitrite concentrations did not exceed the Finnish statutory limit for nitrite (0.15 mgN l^{-1}); the highest concentrations in the obligatory monitoring data were 85% of the limit, and in the sampling campaign data they were 78%. However, the earlier Finnish limit of 0.03 mgN l^{-1} from 1994 [38] was exceeded in 70% of the obligatory monitoring data and in 50% of the sampling campaign data. The lower limit is still use, for example, in Denmark [39]. The median of the obligatory monitoring data was 0.052 mgN l^{-1}, which suggests that roughly half of the consumers in the area were exposed to concentrations of this level or higher. To perform a more accurate epidemiological assessment of the population exposed to nitrite, a study combining the spatial population data with the spatial nitrite data is required.

4. Conclusions

We studied the seasonal variation of nitrite concentrations in a DWDS with monochloramine disinfection in the Helsinki Metropolitan Area. In Finland, tap water is the main source of drinking water, and thus nitrite in tap water increases the nitrite exposure. We used two methods to inspect the seasonal variation of nitrite concentrations: comparing nitrite time series to the water temperature time series and calculating seasonal indices of the nitrite concentrations. The main drivers of nitrite seasonality were the temperature and the water age. We observed that with low water ages (median: 6.7 h), the highest nitrite exposure occurred during the summer months and with higher water ages (median: 31 h) during the winter months. With the highest water age (190 h), nitrite concentrations were the lowest. The dense population closer to the WTP was exposed to higher nitrite concentrations than the scattered population receiving stagnating drinking water. At a low temperature, the winter maxima were caused by the decelerated ammonium oxidation. The correlation inspection of nitrite, ammonium, and nitrate revealed that the dominant reaction at low water ages was ammonium oxidation into nitrite, and at high water ages, it was nitrite oxidation into nitrate. Denitrification did not occur significantly in the DWDS.

These results help to understand where and when nitrite is formed in the DWDS and direct monitoring appropriately to gain exact knowledge of nitrite exposure. Also, possible future changes in the treatment process and additional disinfection measures can be designed appropriately to minimize extra nitrite exposure.

Supplementary Materials: The following are available online at http://www.mdpi.com/1660-4601/15/8/1756/s1, Section S1. The Analytical Methods: Table S1; Section S2. Additional Methods for Evaluating the Seasonality of Nitrite Concentrations: Figures S1 and S2.

Author Contributions: The original idea for this research was conceived by R.V. and P.-L.R. The study was designed by P.-L.R., M.M. K.-T. and M.A. The research was conducted by P.-L.R., and the analysis of the results was executed by P.-L.R. and I.M. P.-L.R. wrote the original manuscript. All authors contributed to writing, reviewing and editing of the article.

Funding: This research was funded by Maa-ja vesitekniikan tuki ry grant numbers 31024 and 35211.

Acknowledgments: We are grateful to the HSY for providing the obligatory monitoring data and analytical services.

Conflicts of Interest: The authors declare no conflict of interest.

References

1. Jaffé, E.R. Methaemoglobinaemia. *Clin. Haematol.* **1981**, *10*, 99–122. [PubMed]
2. Mitchell, J. *Ingested Nitrate and Nitrite and Cyanobacterial Peptide Toxins*; International Agency for Research on Cancer: Lyon, France, 2010; 464p, ISBN 978-92-832-1294-2.
3. AWWA Staff. *Water Chlorination/Chloramination Practices and Principles*, 2nd ed.; American Water Works Association: Denver, CO, USA, 2005; 188p, ISBN 1-58321-408-9.
4. Wilczak, A.; Jacangelo, J.G.; Marcinko, J.P.; Odell, L.H. Occurrence of nitrification in chloraminated distribution systems. *J. AWWA* **1996**, *88*, 74–85. [CrossRef]
5. Zhang, Y.; Love, N.; Edwards, M. Nitrification in Drinking Water Systems. *Crit. Rev. Environ. Sci. Technol.* **2009**, *39*, 153–208. [CrossRef]
6. Schullehner, J.; Stayner, L.; Hansen, B. Nitrate, Nitrite, and Ammonium Variability in Drinking Water Distribution Systems. *Int. J. Environ. Res. Public Health* **2017**, *14*. [CrossRef] [PubMed]
7. Finnish Ministry of Social Affairs and Health. Sosiaali-ja terveysministeriön asetus talousveden laatuvaatimuksista ja valvontatutkimuksista. 2015; 1352/2015. Available online: http://www.finlex.fi/fi/laki/alkup/2015/20151352 (accessed on 19 May 2017).
8. European Council. Council Directive 98/83/EC, of 3 November 1998, on the Quality of Water Intended for Human Consumption. L 330/32. 1998. Available online: http://eur-lex.europa.eu/legal-content/EN/TXT/?uri=CELEX:31998L0083 (accessed on 19 May 2017).
9. Wolfe, R.L.; Means, E.G.; Davis, M.K.; Barrett, S.E. Biological Nitrification in Covered Reservoirs Containing Chloraminated Water. *J. AWWA* **1988**, *80*, 109–114. [CrossRef]
10. Wolfe, R.L.; Lieu, N.I.; Izaguirre, G.; Means, E.G. Ammonia-Oxidizing Bacteria in a Chloraminated Distribution System: Seasonal Occurrence, Distribution, and Disinfection Resistance. *Appl. Environ. Microbiol.* **1990**, *56*, 451–462. [PubMed]
11. Ike, N.R.; Wolfe, R.L.; Means, E.G. Nitrifying Bacteria in a Chloraminated Drinking Water System. *Water Sci. Technol.* **1988**, *20*, 441–444. [CrossRef]
12. Pinto, A.J.; Schroeder, J.; Lunn, M.; Sloan, W.; Raskin, L. Spatial-Temporal Survey and Occupancy-Abundance Modeling to Predict Bacterial Community Dynamics in the Drinking Water Microbiome. *mBio* **2014**, *5*. [CrossRef] [PubMed]
13. Stanish, L.F.; Hull, N.M.; Robertson, C.E.; Harris, J.K.; Stevens, M.J.; Spear, J.R.; Pace, N.R. Factors Influencing Bacterial Diversity and Community Composition in Municipal Drinking Waters in the Ohio River Basin, USA. *PLoS ONE* **2016**, *11*. [CrossRef] [PubMed]
14. Zeng, T.; Mitch, W.A. Impact of Nitrification on the Formation of *N*-Nitrosamines and Halogenated Disinfection Byproducts within Distribution System Storage Facilities. *Environ. Sci. Technol.* **2016**, *50*, 2964–2973. [CrossRef] [PubMed]
15. Woods, G.C.; Trenholm, R.A.; Hale, B.; Campbell, Z.; Dickenson, E.R.V. Seasonal and spatial variability of nitrosamines and their precursor sources at a large-scale urban drinking water system. *Sci. Total Environ.* **2015**, *520*, 120–126. [CrossRef] [PubMed]
16. UNESDA. *Statistics on the Consumption of Non-Alcoholic Beverages in Europe*; Excel File; Union of European Soft Drinks Associations: Brussels, Belgium, 2017; Available online: https://www.unesda.eu/products-ingredients/consumption/ (accessed on 31 July 2018).
17. Helsinki Region Environmental Services Authority HSY. *Annual Report 2015*; HSY: Helsinki, Finland, 2016. Available online: https://julkaisu.hsy.fi/vuosikertomus_2015.pdf (accessed on 31 July 2018).

18. Vahala, R.; Laukkanen, R. Nitrification in GAC-Filtered, UV-Disinfected and chloraminated distribution system. In Proceedings of the Specialized Conference on Drinking Water Distribution with or without Disinfectant Residual, Mülheim an der Ruhr, Germany, 28–30 September 1998.

19. Rantanen, P.L.; Keinänen-Toivola, M.M.; Ahonen, M.; Mellin, I.; Zhang, D.Y.; Laakso, T.; Vahala, R. The Spatial Distribution of Nitrite Concentrations in a Large Drinking Water Distribution System in Finland. *J. Water Res. Prot.* **2017**, *9*, 1026–1042. [CrossRef]

20. Helsinki Region Environmental Services Authority HSY. *Pitkäkoski, Talousvesi 2010—2015*; Excel File; Helsinki Region Environmental Services Authority HSY: Helsinki, Finland, 2016.

21. Kalso, S. *Drinking Water Analysis Reports 2010–2013*; Metropolilab, HSY Vesi: Helsinki, Finland, 2013.

22. Roeselers, G.; Coolen, J.; van der Wielen, P.W.; Jaspers, M.C.; Atsma, A.; de Graaf, B.; Schuren, F. Microbial biogeography of drinking water: Patterns in phylogenetic diversity across space and time. *Environ. Microbiol.* **2015**, *17*, 2505–2514. [CrossRef] [PubMed]

23. Laitala, R. *Water Age with Mean Daily Consumption in Present Situation in the Calculation Model of HSY's Drinking Water Distribution System*; Excel File; Pöyry Finland Oy: Vantaa, Finland, 2015.

24. Serrano, M.; Montesinos, I.; Cardador, M.J.; Silva, M.; Gallego, M. Seasonal evaluation of the presence of 46 disinfection by-products throughout a drinking water treatment plant. *Sci. Total Environ.* **2015**, *517*, 246–258. [CrossRef] [PubMed]

25. Fleming, K.K.; Harrington, G.W.; Noguera, D.R. Nitrification potential curves: A new strategy for nitrification prevention. *J. Am. Works Assoc.* **2005**, *97*, 90–99. [CrossRef]

26. Brendstrup, B.; Hylleberg, S.; Nielsen, M.O.; Skipper, L.; Stentoft, L. Seasonality in Economic Models. *Macroecon. Dyn.* **2004**, *8*, 362–394. [CrossRef]

27. Hyndman, R.J.; Athanasopoulos, G. *Forecasting: Principles and Practice*, 2nd ed.; OTexts: Melbourne, Australia, 2013.

28. Zhang, Y.; Edwards, M. Accelerated Chloramine Decay and Microbial Growth by Nitrification in Premise Plumbing. *J. AWWA* **2009**, *101*, 51–62. [CrossRef]

29. Vahala, R.; Niemi, R.M.; Kiuru, H.; Laukkanen, R. The effect of GAC filtration on bacterial regrowth and nitrification in a simulated water main. *J. Appl. Microbiol.* **1998**, *85*, 178S–185S. [CrossRef] [PubMed]

30. Stark, J.M. Modeling the temperature response of nitrification. *Biogeochemistry* **1996**, *35*, 433–445. [CrossRef]

31. Ekama, G.A.; Takács, I. Modeling. In *Activated Sludge—100 Years and Counting*, 1st ed.; Jenkins, D., Wanner, J., Eds.; IWA Publishing: London, UK, 2014; pp. 271–291, ISBN 9781780404943.

32. Harrington, G.W.; Noguera, D.R.; Kandou, A.I.; Vanhoven, D.J. Pilot-Scale Evaluation of Nitrification Control Strategies. *J. AWWA* **2002**, *94*, 78–89. [CrossRef]

33. Lipponen, M.T.T.; Suutari, M.H.; Martikainen, P.J. Occurrence of nitrifying bacteria and nitrification in Finnish drinking water distribution systems. *Water Res.* **2002**, *36*, 4319–4329. [CrossRef]

34. Nagymate, Z.; Homonnay, Z.G.; Marialigeti, K. Investigation of Archaeal and Bacterial community structure of five different small drinking water networks with special regard to the nitrifying microorganisms. *Microbiol. Res.* **2016**, *188–189*, 80–89. [CrossRef] [PubMed]

35. Li, X.M.; Wang, D.B.; Yang, Q.; Zheng, W.; Cao, J.B.; Yue, X.; Shen, T.T.; Zeng, G.M.; Deng, J.H. Excess nitrogen accumulation in activated sludge in sequencing batch reactor with a single-stage oxic process. *Water Sci. Technol.* **2009**, *59*, 573–582. [CrossRef] [PubMed]

36. Wagner, J.; Guimarães, L.B.; Akaboci, T.R.V.; Costa, R.H.R. Aerobic granular sludge technology and nitrogen removal for domestic wastewater treatment. *Water Sci. Technol.* **2015**, *71*, 1040–1046. [CrossRef] [PubMed]

37. Jurmu, J. Effect of Prefiltration on Natural Organic Matter Removal by Nanofiltration in Drinking Water Treatment. Master's Thesis, Aalto University, Espoo, Finland, 2016.

38. Finnish Ministry of Social Affairs and Health. Sosiaali-ja Terveysministeriön Päätös Talousveden Laatuvaatimuksista ja Valvontatutkimuksista. 74/1994. 1994. Available online: http://www.finlex.fi/fi/laki/alkup/1994/19940074 (accessed on 31 July 2018).

39. Danish Environmental Ministry. Bekendtgørelse om Vandkvalitet og Tilsyn Med Vandforsyningsanlæg. 2015; BEK nr. 1310, j.nr. NST-400-00073. Available online: www.retsinformation.dk (accessed on 31 May 2017).

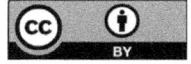

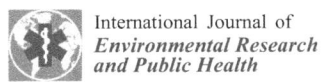

Article

Stability of Major Geogenic Cations in Drinking Water—An Issue of Public Health Importance: A Danish Study, 1980–2017

Kirstine Wodschow [1,2,*], Birgitte Hansen [2], Jörg Schullehner [2,3] and Annette Kjær Ersbøll [1]

[1]   National Institute of Public Health, University of Southern Denmark, 1455 Copenhagen K, Denmark;
      ake@si-folkesundhed.dk
[2]   Department of Groundwater and Quaternary Geological Mapping, Geological Survey of Denmark and
      Greenland, 8000 Aarhus C, Denmark; bgh@geus.dk
[3]   National Centre for Register-based Research, Department of Economics and Business Economics,
      Aarhus BSS, Aarhus University, 8210 Aarhus V, Denmark; jsc@geus.dk
*   Correspondence: ikwo@si-folkesundhed.dk; Tel.: +45-6550-7758

Received: 14 May 2018; Accepted: 4 June 2018; Published: 8 June 2018

Abstract: Concentrations and spatial variations of the four cations Na, K, Mg and Ca are known to some extent for groundwater and to a lesser extent for drinking water. Using Denmark as case, the purpose of this study was to analyze the spatial and temporal variations in the major cations in drinking water. The results will contribute to a better exposure estimation in future studies of the association between cations and diseases. Spatial and temporal variations and the association with aquifer types, were analyzed with spatial scan statistics, linear regression and a multilevel mixed-effects linear regression model. About 65,000 water samples of each cation (1980–2017) were included in the study. Results of mean concentrations were 31.4 mg/L, 3.5 mg/L, 12.1 mg/L and 84.5 mg/L for 1980–2017 for Na, K, Mg and Ca, respectively. An expected west-east trend in concentrations were confirmed, mainly explained by variations in aquifer types. The trend in concentration was stable for about 31–45% of the public water supply areas. It is therefore recommended that the exposure estimate in future health related studies not only be based on a single mean value, but that temporal and spatial variations should also be included.

Keywords: drinking water; exposure assessment; sodium; potassium; magnesium; calcium; spatial variations; Denmark

1. Introduction

1.1. Geogenic Elements in Drinking Water

Drinking water based on groundwater resources contains geogenic elements which may be important long-term exposures to humans and may result in both harmful (e.g., arsenic) or beneficial (e.g., magnesium and calcium) health effects [1]. Concentrations of the elements in drinking water can be altered during water extraction and water treatment (e.g., aeration) at the waterworks, and the concentrations in drinking water are therefore not completely equal to concentrations found in groundwater.

1.2. Selected Cations

This study focusses on the four major cations in groundwater: sodium (Na), potassium (K), magnesium (Mg) and calcium (Ca) which are all geogenic and important for human health.

The selected cations have all been related to cardiovascular diseases. For several decades, the positive association between high Na concentration in drinking water and increased risk of hypertension (HTN) has been studied [2]. In a recent study, it was argued that the association might be overstated and more complex than previously assumed [3], while the World Health Organization (WHO) concludes that the association is not conclusive [4]. Dietary K has been found to have a protective effect on systolic blood pressure in women, and the Na:K ratio in diet has been found to be associated with systolic blood pressure in both men and women [3].

In a systematic review of the association between cardiovascular disease and drinking water (including studies on Mg and Ca) in 2008, Catling et al. [5] found an association between increased Mg in water and a small reduction in cardiovascular mortality, but the evidence for an association between Ca and cardiovascular mortality was limited.

A taste-related limit of 200 mg/L Na is recommended by WHO and, for that reason, the Danish drinking water quality specification is 175 mg/L [6]. WHO has not proposed guideline values for neither K, Ca nor Mg [1]. However, national limits have earlier been 10 mg/L for K, 50 mg/L for Mg and for Ca, the concentration should not exceed 200 mg/L [7].

Several studies have focused on defining baseline concentrations in groundwater (including major cations), e.g., for a chalk aquifer around Copenhagen [8] and in the United Kingdom [9], a coastal aquifer in South Africa [10] and a European project *"Natural baseline quality in European aquifers: a basis for aquifer management for the purpose of monitoring ground water quality"* [11]. Furthermore, the geochemistry of bottled water has been studied in e.g., Europe [12], Scandinavia [13] and Germany [14]. The typical ion concentration levels in drinking water are therefore known to some extent on a larger scale. In Denmark, concentrations of Na, K, Mg and Ca in the latest groundwater samples ranged from 5.6–10,000 mg/L, 0.45–120 mg/L, 0–855 mg/L and 2.5–820 mg/L, respectively [15].

1.3. Origin of the Four Major Cations in Drinking Water

All tap water in Denmark is groundwater based [16] with the exception of a single small island (north-east of Bornholm, with around 80 consumers, see Figure 1 for a map of Denmark).

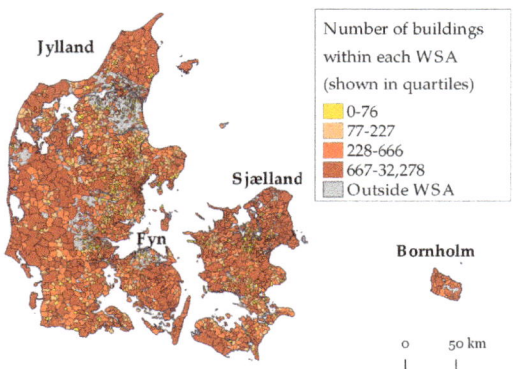

Figure 1. Public water supply areas (WSAs) (*N* = 2813 WSAs) in Denmark colored according to number of buildings within each WSA.

The following is a list of the three most important aquifers in terms of extracted water volume: (1) Quaternary sand and gravel glacial deposits, (2) limestone and chalk from Upper Cretaceous and Danian, (3) and, quartz sand and micaceous sand from Upper Tertiary, with a distribution of approximately 58%, 24% and 10%, respectively [17]. Bornholm is the only place in Denmark where bedrock is present at the surface and used as an aquifer [17]. Since the western part of Denmark was not covered by ice during the latest Ice Age (Weichsel), the aquifers in this area have undergone a longer period of chemical weathering resulting in significant deeper acidification depth, and differences in the geochemical content of the groundwater, e.g., the content of Ca and Mg [17].

Na (atomic number 11) and K (atomic number 19) are alkali metals and occur in nature in the +1 oxidation state. In many rock-forming minerals, Na and K occur as important constituents [12], in Denmark mainly in feldspars $(Na, K, Ca, Ba)(Al, Si)_4O_8)$, micas (ex. biotite $K(Mg, Fe, Al)_2Si_4O_{10}(OH)_2)$ and on cation exchange sites on clay minerals $(Al_4Si_4O_{10}(OH)_8O)$. Furthermore, Na occurs in halite $(NaCl)$ or in porewater of old marine deposits. Groundwater recharge also contains Na due to e.g., atmospheric deposition, de-icing salt or artificial fertilizers [12,18].

Mg (atomic number 12) and Ca (atomic number 20) are chemically alkaline earth metals and occur in nature in a +2 oxidation state [12]. Mg and Ca are found in several minerals, where carbonates are the main mineral source in groundwater, since they are ubiquitous and have high dissolution kinetics [12]. In Denmark, the main sources are calcite $(CaCO_3)$ where Mg can substitute for Ca $(MgCO_3)$ [12,17], which are found both in small gravels in the Quaternary glacial deposits and as the major minerals in limestone. Furthermore, Ca and Mg as well as Na can be found on cation exchange sites on clay minerals, e.g., smectite [17].

1.4. Processes That Influence Concentration Levels

Chemical constituents are slowly infiltrated to or released in the aquifer, and the rate and amount of geochemical change is, among others, depending on groundwater recharge changes, anthropogenic input to the soil surface, atmospheric deposition, top soil type, water residence time and chemical weathering. In a Danish context, the three main processes in the aquifers regarding the four major cations are the carbonate system, solubility of minerals and cation exchange.

The carbonate system is a buffer system against acid entering a carbonate rich aquifer and in relation to Ca, the governing equation is: $CaCO_3 + H^+ \leftrightarrow Ca^{2+} + HCO_3^-$. The equilibrium is controlled by CO_2, pH and the amount of available calcite. If the calcite buffer is depleted and acid (e.g., from oxidation processes) enters the aquifer, the pH can change, resulting in "aggressive water", which is found in western Denmark [19].

Clay minerals and organic material have the largest cation exchange capacity (CEC) and cations are exchanged according to concentrations in the water and the affinity order: $Al^{3+} > Ca^{2+} > Mg^{2+} > K^+ > Na^+ > Li^+$ [20]. Aquifers protected by thick clay layers, or layers with high levels of organic material, calcium carbonate or magnesium carbonate result in Na enriched water.

These processes can be anthropogenically enhanced, unintentional and intentional. During water abstraction, there is a risk of water table drawdown resulting in increased pyrite oxidation and thereby increasing Ca and Mg concentrations due to production of acidification. Furthermore, over exploitation can lead to intrusion of recent sea water or deeper connate water, resulting in increased Na concentrations [8].

At the waterworks, concentrations can be changed during normal water treatment, e.g., where pH is controlled during treatment of acid water or in advanced water treatment as e.g., water softening.

1.5. Drinking Water in Denmark and Exposure Assessment

The water supply structure in Denmark is mainly decentralized [16]. A total of 97% of the Danish population are supplied with tap water from about 2600 public water supplies and 3% are supplied with water from private smaller waterworks defined as wells serving less than 10 households [21]. Simple water treatment is sufficient at most waterworks; further, in 2012, only 74 waterworks had a permit for advanced water treatment of which only one was for water softening [22]. The drinking water quality is analyzed between 1/3 and 12 times per year, depending on the yearly amount of water abstraction [6]. Water samples are collected and analyzed by certified laboratories, that are required to report the analyses to the national database for groundwater and drinking water wells (Jupiter). The municipalities are the governmental supervisory authority and have to approve the analyses in Jupiter before they are publicly available [6]. Each waterworks supplies one to several administrative water supply areas (WSAs), and, furthermore, each WSA can be supplied by one to several waterworks. The decentralized water supply structure; close to 100% groundwater based drinking water; low consumption of bottle water [23]; and the relatively high number of drinking water samples registered in one national database are advantages in studies of drinking water and health, see e.g., [24–29].

1.6. Aim of the Study

The concentration levels of Na, K, Mg and Ca in groundwater and drinking water in Denmark are known due to comprehensive monitoring, and collection in one single national database (Jupiter). When drinking water is used as exposure for diseases, it is important, especially for long term epidemiological studies, to know both the spatial and the temporal variations in exposure. However, the spatial variations and the stability of the concentrations across time in exclusively drinking water have not been studied before in a national Danish context. The aim of the present study is to examine the spatial and temporal changes in drinking water concentration of Na, K, Mg and Ca. The results will contribute with new knowledge for future studies in the field of environmental exposure assessment and impact on public health. Furthermore, the study contributes to the discussion on health effects of water softening, which has been requested lately by the consumers in Denmark [30], though possible health effects are not conclusive [31].

2. Materials and Methods

2.1. Study Design and Drinking Water Samples

Data on drinking water concentrations between 2 September 1892 and 29 June 2017 were extracted in end of June 2017 from the Jupiter database, administered by Geological Survey of Denmark and Greenland (GEUS). On waterworks-level, the database includes information on yearly water abstraction and water samples from both private and public waterworks [32] (See supplemental materials, Figure S1, for details on the data management workflow).

Data were restricted to year 1980–2017, public waterworks and to drinking water samples after end treatment at the waterworks. A nationwide study on nitrate exposure from drinking water in Denmark was conducted in 2014 by Schullehner and Hansen [33], in which 2816 existing public WSAs were collected. In the present study, data have been updated to 2813 public WSAs.

In the Jupiter database, each drinking water sample is linked to a waterworks by a WaterworksID. For each WaterworksID a time series for each cation was created, and extremely low or high values (e.g., 0 mg/L and >200 mg/L difference in Ca concentration between the extreme value and the rest of the measurements at the waterworks) were manually validated. All analysis reports are stored in the Jupiter database. In case of extremely high or low concentrations these analysis reports were investigated for possible errors in decimal place. Furthermore, Na and K concentrations were compared with chloride (Cl) concentrations, and Mg and Ca concentrations where compared, since they are expected to be correlated. Extreme concentrations were excluded when no explanation was found for the measured concentration or when an error in decimal place was noticed.

Waterworks were linked to WSAs by spatial join in Quantum GIS version 2.18.14 (Quantum GIS, open source) [34]. When waterworks were located outside of the WSA, waterworks were manually linked based on information from the respective water supply companies and water supply plans from the municipalities [27]. Waterworks with no coordinates but with >10 drinking samples were manually matched to a WSA, by searching water supply plans and supply company webpages. Each waterworks distributes water to at least one WSA and each WSA can be supplied by several waterworks.

Difference in cation concentrations between water samples from waterworks and water samples from water pipes were compared in a scatterplot and tested with a multilevel mixed-effects linear regression model adjusted for date and waterworks were entered as a random effect. Due to a right skewed distribution of Na, K, and Mg, concentrations for these three cations were square-root transformed prior to the analyses.

To compare drinking water concentrations of Na, Ca, K and Mg, WSAs were linked to their primary groundwater aquifer type. In 1996, GEUS initiated the development of a National Hydrological Model (DK-model) [35]. (For description of latest release of the model, see [36]). The geology is discretized in a 100 m × 100 m grid and the model consists of 16 hydro stratigraphic layers [37]. In the present study, the layers are simplified into the following four aquifer types: (1) Pre-quaternary hard rock (Hard rock) on the island of Bornholm, (2) Quaternary sandy deposits (Qs), (3) Tertiary sandy deposits (Ts), (4) and, Tertiary/Cretaceous limestone (Ls). The model contains lithological and hydrological information from wells in the national Jupiter database. An aquifer type was estimated in the model for 137,971 screened wells. After linking wells to waterworks based on ID number in the database, the primary aquifer was assigned to each waterworks. When more than one aquifer type was present, the primary aquifer was assigned as the one where ≥80% of the intakes were in, otherwise all respective aquifer types to the waterworks were listed. For WSAs supplied by >1 waterworks with different aquifer types, all aquifer types were kept.

2.2. Yearly Mean Concentration of the Major Cations

For each WSA and cation a yearly mean concentration was calculated. First, a yearly mean was calculated for each waterworks and year, for the period from oldest to youngest water sample for the given waterworks, starting in 1980. Then, for WSAs supplied by >1 waterworks, mean yearly concentration weighted by the yearly water extraction volume from each waterworks was calculated [24]. For waterworks supplying >1 WSA, the extracted water volume was divided by number of respective WSAs.

2.3. Spatial Clustering of the Cation Concentrations: Na, K, Mg and Ca

For selected years (1980, 1990, 2000, 2010, 2015 and mean 2011–2015), areas with significant high or low concentrations were identified using yearly mean concentrations for each of the cations Na, K, Mg and Ca. Spatial scan statistics with a normal probability model was used to evaluate significance and approximate location of clusters [38]. An elliptic search window, 999 Monte Carlo replications and a maximum spatial cluster size of alternating 10%, 25% and 50% of the WSAs were applied in the analyses. The cluster analyses were based on centroids of WSAs. Due to a right skewed distribution of Na, K, and Mg, concentrations were square-root transformed prior to the cluster analyses. The cluster analyses were performed using the SaTScan™ software package v. 9.4.4.; (SaTScan™, Boston, MA, USA; https://www.satscan.org/).

2.4. Drinking Water and Aquifers

The association between type of aquifer and concentrations of Na, K, Mg and Ca was analyzed using a multilevel mixed-effects linear regression model. The association was adjusted for calendar year and WSA was included as a random effect. The analyses were followed by a pairwise comparison of the estimated marginal means to rank the aquifer types according to mean concentrations. Due to a skewed distribution of the concentration of Na, K, Mg and Ca, different transformations were considered including log, Box-Cox, square-root and rank transformation. Prior to the analyses, drinking water concentration for each cation was square-root transformed to obtain nearly normal distributed data. The analyses are limited to WSAs that are assigned with only one aquifer type.

2.5. Temporal Trends in the Cation Concentrations: Na, K, Mg and Ca

To evaluate if the concentrations of Na, K, Mg and Ca were stable in the study period at WSA level, a temporal trend analysis was performed. Initially, scatterplots of concentration versus date of drinking water sample were created at WSA level for each cation. Each WSA was afterwards categorized into one of six trend categories (See supplemental materials, Figure S2, for further specifications of trend categories):

Too few: Less than 3 drinking water samples.

Constant: Concentration interval < standard deviation of the concentration for all samples, excluding the 10% lowest and 10% highest measured concentrations. Furthermore, no significant increase or decrease in concentration during the study period.

Significant increase/decrease: Significant increase or decrease in concentration during the study period. Categorized based on linear regression where 95% confidence intervals of the trends were calculated and the null hypothesis (no trend over time) was significant ($\alpha = 0.05$) and a degree of determination, $R^2 > 0.1$

Change-point: Two or more different, but constant concentration levels or a significant change-point was observed (two connected regression lines). The change-point analysis was performed using two analyses. First, a Bayesian analysis with Markov chain Monte Carlo simulation of a change point regression model estimating the change point, and two slopes [39]. Secondly, the difference in concentration means before and after the change-point was tested with a *t*-test.

Parallel: Two or more constant concentration levels occurring at the same time were detected visually. Only WSAs which were not earlier categorized were included in the visual analysis.

Fluctuating: WSAs that do not fit into categories 1–5.

3. Results

3.1. Descriptive Results

The total number of drinking water samples per year (1980–2016) for Na, K, Mg and Ca increased from 1980 to 2002, from where on it was approximately stable until 2016, at a level of roughly 2000 drinking water samples per year per cation (Figure 2). Data for 2017 were only available for the first six months of 2017 and therefore omitted in the figure. For a period from 1988 to 2001, Ca was measured more frequently than the other cations, according to law [40,41]. Each year, the concentrations were measured at up to 1,900 different WSAs (Ca in 2001). Total number of WSAs was 2813.

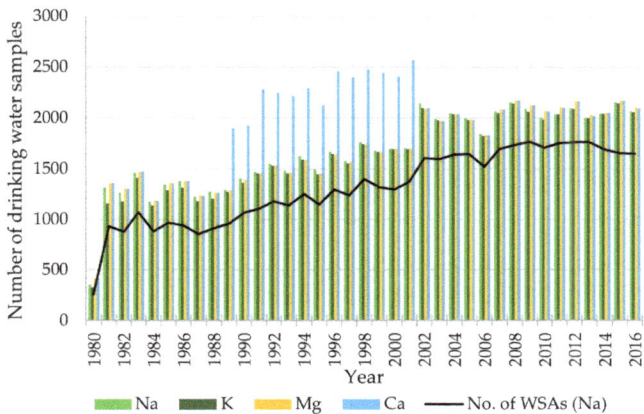

Figure 2. Number of drinking water samples per year for Na, K, Mg and Ca and number of water supply areas (WSAs) with water samples, 1980–2016.

The mean concentrations of the cations Na, K, Mg and Ca were 31.4 mg/L, 3.5 mg/L, 12.1 mg/L and 84.5 mg/L (Table 1). A total of 21, 30, 21 and 65 water samples were excluded as outliers for Na, K, Mg and Ca, respectively. Ca concentrations are normally distributed, whereas concentrations of Na, K and Mg are right skewed.

Table 1. Descriptive analysis of selected geogenic cations in drinking water in Denmark (1980–2017) given by means of number of drinking water samples, mean, median, 2.5% and 97.5% percentiles of the concentration for each of the cations Na, K, Mg and Ca.

Cation	No. of			Concentration (mg/L)			
	Samples	**Waterworks**	**Samples Excluded**	**Mean**	**Median**	**2.5%**	**97.5%**
Na	62,708	3724	20	31.4	20	9.1	130
K	61,581	3710	30	3.5	2.8	0.9	9.9
Mg	62,941	3724	21	12.1	9.8	2.8	35
Ca	72,561	3807	65	84.5	85	28.2	148

Waterworks have been linked for 2539, 2537, 2539, and 2549 WSAs with concentrations of Na, K, Mg, and Ca, respectively. A total of 99% of the waterworks have been assigned to a WSA. The 1% missing was due to lack of geographical coordinates of the waterworks.

3.2. Spatial Variations in Drinking Water Na, K, Mg and Ca

Spatial variations in yearly mean Na, K, Mg and Ca concentrations in drinking water for each WSA (2011–2015) are shown in Figure 3a–d. Elliptic clusters of statistical ($p \leq 0.004$) high or low concentrations overlaid on the maps are presented.

The geographical variation in all four cations are similar, with generally higher concentrations in the eastern part of Denmark (Sjælland and southern islands) and lower concentrations in the western part of Denmark. Furthermore, higher concentrations of Na and Mg are present in the northernmost part of Denmark and Na concentrations tend to be higher along the west coast of Denmark compared to the other cations. Notice the large concentration interval in the upper quartiles. For seven WSAs, the mean Na concentration is above the national recommended upper limit of 175 mg/L.

Number of WSAs included in the clusters, mean concentrations and *p*-values for cluster analyses of Na, K, Mg and Ca are presented in Table 2 (See supplemental materials, Table S1, for analyses results of transformed data). Change in number of included WSAs from 25% to 10% and 50%, respectively, in the cluster analyses did not change the overall results. Two significant clusters, one hot spot and one cold spot have been identified for all four cations, which enforced the earlier findings of an east–west pattern in concentrations. For Na, K and Mg the cold spot clusters are larger than the hot spot clusters, which underlines the earlier results of a right skewed distribution. Geographical extent of clusters for 1994, 2004 and 2014 resulted in similar east-west patterns (Figure 3a–d).

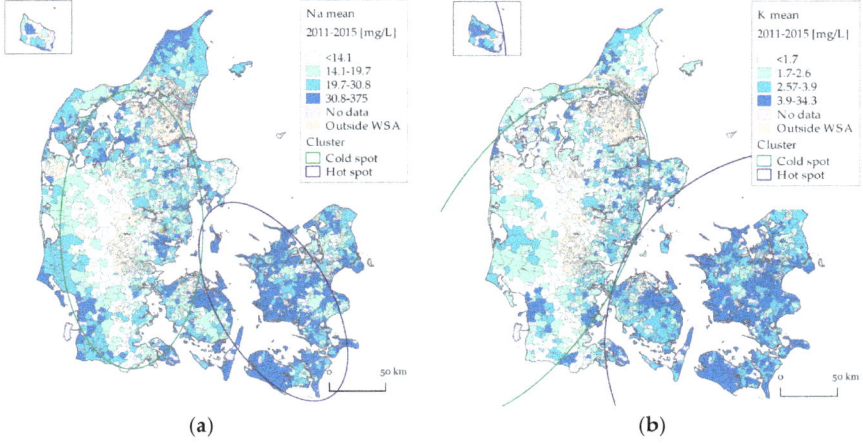

(a) (b)

Figure 3. *Cont.*

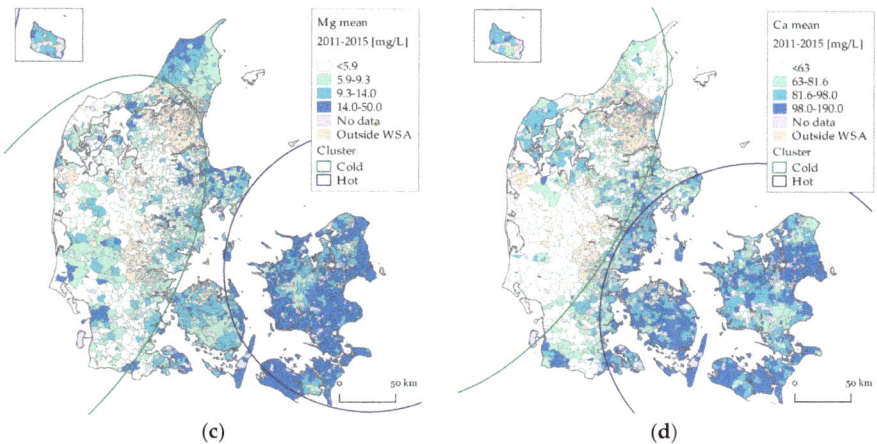

Figure 3. Spatial distribution of mean concentration of (**a**) Na; (**b**) K; (**c**) Mg; and (**d**) Ca, 2011–2015. Concentrations are shown in quartiles. In (**b**), Bornholm is included in the hot spot cluster.

Table 2. Statistical significant clusters ($p \leq 0.05$) of high (hot spot) and low concentrations (cold spot) of Na, K, Mg and Ca in drinking water. Up to 50% of the data points were included in the clusters, 2011–2015.

Cation	Type of Cluster	No. of WSAs		Mean Concentration (mg/L)		*p*-Value
		In Cluster	Total	Inside Cluster	Outside Cluster	
Na	Hot	500	2345	47.98	23.09	$\leq$0.001
Na	Cold	1156	2345	20.74	35.83	0.002
K	Hot	902	2344	4.35	2.42	$\leq$0.001
K	Cold	1154	2344	2.26	4.03	0.003
Mg	Hot	693	2345	18.19	8.14	$\leq$0.001
Mg	Cold	1171	2345	7.02	15.19	$\leq$0.001
Ca	Hot	1155	2344	96.24	66.48	$\leq$0.001
Ca	Cold	894	2344	63.86	91.78	$\leq$0.001

3.3. Aquifer Types Associated with Drinking Water Quality

An aquifer type has been assigned for 2543 WSAs and the geographical range and number of WSAs for each aquifer type are presented in Figure 4. The results reflect the general geology in Denmark. Limestone and chalk dominates the eastern part of Sjælland, and the mid north of Jylland, whereas Quaternary sand and Tertiary sand dominates large parts of Fyn and Jylland. Bornholm is the only place in Denmark where the aquifer is in hard rock. For 696 WSAs, drinking water was extracted from more than one type of aquifer.

The association between the four main aquifer types and drinking water concentrations of Na, K, Mg and Ca is shown in Table 3. For all four cations, the pairwise comparison of estimated marginal means showed that the mean concentration in Tertiary/Cretaceous limestone was higher than the mean concentration in Quaternary sand (*p*-value $\leq$ 0.001), which again was higher than the mean concentration in Tertiary sand (*p*-value $\leq$ 0.001). The mean concentration of the K cation in the Hard rock aquifer was significantly higher than in the three other aquifers. For Mg, the concentration in Tertiary/Cretaceous limestone and Hard rock aquifer was higher than in the two sand aquifers. For Ca, the mean concentration was significantly lower in the Tertiary sand aquifer compared to the mean concentration in the three other types of aquifers. For Na, the mean concentration in the Hard rock aquifer was not significantly different from the mean concentrations in any of the other aquifers (*p*-value > 0.1). Same overall results were obtained on log, square root and rank transformed data.

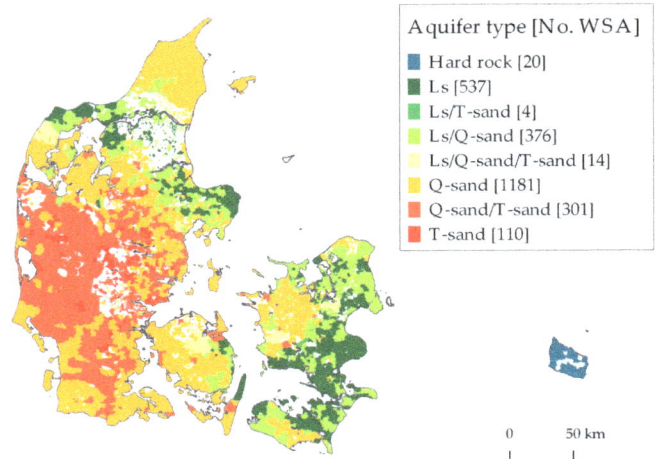

Figure 4. WSAs linked to main aquifer types in Denmark average 1980–2017. Ls = Tertiary/Cretaceous limestone, T-sand = Tertiary sand, Q-sand = Quaternary sand.

Table 3. Comparison of mean drinking water concentrations of Na, K, Mg and Ca between the four main aquifer types.

Type of Aquifers	No. WSAs [2]	Concentration (mg/L)			
		Na	**K**	**Mg**	**Ca**
		Mean (*SD*)	Mean (*SD*)	Mean (*SD*)	Mean (*SD*)
Tertiary/Cretaceous limestone (1)	528	37.8 (38.0)	4.2 (3.6)	18.1 (10.5)	95.5 (28.4)
Quaternary sand (2)	1157	28.6 (27.2)	3.2 (2.5)	9.4 (5.0)	86.5 (27.2)
Tertiary sand (3)	110	17.5 (11.1)	2.2 (1.5)	6.7 (3.0)	63.8 (27.0)
Hard rock (4)	20	24.6 (15.1)	6.2 (5.2)	13.3 (5.5)	89.8 (21.4)
Order of aquifers [1]	-	1 > 2 > 3	4 > 1 > 2 > 3	1 > 2 > 3 4 > 2 > 3	1 > 2 > 3 4 > 3

[1] The order of aquifers is based on pairwise comparisons of estimated marginal means. An aquifer type is only listed where the difference in mean concentrations was significant (*p*-value $\leq$ 0.001); [2] Count of WSAs is only presented for Na.

3.4. Temporal Variations in Drinking Water cancentrations of Na, K, Mg and Ca

On a national scale the temporal variation in mean yearly concentration for all four cations is constant (1980–2016) (Figure 5). Percentage of total number of WSAs (2813) increases from the year 1980 to about 2002, from where on the yearly percentage of WSAs with samples is stable at about 60% of the total number of WSAs.

The result of the trend categorization shows that the number of WSAs in each category (*Too few*, *Constant*, *Decreasing/increasing*, *Change-point*, *Parallel* and *Fluctuating*) is similar for all four cations (Table 4). Between 25–41 WSAs have less than three samples, and were therefore categorized as *Too few*. The concentration trend is categorized as *Constant* for about 31% to 45% of WSAs. Twenty-two to 33% of the WSAs were categorized as *Decreasing/increasing* of which the change was more than ± the difference between the 25th and the 75th fractile for only 103, 79, 46, and 71 WSAs for Na, K, Mg and Ca, respectively (differences were 0.52 mg/L for Na, 0.07 mg/L for K, 0.27 mg/L for Mg and 1.07 mg/L for Ca). Just 2% to 4% of the WSAs are categorized as *Change-point* and 2% to 6% are categorized as *Parallel* trend. The second largest category is *Fluctuating* and 20% to 31% of the WSAs are in this group.

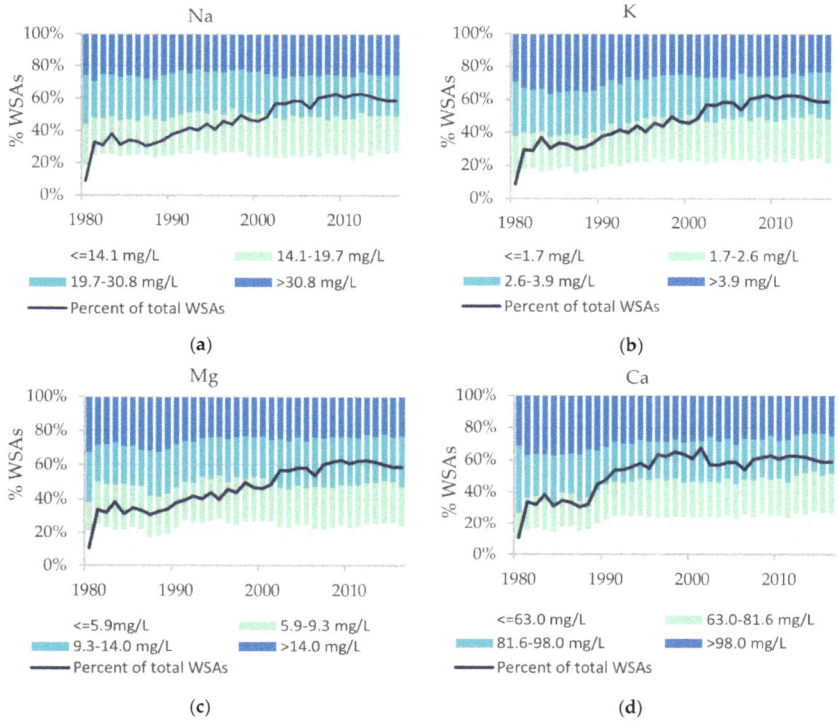

Figure 5. Temporal variations in yearly mean concentration at water supply area (WSA) level 1980–2016: (**a**) Na; (**b**) K; (**c**) Mg; (**d**) Ca. Concentration intervals are equal to quartiles of mean yearly concentration 2011–2015.

Table 4. Categorization of drinking water concentrations of Na, K, Mg and Ca at water supply area (WSA) level according to the temporal distribution ranked in trend categories.

Cation	Total WSA	Too Few *n* (%)	Constant *n* (%)	Decreasing/ Increasing *n* (%)	Change-Point *n* (%)	Parallel *n* (%)	Fluctuating *n* (%)
Na	2539	41 (1.6)	1136 (44.7)	723 (28.5)	56 (2.2)	86 (3.4)	497 (19.6)
K	2537	41 (1.6)	925 (36.5)	551 (21.7)	100 (3.9)	134 (5.3)	786 (31.0)
Mg	2539	42 (1.7)	1003 (39.5)	675 (26.6)	76 (3.0)	64 (2.5)	679 (26.7)
Ca	2549	25 (1.0)	786 (30.8)	831 (32.6)	103 (4.0)	148 (5.8)	656 (25.7)

4. Discussion

4.1. Key Findings

The mean drinking water concentrations of Na, K, Mg and Ca for the period 1980–2017 are 31.4 mg/L, 3.5 mg/L, 12.1 mg/L and 84.5 mg/L, respectively. We found statistically significant geographical variations in all four cations, with higher concentrations in the east Denmark and lower in west. The pattern reflects the general geological structures in Denmark. We found that the concentrations were constant, or with only a little increase or decrease per year for about 60% of the WSAs.

4.2. Comparison with Similar Studies

Median concentrations in comparison with concentrations found in selected studies are presented in Table 5. Our results are comparable with the median concentrations found in a similar sandy aquifer type in North Germany [42]. Compared to the concentrations in chalk in Denmark, both K, Mg and Ca are relatively lower, which underlines the finding of generally higher concentrations in chalk/limestone compared to Tertiary sandy aquifers.

Table 5. Median concentration (mg/L) of the four cations in the present study in comparison to other studies.

Cation	Concentration (mg/L)						
	Present Study	European Tap Water [43] [1]	European Bottled Water [43] [1]	Copenhagen Baseline (Chalk) [8]	North Germany Groundwater [42]	UK Chalk [44]	Groundwater Slovakia [45] [2]
Na	20.0	9.47	17.8	19	19.3	36	20.34
K	2.8	1.6	2.5	4	3.4	6.8	11.10
Mg	9.8	9.61	18.9	19	9.1	19	28.29
Ca	85.0	59.5	76.3	114	71	57	93.56

[1] Euro Geo Surveys (EGS) 2010, in [43]; [2] Concentration given as mean value.

The geographical patterns in the drinking water concentrations of Na, K, Mg and Ca are similar to known concentration levels in groundwater, with higher concentrations in eastern Denmark and lower concentrations at the glacial outwash plain in the west. The results correspond to an earlier study on geogenic elements, where higher concentrations of iodine, lithium and strontium were found in eastern Denmark and lower concentrations in the west [46]. (High concentrations of iodine were, however, also found in the northernmost part of Denmark).

The slightly increased Na concentrations along the west coast of Jylland may be caused by high atmospheric deposition, flooding or saltwater intrusion in the aquifers. However, increased Na concentrations are not found specifically in coastal regions but also inland, where Na concentrations in groundwater are primarily caused by residual saltwater in marine deposits as e.g., chalk [8]. Furthermore, saltwater intrusion is expected to be most relevant in the distance of 200–300 meters from the coastline, and the size of the WSA might therefore weaken a possible relation.

About 90% of the WSAs categorized as *Constant* trend are only supplied by one waterworks, whereas about 40% of the WSAs categorized as *Fluctuating*, are supplied by >1 waterworks (see Supplementary Data, Table S2). The variation in concentrations, are thereby firstly explained by changes in active extraction wells or change in the water supply structure, compared to natural changes in the aquifers.

4.3. Limitations

4.3.1. Validity of Drinking Water Quality Data

During this study, misclassified concentration levels have been found and e.g., data on yearly extracted water volume are not complete. Lack of validation might influence the result, by blurring correct patterns and over or under estimation of concentrations. Compared to the high number of samples, this is expected to have a minor effect on the results.

The geographical variations of WSAs with assigned concentrations were analyzed, and the missing data were linked with specific geographical regions. Until around year 2000 there were no water samples from the former counties in southern Denmark, northern Denmark and west Sjælland. Water samples do exist before 2000, but no registration on sample purpose is listed in the database. Schullehner et al. [33] included nitrate samples not registered as drinking water samples. This would be incorrect in the present study where Ca can change during water treatment. The unequal geographical distribution of number and interval of water samples reduces the certainty of the temporal variations results and the distribution of trend categories.

However, no association between the number of WSAs with water samples and the overall change in concentrations has been found, and the estimated trends are therefore assessed as a reliable indicator for the general trend in concentrations in drinking water.

The trend category *Parallel* is partly subjectively estimated, and the estimated number of WSAs in the group is therefore an approximation. Statistically based criteria have been set up for the other categories, and it is expected that the overall tendency will not change.

4.3.2. Water Samples from Waterworks or Water Pipe

Drinking water samples taken at the outlet of waterworks, in the water pipe system, and at the inlet to households were included in the study. Comparison of the groups for each cation showed no visual difference. The results from the multilevel mixed-effects linear regression model showed, that the mean concentrations were significantly different between the two groups for Na (*p*-value = 0.003) and Mg (*p*-value = 0.001). For both cations, the mean concentration was lowest in the water pipe system (5.4 mg/L for Na and 4.27 mg/L for Mg) compared to the waterworks, although only 146 and 148 measurements, respectively, were included in the analyses. For Mg, the difference was not statistically significant when the waterworks with highest concentrations (>40 mg/L) were excluded from the analysis, *p*-value = 0.132. Due to the low number of measurements and the fact that a small variation is expected because of time lag between the water samples at each waterworks, water samples from both waterworks and water pipes are included in the study.

4.3.3. Public and Private Waterworks

A total of 2444, 1249, 1284 and 1448 samples from private wells exist for Ca, Na, Mg and K, respectively. Concentration levels have visually been compared with concentration levels at nearest public WSA, and the concentrations were estimated to be similar. Schullehner et al. [33] found significantly higher concentrations of nitrate in private wells, which are mainly explained by higher agricultural nitrate pollution of the private wells compared to the public waterworks.

4.3.4. Classification of Groundwater Aquifers

Classification of aquifers is based on a model, and uncertainties thereby exist. Although only WSAs assigned with one aquifer type are included in the regression analyses, the aquifer type is still an approximation to the aquifer type from which 80% of the water is extracted. The analyses have been tested on only WSAs categorized as a *Constant* trend. However, this resulted in too few observations in both Tertiary sand and Hard rock for the analyses to be valid.

4.3.5. Accuracy of Concentration Estimate

WSAs are assumed constant in time, which is a necessary simplification of reality. The misclassification of WSAs is expected to have a larger influence in areas with larger population growth compared to more rural areas. On the other hand, several of the well-fields to the WSAs for the capital are more than 30 years old. A larger change is found in the rural areas, where there is a tendency to change from private wells to public water supply. Since the geographical variations indicate that drinking water concentrations in a WSA are similar to neighboring WSAs the issue seems less important.

4.4. Strengths

Compared to other countries, the large number of water samples is an asset for the study. It results in a unique data set, for which the major cations otherwise might not be regularly measured and registered in a national database. The decentralized water supply structure, close to 100% groundwater based drinking water, low consumption of bottled water and the relatively high number of drinking water samples are advantages in studies of drinking water and health (see e.g., [24–27]). This has proven to be useful in the present study where the cation concentrations have not been studied at this detailed level earlier.

Furthermore, the well-researched geology in Denmark is a strength for the study, improving the understanding of the mechanisms controlling the drinking water concentrations, and thereby revealing an opportunity for in future studies to define exposure variable concentrations based on the knowledge of geology and not only based on similar concentrations in the neighborhood.

5. Conclusions

Yearly mean concentrations (2011–2015) of the major cations Na, K, Mg and Ca in drinking water in Denmark are estimated at 31.4 mg/L, 3.5 mg/L, 12.1 mg/L and 84.5 mg/L, respectively. A strong association has been found between aquifer types and drinking water concentrations, with decreasing concentration in the order of Tertiary/Cretaceous limestone, Quaternary sand and Tertiary sand. Our study shows that the concentrations of Na, K, Mg and Ca in drinking water are constant in time for about 31% to 45% WSAs. Where concentrations vary, the main explanation is that several waterworks are supplying the same WSA. In future studies, concentrations of Na, K, Mg and Ca in drinking water can be reasonably estimated as a yearly mean, despite lack of concentrations in space and time with a few exceptions. However, precaution must be applied when estimating correct exposure for drinking water consumers in about 23−36% of WSAs where concentrations have been identified as fluctuating or with two parallel concentration levels.

Supplementary Materials: The following are available online at http://www.mdpi.com/1660-4601/15/6/1212/s1, Figure S1: Workflow, Figure S2: Description and selected illustrations of the different trends in concentration, Table S1: Statistical significant clusters, Table S2: Comparison between number of waterworks and trend in concentration.

Author Contributions: The linking of the different data sources and the trend categorization was done by K.W. in discussion with A.K.E., B.H. and J.S. The analyses on aquifers and cluster analyses were done by K.W. in association with A.K.E. A.K.E. did the change-point analyses. K.W. drafted the article and A.K.E., B.H. and J.S. have all equally participated with valuable corrections, ideas and suggestions.

Acknowledgments: We would like to thank Lars Troldborg at GEUS who has kindly delivered data on aquifer types, extracted from the National Groundwater Resource Model.

Conflicts of Interest: The authors declare no conflict of interest.

References

1. World Health Organization (WHO). *Guidelines for Drinking-Water Quality: Fourth Edition Incorporating the First Addendum*; World Health Organization: Geneva, Switzerland, 2017.
2. Talukder, M.R.; Rutherford, S.; Huang, C.; Phung, D.; Islam, M.Z.; Chu, C. Drinking water salinity and risk of hypertension: A systematic review and meta-analysis. *Arch. Environ. Occup. Health* **2017**, *72*, 126–138. [CrossRef] [PubMed]
3. Lelong, H.; Galan, P.; Kesse-Guyot, E.; Fezeu, L.; Hercberg, S.; Blacher, J. Relationship Between Nutrition and Blood Pressure: A Cross-Sectional Analysis from the NutriNet-Santé Study, a French Web-based Cohort Study. *Am. J. Hypertens.* **2015**, *28*, 362–371. [CrossRef] [PubMed]
4. World Health Organization (WHO). *Sodium in Drinking-Water—Backgrond Document for the Development of WHO Guidelines for Drinking-Water Quality*; World Health Organization: Geneva, Switzerland, 2003.
5. Catling, L.A.; Abubakar, I.; Lake, I.R.; Swift, L.; Hunter, P.R. A systematic review of analytical observational studies investigating the association between cardiovascular disease and drinking water hardness. *J. Water Health* **2008**, *6*, 433–442. [CrossRef] [PubMed]
6. Ministry of Environment and Food. *BEK nr. 1147 af 24/10/2017. Bekendtgørelse om Vandkvalitet og Tilsyn med Vandforsyningsanlæg (Ministerial Order No. 1147 of 24/10/2017 on Water Quality and Supervision of Water Supply Facilities)*; Ministry of Environment and Food: Copenhagen, Denmark, 2017. Available online: https://www.retsinformation.dk/forms/r0710.aspx?id=194227 (accessed on 6 June 2018). (In Danish)

7.   Ministry of Environment and Food. *BEK nr. 802 af 01/06/2016. Bekendtgørelse om Vandkvalitet og Tilsyn med Vandforsyningsanlæg (Ministerial Order No. 802 of 01/06/2016 on Water Quality and Supervision of Water Supply Facilities)*; Ministry of Environment and Food: Copenhagen, Denmark, 2016. Available online: https://www.retsinformation.dk/Forms/R0710.aspx?id=180348 (accessed on 6 June 2018). (In Danish)

8.   Hinsby, K.; Jensen, T.F.; Bidstrup, T. *European Reference Aquifers: The Limestone Aquifers around Copenhagen, Denmark*; GEUS: Copenhagen, Denmark, 2003; pp. 1–18.

9.   Edmunds, W.M.; Cook, J.M.; Darling, W.G.; Kinniburgh, D.G.; Miles, D.L.; Bath, A.H.; Morgan-Jones, M.; Andrews, J.N. Baseline geochemical conditions in the Chalk aquifer, Berkshire, UK: A basis for groundwater quality management. *Appl. Geochem.* **1987**, *2*, 251–274. [CrossRef]

10. Bjorkenes, M.S.; Haldorsen, S.; Mulder, J.; Kelbe, B.; Ellery, F. Baseline groundwater quality in the coastal aquifer of St. Lucia, South Africa. In *Urban Groundwater Management and Sustainability*; Tellam, J.H., Rivett, M.O., Israfilov, R.G., Herringshaw, L.G., Eds.; Springer: Dordrecht, The Netherlands, 2006; Volume 74, pp. 233–240.

11. Eugris Baseline Natural Baseline Quality in European Aquifers: A Basis for Aquifer Management. Available online: http://www.eugris.info/DisplayProject.asp?P=4163 (accessed on 19 April 2018).

12. Reimann, C.; Birke, M. *Geochemistry of European Bottled Water*; Gebr. Borntraeger Verlagsbuchhandlung: Stuttgart, Germany, 2010.

13. Frengstad, B.S.; Lax, K.; Tarvainen, T.; Jaeger, O.; Wigum, B.J. The chemistry of bottled mineral and spring waters from Norway, Sweden, Finland and Iceland. *J. Geochem. Explor.* **2010**, *107*, 350–361. [CrossRef]

14. Birke, M.; Rauch, U.; Harazim, B.; Lorenz, H.; Glatte, W. Major and trace elements in German bottled water, their regional distribution, and accordance with national and international standards. *J. Geochem. Explor.* **2010**, *107*, 245–271. [CrossRef]

15. GEUS Grundvandsanalyser (Groundwater Samples). Available online: http://data.geus.dk/geusmap/?lang=da&mapname=grundvand&#zoom=6&lat=6221704.9737511&lon=623976.22954561&visiblelayers=Topografisk&filter=&layers=mc_analyse&mapname=grundvand&filter=&epsg=25832&mode=map&map_imagetype=png&oldmapname=jupiter&mc_analyse_filter=stofnr.num%253D2081%2526seneste_analysevaerdi.min%253D&wkt= (accessed on 5 April 2018). (In Danish)

16. Thorling, L.; Ditlefsen, C.; Ernstsen, E.; Hansen, B.; Johnsen, A.R.; Troldborg, L. *Grundvand Status og Udvikling 1989–2016 (Groundwater Status and Trend 1989–2016)*; GEUS: Copenhagen, Denmark, 2018. (In Danish)

17. Sørensen, I. Geologi (Geology). In *Vandforsyning (Water Supply)*; Rump, T., Ed.; Nyt Teknisk Forlag: Copenhagen, Denmark, 2014; Volume 3, p. 784. (In Danish)

18. Labadia, C.F.; Buttle, J.M. Road salt accumulation in highway snow banks and transport through the unsaturated zone of the Oak Ridges Moraine, southern Ontario. *Hydrol. Process.* **1996**, *10*, 1575–1589. [CrossRef]

19. Ramsey, L. Grundvandskvalitet (Groundwater quality). In *Vandforsyning (Water Supply)*; Rump, T., Ed.; Nyt Teknisk Forlag: Copenhagen, Denmark, 2014; Volume 3, p. 784. (In Danish)

20. Appelo, C.A.J.; Postma, D. *Geochemistry, Groundwater and Pollution*, 2nd ed.; A.A. Balkema Publishers: Leiden, The Netherlands, 2005.

21. Danish Environmental Protection Agency Hvem Leverer Drikkevandet? (Who Delivers the Drinkingwater?). Available online: http://mst.dk/natur-vand/vand-i-hverdagen/drikkevand/hvem-leverer-drikkevandet/ (accessed on 21 March 2018). (In Danish)

22. Ministry of Environment and Food of Denmark—The Danish Nature Agency Videregående vandbehandling. *Kortlægning af Kommunernes Tilladelser (Advanced Water Treatment. Analysis of Permits Governed by the Municipalities)*; The Danish Nature Agency: Copenhagen, Denmark, 2012; p. 170. (In Danish)

23. European Federation of Bottled Water Key Statistics: Consumption of Water in the EU. Available online: http://www.efbw.org/index.php?id=90 (accessed on 3 May 2018).

24. Baastrup, R.; Sorensen, M.; Balstrom, T.; Frederiksen, K.; Larsen, C.L.; Tjonneland, A.; Overvad, K.; Raaschou-Nielsen, O. Arsenic in drinking-water and risk for cancer in Denmark. *Environ. Health Perspect.* **2008**, *116*, 231–237. [CrossRef] [PubMed]

25. Monrad, M.; Ersboll, A.K.; Sorensen, M.; Baastrup, R.; Hansen, B.; Gammelmark, A.; Tjonneland, A.; Overvad, K.; Raaschou-Nielsen, O. Low-level arsenic in drinking water and risk of incident myocardial infarction: A cohort study. *Environ. Res.* **2017**, *154*, 318–324. [CrossRef] [PubMed]

26. Knudsen, N.; Schullehner, J.; Hansen, B.; Jørgensen, L.F.; Kristiansen, S.M.; Voutchkova, D.D.; Gerds, T.A.; Andersen, P.K.; Bihrmann, K.; Grønbæk, M.; et al. Lithium in Drinking Water and Incidence of Suicide: A Nationwide Individual-Level Cohort Study with 22 Years of Follow-Up. *Int. J. Environ. Res. Public Health* **2017**, *14*, 627. [CrossRef] [PubMed]

27. Schullehner, J. Nitrate in Drinking Water and Public Health Effects—The Example of Colorectal Cancer. Ph.D. Thesis, Department of Public Health, Aarhus University, Aarhus, Denmark, August 2016.

28. Kessing, L.V.; Gerds, T.A.; Knudsen, N.N.; Jorgensen, L.F.; Kristiansen, S.M.; Voutchkova, D.; Ernstsen, V.; Schullehner, J.; Hansen, B.; Andersen, P.K.; et al. Association of Lithium in Drinking Water with the Incidence of Dementia. *JAMA Psychiatry* **2017**, *74*, 1005–1010. [CrossRef] [PubMed]

29. Kessing, L.V.; Gerds, T.A.; Knudsen, N.N.; Jorgensen, L.F.; Kristiansen, S.M.; Voutchkova, D.; Ernstsen, V.; Schullehner, J.; Hansen, B.; Andersen, P.K.; et al. Lithium in drinking water and the incidence of bipolar disorder: A nation-wide population-based study. *Bipolar. Disord.* **2017**, *19*, 563–567. [CrossRef] [PubMed]

30. Ministry of Environment and Food of Denmark—The Danish Nature Agency. *Blødt vand i en Cirkulær Økonomi (Soft Water in A Circular Economy)*; Danish Nature Agency: Copenhagen, Denmark, 2017; p. 81. (In Danish)

31. World Health Organization (WHO). *Hardness in Drinking-Water. Background Document for Development of WHO Guidelines for Drinking-Water Quality*; World Health Organization: Geneva, Switzerland, 2011.

32. Hansen, M.; Pjetursson, B. Free, online Danish shallow geological data. *Geol. Surv. Den. Greenl. Bull.* **2011**, *23*, 53–56.

33. Schullehner, J.; Hansen, B. Nitrate exposure from drinking water in Denmark over the last 35 years. *Environ. Res. Lett.* **2014**, *9*, 9. [CrossRef]

34. QGIS Development Team. QGIS Geographic Information System. Open Source Geospatial Foundation. 2016. Available online: https://www.qgis.org/en/site/ (accessed on 6 June 2018).

35. Henriksen, H.J.; Troldborg, L.; Nyegaard, P.; Sonnenborg, T.O.; Refsgaard, J.C.; Madsen, B. Methodology for construction, calibration and validation of a national hydrological model for Denmark. *J. Hydrol.* **2003**, *280*, 52–71. [CrossRef]

36. Højberg, A.J.; Stisen, S.; Olsen, M.; Troldborg, L.; Uglebjerg, T.; Jørgensen, L. *DK-model2014—Model Opdatering og Kalibrering. GEUS Rapport 2015/8 (DK-model2014—Model Update and Calibration. GEUS Report 2015/8)*; GEUS: Copenhagen, Denmark, 2015. (In Danish)

37. Troldborg, L.; Sørensen, B.L.; Kristensen, M.; Mielby, S. *Afgrænsning af Grundvandsforekomster: Tredje Revision af Grundvandsforekomster i Danmark*; GEUS: Copenhagen, Denmark, 2014.

38. Kulldorff, M.; Huang, L.; Konty, K. A scan statistic for continuous data based on the normal probability model. *Int. J. Health Geogr.* **2009**, *8*, 58. [CrossRef] [PubMed]

39. Carlin, B.P.; Gelfand, A.E.; Smith, A.F.M. Hierarchical Bayesian—Analysis of Changepoint Problems. *J. R. Stat. Soc. Ser. C Appl. Stat.* **1992**, *41*, 389–405. [CrossRef]

40. Ministry of Environment and Food. *BEK nr. 515 af 29/08/1988. Bekendtgørelse om Vandkvalitet og Tilsyn med Vandforsyningsanlæg (Ministerial Order No. 515 of 29/08/1988 on Water Quality and Supervision of Water Supply Facilities)*; Ministry of Environment and Food: Copenhagen, Denmark, 1988. Available online: https://www.retsinformation.dk/Forms/R0710.aspx?id=48476 (accessed on 6 June 2018). (In Danish)

41. Ministry of Environment and Food. *BEK nr. 871 af 21/09/2001. Bekendtgørelse om Vandkvalitet og Tilsyn med Vandforsyningsanlæg (Ministerial Order No. 871 of 21/09/2001 on Water Quality and Supervision of Water Supply Facilities)*; Ministry of Environment and Food: Copenhagen, Denmark, 2001. Available online: https://www.retsinformation.dk/Forms/R0710.aspx?id=12524 (accessed on 6 June 2018). (In Danish)

42. Wendland, F.; Blum, A.; Coetsiers, M.; Gorova, R.; Griffioen, J.; Grima, J.; Hinsby, K.; Kunkel, R.; Marandi, A.; Melo, T.; et al. European aquifer typology: A practical framework for an overview of major groundwater composition at European scale. *Environ. Geol.* **2008**, *55*, 77–85. [CrossRef]

43. Birke, M.; Reimann, C.; Demetriades, A.; Rauch, U.; Lorenz, H.; Harazim, B.; Glatte, W. Determination of major and trace elements in European bottled mineral water—Analytical methods. *J. Geochem. Explor.* **2010**, *107*, 217–226. [CrossRef]

44. Edmunds, W.M.; Shand, P.; Hart, P.; Ward, R.S. The natural (baseline) quality of groundwater: A UK pilot study. *Sci. Total Environ.* **2003**, *310*, 25–35. [CrossRef]

45. Rapant, S.; Cveckova, V.; Fajcikova, K.; Sedlakova, D.; Stehlikova, B. Impact of Calcium and Magnesium in Groundwater and Drinking Water on the Health of Inhabitants of the Slovak Republic. *Int. J. Environ. Res. Public Health* **2017**, *14*, E278. [CrossRef] [PubMed]

46. Voutchkova, D.; Schullehner, J.; Knudsen, N.; Jørgensen, L.; Ersbøll, A.; Kristiansen, S.; Hansen, B. Exposure to Selected Geogenic Trace Elements (I, Li, and Sr) from Drinking Water in Denmark. *Geosciences* **2015**, *5*, 45. [CrossRef]

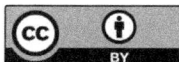

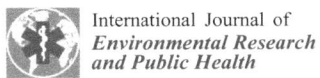

Article

An Assessment of Current and Past Concentrations of Trihalomethanes in Drinking Water throughout France

Magali Corso [1,*], Catherine Galey [1], René Seux [2] and Pascal Beaudeau [1]

[1]   French National Public Health Agency, 94415 Saint-Maurice, France;
       catherine.galey@santepubliquefrance.fr (C.G.); pascal.beaudeau@santepubliquefrance.fr (P.B.)
[2]   French School of Public Health (EHESP), 35043 Rennes, France; rene.seux0637@orange.fr
*   Correspondence: magali.corso@santepubliquefrance.fr; Tel.: +33-(0)1-41-79-68-84

Received: 11 June 2018; Accepted: 28 July 2018; Published: 6 August 2018

Abstract: In France, 95% of people are supplied with chlorinated tap water. Due to the presence of natural organic matter that reacts with chlorine, the concentrations of chlorination by-products (CBPs) are much higher in chlorinated water produced from surface water than from groundwater. Surface water supplies 33% of the French population. Until the 1980s, almost all surface water utilities pre-chlorinated water at the intake. Pre-chlorination was then gradually banned from 1980 to 2000. Trihalomethanes (THMs) are the only regulated CBP in France. Since 2003, THMs have been monitored at the outlet of all utilities. This study assessed current (2005–2011) and past (1960–2000) exposure of the French population to THMs. We developed an original method to model THM concentrations between 1960 and 2000 according to current concentrations of THMs, concentration of total organic carbon in raw and finished water, and the evolution of water treatments from 1960 onward. Current and past mean exposure of the French population to THMs was estimated at 11.7 $\mu g \cdot L^{-1}$ and 17.3 $\mu g \cdot L^{-1}$, respectively. In the past, approximately 10% of the French population was exposed to concentrations >50 $\mu g \cdot L^{-1}$ vs. 1% currently. Large variations in exposure were observed among France's 100 administrative districts, mainly depending on the water origin (i.e., surface vs. ground), ranging between 0.2 and 122.1 $\mu g \cdot L^{-1}$ versus between 1.8 and 38.6 $\mu g \cdot L^{-1}$ currently.

Keywords: chlorination by-product; France; environmental exposure; organic matter; tap water; trihalomethanes

1. Introduction

Today, almost all the French population is supplied with chlorinated tap water. Chlorination can interact with organic matter dissolved in the water, leading to the formation of unwanted and potentially toxic chlorination by-products (CBPs). The first CBPs were identified in drinking water in the early 1970s with the detection of chloroform and other organohalides [1]. As analytical methods improved, the number of CBPs identified in tap water increased considerably and now includes over 750 substances [2]. The toxicity of several of these substances has been evaluated, and some, including chloroform, bromodichloromethane, and dichloroacetic acid, are considered possible carcinogens for humans (group 2B) by the International Agency for Research on Cancer (IARC) [3].

In France, approximately 33% of the population is supplied by large drinking water treatment plants (DWTPs) fed by surface water, and 67% by smaller DWTPs fed by groundwater [4,5]. Because of its higher organic matter, surface water has a greater potential for CBP formation than groundwater. Some karstic and alluvial groundwater bodies influenced by surface water may also contain a non-negligible amounts of organic matter. The CBP formation potential depends mainly on the effectiveness of the treatment process used to eliminate organic matter, as well as on the chlorination process. Prechlorination of surface water—banned in France since 2000—required higher doses of chorine than chlorination at the outlet of the DWTP and was therefore responsible for the development of many more CBPs.

The population's main source of exposure to CBP is tap water, through ingestion, inhalation, and skin absorption [6]. The latter two are responsible for the greatest exposure to most CBPs, especially trihalomethanes (THMs), the exposure to which mainly occurs during showers and baths [7]. THMs are the most common CBPs, and the first to have been studied and regulated. The regulatory limit has been set at 100 $\mu g \cdot L^{-1}$ in France since 2008, while in the U.S. and Quebec, it is 80 $\mu g \cdot L^{-1}$. In Europe, they are the only regulated CBP. THM analytical data are widely used as indicators of exposure to CBPs in tap water. Many studies have shown a link between THM concentrations in tap water and bladder cancer in men, a link confirmed by meta-analyses [8,9] and pooled analyses [9,10] of the most robust studies. The average THM concentration, as measured at the consumer's tap or at the outlet of DWTP, is the indicator most often used in epidemiological studies [11–14]. Using the data from a Spanish case-control study, Salas showed that average concentration over forty years was the most appropriate THM-based indicator for studying the risk of bladder cancer [15].

We used the updated exposure-risk function published in 2011 by Costet et al. [9] to conduct a quantitative health impact assessment of CBP in water intended for human consumption in France [16]. This paper describes the levels of THMs and their trend in French water distribution systems between 1960 and 2011, and the use of water monitoring data for past (1960–2000) exposure assessment.

2. Materials and Methods

The geographical unit we used to determine the population's exposure to CBP was the water distribution zone (WDZ). WDZs are fed by one or more DWTP. The water quality data used come from samples collected from DWTP water.

Since THM data were not available before 2000, past concentrations were modelled. For this purpose, we developed methods that account for changes that occurred in treatment practices from 1960 onwards for both ground and surface water.

After estimating mean concentrations for 1960–2000 and 2005–2011 for all WDZs throughout France, we calculated administrative district (called département in France) and national averages, by weighting WDZ values by the size of the population supplied.

2.1. Water Data

DWTP data (location, type of water used, treatment facilities, towns and populations served) and water analytical data were extracted from the national database SISE-Eaux, which is used to monitor tap-water quality. The THM concentration data used in this study came from samples taken at the outlet of all DWTPs under regulatory monitoring from 2005 to 2011. From the SISE-Eaux database, we extracted 88,350 THM analyses from 13,732 DWTPs. Analysis of THMs was performed with a gas chromatography and mass spectrometry system by a static headspace technique (HS-GC-MS) according to the ISO 20595 standard [17]; or with a Purge and Trap and gas chromatography system according to the ISO 15680 standard [18] (Water quality—Determination of selected highly volatile organic compounds in water—Method using gas chromatography and mass spectrometry by static headspace technique (HS-GC-MS)) adapted to THM concentration measurement in tap water following the ISO 5725 standard [19].

The drinking water produced in France from surface water has always undergone post-chlorination. That is not the case for groundwater, a significant proportion being distributed without chlorination before 2003. In 2003, health authorities promoted post-chlorination [20] of groundwater and it was gradually implemented into all of France's DWTPs.

To identify when water chlorination of a given groundwater DWTP commenced, we looked for the earliest chlorine-free analyses in SISE-Eaux. Since no chlorination data were available before 2000, we assumed that DWTPs with no chlorine analysis after 2000 were not equipped with chlorination facilities before 2000. When data were available for the period 2000–2003, we assumed that, for the 1960–2000 period, the serviced population was supplied with chlorinated water. Approximately 130,000 samples of free chlorine were collected in 9400 DWTP supplied with groundwater between 2000 and 2003, i.e., 66% of these DWTP and 90% of the total population supplied with groundwater.

Our method to model the past concentrations of THMs (see section "Estimating past average concentrations of THM") also necessitated having total organic carbon (TOC) data. A total of 33,496 TOC values taken from analyses of raw water, and 68,604 from analyses of treated water, were extracted from the SISE-Eaux database.

2.2. Processing of the THM Measurements below the Limit of Quantification

Seventy-seven percent of the THM analyses had at least one compound whose concentration was below the limit of quantification (LQ). For 37% of the THM analyses, all the parameters measured were below the LQ. We therefore produced two estimates of average concentration per DWTP, a high and a low estimate calculated by assigning to the values below the LQ the LQ value or zero, respectively. The mean estimate, as referred in the "Results section", is the average of the low and high estimates.

2.3. Correction for the Seasonality of THM Concentrations

The combination of seasonal effects of both sampling frequency and THM concentrations resulted in potential bias in the assessment of THM average concentrations that we analyzed and corrected. As the seasonal effect on THM concentration varies depending on local climate, we firstly modeled by a spline function the seasonal variations at the district level, using available THM data for all DWTPs fed by surface water in the district. We then weighted the THM measurements made for each DWTP.

2.4. Estimating the Current Average Concentrations of THM

The current exposure of the population living in a given WDZ was defined as the average THM concentration of water for each DWTP feeding this WDZ for the 2005–2011 period. Data were corrected for seasonal variations affecting both THM concentrations and sampling plans. The latter were developed at the district level (i.e., smaller than the WDZ level) and possibly did not target same seasons. Accordingly, to correct for this, we calculated the average seasonal component of THM concentrations at the district level and referred to this distribution to correct the available data sample at the WDZ scale. Average concentrations of THM in the WDZs were estimated as the average of all selected concentration measurements.

2.4.1. Estimating Past Average Concentrations of THM in Treated Surface Water

Two different methods were used to estimate THM levels in treated surface water. Both take into account the greater exposure to THM at the outlet of DWTP caused by prechlorination (vs. postchlorination) prior to 2000. We assumed that all DWTP ran prechlorination before 1960 and gradually stopping it from 1980 onwards, before it was finally banned in 2000.

The first method (Method 1) was used by Chevrier et al. in their case-control study [12]. It uses the results of a pilot experiment reproducing types of treatment facilities in use before 2000, and focuses on the impact of different chlorination practices on THM formation. Average concentrations of THM ranging from 0 to 78 $\mu g \cdot L^{-1}$ were found for the eight (i.e., four each for ground and surface water) most common combinations of treatments. Two of these combinations prevailed in DWTP using surface water: (i) treatment including both pre-chlorination and post-chlorination and (ii) post-chlorination but no pre-chlorination. The average THM concentration was estimated, respectively, at 78.3 $\mu g \cdot L^{-1}$ and 31.8 $\mu g \cdot L^{-1}$ (i.e., 2.5 times lower).

We chose this ratio (2.5) of THM concentrations ($THM_{2005-2011}$) to estimate past values $THM_{pre-chlo}$ (i.e., before pre-chlorination was banned) from the current value $THM_{2005-2011}$.

$$\text{THM}_{pre\_chlo} = \text{THM}_{2005-2011} \times 2.5 \tag{1}$$

The second method (Method 2) is an original method which we developed. It is based on the observed correlation between THM concentrations and TOC concentrations [21,22]. We estimated past concentrations $\text{THM}_{pre-chlo}$ to be the product of the current concentration ($\text{THM}_{2005-2011}$) and the ratio between TOC concentrations in raw (TOC_{RW}) and treated water (TOC_{TW}):

$$\frac{\text{THM}_{pre-chlo}}{\text{THM}_{2005-2011}} = \frac{\text{TOC}_{RW}}{\text{TOC}_{TW}} \rightarrow \text{THM}_{pre-chlo} = \text{THM}_{2005-2011} \times \frac{\text{TOC}_{RW}}{\text{TOC}_{TW}} \tag{2}$$

Method 2 assumes:

(1) The constancy of the organic matter content of raw water;
(2) The constancy of the ratio of the THM concentration at the outlet of the DWTP to the TOC concentration at the chlorine injection point, irrespective of the location of the chlorine injection point. This implies that:

    (a) The qualitative composition of organic matter responsible for THM formation did not differ between raw and treated water, despite the huge reduction seen in the amount of organic matter.

    (b) Chlorine was not a limiting factor of THM formation, either in pre- or post-chlorination. We assumed that raw water quality remained stable from 1960 onward and that TOC at the chlorine injection point determined the total amount of THM produced.

The average THM concentration for each DWTP from 1960 to 2000 ($\text{THM}_{1960-2000}$) was calculated by using the average of $\text{THM}_{pre-chlo}$ and $\text{THM}_{2005-2011}$, weighted by the number of years with and without pre-chlorination. As data for year t, when pre-chlorination was banned for a given DWTP, were not available for all DWTP, t was randomly chosen for each DWTP following a uniform distribution between 1980 and 2000:

$$\text{THM}_{1960-2000} = \left(\text{THM}_{pre-chlo} \times (t-1960)\right) + (\text{THM}_{2005-2011} \times (2000-t)) \tag{3}$$

2.4.2. Estimating Past THM Levels in Treated Groundwater

Whether chlorination occurred before 2003 or not was determined by the presence or not of measurements of free chlorine in the SISE-Eaux database from 2000 to 2003. We assumed that past chlorination practices were similar to current ones and that the content of organic matter of raw water did not significantly change over the study period, and therefore that $\text{THM}_{1960-2000} = \text{THM}_{2005-2011}$. If no residual chlorine measurements were available, we assumed that the water was not chlorinated (i.e., neither pre- nor post-) before 2003 ($\text{THM}_{1960-2000} = 0$).

2.5. Calculating National and District Averages

Once the estimating concentrations of THMs for 1960–2000 and 2005–2011 were determined for each DWTP, we calculated district and national averages weighted by the size of the population.

3. Results

The sampling plan, elaborated at the district level, shew seasonal variations in sampling frequency with high density in spring and fall and lower density in summer and winter (Figure 1).

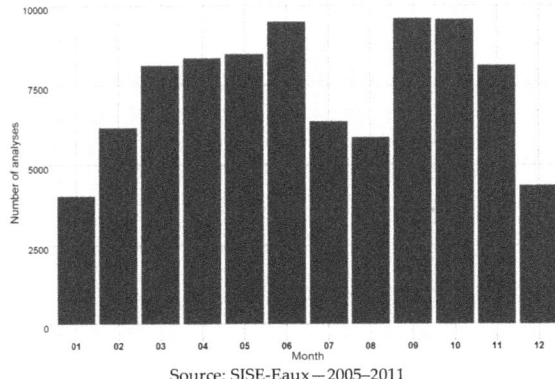

Source: SISE-Eaux—2005–2011

Figure 1. Number of samples for the measurement of THM, per month (13,732 DWTP). THM: trihalomethanes.

The average current THM concentrations in France (11.7 g·L^{-1}) depend on the nature of the resource (10.3 for groundwater origin vs. 20.3 μg·L^{-1} for surface water origin) in direct relation with their content in organic matter). TOC in raw surface water ranged 0.2–15.0 mg·L^{-1} (median = 1.8 average = 2.7) and TOC in corresponding finished water ranged 0.2–5.7 mg·L^{-1} (median = 1.2 average = 1.3). THM concentrations in water of surface origin peaked in summer (Figure 2) and linearly decreased during the period 2005–2011(Figure 2), since THM concentration in finished groundwater remained quite stable across seasons and years.

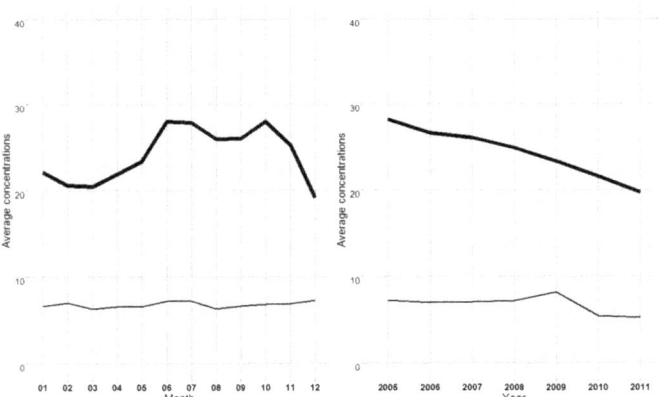

Figure 2. Average THM concentrations of (μg·L^{-1}), by month and year depending on the nature of the water (line in bold: surface water; thin line: groundwater).

With regard to past exposure, Method 1 and Method 2 yielded similar average THM concentration estimates in France (17.3 and 17.5 μg·L^{-1}, respectively), reflecting a dramatic decrease in comparison with current exposure (Table 1).

The two methods used to estimate past contamination yielded similar average contamination estimates. Method 2 saw a slightly lower prevalence of low concentrations (35% vs. 36%) and a slightly higher estimate of high concentrations (8% vs. 7%). (Table 2).

Table 1. Average concentrations of THM in finished water (2005–2011), France.

THM (in $\mu g \cdot L^{-1}$)	Sources		
	Groundwater	Surface Water	Total
	Mean (min; max)	Mean (min; max)	Mean (min; max)
2005–2011	10.3 (8.6; 11.9)	20.3 (18.9; 21.6)	11.7 (10.3; 13.2)
1960–2000 (Method 1)	8.9 (7.5; 10.2)	43.8 (41.0; 46.7)	17.5 (15.8; 19.2)
1960–2000 (Method 2)		39.0 (36.6; 41.4)	17.3 (15.7; 18.9)

Sources: SISE-Eaux, French Ministry of Health.

Table 2. Distribution of the French population in terms of current and past exposure to THM (in %).

THM ($\mu g \cdot L{-}1$)	Ground Water				Surface Water				Total			
	0–5	5–25	25–50	>50	0–5	5–25	25–50	>50	0–5	5–25	25–50	>50
2005–2011	29%	66%	5%	0%	8%	42%	45%	5%	32%	58%	9%	1%
1960–2000 (Method 1)	36%	59%	5%	0%	4%	21%	46%	28%	35%	43%	15%	8%
1960–2000 (Method 2)					6%	26%	44%	24%	36%	44%	13%	7%

Sources: SISE-Eaux, French Ministry of Health.

THM concentrations decreased by one third between 1960–2000 and 2005–2011. This decrease was driven by a fall in concentrations in the most contaminated districts. One percent of the population was exposed to concentrations over 50 $\mu g \cdot L^{-1}$ in 2005–2011, compared with 8% in 1960–2000. This can be attributed to treatment progress: the banning of pre-chlorination and further removal of organic matter prior to post-chlorination.

For groundwater, a slight increase in average concentrations of THM between 1960–2000 and 2005–2011 was observed (Table 2), linked to the roll-out of post-chlorination.

Large variations in exposure were observed between France's 100 (at the time of the study) administrative districts, these spatial variations broadly remaining unchanged throughout the study period (Figure 3). The districts with the highest THM concentrations were in western France (Vendée with 38.6 $\mu g \cdot L^{-1}$; Morbihan and Ille-et-Vilaine with 34.5 $\mu g \cdot L^{-1}$), in North-Eastern France, (Meurthe-et-Moselle with 28.2 $\mu g \cdot L^{-1}$), and overseas (Guyane with 31.1 $\mu g \cdot L^{-1}$; and Martinique with 22.3 $\mu g \cdot L^{-1}$). This disparity essentially reflects the proportion of the population supplied with surface water. Current THM contaminations may thus be worse than past contamination in districts where groundwater is mainly used as a drinking water resource, because of the implementation of chlorination between the two periods considered. Indeed, among the 31 districts where the THM concentration increased, all except one were mainly fed by groundwater (>75% of the distributed flow). Within this category, the difference between past and current THM average concentrations ranged from 0 to 7.7 $\mu g \cdot L^{-1}$, with a mean of 0.9 $\mu g \cdot L^{-1}$ and a median of 0.4 $\mu g \cdot L^{-1}$. In contrast, among the districts where water quality improved ($N = 67$), the difference ranged from 0 to 40.7 $\mu g \cdot L^{-1}$, with a mean of 9.0 $\mu g \cdot L^{-1}$ and a median of 6.8 $\mu g \cdot L^{-1}$, the greatest improvements being associated with more than 50% of the production provided by surface water.

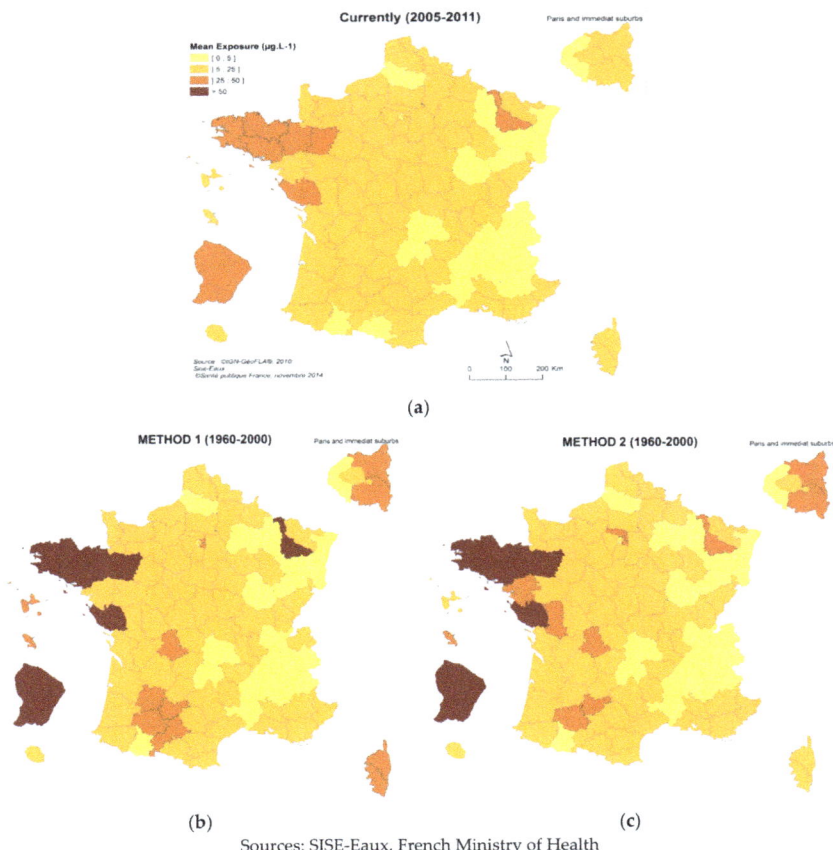

Sources: SISE-Eaux, French Ministry of Health

Figure 3. Average THM concentrations in the 100 French districts. (**a**) Current concentrations (2005–2011); (**b**) Past concentrations (1960–2000, Method 1); (**c**) Past concentrations (1960–2000, Method 2).

4. Discussion

4.1. Added Value of Method 2

THM concentrations gathered between 2005 and 2011 provided estimates for current exposure to CBP. In France, current concentrations should not be used as an estimate of past exposure since important changes in the treatment processes driving THM concentrations have occurred in the last few decades. However, these estimates can be useful for predicting the future impact and testing the potential effects of management actions, such as lowering the regulatory limit value for THM concentrations in tap water.

To reconstruct the past exposure of the French population to CBP, we used two methods that explicitly accounted for changes in water treatment methods. This helped estimate exposure over a long period in the absence of past THM measurements. In particular, these methods took the end of pre-chlorination of surface water into account. This element is critical, because ending pre-chlorination resulted in a 50% decrease in CBP exposure. The first method consisted in applying an overall increase coefficient to current exposure, as a proxy of past exposure associated with the presence of pre-chlorination. However, this method did not account for actual levels of organic matter in the surface resources nor for the capacity of the treatment to reduce TOC concentration in water. We therefore developed a second method which, like the first, relied on the reconstruction of the history of changes in treatment, but importantly accounted for local specificities, i.e., the content of organic matter in local resources measured by evaluating the TOC in raw water and the capacity of local treatment to reduce the TOC. This was measured using the ratios of TOC in raw and finished water. TOC data are available in the SISE-Eaux database from 2000 onward for all DWTP that use surface water. Method 2 assumed that TOC data measured at the chlorine injection point roughly determine the amount of THM formed. Some data and studies support this hypothesis [21]. The fact that Method 2 yielded a national level estimate for exposure similar to the one obtained through pilot simulation (Method 1) is in favors of its validity at a national level. Furthermore, Method 2 provided a more contrasted and realistic distribution of exposure than Method 1, due to the spread of the DWTP TOC_{RW}/TOC_{TW}, the 25th and 75th percentiles of which being, respectively, 1.06 and 2.55.

Estimates of past THM levels were reassessed in the USA, for a case-control epidemiologic study conducted in Iowa [23]. In the original analysis, surface water treatment plants were assigned one of two possible THM levels depending on the point of chlorination. The reassessment considered multiple treatment/disinfection scenarios and water quality parameters with actual DBP measurements, in order to develop estimates of past levels. As in Method 2, the water quality and treatments impacting DBP formation were taken into account. We therefore recommend Method 2 for estimating past exposure in France, in the absence of THM data.

4.2. Uncertainties Due to Data

The main sources of uncertainty affecting estimates of past THM contamination levels in distributed water stem from the hypothesis made on the model of reconstruction of past exposure. This hypothesis cannot be validated given the absence of THM data for DWTP that included pre-chlorination, and the gaps and uncertainties in the data detailed below.

4.2.1. THM Limits of Quantification

Thirty seven percent of THM analyses had at least one compound whose concentration was below the limit of quantification and were thus categorized < LQ (Limits of Quantification). We observed large gaps between low and high exposure estimates for the least contaminated DWTP. The effect of these censored data was taken into account in the confidence intervals and exposure estimates.

4.2.2. Point of Collection of Water Samples for THM Analysis

We estimated exposure as the mean THM concentration at the outlet of the DWTP. With current chlorination practices, THM concentrations increase during water transit in distribution networks. Within a single WDZ, the THM concentration can increase by a mean factor of 2 to 6 from the outlet of DWTP to consumers' taps [24], and this partly depends on the time for water transit. Consequently drinking water THM is greatly underestimated, especially in widespread networks and networks supplied with water containing high levels of organic matter, i.e., mainly networks supplied with surface water, where re-chlorination stations maintain a chlorine residual everywhere within the distribution network. Thus, the greatest increase in THM concentration from DWTP to taps is seen in rural districts served by a few, spread out WDZs fed by surface water (e.g., in the Loire-Atlantique district), while the lowest increases are seen where populations are dense and distribution networks compact.

4.2.3. Uncertainty about Treatment Evolution

Due to the lack of easy-to-obtain information about the dates of implementation and of cessation of pre-chlorination at the DWTP level, we assumed that all DWTP treating surface water used pre-chlorination from 1960 to 1980. We randomly generated the date of cessation within the next 20-year period of time (i.e., 1980–2000). Several simulated dates resulted in variations under 3%

between the estimates and the average past exposure of the French population supplied with surface water. This relative insensitivity of exposure to simulated dates of pre-chlorination cessation at the national level does not imply insensitivity at the district level, given the smaller number of DWTP involved. Maximum uncertainty was found for districts supplied by a small number of WDZ (e.g., in the Loire-Atlantique district, supplied by only 9 WDZ).

In addition to the uncertainty about the period when pre-chlorination prevailed, we identified two categories of water systems for which high uncertainty hindered the assessment of past THM concentrations. The use of a common model for all WDZ fed by groundwater is questionable in the case of groundwater influenced by surface water. This category covers karstic and shallow alluvial aquifers. In the case of karstic water, clarification facilities may have been implemented during the time period considered for exposure to cope with turbidity spates. Since the vulnerability of aquifers to surface water influence is not clearly labelled in the SISE-Eaux database, no specific processing has been implemented in model 2. Ozonation also may change the quantity and the quality of the residual organic matter. The presence of ozonation could reduce the risk of bladder cancer associated with THM [12]. Again, among the WDZ fed by surface water, we cannot distinguish in the SISE-Eaux database those whose treatment includes ozonation from those that do not. Accordingly, it would be worth it to collect additional information on treatment evolution within the sectors included in an epidemiological study, in particular the actual date when prechlorination stopped, the presence of ozonation, and the implementation of clarification facilities for WDZ fed by karst groundwater.

4.2.4. Existence of Multiple Water Resources

Twenty-five percent of WDZ and 42% of the French population are supplied by several DWTPs. Twelve percent of the population is supplied by more than three DWTPs. However, the contamination of one WDZ is estimated as the arithmetic average of the concentration for all DWTPs feeding into that WDZ, without weighting it by the volume of water supplied by the DWTP, creating a bias. This resulting bias is nevertheless moderated by the fact that the greater the volume supplied by the DWTP, the greater the frequency of regulatory sampling.

4.2.5. Low Frequency of THM Analyses

The annual number of analyses required by regulations is low for DWTPs serving fewer than 500 inhabitants (between 0.1 and 0.5 analyses per year). The average THM concentrations over the period from 2005–2011 were estimated based on one to four analyses, leading to very imprecise mean contamination estimates, given the variations in concentrations over time. However, the corresponding population accounted for only 3% of the French population, almost all exclusively (98%) supplied with groundwater with very low levels of contamination, which remains quite consistent throughout the year. The bias that this introduced in average contamination estimates was therefore negligible at the district and national levels. The problem is more serious for DWTPs that supply water to between 500 and 4999 inhabitants. Even though a higher number of measurements was available for these DWTPs (one per year, seven over the studied period), the population supplied represented only 22% of the whole French population, 19% of whom being supplied only surface water. For DWTPs supplying water to over 5000 inhabitants, the number of samples (5–12 samples per year) provided an acceptable accuracy in average contamination assessment at the district level.

4.2.6. Non-Random THM Sampling Strategy

Current French regulations establish the annual number of analyses that must be collected, without specifying how these analyses should be distributed throughout the year. Sampling strategies differ noticeably from one district to another, based on the choices of health authorities' district representatives. Data show that some local authorities search for the maximum THM concentrations, leading to over-represented summer measurements, while others avoid conducting sampling campaigns during the summer. The average concentration estimates are subject to biases resulting from the combination of seasonal variations of concentrations and district sampling practices. We controlled for this potential bias in DWTPs fed by surface water, by correcting the measured concentrations for seasonal variations modelled at the district level.

4.2.7. Conclusion: Uncertainties that Matter

THM data related to surface water resources were corrected for by using non-random THM sampling strategy. Inaccuracy due to censored analyses (<LQ) was incorporated into the confidence intervals. The main source of non-corrected uncertainty affecting estimates of past THM contamination in distributed water was the date when pre-chlorination of the DWTP ended. This resulted in possibly large errors in mean contamination estimates at the WDZ level, moderate errors at the district level, and a negligible error at the national level.

4.3. Ways Forward

4.3.1. Water Quality Management

Results from Method 2 suggest that THM exposure halved between 1960–2000 and 2005–2011, in direct correlation with the end of pre-chlorination of surface water. This change in treatment firstly translated into a dramatic decrease in extreme exposure: from 7% to 1% for those exposed to more than $50~\mu g \cdot L^{-1}$, and from 24% to 5% for those whose tap water came from surface water resources. The decrease in exposure continued over the 2005–2011 period despite reinforced disinfection procedures. This demonstrates the efforts of water operators to reduce soluble organic matter in water before chlorination [25] and adapt their strategy to maintain residual chlorine in the distribution network in a more parsimonious way (i.e., by injecting less chlorine at the outlet of the DWTP and counterbalancing this cut with appropriate re-chlorination points within the WDZ).

4.3.2. From Exposure to Health Impact

Accurately estimating past exposure is a major limitation for retrospective epidemiological studies focusing on cancer and diseases with long incubation periods. We developed a new method to estimate past THM contamination of tap water across France. The present study's greatest limitation is inaccuracy about exposure to THM in surface water-fed WDZs. This problem is the result of not knowing exactly when pre-chlorination for specific WDZs was abandoned. However, this inaccuracy decreases appreciably at the district level, due to the law of large numbers, and becomes negligible when assessing the national average exposure. Accordingly, this method is suitable for epidemiological studies and health impact assessments in France, depending on the geographical scale considered. More specifically, it is only a limitation for epidemiological studies requiring the estimation of exposure to the DWZ. For health impact assessments at a larger geographical scale, this limitation is greatly reduced.

Besides the limitation arising from not knowing when pre-chlorination was abandoned, our choice to consider THM samples at the outlet of the DWTP clearly led to a systematic underestimation of exposure levels. Having said that, most epidemiological studies [11–13] also consider these data for the same practical reasons which guided our choice: data availability and representativeness. However, when carrying out a health impact assessment, replicating the exposure assessment design formerly used in epidemiological studies selected to build the concentration-risk function, means that unbiased risk estimates can be made. In other words, unbiased risk estimates may be assessed from our biased exposure estimate, provided that the methods used for exposure assessment are homogenous between both the Health Impact Assessment and the studies selected to build the concentration-risk function formulation.

Estimating past exposure is a challenge faced by all epidemiological studies dealing with long exposure outcomes. Our study points out the crucial importance of considering the evolution of treatments in past exposure modeling. It could be adapted to other countries, for example, countries in the European Community, which share a common framework for water management and quality monitoring. The exposure of the population is however the result of a combination of the contamination of tap water and the user behavior. People are exposed more to THMs through showering and bathing than drinking tap water [14]. However, consumer behavior may have evolved during the time period considered for exposure assessment. In particular, the time given to bathing and showering has most likely increased from 1960 to nowadays, resulting in more exposure to constant contamination. Consequently, THM concentration at the outlet of DWTP may be considered an indicator of the contamination at the consumer's tap but only a proxy of exposure, if the changes in exposure behaviors are ignored.

5. Conclusions

In this article, we assess the current and past concentrations of THMs from data collected in the framework of European regulations. We observed a dramatic decrease in tap water contamination by THMs in France, with an average concentration of 11.7 µg·L^{-1} in 2005–2011, vs. 17.3 µg·L^{-1} in 1960–2000. The population supplied with surface water was two times less potentially exposed in 2011 than in 1960, but still two times more exposed than the population supplied with groundwater. Geographical inequalities remained due to the type of resources operated.

Our study confirms the crucial importance of considering the evolution of treatments in the past exposure modeling. It proposes an alternative approach to measuring past exposure of the French population to THMs, based not only on historical treatment method changes impacting THM formation, something previously done elsewhere, but also on the organic content in water resources. The model can be used for health impact assessment at the country and district levels. At the WDZ level, our estimates were inaccurate due to a lack of knowledge about local treatment changes. This is the main way forward to improve the specificity of model 2 for an epidemiological use.

Author Contributions: Writing—original draft, M.C.; Writing—review and editing, M.C., C.G., R.S. and P.B.

Funding: This research received no external funding.

Acknowledgments: We would like to thank the services of the French Ministry of Health for access to the water quality regulatory database SISE-EAUX.

Conflicts of Interest: The authors declare no conflict of interest.

References

1. Bellar, T.A.L.J.J.; Kroner, R.C. The occurence of organohalides in chlorinated drinking water. *J. Am. Water Work Assoc.* **1974**, *66*, 703. [CrossRef]
2. Wagner, E.D.; Plewa, M.J. CHO cell cytotoxicity and genotoxicity analyses of disinfection by-products: An updated review. *J. Environ. Sci. (China)* **2017**, *58*, 64–76. [CrossRef] [PubMed]
3. IARC. *Some Chemicals that Cause Tumours of the Kidney or Urinary Bladder in Rodents and Some Other Substances*; IARC: Lyon, France, 1999; Available online: https://monographs.iarc.fr/iarc-monographs-on-the-evaluation-of-carcinogenic-risks-to-humans-48/ (accessed on 20 November 2017).
4. Ministry of Health. L'Eau Potable en France 2005–2006; 2008; p. 63. Available online: http://solidarites-sante.gouv.fr/IMG/pdf/bilanqualite_05_06.pdf (accessed on 20 November 2017).
5. Ministry of Health. La Qualité de L'Eau du Robinet en France—Données 2012; 2014; p. 55. Available online: http://solidarites-sante.gouv.fr/IMG/pdf/rapport_qualite_eau_du_robinet_2012_dgs.pdf (accessed on 20 November 2017).
6. Villanueva, C.M.; Cantor, K.P.; Grimalt, J.O.; Castano-Vinyals, G.; Malats, N.; Silverman, D.; Tardon, A.; Garcia-Closas, R.; Serra, C.; Carrato, A.; et al. Assessment of lifetime exposure to trihalomethanes through different routes. *Occup. Environ. Med.* **2006**, *63*, 273–277. [CrossRef] [PubMed]
7. Xu, X.; Weisel, C.P. Dermal uptake of chloroform and haloketones during bathing. *J. Expo. Anal. Environ. Epidemiol.* **2005**, *15*, 289–296. [CrossRef] [PubMed]

8. Villanueva, C.M.; Fernandez, F.; Malats, N.; Grimalt, J.O.; Kogevinas, M. Meta-analysis of studies on individual consumption of chlorinated drinking water and bladder cancer. *J. Epidemiol. Community Health* **2003**, *57*, 166–173. [CrossRef] [PubMed]
9. Costet, N.; Villanueva, C.M.; Jaakkola, J.J.; Kogevinas, M.; Cantor, K.P.; King, W.D.; Lynch, C.F.; Nieuwenhuijsen, M.J.; Cordier, S. Water disinfection by-products and bladder cancer: Is there a European specificity? A pooled and meta-analysis of European case-control studies. *Occup. Environ. Med.* **2011**, *68*, 379–385. [CrossRef] [PubMed]
10. Villanueva, C.M.; Cantor, K.P.; Cordier, S.; Jaakkola, J.J.; King, W.D.; Lynch, C.F.; Porru, S.; Kogevinas, M. Disinfection byproducts and bladder cancer: A pooled analysis. *Epidemiology* **2004**, *15*, 357–367. [CrossRef] [PubMed]
11. Cantor, K.P.; Lynch, C.F.; Hildesheim, M.E.; Dosemeci, M.; Lubin, J.; Alavanja, M.; Craun, G. Drinking water source and chlorination byproducts. I. Risk of bladder cancer. *Epidemiology* **1998**, *9*, 21–28. [CrossRef] [PubMed]
12. Chevrier, C.; Junod, B.; Cordier, S. Does ozonation of drinking water reduce the risk of bladder cancer? *Epidemiology* **2004**, *15*, 605–614. [CrossRef] [PubMed]
13. King, W.D.; Marrett, L.D. Case-control study of bladder cancer and chlorination by-products in treated water (Ontario, Canada). *Cancer Causes Control* **1996**, *7*, 596–604. [CrossRef] [PubMed]
14. Villanueva, C.M.; Cantor, K.P.; Grimalt, J.O.; Malats, N.; Silverman, D.; Tardon, A.; Garcia-Closas, R.; Serra, C.; Carrato, A.; Castano-Vinyals, G.; et al. Bladder cancer and exposure to water disinfection by-products through ingestion, bathing, showering, and swimming in pools. *Am. J. Epidemiol.* **2007**, *165*, 148–156. [CrossRef] [PubMed]
15. Salas, L.A.; Cantor, K.P.; Tardon, A.; Serra, C.; Carrato, A.; Garcia-Closas, R.; Rothman, N.; Malats, N.; Silverman, D.; Kogevinas, M.; et al. Biological and statistical approaches for modeling exposure to specific trihalomethanes and bladder cancer risk. *Am. J. Epidemiol.* **2013**, *178*, 652–660. [CrossRef] [PubMed]
16. Corso, M.; Galey, C.; Beaudeau, P. Health Impact Assessment of Chlorination By-Products in Water Intended for Human Consumption. Available online: http://invs.santepubliquefrance.fr/Publications-et-outils/ Rapports-et-syntheses/Environnement-et-sante/2017/Evaluation-quantitative-de-l-impact-sanitaire-des-sous-produits-de-chloration-dans-l-eau-destinee-a-la-consommation-humaine-en-France (accessed on 20 November 2017).
17. ISO 20595. *Water Quality—Determination of Selected Highly Volatile Organic Compounds in Water—Method Using Gas Chromatography and Mass Spectrometry by Static Headspace Technique (HS-GC-MS)*; International Organization for Standardization: Geneva, Switzerland, 2018.
18. International Organization for Standardization ISO 15680, 2003. Water Quality e Gas-Chromatographic Determination of a Number of Monocyclic Aromatic Hydrocarbons, Naphthalene and Several Chlorinated Compounds Using Purge-and-Trap and Thermal Desorption. Available online: https://www.iso.org/obp/ ui/#iso:std:iso:15680:ed-1:v1:fr (accessed on 20 November 2017).
19. International Organization for Standardization ISO 5725. *Accuracy (Trueness and Precision) of Measurement Methods and Results—Part 1: General Principles and Definitions*; International Organization for Standardization: Geneva, Switzerland, 1994.
20. Ministry of Health, Circulaire DGS/SD7A n 2003-524/DE/19-03 du 7 Novembre 2003 Relative Aux Mesures A Mettre en Oeuvre en Matière de Protection des Systèmes D'Alimentation en eau Destinée à la Consommation Humaine, y Compris les Eaux Conditionnées, Dans le Cadre de L'Application du Plan Vigipirate (Internet). Available online: http://circulaires.legifrance.gouv.fr/pdf/2009/04/cir_19331.pdf (accessed on 20 November 2017).
21. Seux, R.; Clement, M. Why Eliminate Organic Matter from Water?—Fundamentals and Processes (Pourquoi éLiminer la Matière Organique des Eaux?—Principes Fondamentaux et Procédés). Available online: https: //slideplayer.fr/slide/1200937/ (accessed on 20 November 2017).
22. Urano, K.; Wada, H.; Takemasa, T. Empirical rate equation for thialomethane formation with chlorination of humic substances in water. *Water Res.* **1983**, *17*, 1797–1802. [CrossRef]
23. Krasner, S.W.; Cantor, K.P.; Weyer, P.J.; Hildesheim, M.; Amy, G. Case study approach to modeling historical disinfection by-product exposure in Iowa drinking waters. *J. Environ. Sci.* **2017**, *58*, 183–190. [CrossRef] [PubMed]

24. Mouly, D.; Joulin, E.; Rosin, C.; Beaudeau, P.; Zeghnoun, A.; Olszewski-Ortar, A.; Munoz, J.F.; Welte, B.; Joyeux, M.; Seux, R.; et al. Variations in trihalomethane levels in three French water distribution systems and the development of a predictive model. *Water Res.* **2010**, *44*, 5168–5179. [CrossRef] [PubMed]
25. Courcier, J.P.; Decerle, D.; Jédor, B.; Thibert, S.; Welté, B. To limit the formation of disinfection by-products. The case of bromate and trihalomethanes in drinking water. *Tech. Sci. Method* **2014**, *6*, 69–83.

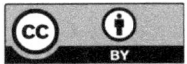

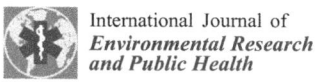

International Journal of
Environmental Research and Public Health

Article

A Physiologically-Based Pharmacokinetic Modeling Approach Using Biomonitoring Data in Order to Assess the Contribution of Drinking Water for the Achievement of an Optimal Fluoride Dose for Dental Health in Children

Keven J. Jean [1,2], Nancy Wassef [1], Fabien Gagnon [1,3] and Mathieu Valcke [1,2,*]

1   Institut National de Santé Publique du Québec (INSPQ), Montréal, QC H2P 1E2, Canada;
    keven.biomed@outlook.com (K.J.J.); nancy.wassef@inspq.qc.ca (N.W.); fabien.gagnon@inspq.qc.ca (F.G.)
2   Département de Santé Environnementale et Santé au Travail, École de Santé Publique de l'Université de
    Montréal (ESPUM), Montréal, QC H3C 3J7, Canada
3   Centre de Recherche du Centre Hospitalier Universitaire de Sherbrooke (CRCHUS), Sherbrooke,
    QC J1H 5N4, Canada
*   Correspondence: mathieu.valcke@inspq.qc.ca; Tel.: +1-514-864-1600 (ext. 3226)

Received: 27 April 2018; Accepted: 21 June 2018; Published: 28 June 2018

Abstract: Due to an optimal fluoride concentration in drinking water advised for caries prevention purposes, the population is now exposed to multiple sources of fluoride. The availability of population biomonitoring data currently allow us to evaluate the magnitude of this exposure. The objective of this work was, therefore, to use such data in order to estimate whether community water fluoridation still represents a significant contribution toward achieving a suggested daily optimal fluoride (external) intake of 0.05 mg/kg/day. Therefore, a physiologically-based pharmacokinetic model for fluoride published in the literature was used and adapted in Excel for a typical 4-year-old and 8-year-old child. Biomonitoring data from the Canadian Health Measures Survey among people living in provinces with very different drinking water fluoridation coverage (Quebec, 2.5%; Ontario, 70% of the population) were analyzed using this adapted model. Absorbed doses for the 4-year-old and 8-year-old children were, respectively, 0.03 mg/kg/day and 0.02 mg/kg/day in Quebec and of 0.06 mg/kg/day and 0.05 mg/kg/day in Ontario. These results show that community water fluoridation contributes to increased fluoride intake among children, which leads to reaching, and in some cases even exceeding, the suggested optimal absorbed dose of 0.04 mg/kg/day, which corresponds to the suggested optimal fluoride intake mentioned above. In conclusion, this study constitutes an incentive to further explore the multiple sources of fluoride intake and suggests that a new balance between them including drinking water should be examined in accordance with the age-related physiological differences that influence fluoride metabolism.

Keywords: biomonitoring; dental health; drinking water; fluoride; pharmacokinetic modeling

---

1. Introduction

Intentional fluoridation of drinking water has been in use as early as the 1950s in order to prevent tooth decay both in children and adults. Based on data extracted from McClure's [1] work, for the past several decades, an intake (that is, an external dose) of 0.05 mg/kg/day of fluoride has been considered to correspond to an "optimal fluoride intake" for caries prevention while minimizing fluorosis risk. It is the underlying population intake target behind the artificial fluoridation of drinking water at a concentration varying between 0.5 mg/L and 1 mg/L. This is now generally considered by many dental health professionals as a key public dental health measure [2]. Such fluoridation is recommended by the World Health Organization and supported by several organizations such as Health Canada, the Canadian Dental Association, the Centers for Disease Control and Prevention (CDC), and the United States Environmental Protection Agency (US EPA) [3]. Fluoride's mechanism of action to prevent caries relies on its effect on tooth enamel, which is mainly composed of hydroxyapatite crystals. Exposure to fluoride results in the substitution of the hydroxy group by the fluoride anion to produce fluoroapatite. At the same time, hydroxyapatite is soluble at a pH of 5.5 and fluoroapatite is soluble at pH 4.5. Lactic acid produced by cariogenic bacteria can cause the pH at the surface of enamel to drop to between 5.5 and 4.5, which causes demineralization of the enamel. Therefore, the caries preventive effect of fluoride stems from its ability to be incorporated into dental enamel and form fluoroapatite, which is resistant to demineralization at a lower pH [4].

In Canada, the proportion of the population with access to intentionally fluoridated water is currently about 37% [3], but interprovincial disparities on this proportion, which do not vary throughout the year as a function of the season (contrary to some other places in the world), is important. Furthermore, approximately 70% of Ontario's population now benefit from this public health measure. The public health concern has decreased from 12% in the early 2000s to less than 2.5% today in the neighboring Province of Quebec [5]. In this context, it is interesting to note that, according to the Ontario Association of Public Health Dentistry (OAPHD), for the 2012–2013 school year, Grade 2 students in Ontario had a mean DMFT index (decayed, missing, or filled teeth due to caries) in primary and permanent teeth (dmft+DMFT) of 2.22 with 50% of students being caries free. This result is based on screening data voluntarily reported by participating public health units to the OAPHD [6]. In Quebec, the Clinical Study on the Oral Health of Quebec Elementary School Students in 2012–2013 revealed, for the same age group, a mean dmft+DMFT of 2.67 with 44% of students being caries-free [7]. It should be recalled that dental caries have a multifactorial etiology and that the study groups were neither sampled nor weighted, according to fluoride exposure.

Proponents of community water fluoridation (CWF) highlight its contribution to address social health disparities [8]. In addition, nearly one in three Canadians does not have dental insurance and cannot receive the treatments needed due to their cost [9]. In Canada, dental caries treatments are second only to mental health problems with regard to societal costs ever since the mid-1970s [10]. Since tooth decay can affect children and adults as well as the elderly, the protective effect of fluoridated water consumption benefits everyone regardless of age. However, overexposure to fluoride during the tooth development can cause dental fluorosis. Mild to severe dental fluorosis is observed more frequently when the concentrations of fluoride in drinking water increase. Chronic exposure to high levels of fluoride may also cause more severe effects such as skeletal fluorosis and bone fractures [3,11–14], but the relevant studies have many limitations inherent to their ecological design. In addition, Health Canada's fluoride expert panel concluded a decade ago that the scientific studies available at the time did not support a link between intentional fluoridation of drinking water and cancer or any other adverse effect than fluorosis [15]. Since that time, further studies have raised some concerns regarding the neurodevelopmental toxicity of fluoride. However, at exposure levels that are generally well above the exposure levels correspond to intentional fluoridation of drinking water [16]. Additional studies have further supported the presumption that drinking water fluoridation is not associated with an increased risk of osteosarcoma [17–21] nor with altered thyroid function [22].

In contrast with the era when the optimal fluoride concentration in drinking water was determined, the population is now exposed to multiple sources of fluoride that contribute to the total daily fluoride intake (TDFI) such as through the use of fluoride toothpaste but also by ingesting a greater variety of foods and beverages as well as existing exposure routes such as soil ingestion and inhalation of residual air concentrations. Therefore, it appears relevant to re-examine the contribution of drinking water fluoride for caries prevention purposes today. The availability of both a physiologically-based pharmacokinetic (PBPK) model for fluoride [23] as well as population biomonitoring data for this element within the Canadian Health Measures

Survey (CHMS) [24], which is combined with the acknowledged disparity between drinking water fluoridation coverage between two provinces mentioned above, represent a unique opportunity in this regard. The considerable statistical weight of the participants from the provinces of Quebec and Ontario within the whole CHMS allows the extraction of data specific to these provinces and considered as reasonably representative of their population's exposure to the measured chemicals including fluoride [25].

The objective of this work was, therefore, to apply a PBPK modeling approach based on fluoride biomonitoring data from two CHMS provinces with very different drinking water fluoridation coverage in order to examine the resulting contribution of drinking water to achieving an optimal dose of fluoride in children from a caries prevention perspective.

2. Materials and Methods

The approach followed here relies on the use of a PBPK model in order to estimate internal exposure in the provinces of Quebec and Ontario using corresponding fluoride biomonitoring data from the second and third cycles (2009–2013) of the CHMS. The obtained doses are then compared to the suggested optimal intake for dental health of 0.05 mg/kg/day. Lastly, the internal dose metrics (IDM) in blood and urine corresponding to the chronic consumption of 0.7 mg/L fluoridated water were compared to the same IDM associated with the suggested optimal intake of 0.05 mg/kg/day.

2.1. PBPK Model Development and Validation

2.1.1. Model Structure

The PBPK modeling approach used in this work is based on the model developed by Rao et al. [23] to simulate the bone kinetics of fluorides for life-long chronic exposure in rats and humans (Figure 1).

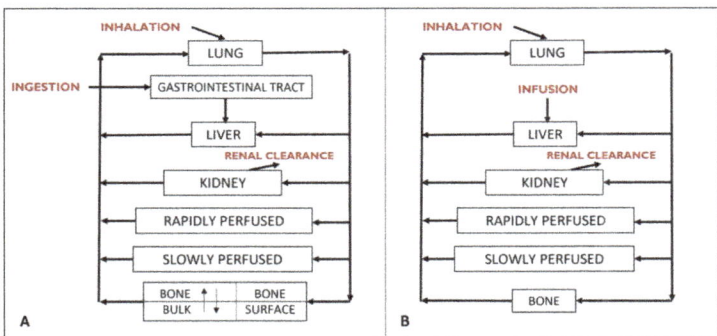

Figure 1. Conceptual diagram of (**A**), the original PBPK model of Rao et al. [23] and (**B**) the PBPK model simplified for the purposes of this work. Each box represents a compartment (an organ or a set of organs). The arrows symbolize the distribution of fluoride through the bloodstream.

The initial model of Rao et al. [23] considers the subdivision of the bone compartment into the surface bone and the inner bulk bone in order to simulate the bone kinetics of fluoride in detail. The original objective of these authors was to model the variation of the bone fluoride concentration for a period of several years. For the purposes of the current work, however, solely the blood and urinary concentrations of fluoride were of interest. In addition, since the model aimed to simulate fluoride's kinetics in children, the targeted population in the current study, in whom there is virtually no bone resorption because of growth, the inclusion of a compartment to consider the mobilization of bone fluoride and its release into the blood circulation was not required. Therefore, the original Rao et al. [23] model was simplified by considering a single bone compartment, which was reproduced in Microsoft Excel™ by Haddad et al. [26] and modified to specifically reflect the kinetics of fluoride in children.

2.1.2. Model Parameters

In order to adapt the model of Rao et al. [23] in children, the fixed values of the physiological parameters used in the original model were replaced by formulas described in the literature [27–30]. These equations allow for accounting the age-specific and body weight-specific variations of blood flow and volume in the child. In doing so, average human equations for both sexes were used because provincial biomonitoring data for the current work were not distinguished by gender. The tissue partition coefficients of the Rao et al. [23] model were applied unchanged. The model considers that fluorides are solely eliminated by renal clearance. Therefore, the plasma clearance formula used by Rao et al. [23] was normalized to body weight to the 0.75th power. In a longitudinal dog study, bone clearance and renal clearance accounted respectively for 90% and 10% of plasma clearance in the pup and 50% each in the mature dog [23]. Assuming this relation is linear, this reasoning was used to draw two lines (0, 90, 18, 50) and (0, 10, 18, 50) whose slopes make it possible to obtain the percentages of the plasma clearance attributable to bone clearance or renal clearance as a function of age. By multiplying these percentages by plasma clearance, values for bone clearance and renal clearance were obtained.

Since the model aims to consider various sources of fluoride exposure such as air, tap water, soil (dust), fluoride toothpaste, food, and beverages (bottled water included), source-specific bioavailability factors were assigned in the model according to available literature [11]. Bioavailability factors of 83%, 100%, 100%, and 40% were used for water [31–33], air [34], fluoride toothpaste [35], and diet [36], respectively. For soil, the same bioavailability factor used for diet was attributed given that the factors influencing its bioavailability are similar. Due to the lack of available data on oral absorption constants from the GI tract in human PBPK models for fluoride, direct infusion in the liver was assumed, which triggers the withdrawal of the GI track compartment from the initial model (Figure 1B). Therefore, any daily dose ingested would be transformed into a minute-based infused dose in the liver over 24 h.

2.1.3. Model Validation

For the purpose of model validation, data described in several published studies [37–41] in which fluoride intake was estimated and its urinary excretion measured were used in order to compare model simulations with observed data for given exposure conditions of specific child subjects. Additionally, among the available studies with measured fluoride intake and excretion in 24-h urine samples, the need for study participants to be aged eight years and under, in accordance with the targeted population for the modeling, was retained as a selection criterion. Since no such studies were found for children in Canada, studies from various countries (Venezuela, Chile, Germany, and United Kingdom) were selected to validate the model. Table 1 shows the five studies selected for fluoride intake and the amount of excreted urinary fluoride they measured.

Table 1. Fluoride intake and urinary fluoride measured in the studies were selected to validate the model.

Age (years)	Children (*n*)	Intake (mg/day)				AuF-24 [1] (mg/day)	Country
		Diet	Toothpaste	Water	Supplement		
4	31	0.560	0.706	0.042	-	0.3682	Venezuela [37]
4	20	0.533	0.254	0.231	-	0.358	Chile [38]
5	61	0.151	0.608	0.407	-	0.3705	UK [39]
5	11	0.092	0.274	0.111	0.455 [2]	0.476	Germany [40]
7	21	0.187	0.606	0.154	-	0.297	UK [41]
7	12	0.229	1.130	0.349	-	0.393	UK [41]

[1] Amount of urinary fluoride excreted in 24 h. [2] Fully absorbed fluoride tablets.

2.2. Exposure Scenarios

2.2.1. Subjects of Interest

Since this study aimed to interpret and use Canadian biomonitoring measures of fluorides, specific PBPK models for children of the corresponding age were built. In doing so, the median age of the two CHMS child age groups, was entered in the generic model described in Section 2.1. Specifically, distinct models for 4-year-old and 8-year-old children were built. Additionally, the 3-year to 5-year age group (median age: 4 years) was selected to evaluate the risk of dental fluorosis. In this age group, permanent teeth are still in development. Although the esthetic effects of dental fluorosis on permanent anterior teeth are generally considered to have taken place from birth to age 3, there was a lack of studies permitting a suitable validation of the model for this group. Complimentarily, the 6-year to 11-year age group (median age: 8 years) was selected in order to bring out insights on the possible age-related physiological differences that influence fluoride metabolism. The 50th percentile values of the World Health Organization (WHO) growth charts adapted for Canada in 2014 [42] were used to determine body weights and heights of the targeted median children. Then, data reflecting the Canadian exposure context were sought. The intake considered for fluoride toothpaste originated from an internal consultant report discovered by Health Canada based on data collected in the early 2000s concerning toothpaste containing between 996 and 1455 ppm of fluoride [11] while air and soil intakes were taken from the INSPQ [43]. Data on food and beverage intake from a survey of fluoride intake in the Canadian diet were also used [11]. With respect to the daily rate of water consumption, direct water consumption from a UK study [44] was selected. This was due to available Canadian data that did not concern the specific ages targeted herein or include indirect water consumption already taken into account by the food and beverage intake. Age-specific parameter values are presented in Table 2.

Table 2. Age-specific fixed parameter values needed to model fluoride exposure.

| Age (year) | Weight (kg) | Height (cm) | Sources of Fluorides | | | | |
			Toothpaste (µg/kg/day)	Diet (µg/kg/day)	Soil (µg/kg/day)	Air (µg/kg/day)	Water (L/day)
4	16	103	40	21	1.19	0.01	0.442
8	25	127	30	17.5	0.21	0.01	0.56

2.2.2. Model Simulations of Internal Dose Metrics of Interest

Continuous fluoride exposure until the steady-state is reached, after approximately 150 days for both arterial blood and urinary fluoride (see example in Figure 2), was simulated with the models. Given that CHMS biomonitoring data, which will be used further, result from spot urine samples, an assumption that the measured urinary fluoride is a consequence of steady-state exposure is made. This presumption is a state-of-the art hypothesis for the interpretation. For instance, Biomonitoring Equivalents (BE) [45] of data was collected in large biomonitoring surveys such as the National Health and Nutrition Examination Survey (NHANES) [46], the German chemical Exposure Study (GERes) [47,48], and CHMS [49] with model-derived or model-simulated exposures.

By entering the available fluoride's external exposure data for Quebec and Ontario as input in the PBPK model, the resulting urinary levels can be compared to the corresponding CHMS values, which exhibit significantly greater population mean urinary fluoride concentration in Ontario as compared to Quebec [25]. Specifically, a 24-h steady state amount of excreted urinary fluoride was obtained by subtracting the simulated amount of urinary fluoride excreted after 149 days of continuous exposure from the same amount excreted after 150 days.

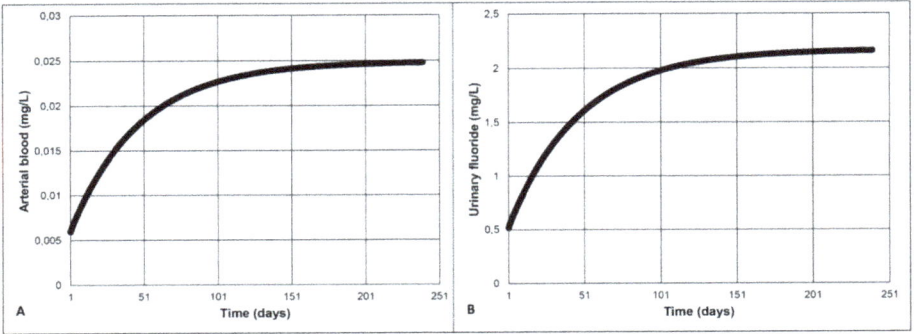

Figure 2. (**A**) Arterial and (**B**) urinary fluoride concentration in a 4-year-old child continuously exposed to 0.7 mg/L of fluoridated water.

2.2.3. Exposure Scenarios Simulated

Three exposure scenarios were considered. In the first scenario, exposure for a 4-year old and an 8-year old child from Ontario is modeled based on intakes listed in Table 2 from air, soil, diet, fluoride toothpaste, and fluoridated water (Figure 3). Since 70% of Ontario's population including children has access to fluoridated water at 0.7 mg/L. An equivalent average fluoride concentration of 0.5 mg/L was calculated assuming that the remaining 30% non-fluoridated water had a concentration of 0.05 mg/L (detection limit). In the second scenario, in the deemed representative of a 4-year old or an 8-year old child in Quebec, it is assumed that the only difference in exposure sources lies in the much lower access to fluoridated water at 0.7 mg/L. Therefore, this second scenario was modeled with 2.5% of the Quebec child population consuming fluoridated water at 0.7 mg/L for an equivalent average of 0.06 mg/L (if 97.5% of inhabitants drink non-fluoridated water at a concentration of 0.05 mg/L).

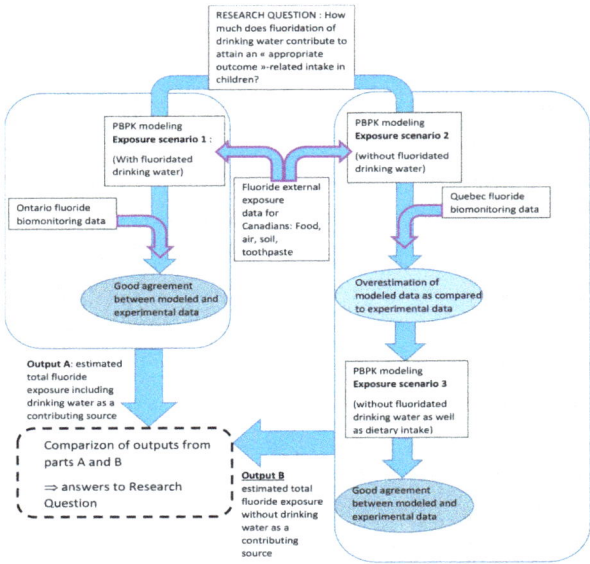

Figure 3. Flow chart describing the methodological rationale underlying the fluoride exposure scenarios simulated by PBPK modeling in order to examine the original research question.

As shown later (see Results), the simulation of the second scenario tends to overestimate the urinary concentration of fluoride. In order to evaluate the contribution of drinking water to TDFI in Quebec, the consistency between input parameters used in the model and reality, presumably reflected accurately by CHMS data, is required. This contribution was evaluated differentially by modeling the daily amounts of urinary fluoride excreted at steady-state levels assuming the exposure conditions present in Ontario vs. Quebec and comparing them to those modeled for the TDFI using available fluoride intake input parameters. Therefore, for determining the contribution of drinking water to the overall fluoride exposure, it was necessary to account for the fact that fluoride concentrations in water may affect those found in foods via cooking and preparation of processed food. Therefore, the third scenario was modeled without fluoride intake from the diet to better reflect the exposure of a 4-year old or an 8-year old child in Quebec.

2.3. Determination of Mean Absorbed Fluoride Dose in Average Children from Quebec and Ontario Using Biomonitoring Data

Since the present work relies in part on biomonitoring data, an absorbed dose is deemed more relevant to work for the purpose of the present study than an intake. Therefore, the calculated total ingested fluoride intake from water and diet were converted into corresponding absorbed doses by applying the relevant bioavailability factors of 83% and 40% presented above (see Appendix A Table A1). A mean resulting absorbed dose across all ages investigated (1–12 years old) of 0.04 mg/kg/day was obtained and was, henceforth, used for the purpose of this work.

Based on the mean and 95th percentile values of urinary concentrations of fluoride measured in the two CHMS provinces, corresponding absorbed doses in Quebec and Ontario could be modeled using the solver complement in Microsoft Excel™. The solver provides a value for a given parameter by modifying one or more model parameters while including constraints as needed. Therefore, CHMS urinary concentrations were converted to excreted amounts of urinary fluoride using daily urinary fluoride excretion rates [50]. The converted CHMS fluoride amount was entered into the solver as a 24-h steady state parameter and the model was only allowed to change the absorbed TDFI parameter while retaining the values and equations for all other parameters. The only constraint in this case was that the TDFI had to be a positive number (greater than zero). The solver then made it possible to determine the absorbed dose associated with the amount of urinary fluoride. The absorbed doses from Quebec and Ontario obtained by using the solver with CHMS urinary fluoride amounts at the mean and 95th percentile values could then be analyzed to determine if (1) the absorbed dose of 0.04 mg/kg/day detailed above was reached in those provinces and (2) the resulting intakes correspond to the total intakes computed in Section 2.2.2 considering different exposure levels via drinking water fluoridation.

2.4. PBPK Model Sensitivity Analyses

In order to know the impact of the variation of each parameter on the predicted internal concentrations of fluoride, a sensitivity analysis of the model parameters was carried out, according to the following formula (Valcke & Krishnan [29]).

$$SI_P = \frac{Aexc_{F_2} - Aexc_{F_i}}{P_2 - P_i} \times \frac{P_i}{Aexc_{F\_i}} \tag{1}$$

where SI_P is the sensitivity index of the parameter "P", $Aexc_{F\_2}$ is the quantity of urinary fluoride excreted over 24 h at a steady-state after reduction of the "P" parameter by 2% of its initial value, $Aexc_{F\_i}$ is the initial value of the quantity of urinary fluoride excreted over 24 h at a steady-state, P_i is the initial value of a parameter "P", and P_2 is its value after being reduced by 2% of its initial value.

3. Results

3.1. Model Validation

For intakes ranging from 0.04 mg/kg/day to 0.08 mg/kg/day in the studies used as validation, the amounts of urinary fluoride predicted by the PBPK model were always greater than the amounts measured (Figure 4). In order to overcome this systematic overestimation by the model, the average ratios "urinary fluoride measured/urinary fluoride modeled" were calculated to obtain the average empirical adjustment factor of 0.43. This factor was incorporated into the final model prior to running the simulation of exposure scenarios and model-based interpretation of biomonitoring data for which the results are presented hereafter in Sections 3.2 and 3.3.

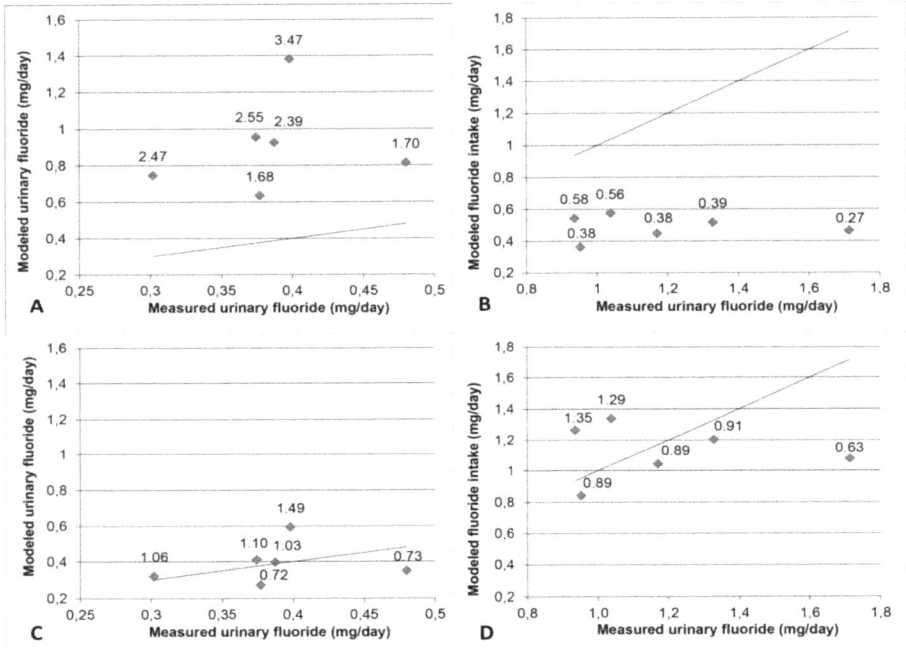

Figure 4. Results of model simulation of exposure data in the literature as a function of experimental biological measures in children aged 4 to 7 years. Each point represents a study while the line represents a perfect agreement. The values at the top of the points represent the ratios between the modeled values and the experimental values. Panels (**A,B**) illustrate, respectively, the over-estimation and underestimation of the modeled values. Panels (**C,D**) show the predicted values around the perfect agreement line when adjusted by multiplying by the adjustment factor of 0.43 in (**C**) and 1/0.43 in (**D**).

3.2. Modeled Exposure Scenarios

Table 3 shows that the modeled urinary concentrations of fluoride for the first scenario are slightly higher than the concentrations measured in Ontario's CHMS participants with ratios of 1.02 and 1.09. For the second scenario, the modeled concentrations were much higher than those measured in Quebec's CHMS participants with ratios of 1.81 and 1.78. This suggests that the modeled exposure for this scenario does not correspond to the actual exposure likely due to one or more sources of fluoride are overestimated for Quebec. The concentrations modeled for exposure in the third scenario approximate the measured concentrations while remaining higher with ratios of 1.47 and 1.41.

Table 3. Urinary fluoride concentrations (mg/L) modeled in a 4-year-old and an 8-year-old child for different exposure scenarios compared with Province-specific CHMS biomonitoring data.

Province	Scenario	Age-Specific Results					
		4 year-old Child			8 year-old Child		
		Model	CHMS	Ratio [1]	Model	CHMS	Ratio [1]
Ontario	1. (Fluoridation of drinking water at 0.7 mg/L)	0.846	0.83	1.02	0.73	0.67	1.09
Quebec	2. (Fluoridation at 0.06 mg/L with dietary intake)	0.708	0.39	1.81	0.605	0.34	1.78
Quebec–modified	3. (Fluoridation at 0.06 mg/L without dietary intake)	0.574		1.47	0.48		1.41

[1] Ratio of the modeled urinary concentration over the CHMS bio-monitored urinary concentration.

Table 4 shows the average absorbed fluoride doses, which were modeled based on CHMS urine concentrations using Microsoft Excel™'s solver complement. In Quebec, it is lower than the suggested optimal absorbed dose of 0.04 mg/kg/day. In Ontario, this dose is reached and even exceeded. However, when looking at the 95th percentile, the suggested optimal absorbed dose is exceeded in both provinces.

Table 4. Absorbed fluoride doses (mg/kg/d) modeled with CHMS biomonitoring data from Quebec and Ontario.

Age	Quebec, Geometric Mean (95th Percentile)	Ontario, Geometric Mean (95th Percentile)
4	0.03 (0.13)	0.06 (0.17)
8	0.02 (0.05)	0.05 (0.12)

3.3. Contribution of Drinking Water to the Total Intake of Fluoride

Figure 5 shows the contribution, based on PBPK model simulations, of different fluoride sources (see Table 2) to total intake as well as amounts or urinary fluoride for Quebec and Ontario converted from CHMS biomonitoring data. The contribution of air and soil is minimal. The most important source is toothpaste followed by fluoridated water at 0.7 mg/L and diet. The TDFI when the water is fluoridated at 0.7 mg/L is above the suggested optimal intake, which is slightly higher than what was measured in Ontario. In Quebec, where the majority of fluoride exposure is through ingestion of fluoride toothpaste, the intake measured by the CHMS is even lower than the modeled intake from fluoride toothpaste.

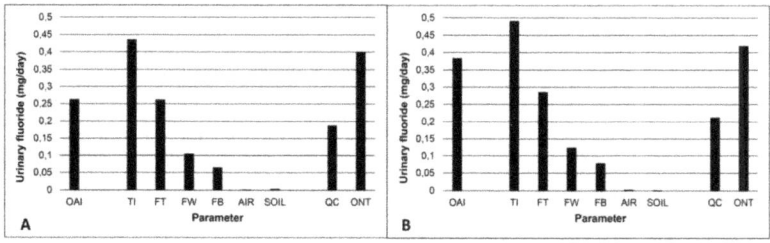

Figure 5. Modelled excreted fluoride over 24 h at a steady-state, according to the different intakes considered in the 4-year-old (**A**) and 8-year-old (**B**) child. The data from Table 2 were used for fluoride sources. These modeled data are compared to CHMS biomonitoring geometric mean data for cycles 2 and 3 combined for Quebec (QC) and Ontario (ONT) for children aged 3–5 years-old (**A**) and 6–11 years-old (**B**). Symbols: OAI: suggested Optimal absorbed intake of 0.04 mg/kg/day. TI: Total (absorbed) intake. FT: Fluoride toothpaste. FW: 0.07 mg/L fluoridated water. FB: Food and beverages.

3.4. Sensitivity Analyses

Figure 6 shows the parameters with the highest sensitivity indexes (SI) in the model. These include body weight, oral absorption fraction, renal clearance, bone volume, and fluoride intake (by using water, food, and toothpaste ingestion). For concision reasons, Figure 6 only includes parameters exhibiting an SI equal to or greater than 0.05.

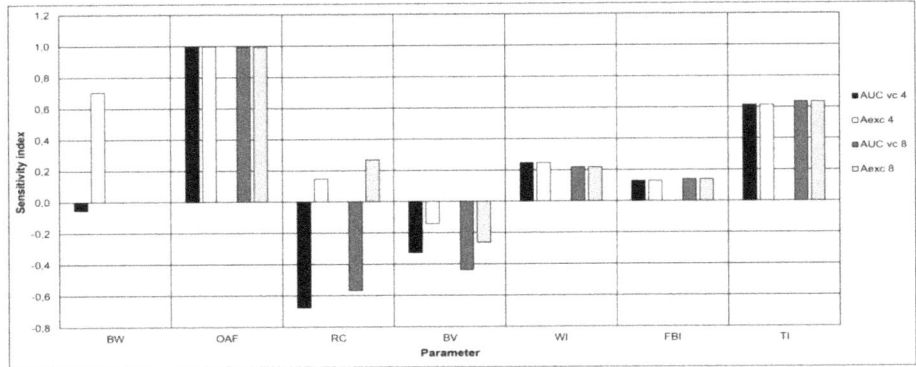

Figure 6. Sensitivity indices of the model parameters above the arbitrarily determined threshold of 0.05. Symbols: BW: Body weight. OAF: Oral absorption fraction. RC: Renal clearance. BV: Bone volume. WI: water intake. FBI: Food and beverages intake. TI: Toothpaste intake. AUC vc 4: Area under the curve of venous concentrations of fluorides over 24 h for a 4-year-old child. AUC vc 8: Area under the curve of venous concentrations of fluorides over 24 h for an 8-year-old child. Aexc 4: Amount of urinary fluorides excreted over 24 h for a 4-year-old child. Aexc 8: Amount of urinary fluorides excreted over 24 h for an 8-year-old child.

4. Discussion

To the best of the author's knowledge, this study is the first of its kind considering a coupled PBPK/biomonitoring data modeling approach to the comparison of fluoride intake in children living in regions with significantly differences in their access to intentionally fluoridated drinking water. PBPK modeling is an extensively used approach in order to interpret population biomonitoring data on chemical exposures [51–58], but it has never been applied to fluoride in this perspective nor has it been applied to fluoride exposure through drinking water from a dental health perspective. Therefore, the comparison made regarding the fluoride intake in children from two Canadian provinces differing in their access to optimally fluoridated water proposes new methodological insights with regard to future fluoride intake assessments.

This study suggests that drinking water fluoride still represents an important contribution for children under 8 years of age to attain the suggested daily optimal fluoride intake to prevent caries, but that a reduction in the intake of fluoride could also be desirable from the perspective of the most exposed children in order to prevent them from exhibiting a total exposure that may exceed toxicological reference values. Such a reduction could still be made while continuing to benefit from the protective effects of fluoride against tooth decay.

Although fluoride is classified as a non-essential mineral, it does have a protective effect against tooth decay. As any other preventive measure, its relevance is directly related to the risk of developing caries. It may not be relevant to use fluorides in populations who are not at risk of developing dental caries. In addition, fluoride's effect being predominantly topical, it is important not to confuse the systemic absorption of fluoride with its topical effect since "topical fluorides" will always have some degree of ingestion and "systemic fluorides" will exert topical effects through saliva and crevicular fluid [59].

The use of an "optimal fluoride dose" based on McClure's work, though controversial, remains the most appropriate population-level estimate for the purposes of this study because there is no other estimate currently available to predict how much fluoride is likely to confer a caries preventive effect while minimizing the risk of developing fluorosis. Although the relevancy of the notion of "optimal fluoride dose" to prevent dental caries exceeds the scope of this paper, it is worth mentioning that it has recently been suggested that the term optimal or "optimum" be dropped in favor of defining a value that provides "appropriate outcomes" for both caries and fluorosis [60]. However, considering the varying levels of caries risk between population subgroups as well as physiological differences affecting fluoride metabolism and absorption, a range of values may be more appropriate for future population level modeling studies [61].

By using the daily urinary fluoride presented in Figure 5, the contribution of drinking water fluoridated at 0.7 mg/L was calculated as 25% of the TDFI. At first glance, it may seem different from what other studies have found. In a US EPA relative source contribution analysis based on a mean exposure scenario in the United States, a relative contribution of 42% was found for children between 4 and 6 years old [62]. However, the fluoride concentration used in their scenario was 0.87 mg/L and the 90th percentile of water consumption (0.943 L/day) was used rather than the mean (0.442 L/day), which can partly explain the difference with the present analysis. Health Canada's assessment [11] based on exposure scenarios using daily Canadian intakes suggests a contribution of water to the TDFI of 48%. Both direct and indirect water consumption were included in that assessment. If only direct water consumption was considered, as is the case in the present study, drinking water contribution would drop to 17%. In another study [63], using a three-day food diary and samples collected from various fluoride sources (tap water, drinks, foods, toothpastes, and tooth-brushing expectorate) consumed by 3–4 year old children residing in the Gaza Strip, water contribution to the TDFI was found to be 12%. The authors of that study mention that very little tap water was used as a drink. Therefore, the lower contribution of water to the TDFI. Estimates of fluoride intake by analysis of various sources with a fluoride ion selective electrode were made in South India in order to assess drinking water contribution to the TDFI, which was evaluated at 39% in 3 year old to 10 year old children [64]. On the other hand, fluoride toothpaste was not included in that assessment nor mentioned in the article. If the fluoride toothpaste intake considered in the current study was added in their contribution assessment, a relative water contribution to the TDFI value of 25% can be obtained. Therefore, the contribution of drinking water to the TDFI of 25%, as found in the present study using model simulations, is rather coherent with the values obtained in the aforementioned studies.

The results obtained here suggest that the difference in exposure levels between children from Quebec and Ontario, brought out by the biomonitoring data, cannot be solely explained by the fluoridated drinking water at 0.7 mg/L. Furthermore, it can be deduced from studying Figure 5 that the difference between the two provinces also appears to result from dietary exposure. Since water is used in the preparation of many foods and beverages, it is to be expected that the concentration of fluoride in drinking water will affect the concentration found in the diet, which can explain the difference between both provinces. Taking into account the halo effect, it would be expected that in Quebec, where only 2.5% of the population has access to fluoridated water, fluoride would still be found in foods imported from Ontario or the United States. For example, it would be found where fluoridation is more prevalent. This effect indicates that foods produced in a fluoridated city will contain a higher fluoride concentration than those produced in a non-fluoridated city where it could be distributed and consumed, which increases the fluoride exposure of non-fluoridated areas' residents and vice-versa [65]. Conversely, modeled dietary intakes do not seem to contribute significantly to the total intake estimated from biomonitoring data in Quebec, according to Figure 5. However, this assertion appears rather uncertain given that modeled data on fluoride levels in foods were taken from a 1969 Nutrition Canada study [11] and may have changed since then based on the population's dietary habits.

The results also suggest that, at age 4, intake from fluoride toothpaste could be sufficient to reach the suggested optimal intake in the specific population of the present study while, at 8 years of age, the contribution from other sources would also be necessary (Figure 5). However, Ontario's modeled intake exceeds the suggested optimal intake and, therefore, it is possible that only a fraction of the contribution from the other sources than fluoride toothpaste (drinking water and food) may be sufficient. These fractions are to be determined. This observation is important given that, although fluoride exposure prevents tooth decay, it may trigger adverse health effects particularly fluorosis if the exposure is too high. Setting a drinking water fluoride concentration limit, therefore, requires an ideal compromise between risk and benefits from a dental health perspective [66]. Still, by applying the bioavailability factors previously mentioned to tolerable daily intakes (TDI) recommended by Health Canada (0.1 mg/kg/day) [3,11,15] and, more recently, Australia and New Zealand (0.20 mg/kg/day) [67], it is possible to compute absorbed TDI values determined to be 0.08 mg/kg/day by Canadian public health authorities and 0.16 mg/kg/day by those from Australia/New Zealand. The CHMS biomonitoring data-derived exposure dose for the mean and 95th percentile of Quebec and Ontario can, therefore, be compared to these absorbed TDIs. This allowed us to evaluate the risk of exceeding TDIs when drinking water contains fluoride at concentrations targeted with the aim of reaching a suggested optimal dose against tooth decay.

When comparing those absorbed TDIs with absorbed doses calculated from CHMS data (see Table 4), it can be noted that, on average, the fluoride intake in Quebec and Ontario is lower than the Canadian TDI. However, at age 4, the 95th percentile in Quebec has an intake greater than the Canadian TDI but lower than the Australia/New Zealand TDI. In Ontario, the 95th percentile exceeds the Canadian TDI at ages 4 and 8 and exceeds the Australia/New Zealand TDI at age 4. Conversely, in a context where water is generally not fluoridated as in Quebec, the TDI of Australia/New Zealand is not exceeded. Likewise in Ontario, where most of the population has access to fluoridated water at a level of 0.7 mg/L, children in the 95th percentile may have an intake greater than the TDI of Australia/New Zealand at age 4 and, therefore, presents a potentially increased risk of severe, otherwise rare, dental fluorosis. Additionally, this TDI is twice as permissible as the Canadian one. Yet, while both TDIs are determined in order to be protective of any adverse health effect including fluorosis, it is noteworthy to recall that any TDI does not necessarily correspond to an exposure over which the prevalence of adverse health effects automatically increases, but rather an exposure below which any effect is likely to occur based on the available weight of evidence. Therefore, we consider whether a fraction of the population exceeding a given TDI should be thought of as a safeguard rather than an absolute threshold. Since the dose is expressed in mg/kg, the fluoride intake would have to increase in proportion to body weight in the long-term to remain at 0.2 mg/kg/day and, therefore, increase risks of adverse effects. Increased monitoring using tools such as the urinary fluoride/creatinine ratio (UF/Cr) of 1.69 mg/g suggested by Zohoori and Maguire [68] in order to detect an excessively high fluoride intake well before the onset of dental fluorosis, could be an alternative for amending the water fluoridation guideline.

This study has some limitations that must be acknowledged. In the first place, the PBPK models used are built based on an original one that has seldom, if ever, been used nor validated since its publication. Therefore, this limits the assessment of its validity. However, the validation process realized herein shows that, when corrected appropriately, it can reproduce experimental data rather well (Figure 4). The models are deterministic and represent theoretical average exposure levels in the two ages considered. They, therefore, do not consider the physiological variations in the individuals of the same age group nor of different ages. Neither did they account for the variations in fluoride concentrations in the different exposure sources contrary to the population biomonitoring data used. This may have contributed in some cases to the lack of agreement between modeled and measured urinary fluoride values. In this line, a systematic overestimation by a factor of about

2.5 of the modeled urinary concentration and, therefore, an underestimation of the associated fluoride intake was observed. The model parameters attributable to such overestimations are revealed by the sensitivity analysis (Figure 6).

First, the bone clearance of the model, related to the bone volume in the model, which exhibits a negative AUC-based sensitivity index, may be too low. As a result, the plasma concentration is overestimated with correspondingly overestimated modeled urine concentration. Since bone clearance was calculated with a two-point line assuming that the relationship was linear (see Methods), it is also possible that the values used are not accurate enough. In addition, the model's overestimation of urinary fluoride could be explained by an excessive modeled renal clearance, which also exhibits a negative AUC-based sensitivity index and a positive Aexc-based one. However, according to the values found in the literature, this does not appear to be the case [8]. Lastly, the absorption fraction appears to be the main contributor to the overestimation. Direct infusion into the liver was considered herein rather than via an intermediate gastrointestinal compartment from which part of the ingested fluoride is absorbed following a rate dictated by an oral absorption constant. The highly model-sensitive correspondent absorption fraction modeled herein (Figure 6) is probably too high as a result. Excessive modeled bioavailability for toothpaste is also a valid explanation. Bioavailability studies are often performed on an empty stomach while tooth brushing is recommended after eating a meal. The ingestion of toothpaste is more likely to happen in the presence of food, which could decrease its true bioavailability. This is supported by a lower modeled Aexc for toothpaste exposure alone than what CHMS data suggests (Figure 5). Unfortunately, the lack of availability of a relevant oral absorption constant and toothpaste bioavailability for different states of stomach emptiness have precluded correcting the model in any other way than applying an empirical modification of the model by a factor of 0.43, which did, however, correct the initial systematic error (Figure 4).

Another limitation related to the fluoride intake may come from dental care or dental hygiene measures other than the use of fluoride toothpaste. Furthermore, this intake was not taken into account in the model due to a lack of data precise enough to be used in the model. However, because professional dental care is provided only a few times each year, it does not appear to be a significant source of long-term exposure, which, in principle, is what is reflected in CHMS biomonitoring data. For other personal fluoride products such as mouthwash, these are not recommended for children under 12 and, therefore, should not affect the estimates in this work. The lack of information on water fluoride levels associated with CHMS biomonitoring data is a source of uncertainty as well.

Two final sources of uncertainties in this study that preclude drawing firm conclusions include the low statistical power of the provincial biomonitoring data for the age groups corresponding to the typical individuals whose exposure was modeled as well as the fact that the child data used to validate the model did not come from Canadian studies despite Canadian biomonitoring data being used in this work. Therefore, since this is the first study of its kind, it needs to be replicated in future studies to validate the findings. In this regard, obtaining more robust data on fluoride levels in foods and their bioavailability in foods for cities with variable levels of fluoride content in the drinking water would improve our assessment particularly with respect to the halo effect of drinking water on food. Probabilistic modeling should be considered, e.g., via Monte Carlo simulations, in order to address the limitation issue related to the inter-individual variability of the various fluoride intakes and of the physiological determinants of its kinetics in children.

5. Conclusions

According to the present model, the currently recommended absorbed fluoride dose of 0.04 mg/kg/day to prevent tooth decay is not attained in Quebec children where drinking water fluoridation is sparse while it is surpassed by children in Ontario where such fluoridation is extended. Since this study is the first of its kind regarding the use of biomonitoring data under a PBPK modeling approach in order to compare fluoride intake in children from two regions differing in their access to intentionally fluoridated water, further research needs to be undertaken in order to confirm these results. In addition, these results are an incentive to further explore the multiple sources of fluoride intake since they suggest that a new balance between them are sought, which is in accordance with the physiological differences that influence fluoride metabolism in each age group. This is important from a public health perspective since the aim is to maximize the number of individuals capable of achieving a daily fluoride intake that provides appropriate outcomes in terms of caries prevention and minimizing the risk of fluorosis.

Author Contributions: M.V. and F.G. conceived and designed the study. K.J.J. performed the study. K.J., F.G., and M.V. analyzed the data. N.W. contributed to the dental health considerations. K.J.J. wrote the first draft of the manuscript. M.V. commented and reviewed the first few drafts of the paper. All authors commented and edited on the following version of the paper until the approval of the final version. M.V. coordinated the overall work and submitted the paper.

Funding: This research received no external funding.

Acknowledgments: In-kind contributions of INSPQ's staff are acknowledged. The authors thank André Lavallière from the Public Health Directorate of Estrie (Sherbrooke, QC, Canada) for his very relevant comments especially regarding the notion of suggested optimal fluoride intake.

Conflicts of Interest: The authors declare no conflict of interest.

Appendix A

Table A1. Absorbed doses calculated from the McClure [1] data on intakes from water and diet [1].

Age (year)	Weight (kg)	Water (mL/day)	Diet (mg/day)	Total (mg/day)	Intake (mg/kg/day)	Absorbed Dose (mg/kg/day) [1]
1 to 3	8 à 16	0.39–0.56	0.027–0.265	0.417–0.825	0.026–0.103 (0.065)	0.036–0.058 (0.047)
4 to 6	13 à 24	0.52–0.745	0.036–0.360	0.556–1.105	0.023–0.085 (0.054)	0.030–0.049 (0.040)
7 to 9	16 à 35	0.65–0.93	0.045–0.450	0.695–1.380	0.020–0.086 (0.053)	0.029–0.048 (0.039)
10 to 12	25 à 54	0.81–1.66	0.056–0.560	0.866–1.725	0.016–0.069 (0.043)	0.023–0.037 (0.031)

[1] Absorbed optimal doses were calculated by multiplying mean water and diet intake by their respective bioavailability factors of 83% and 40% and dividing that total absorbed dose by the mean weight for that age group.

References

1. McClure, F.J. Ingestion of fluoride and dental caries: Quantitative relations based on food and water requirements of children one to twelve years old. *Am. J. Dis. Child.* **1943**, *66*, 362–369. [CrossRef]
2. Galagan, D.J.; Vermillion, J.R. Determining optimum fluoride concentrations. *Public Health Rep.* **1957**, *72*, 491–493. [CrossRef] [PubMed]
3. Health Canada. Fluoride and Oral Health. Available online: https://www.canada.ca/en/health-canada/services/healthy-living/your-health/environment/fluorides-human-health.html (accessed on 26 April 2018).
4. Buzalaf, M.A.R.; Pessan, J.P.; Honório, H.M.; ten Cate, J.M. Mechanisms of Action of Fluoride for Caries Control. In *Fluoride and the Oral Environment*; Buzalaf, M.A.R., Ed.; Karger: Basel, Switzerland, 2011; Volume 22, pp. 20–36.
5. Public Health Agency of Canada. *The State of Community Water Fluoridation across Canada*; Public Health Agency of Canada: Ottawa, ON, Canada, 2017; p. 13. Available online: https://www.canada.ca/content/dam/hc-sc/documents/services/publications/healthy-living/community-water-fluoridation-across-canada-2017/community-water-fluoridation-across-canada-2017-eng.pdf (accessed on 26 June 2018).
6. Ontario Association of Public Health Dentistry. Mean dmft+DMFT and % Caries Free JK, SK and Grade 2 Children from Participating Ontario Health Units 2003 to 2014. In *Wellington-Dufferin-Guelph Public Health, Oral Health Status Report*; Ontario Association of Public Health Dentistry: Guelph, ON, Canada, 2015; p. 34. Available online: https://www.wdgpublichealth.ca/sites/default/files/file-attachments/report/hs_report_2015-oral-health-in-wdg-fullreport_access.pdf (accessed on 26 June 2018).

7.   Galarneau, C.; Arpin, S.; Boiteau, V.; Dube, M.A.; Hamel, D.; Wassef, N. *Étude Clinique sur l'État de Santé Buccodentaire des Élèves Québécois du Primaire 2012–2013 (ÉCSBQ)—Rapport National*, 2nd ed.; Institut National de Santé Publique du Québec: Montréal, QC, Canada, 2018; p. 181. Available online: https://www.inspq.qc.ca/sites/default/files/publications/2034_sante_buccodentaire_primaire.pdf (accessed on 6 June 2018).

8.   Institut National de Santé Publique du Qubec (INSPQ). *Avis sur un Projet de Fluoration de l'Eau Potable*; INSPQ: Montreal, QC, Canada, 2011; p. 13. Available online: https://www.inspq.qc.ca/publications/1278 (accessed on 13 February 2018).

9.   Health Canada; Canadian Health Measures Survey (CHMS). Oral Health Statistics 2007–2009. Available online: https://www.canada.ca/en/health-canada/services/healthy-living/reports-publications/oral-health/canadian-health-measures-survey.html (accessed on 26 April 2018).

10.   Canadian Institute of Health Information. *National Health Expenditure Trends, 1975 to 2016*; Canadian Institute for Health Information: Ottawa, ON, Canada, 2016; p. 44. Available online: https://secure.cihi.ca/free_products/NHEX-Trends-Narrative-Report_2016_EN.pdf (accessed on 13 February 2018).

11.   Health Canada. *Guidelines for Canadian Drinking Water Quality: Guideline Technical Document—Fluoride*; Minsitry of Health: Ottawa, ON, Canada, 2010; p. 104. Available online: https://www.canada.ca/content/dam/canada/health-canada/migration/healthy-canadians/publications/healthy-living-vie-saine/water-fluoride-fluorure-eau/alt/water-fluoride-fluorure-eau-eng.pdf (accessed on 13 February 2018).

12.   Cauley, J.A.; Murphy, P.A.; Riley, T.J.; Buhari, A.M. Effects of fluoridated drinking water on bone mass and fractures: The study of osteoporotic fractures. *J. Bone Min. Res.* **1995**, *10*, 1076–1086. [CrossRef] [PubMed]

13.   Karagas, M.R.; Baron, J.A.; Barrett, J.A.; Jacobsen, S.J. Patterns of fracture among the United States elderly: Geographic and fluoride effects. *Ann. Epidemiol.* **1996**, *6*, 209–216. [CrossRef]

14.   Leone, N.C.; Stevenson, C.A.; Hilbish, T.F.; Sosman, M.C. A roentgenologic study of a human population exposed to high-fluoride domestic water; a ten-year study. *Am. J. Roentgenol. Radium Ther. Nucl. Med.* **1955**, *74*, 874–885. [PubMed]

15.   Health Canada.   Findings and Recommendations of the Fluoride Expert Panel (January 2007). https://www.canada.ca/en/health-canada/services/environmental-workplace-health/reports-publications/water-quality/findings-recommendations-fluoride-expert-panel-january-2007.html (accessed on 26 April 2018).

16.   Choi, A.L.; Sun, G.; Zhang, Y.; Grandjean, P. Developmental fluoride neurotoxicity: A systematic review and meta-analysis. *Environ. Health Perspect.* **2012**, *120*, 1362–1368. [CrossRef] [PubMed]

17.   Comber, H.; Deady, S.; Montgomery, E.; Gavin, A. Drinking water fluoridation and osteosarcoma incidence on the island of Ireland. *Cancer Causes Control* **2011**, *22*, 919–924. [CrossRef] [PubMed]

18.   Levy, M.; Leclerc, B.S. Fluoride in drinking water and osteosarcoma incidence rates in the continental United States among children and adolescents. *Cancer Epidemiol.* **2012**, *36*, e83–e88. [CrossRef] [PubMed]

19.   Blakey, K.; Feltbower, R.G.; Parslow, R.C.; James, P.W.; Gómez Pozo, B.; Stiller, C.; Vincent, T.J.; Norman, P.; McKinney, P.A.; Murphy, M.F.; et al.   Is fluoride a risk factor for bone cancer?   Small area analysis of osteosarcoma and Ewing sarcoma diagnosed among 0–49-year-olds in Great Britain, 1980–2005. *Int. J. Epidemiol.* **2014**, *43*, 224–234. [CrossRef] [PubMed]

20.   Rebhun, R.B.; Kass, P.H.; Kent, M.S.; Watson, K.D.; Withers, S.S.; Culp, W.T.N.; King, A.M. Evaluation of optimal water fluoridation on the incidence and skeletal distribution of naturally arising osteosarcoma in pet dogs. *Vet. Comp. Oncol.* **2017**, *15*, 441–449. [CrossRef] [PubMed]

21.   Archer, N.P.; Napier, T.S.; Villanacci, J.F. Fluoride exposure in public drinking water and childhood and adolescent osteosarcoma in Texas. *Cancer Causes Control* **2016**, *27*, 863–868. [CrossRef] [PubMed]

22.   Barberio, A.M.; Hosein, F.S.; Quiñonez, C.; McLaren, L. Fluoride exposure and indicators of thyroid functioning in the Canadian population: Implications for community water fluoridation. *J. Epidemiol. Community Health* **2017**, *71*, 1019–1025. [CrossRef] [PubMed]

23.   Rao, H.V.; Beliles, R.P.; Whitford, G.M.; Turner, C.H. A physiologically based pharmacokinetic model for fluoride uptake by bone. *Regul. Toxicol. Pharmacol.* **1995**, *22*, 30–42. [CrossRef] [PubMed]

24.   Statistics Canada. Canadian Health Measures Survey (CHMS). Available online: http://www23.statcan.gc.ca/imdb/p2SV.pl?Function=getSurvey&Id=251160 (accessed on 26 April 2018).

25. Institut National de Santé Publique du Québec (INSPQ). *Extraction et Comparaison des Données Provinciales de Biosurveillance des Substances Chimiques de l'Environnement pour le Québec et l'Ontario Issues de l'Enquête Canadienne sur les Mesures de Santé*; Unpublished Report; Institut National de Santé Publique du Québec: Montreal, QC, Canada, 2016; p. 86.

26. Haddad, S.; Pelekis, M.; Krishnan, K. A methodology for solving physiologically based pharmacokinetic models without the use of simulation softwares. *Toxicol. Lett.* **1996**, *85*, 113–126. [CrossRef]

27. Price, K.; Haddad, S.; Krishnan, K. Physiological modeling of age-specific changes in the pharmacokinetics of organic chemicals in children. *J. Toxicol. Environ. Health A* **2003**, *66*, 417–433. [CrossRef] [PubMed]

28. Price, P.S.; Conolly, R.B.; Chaisson, C.F.; Gross, E.A.; Young, J.S.; Mathis, E.T.; Tedder, D.R. Modeling interindividual variation in physiological factors used in PBPK models of humans. *Crit. Rev. Toxicol.* **2003**, *33*, 469–503. [CrossRef] [PubMed]

29. Valcke, M.; Krishnan, K. Evaluation of the impact of the exposure route on the human kinetic adjustment factor. *Regul. Toxicol. Pharmacol.* **2011**, *59*, 258–269. [CrossRef] [PubMed]

30. Haddad, S.; Tardif, G.C.; Tardif, R. Development of physiologically based toxicokinetic models for improving the human indoor exposure assessment to water contaminants: Trichloroethylene and trihalomethanes. *J. Toxicol. Environ. Health A* **2006**, *69*, 2095–2136. [CrossRef] [PubMed]

31. Whitford, G.M. Fluoride metabolism and excretion in children. *J. Public Health Dent.* **1999**, *59*, 224–228. [CrossRef] [PubMed]

32. Ekstrand, J.; Ziegler, E.E.; Nelson, S.E.; Fomon, S.J. Absorption and retention of dietary and supplemental fluoride by infants. *Adv. Dent. Res.* **1994**, *8*, 175–180. [CrossRef] [PubMed]

33. Trautner, K.; Siebert, G. An experimental study of bio-availability of fluoride from dietary sources in man. *Arch. Oral Biol.* **1986**, *31*, 223–228. [CrossRef]

34. McIvor, M.E. Acute fluoride toxicity. Pathophysiology and management. *Drug Saf.* **1990**, *5*, 79–85. [CrossRef] [PubMed]

35. Ekstrand, J.; Ehrnebo, M. Absorption of fluoride from fluoride dentifrices. *Caries Res.* **1980**, *14*, 96–102. [CrossRef] [PubMed]

36. Yadav, A.K.; Kaushik, C.P.; Haritash, A.K.; Singh, B.; Raghuvanshi, S.P.; Kansal, A. Determination of exposure and probable ingestion of fluoride through tea, toothpaste, tobacco and pan masala. *J. Hazard. Mater.* **2007**, *142*, 77–80. [CrossRef] [PubMed]

37. Héctor, F.; Acevedo, A.; Margaret, P.; Anthony, V.; Rojas-Sanchez, F. Fluoride intake and urinary fluoride excretion in children attending a daycare center in Maracay, Aragua state, Venezuela. *J. Dent. Oral Hyg.* **2009**, *1*, 27–35.

38. Villa, A.; Anabalon, M.; Cabezas, L. The fractional urinary fluoride excretion in young children under stable fluoride intake conditions. *Community Dent. Oral Epidemiol.* **2000**, *28*, 344–355. [CrossRef] [PubMed]

39. Omid, N.; Maguire, A.; O'Hare, W.T.; Zohoori, F.V. Total daily fluoride intake and fractional urinary fluoride excretion in 4- to 6-year-old children living in a fluoridated area: Weekly variation? *Community Dent. Oral Epidemiol.* **2017**, *45*, 12–19. [CrossRef] [PubMed]

40. Haftenberger, M.; Viergutz, G.; Neumeister, V.; Hetzer, G. Total fluoride intake and urinary excretion in German children aged 3–6 years. *Caries Res.* **2001**, *35*, 451–457. [CrossRef] [PubMed]

41. Zohoori, F.V.; Walls, R.; Teasdale, L.; Landes, D.; Steen, I.N.; Moynihan, P.; Omid, N.; Maguire, A. Fractional urinary fluoride excretion of 6–7-year-old children attending schools in low-fluoride and naturally fluoridated areas in the UK. *Br. J. Nutr.* **2013**, *109*, 1903–1909. [CrossRef] [PubMed]

42. Dietitians of Canada. WHO Growth Charts Set 2. Available online: https://www.dietitians.ca/Dietitians-Views/Prenatal-and-Infant/WHO-Growth-Charts/WHO-Growth-Charts-Set-2.aspx (accessed on 26 April 2018).

43. Institut National de Santé Publique du Québec, Fluorures. Available online: https://www.inspq.qc.ca/eau-potable/fluorures (accessed on 26 April 2018).

44. Ipsos MORI Social Research Institute. *Tap Water Drinking Behaviour: A Study of Children Aged 0–15*; DEFRA Drinking Water Inspectorate: London, UK, 2012; p. 84. Available online: http://dwi.defra.gov.uk/research/completed-research/reports/DWI70_2_251.pdf (accessed on 31 May 2018).

45. Hays, S.M.; Becker, R.A.; Leung, H.W.; Aylward, L.L.; Pyatt, D.W. Biomonitoring equivalents: A screening approach for interpreting biomonitoring results from a public health risk perspective. *Regul. Toxicol. Pharmacol.* **2007**, *47*, 96–109. [CrossRef] [PubMed]

46. Centers for Disease Control and Prevention. *Fourth National Report on Human Exposure to Environmental Chemicals*; Centers for Disease Control and Prevention, Department of Health and Human Services: Atlanta, GA, USA, 2009; p. 530. Available online: https://www.cdc.gov/exposurereport/pdf/fourthreport.pdf (accessed on 16 April 2018).

47. Umweltbundesamt (UBA). German Environmental Survey, GerES 2014–2017. Available online: https://www.umweltbundesamt.de/en/topics/health/assessing-environmentally-related-health-risks/ german-environmental-surveys/german-environmental-survey-2014-2017-geres-v#textpart-1 (accessed on 31 May 2018).

48. Becker, K.; Conrad, A.; Kirsch, N.; Kolossa-Gehring, M.; Schulz, C.; Seiwert, M.; Seifert, B. German Environmental Survey (GerES): Human biomonitoring as a tool to identify exposure pathways. *Int. J. Hyg. Environ. Health* **2007**, *210*, 267–269. [CrossRef] [PubMed]

49. Health Canada. *Fourth Report on Human Biomonitoring of Environmental Chemicals in Canada*; Health Canada: Ottawa, ON, Canada, 2017; p. 247. Available online: https://www.canada.ca/content/dam/ hc-sc/documents/services/environmental-workplace-health/reports-publications/environmental-contaminants/fourth-report-human-biomonitoring-environmental-chemicals-canada/fourth-report-human-biomonitoring-environmental-chemicals-canada-fra.pdf (accessed on 15 March 2018).

50. Aylward, L.L.; Hays, S.M.; Vezina, A.; Deveau, M.; St-Amand, A.; Nong, A. Biomonitoring Equivalents for interpretation of urinary fluoride. *Regul. Toxicol. Pharmacol.* **2015**, *72*, 158–167. [CrossRef] [PubMed]

51. Aylward, L.L.; Kirman, C.R.; Blount, B.C.; Hays, S.M. Chemical-specific screening criteria for interpretation of biomonitoring data for volatile organic compounds (VOCs)—Application of steady-state PBPK model solutions. *Regul. Toxicol. Pharmacol.* **2010**, *58*, 33–44. [CrossRef] [PubMed]

52. Brown, K.; Phillips, M.; Grulke, C.; Yoon, M.; Young, B.; McDougall, R.; Leonard, J.; Lu, J.; Lefew, W.; Tan, Y.M. Reconstructing exposures from biomarkers using exposure-pharmacokinetic modeling—A case study with carbaryl. *Regul. Toxicol. Pharmacol.* **2015**, *73*, 689–698. [CrossRef] [PubMed]

53. Clewell, H.J.; Tan, Y.M.; Campbell, J.L.; Andersen, M.E. Quantitative interpretation of human biomonitoring data. *Toxicol. Appl. Pharmacol.* **2008**, *231*, 122–133. [CrossRef] [PubMed]

54. Liao, K.H.; Tan, Y.M.; Clewell, H.J., 3rd. Development of a screening approach to interpret human biomonitoring data on volatile organic compounds: Reverse dosimetry on biomonitoring data for trichloroethylene. *Risk Anal.* **2007**, *27*, 1223–1236. [CrossRef] [PubMed]

55. Lyons, M.A.; Yang, R.S.; Mayeno, A.N.; Reisfeld, B. Computational toxicology of chloroform: Reverse dosimetry using Bayesian inference, Markov chain Monte Carlo simulation, and human biomonitoring data. *Environ. Health Perspect.* **2008**, *116*, 1040–1046. [CrossRef] [PubMed]

56. McNally, K.; Cotton, R.; Cocker, J.; Jones, K.; Bartels, M.; Rick, D.; Price, P.; Loizou, G. Reconstruction of Exposure to m-Xylene from Human Biomonitoring Data Using PBPK Modelling, Bayesian Inference, and Markov Chain Monte Carlo Simulation. *J. Toxicol.* **2012**, *2012*, 760281. [CrossRef] [PubMed]

57. Tan, Y.M.; Liao, K.H.; Conolly, R.B.; Blount, B.C.; Mason, A.M.; Clewell, H.J. Use of a physiologically based pharmacokinetic model to identify exposures consistent with human biomonitoring data for chloroform. *J. Toxicol. Environ. Health A* **2006**, *69*, 1727–1756. [CrossRef] [PubMed]

58. Timchalk, C.; Poet, T.S. Development of a physiologically based pharmacokinetic and pharmacodynamic model to determine dosimetry and cholinesterase inhibition for a binary mixture of chlorpyrifos and diazinon in the rat. *Neurotoxicology* **2008**, *29*, 428–443. [CrossRef] [PubMed]

59. Buzalaf, M.A.R.; Whitford, G.M. Fluoride Metabolism. In *Fluoride and the Oral Environment*; Buzalaf, M.A.R., Ed.; Karger: Basel, Switzerland, 2011; Volume 22, pp. 20–36.

60. Zohoori, F.V. Summary of General Discussion and Conclusions. *Adv. Dent. Res.* **2018**, *29*, 183–185. [CrossRef] [PubMed]

61. Buzalaf, M.A.R. Review of Fluoride Intake and Appropriateness of Current Guidelines. *Adv. Dent. Res.* **2018**, *29*, 157–166. [CrossRef] [PubMed]

62. Health and Ecological Criteria Division Office of Water. *Fluoride: Exposure and Relative Source Contribution Analysis*; U.S. Environmental Protection Agency: Washington, DC, USA, 2010; p. 210.

63. Abuhaloob, L.; Maguire, A.; Moynihan, P. Total daily fluoride intake and the relative contributions of foods, drinks and toothpaste by 3- to 4-year-old children in the Gaza Strip—Palestine. *Int. J. Paediatr. Dent.* **2015**, *25*, 127–135. [CrossRef] [PubMed]

64. Viswanathan, G.; Gopalakrishnan, S.; Siva Ilango, S. Assessment of water contribution on total fluoride intake of various age groups of people in fluoride endemic and non-endemic areas of Dindigul District, Tamil Nadu, South India. *Water Res.* **2010**, *44*, 6186–6200. [CrossRef] [PubMed]

65. American Dental Association. *Fluoridation Facts—2018 Edition*; American Dental Association: Washington, DC, USA, 2018; p. 114.

66. Institute of Medecine. *Dietary Reference Intakes for Calcium, Phosphorus, Magnesium, Vitamin D, and Fluoride*; The National Academies Press: Washington, DC, USA, 1997; p. 432.

67. Expert Working Group for Fluoride. *Australian and New Zealand Nutrient Reference Values for Fluoride*; Australian Government Department of Health; The New Zealand Ministry of Health: Thorndon, New Zealand, 2017; p. 97.

68. Zohoori, F.V.; Maguire, A. Determining an Upper Reference Value for the Urinary Fluoride-Creatinine Ratio in Healthy Children Younger than 7 Years. *Caries Res.* **2017**, *51*, 283–289. [CrossRef] [PubMed]

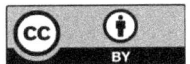

International Journal of
Environmental Research and Public Health

MDPI

Review

Drinking Water Nitrate and Human Health: An Updated Review

Mary H. Ward [1,*], Rena R. Jones [1], Jean D. Brender [2], Theo M. de Kok [3], Peter J. Weyer [4], Bernard T. Nolan [5], Cristina M. Villanueva [6,7,8,9] and Simone G. van Breda [3]

[1] Occupational and Environmental Epidemiology Branch, Division of Cancer Epidemiology and Genetics, National Cancer Institute, 9609 Medical Center Dr. Room 6E138, Rockville, MD 20850, USA; rena.jones@nih.gov
[2] Department of Epidemiology and Biostatistics, Texas A&M University, School of Public Health, College Station, TX 77843, USA; jdbrender@sph.tamhsc.edu
[3] Department of Toxicogenomics, GROW-school for Oncology and Developmental Biology, Maastricht University Medical Center, P.O Box 616, 6200 MD Maastricht, The Netherlands; t.dekok@maastrichtuniversity.nl (T.M.d.K.); s.vanbreda@maastrichtuniversity.nl (S.G.v.B.)
[4] The Center for Health Effects of Environmental Contamination, The University of Iowa, 455 Van Allen Hall, Iowa City, IA 52242, USA; peter-weyer@uiowa.edu
[5] U.S. Geological Survey, Water Mission Area, National Water Quality Program, 12201 Sunrise Valley Drive, Reston, VA 20192, USA; btnolan@usgs.gov
[6] ISGlobal, 08003 Barcelona, Spain; cvillanueva@isiglobal.org
[7] IMIM (Hospital del Mar Medical Research Institute), 08003 Barcelona, Spain
[8] Department of Experimental and Health Sciences, Universitat Pompeu Fabra (UPF), 08003 Barcelona, Spain
[9] CIBER Epidemiología y Salud Pública (CIBERESP), 28029 Madrid, Spain
[*] Correspondence: wardm@mail.nih.gov

Received: 17 May 2018; Accepted: 14 July 2018; Published: 23 July 2018

Abstract: Nitrate levels in our water resources have increased in many areas of the world largely due to applications of inorganic fertilizer and animal manure in agricultural areas. The regulatory limit for nitrate in public drinking water supplies was set to protect against infant methemoglobinemia, but other health effects were not considered. Risk of specific cancers and birth defects may be increased when nitrate is ingested under conditions that increase formation of *N*-nitroso compounds. We previously reviewed epidemiologic studies before 2005 of nitrate intake from drinking water and cancer, adverse reproductive outcomes and other health effects. Since that review, more than 30 epidemiologic studies have evaluated drinking water nitrate and these outcomes. The most common endpoints studied were colorectal cancer, bladder, and breast cancer (three studies each), and thyroid disease (four studies). Considering all studies, the strongest evidence for a relationship between drinking water nitrate ingestion and adverse health outcomes (besides methemoglobinemia) is for colorectal cancer, thyroid disease, and neural tube defects. Many studies observed increased risk with ingestion of water nitrate levels that were below regulatory limits. Future studies of these and other health outcomes should include improved exposure assessment and accurate characterization of individual factors that affect endogenous nitrosation.

Keywords: drinking water; nitrate; cancer; adverse reproductive outcomes; methemoglobinemia; thyroid disease; endogenous nitrosation; *N*-nitroso compounds

1. Introduction

Since the mid-1920s, humans have doubled the natural rate at which nitrogen is deposited onto land through the production and application of nitrogen fertilizers (inorganic and manure), the combustion of fossil fuels, and replacement of natural vegetation with nitrogen-fixing crops such as soybeans [1,2]. The major anthropogenic source of nitrogen in the environment is nitrogen fertilizer, the application of which increased exponentially after the development of the Haber–Bosch process in the 1920s. Most synthetic fertilizer applications to agricultural land occurred after 1980 [3]. Since approximately half of all applied nitrogen drains from agricultural fields to contaminate surface and groundwater, nitrate concentrations in our water resources have also increased [1].

The maximum contaminant level (MCL) for nitrate in public drinking water supplies in the United States (U.S.) is 10 mg/L as nitrate-nitrogen (NO_3-N). This concentration is approximately equivalent to the World Health Organization (WHO) guideline of 50 mg/L as NO_3 or 11.3 mg/L NO_3-N (multiply NO_3 mg/L by 0.2258). The MCL was set to protect against infant methemoglobinemia; however other health effects including cancer and adverse reproductive outcomes were not considered [4]. Through endogenous nitrosation, nitrate is a precursor in the formation of *N*-nitroso compounds (NOC); most NOC are carcinogens and teratogens. Thus, exposure to NOC formed after ingestion of nitrate from drinking water and dietary sources may result in cancer, birth defects, or other adverse health effects. Nitrate is found in many foods, with the highest levels occurring in some green leafy and root vegetables [5,6]. Average daily intakes from food are in the range of 30–130 mg/day as NO_3 (7–29 mg/day NO_3-N) [5]. Because NOC formation is inhibited by ascorbic acid, polyphenols, and other compounds present at high levels in most vegetables, dietary nitrate intake may not result in substantial endogenous NOC formation [5,7].

Studies of health effects related to nitrate exposure from drinking water were previously reviewed through early 2004 [8]. Further, an International Agency for Research on Cancer (IARC) Working Group reviewed human, animal, and mechanistic studies of cancer through mid-2006 and concluded that ingested nitrate and nitrite, under conditions that result in endogenous nitrosation, are probably carcinogenic [5]. Here, our objective is to provide updated information on human exposure and to review mechanistic and health effects studies since 2004. We summarize how the additional studies contribute to the overall evidence for health effects and we discuss what future research may be most informative.

2. Drinking Water Nitrate Exposures in the United States and Europe

Approximately 45 million people in the U.S. (about 14% of the population) had self-supplied water at their residence in 2010 [9]. Almost all (98%) were private wells, which are not regulated by the U.S. Environmental Protection Agency (EPA). The rest of the population was served by public water supplies, which use groundwater, surface water, or both. The U.S. Geological Survey's National Water Quality Assessment (USGS-NAWQA) Project [10] sampled principal groundwater aquifers used as U.S. public and private drinking water supplies in 1988–2015. Nitrate levels in groundwater under agricultural land were about three times the national background level of 1 mg/L NO_3-N (Figure 1) [11]. The mixed land use category mostly had nitrate concentrations below background levels reflecting levels in deeper private and public water supply wells. Based on the NAWQA study, it was estimated that 2% of public-supply wells and 6% of private wells exceeded the MCL; whereas, in agricultural areas, 21% of private wells exceeded the MCL [10]. The USGS-NAWQA study also revealed significant decadal-scale changes in groundwater nitrate concentrations among wells sampled first in 1988–2000 and again in 2001–2010 for agricultural, urban, and mixed land uses [12]. More sampling networks had increases in median nitrate concentration than had decreases.

A study of U.S. public water supplies (PWS) using data from EPA's Safe Drinking Water Information System estimated that the percentage of PWS violating the MCL increased from 0.28 to 0.42% during 1994–2009; most increases were for small to medium PWS (<10,000 population served) using groundwater [13]. As a result of increasing nitrate levels, some PWS have incurred expensive upgrades to their treatment systems to comply with the regulatory level [14–16].

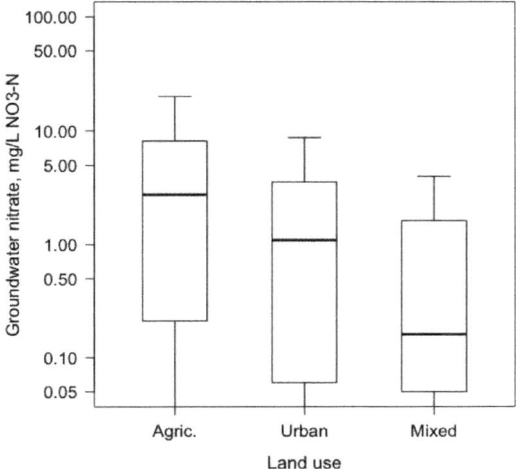

Figure 1. Boxplots of nitrate concentrations in shallow groundwater beneath agricultural and urban land uses, and at depths of private and public drinking water supplies beneath mixed land use. The number of sampled wells were 1573 (agricultural land), 1054 (urban), and 3417 (mixed). The agricultural and urban wells were sampled to assess land use effects, whereas the mixed category wells were sampled at depths of private and public supplies. Median depths of wells in the agricultural, urban, and mixed categories were 34, 32, and 200 feet, respectively. The height of the upper bar is 1.5 times the length of the box, and the lower bound was truncated at the nitrate detection limit of 0.05 mg/L NO_3-N.

In Europe, the Nitrates Directive was set in 1991 [17,18] to reduce or prevent nitrate pollution from agriculture. Areas most affected by nitrate pollution are designated as 'nitrate vulnerable zones' and are subject to mandatory Codes of Good Agricultural Practice [18]. The results of compliance with this directive have been reflected in the time trends of nitrate in some countries. For example, nitrate levels in groundwater in Denmark increased in 1950–1980 and decreased since the 1990s [19]. Average nitrate levels in groundwater in most other European countries have been stable at around 17.5 mg/L NO_3 (4 mg/L NO_3-N) across Europe over a 20-year period (1992–2012), with some differences between countries both in trends and concentrations. Average concentrations are lowest in Finland (around 1 mg/L NO_3 in 1992–2012) and highest in Malta (58.1 mg/L in 2000–2012) [20]. Average annual nitrate concentrations at river monitoring stations in Europe showed a steady decline from 2.7 NO_3-N in 1992 to 2.1 mg/L in 2012 [20], with the lowest average levels in Norway (0.2 mg/L NO_3-N in 2012) and highest in Greece (6.6 mg/L NO_3-N in 2012).

Levels in finished public drinking water have been published only for a few European countries. Trends of nitrate in drinking water supplies from 1976 to 2012 in Denmark showed a decline in public supplies but not in private wells [21]. In Spain, median concentrations were 3.5 mg/L NO_3 (range: 0.4–66.8) in 108 municipalities in 2012 [22], and 4.2 mg/L (range: <1–29) in 11 provinces in 2010 [23]. Levels in other countries included a median of 0.18 mg/L (range: <0.02–7.9) in Iceland in 2001–2012 [24], a mean of 16.1 mg/L (range: 0.05–296 mg/L) in Sicily, Italy in 2004–2005 [25] and a range from undetected to 63.3 mg/L in Deux-Sèvres, France in in 2005–2009 [26].

Nitrate levels in bottled water have been measured in a few areas of the EU and the U.S. and have been found to be below the MCL. In Sicily, the mean level was 15.2 mg/L NO_3(range: 1.2–31.8 mg/L) in 16 brands [25] and in Spain, the median level was 5.2 mg/L NO_3 (range: <1.0–29.0 mg/L) in 9 brands [23]. In the U.S., a survey of bottle water sold in 42 Iowa and 32 Texas communities found varying but generally low nitrate levels. Nitrate concentrations ranged from below the limit of detection (0.1 mg/L NO$_3$-N) to 4.9 mg/L NO$_3$-N for U.S. domestic spring water purchased in Texas.

There are few published studies of nitrate concentrations in drinking water outside the U.S. and Europe. Nitrate concentrations in groundwater were reported for Morocco, Niger, Nigeria, Senegal, India-Pakistan, Japan, Lebanon, Philippines and Turkey with maximum levels in Senegal (median 42.9 mg/L NO$_3$-N) [5]. In India, nitrate in drinking water supplies is particularly high in rural areas, where average levels have been reported to be 45.7 mg/L NO$_3$ [27,28] and 66.6 mg/L NO$_3$ [28]; maximum levels in drinking water exceeded 100 mg/L NO$_3$ in several regions [27,29]. Extremely high levels of nitrate have been reported in The Gaza Strip, where nitrate reached concentrations of 500 mg/L NO$_3$ in some areas, and more than 50% of public-supply wells had nitrate concentrations above 45 mg/L NO$_3$ [30].

3. Exposure Assessment in Epidemiologic Studies

With the implementation of the Safe Drinking Water Act in 1974, more than 40 years of monitoring data for public water supplies in the U.S. provide a framework of measurements to support exposure assessments. Historical data for Europe are more limited, but a quadrennial nitrate reporting requirement was implemented as part of the EU Nitrates Directive [17,18]. In the U.S., the frequency of sampling for nitrate in community water systems is stipulated by their sources (ground versus surface waters) and whether concentrations are below the MCL, and historically, by the size of the population served and vulnerability to nitrate contamination. Therefore, the exposure assessment for study participants who report using a public drinking water source may be based on a variable number of measurements, raising concerns about exposure misclassification. In a study of bladder cancer risk in Iowa, associations were stronger in sensitivity analyses based on more comprehensive measurement data [31]. Other studies have restricted analyses to subgroups with more complete or recent measurements [32–35], with implications for study power and possible selection biases. Sampling frequency also limits the extent to which temporal variation in exposure can be represented within a study population, such as the monthly or trimester-based estimates of exposure most relevant for etiologic investigations of adverse reproductive outcomes. In Denmark, limited seasonal variation in nitrate monitoring data suggested these data would sufficiently capture temporal variation for long-term exposure estimates [36]. Studies have often combined regulatory measurements with questionnaire and ancillary data to better characterize individual variation in nitrate exposure, such as to capture changes in water supply characteristics over time or a participant's duration at a drinking water source [31,33,37,38]. Most case-control studies of drinking water nitrate and cancer obtained lifetime residence and drinking water source histories, whereas cohort studies typically have collected only the current water source. Many studies lacked information about study participants' water consumption, which may be an important determinant of exposure to drinking water contaminants [39].

Due to sparse measurement data, exposures for individuals served by private wells are more difficult to estimate than exposures for those on public water supplies. However, advances in geographic-based modeling efforts that incorporate available measurements, nitrogen inputs, aquifer characteristics, and other data hold promise for this purpose. These models include predictor variables describing land use, nitrogen inputs (fertilizer applications, animal feeding operations), soils, geology, climate, management practices, and other factors at the scale of interest. Nolan and Hitt [40] and Messier et al. [41] used nonlinear regression models with terms representing nitrogen inputs at the land surface, transport in soils and groundwater, and nitrate removal by processes such as denitrification, to predict groundwater nitrate concentration at the national scale and for North Carolina, respectively. Predictor variables in the models included N fertilizer and manure, agricultural or forested land use, soils, and, in Nolan and Hitt [40], water-use practices and major geology. Nolan and Hitt [40] reported a training R^2 values of 0.77 for a model of groundwater used mainly for private supplies and Messier, Kane, Bolich and Serre [41] reported a cross-validation testing R^2 value of 0.33 for a point-level private well model. These and earlier regression approaches for groundwater nitrate [42–46] relied on predictor variables describing surficial soils and activities at the land surface, because conditions at depth in the aquifer typically are unknown. Redox conditions in the aquifer and the time since water entered the subsurface (i.e., groundwater age) are two of the most important factors affecting groundwater nitrate, but redox constituents typically are not analyzed, and age is difficult to measure. Even if a well has sufficient data to estimate these conditions, the data must be available for all wells in order to predict water quality in unsampled areas. In most of the above studies, well depth was used as a proxy for age and redox and set to average private or public-supply well depth for prediction.

Recent advances in groundwater nitrate exposure modeling have involved machine-learning methods such as random forest (RF) and boosted regression trees (BRT), along with improved characterization of aquifer conditions at the depth of the well screen (the perforated portion of the well where groundwater intake occurs). Tree-based models do not require data transformation, can fit nonlinear relations, and automatically incorporate interactions among predictors [47]. Wheeler et al. [48] used RF to estimate private well nitrate levels in Iowa. In addition to land use and soil variables, predictor variables included aquifer characteristics at the depth of the well screen, such as total thickness of fine-grained glacial deposits above the well screen, average and minimum thicknesses of glacial deposits near sampled wells, and horizontal and vertical hydraulic conductivities near the wells. Well depth, landscape features, nitrogen sources, and aquifer characteristics ranked highly in the final model, which explained 77% and 38% of the variation in training and hold-out nitrate data, respectively.

Ransom et al. [49] used BRT to predict nitrate concentration at the depths of private and public-supply wells for the Central Valley, California. The model used as input estimates of groundwater age at the depth of the well screen (from MODFLOW/MODPATH models) and depth-related reducing conditions in the groundwater. These estimates were generated by separate models and were available throughout the aquifer. Other MODFLOW-based predictor variables comprised depth to groundwater, and vertical water fluxes and the percent coarse material in the uppermost part of the aquifer where groundwater flow was simulated by MODFLOW. Redox variables were top-ranked in the final BRT model, which also included land use-based N leaching flux, precipitation, soil characteristics, and the MODFLOW-based variables described above. The final model retained 25 of an initial 145 predictor variables considered, had training and hold-out R^2 values of 0.83 and 0.44 respectively, and was used to produce a 3D visualization of nitrate in the aquifer. These studies show that modeling advances and improved characterization of aquifer conditions at depth are increasing our ability to predict nitrate exposure from drinking water supplied by private wells.

4. Nitrate Intake and Endogenous Formation of *N*-Nitroso Compounds

Drinking water nitrate is readily absorbed in the upper gastrointestinal tract and distributed in the human body. When it reaches the salivary glands, it is actively transported from blood into saliva and levels may be up to 20 times higher than in the plasma [50–53]. In the oral cavity 6–7% of the total nitrate can be reduced to nitrite, predominantly by nitrate-reducing bacteria [52,54,55]. The secreted nitrate as well as the nitrite generated in the oral cavity re-enter the gastrointestinal tract when swallowed.

Under acidic conditions in the stomach, nitrite can be protonated to nitrous acid (HNO_2), and subsequently yield dinitrogen trioxide (N_2O_3), nitric oxide (NO), and nitrogen dioxide (NO_2). Since the discovery of endogenous NO formation, it has become clear that NO is involved in a wide range of NO-mediated physiological effects. These comprise the regulation of blood pressure and blood flow by mediating vasodilation [56–58], the maintenance of blood vessel tonus [59], the inhibition of platelet adhesion and aggregation [60,61], modulation of mitochondrial function [62] and several other processes [63–66].

On the other hand, various nitrate and nitrite derived metabolites such as nitrous acid (HNO_2) are powerful nitrosating agents and known to drive the formation of NOC, which are suggested to be the causal agents in many of the nitrate-associated adverse health outcomes. NOC comprise *N*-nitrosamines and *N*-nitrosamides, and may be formed when nitrosating agents encounter *N*-nitrosatable amino acids, which are also from dietary origin. The nitrosation process depends on the reaction mechanisms involved, on the concentration of the compounds involved, the pH of the reaction environment, and further modifying factors, including the presence of catalysts or inhibitors of *N*-nitrosation [66–69].

Endogenous nitrosation can also be inhibited, for instance by dietary compounds like vitamin C, which has the capacity to reduce HNO_2 to NO; and alpha-tocopherol or polyphenols, which can reduce nitrite to NO [54,70–72]. Inhibitory effects on nitrosation have also been described for dietary flavonoids such as quercetin, ferulic and caffeic acid, betel nut extracts, garlic, coffee, and green tea polyphenols [73,74]. Earlier studies showed that the intake of 250 mg or 1 g ascorbic acid per day substantially inhibited *N*-nitrosodimethylamine (NDMA) excretion in 25 women consuming a fish meal rich in amines (nitrosatable precursors) for seven days, in combination with drinking water containing nitrate at the acceptable daily intake (ADI) [75]. In addition, strawberries, garlic juice, and kale juice were shown to inhibit NDMA excretion in humans [76]. The effect of these fruits and vegetables is unlikely to be due solely to ascorbic acid. Using the *N*-nitrosoproline (NPRO) test, Helser et al. [77] found that ascorbic acid only inhibited nitrosamine formation by 24% compared with 41–63% following ingestion of juices (100 mL) made of green pepper, pineapple, strawberry or carrot containing an equal total amount of ascorbic acid.

The protective potential of such dietary inhibitors depends not only on the reaction rates of *N*-nitrosatable precursors and nitrosation inhibitors, but also on their biokinetics, since an effective inhibitor needs to follow gastrointestinal circulation kinetics similar to nitrate [78]. It has been argued that consumption of some vegetables with high nitrate content, can at least partially inhibit the formation of NOC [79–81]. This might apply for green leafy vegetables such as spinach and rocket salad, celery or kale [77] as well as other vegetables rich in both nitrate and natural nitrosation inhibitors. Preliminary data show that daily consumption of one bottle of beetroot juice containing 400 mg nitrate (the minimal amount advised for athletes to increase their sports performances) for one day and seven days by 29 young individuals results in an increased urinary excretion of apparent total nitroso compounds (ATNC), an effect that can only be partially inhibited by vitamin C supplements (1 g per day) [82].

Also, the amount of nitrosatable precursors is a key factor in the formation of NOC. Dietary intakes of red and processed meat are of particular importance [83–87] as increased consumption of red meat (600 vs. 60 g/day), but not white meat, was found to cause a three-fold increase in fecal NOC levels [85]. It was demonstrated that heme iron stimulated endogenous nitrosation [84], thereby providing a possible explanation for the differences in colon cancer risk between red and white meat consumption [88]. The link between meat consumption and colon cancer risk is even stronger for nitrite-preserved processed meat than for fresh meat leading an IARC review to conclude that processed meat is carcinogenic to humans [89].

In a human feeding study [90], the replacement of nitrite in processed meat products by natural antioxidants and the impact of drinking water nitrate ingestion is being evaluated in relation to fecal excretion of NOC, accounting for intakes of meat and dietary vitamin C. A pilot study demonstrated that fecal excretion of ATNC increased after participants switched from ingesting drinking water with low nitrate levels to drinking water with nitrate levels at the acceptable daily intake level of 3.7 mg/kg. The 20 volunteers were assigned to a group consuming either 3.75 g/kg body weight (maximum 300 g per day) red processed meat or fresh (unprocessed) white meat. Comparison of the two dietary groups showed that the most pronounced effect of drinking water nitrate was observed in the red processed meat group. No inhibitory effect of vitamin C intake on ATNC levels in feces was found (unpublished results).

5. Methemoglobinemia

The physiologic processes that can lead to methemoglobinemia in infants under six months of age have been described in detail previously [8,91]. Ingested nitrate is reduced to nitrite by bacteria in the mouth and in the infant stomach, which is less acidic than adults. Nitrite binds to hemoglobin to form methemoglobin, which interferes with the oxygen carrying capacity of the blood. Methemoglobinemia is a life-threatening condition that occurs when methemoglobin levels exceed about 10% [8,91]. Risk factors for infant methemoglobinemia include formula made with water containing high nitrate levels, foods and medications that have high nitrate levels [91,92], and enteric infections [93]. Methemoglobinemia related to high nitrate levels in drinking water used to make infant formula was first reported in 1945 [94]. The U.S. EPA limit of 10 mg/L NO_3-N was set as about one-half the level at which there were no observed cases [95]. The most recent U.S. cases related to nitrate in drinking water were reported by Knobeloch and colleagues in the late 1990s in Wisconsin [96] and were not described in our prior review. Nitrate concentrations in the private wells were about two-times the MCL and bacterial contamination was not a factor. They also summarize another U.S. case in 1999 related to nitrate contamination of a private well and six infant deaths attributed to methemoglobinemia in the U.S. between 1979–1999 only one of which was reported in the literature [96,97]. High incidence of infant methemoglobinemia in eastern Europe has also been described previously [98,99]. A 2002 WHO report on water and health [100] noted that there were 41 cases in Hungary annually, 2913 cases in Romania from 1985–1996 and 46 cases in Albania in 1996.

Results of several epidemiologic studies conducted before 2005 that examined the relationship between nitrate in drinking water and levels of methemoglobin or methemoglobinemia in infants have been described previously [8]. Briefly, nitrate levels >10 mg/L NO_3-N were usually associated with increased methemoglobin levels but clinical methemoglobinemia was not always present. Since our last review, a cross-sectional study conducted in Gaza found elevated methemoglobin levels in infants on supplemental feeding with formula made from well water in an area with the highest mean nitrate concentration of 195 mg/L NO_3 (range: 18–440) compared to an area with lower nitrate concentration (mean: 119 mg/L NO_3; range 18–244) [101]. A cross-sectional study in Morocco found a 22% increased risk of methemoglobinemia in infants in an area with drinking water nitrate >50 mg/L (>11 as NO_3-N) compared to infants in an area with nitrate levels <50 mg/L nitrate [102]. A retrospective cohort study in Iowa of persons (aged 1–60 years) consuming private well water with nitrate levels <10 mg/L NO_3-N found a positive relationship between methemoglobin levels in the blood and the amount of nitrate ingestion [103]. Among pregnant women in rural Minnesota with drinking water supplies that were mostly ≤3 mg/L NO_3-N, there was no relationship between water nitrate intake and women's methemoglobin levels around 36 weeks' gestation [104].

6. Adverse Pregnancy Outcomes

Maternal drinking water nitrate intake during pregnancy has been investigated as a risk factor for a range of pregnancy outcomes, including spontaneous abortion, fetal deaths, prematurity, intrauterine growth retardation, low birth weight, congenital malformations, and neonatal deaths. The relation between drinking water nitrate and congenital malformations in offspring has been the most extensively studied, most likely because of the availability of birth defect surveillance systems around the world.

Our earlier review focused on studies of drinking water nitrate and adverse pregnancy outcomes published before 2005 [8]. In that review, we cited several studies on the relation between maternal exposure to drinking water nitrate and spontaneous abortion including a cluster investigation that suggested a positive association [105] and a case-control study that found no association [106]. These studies were published over 20 years ago. In the present review, we were unable to identify any recently published studies on this outcome. In Table 1, we describe the findings of studies published since 2004 on the relation between drinking water nitrate and prematurity, low birthweight, and congenital malformations. We report results for nitrate in the units (mg/L NO_3 or NO_3-N) that were reported in the publications. In a historic cohort study conducted in the Deux-Sèvres district (France), Migeot et al. [26] linked maternal addresses from birth records to community water system measurements of nitrate, atrazine, and other pesticides. Exposure to the second tertile of nitrate (14–27 mg/L NO_3) without detectable atrazine metabolites was associated with small-for-gestational age births (Odds Ratio (OR) 1.74, 95% CI 1.1, 2.8), but without a monotonic increase in risk with exposures. There was no association with nitrate among those with atrazine detected in their drinking water supplies. Within the same cohort, Albouy-Llaty and colleagues did not observe any association between higher water nitrate concentrations (with or without the presence of atrazine) and preterm birth [107].

Stayner and colleagues also investigated the relation between atrazine and nitrate in drinking water and rates of low birth weight and preterm birth in 46 counties in four Midwestern U.S. states that were required by EPA to measure nitrate and atrazine monthly due to prior atrazine MCL violations [108]. The investigators developed county-level population-weighted metrics of average monthly nitrate concentrations in public drinking water supplies. When analyses were restricted to counties with less than 20% private well usage (to reduce misclassification due to unknown nitrate levels), average nitrate concentrations during the pregnancy were associated with increased rates of very low birth weight (<1.5 kg Rate Ratio $(RR)_{per\,1\,ppm}$ = 1.17, 95% CI 1.08, 1.25) and very preterm births (<32 weeks $RR_{per\,1\,ppm}$ = 1.08, 95% CI 1.02, 1.15) but not with low birth weight or preterm birth overall.

In record-based prevalence study in Perth Australia, Joyce et al. mapped births to their water distribution zone and noted positive associations between increasing tertiles of nitrate levels and prevalence of term premature rupture of membranes (PROM) adjusted for smoking and socioeconomic status [109]. Nitrate concentrations were low; the upper tertile cut point was 0.350 mg/L and the maximum concentration was 1.80 mg/L NO_3-N. Preterm PROM was not associated with nitrate concentrations.

Among studies of drinking water nitrate and congenital malformations, few before 2005 included birth defects other than central nervous system defects [8]. More recently, Mattix et al. [110] noted higher rates of abdominal wall defects (AWD) in Indiana compared to U.S. rates for specific years during the period 1990–2002. They observed a positive correlation between monthly AWD rates and monthly atrazine concentrations in surface waters but no correlation with nitrate levels. Water quality data were obtained from the USGS-NAWQA project that monitors agricultural chemicals in streams and shallow groundwater that are mostly not used as drinking water sources. A case-control study of gastroschisis (one of the two major types of AWD), in Washington State [111] also used USGS-NAWQA measurements of nitrate and pesticides in surface water and determined the distance between maternal residences (zip code centroids) and the closest monitoring site with concentrations above the MCL for nitrate, nitrite, and atrazine. Gastroschisis was not associated with maternal proximity to surface water above the MCL for nitrate (>10 mg/L NO_3-N) or nitrite (>1 mg/L NO_2-N) but there was a positive relationship with proximity to sites with atrazine concentrations above the MCL. In a USA-wide study, Winchester et al. [112] linked the USGS-NAWQA monthly surface water nitrate and pesticide concentrations computed for the month of the last menstrual period with monthly rates of 22 types of birth defects in 1996–2002. Rates of birth defects among women who were estimated to have conceived during April through July were higher than rates among women conceiving in other months. In multivariable models that included nitrate, atrazine, and other pesticides, atrazine (but not nitrate or other pesticides) was associated with several types of anomalies. Nitrate was associated with birth defects in the category of "other congenital anomalies" (OR 1.18, 95% CI 1.14, 1.21); the authors did not specify what defects were included in this category. None of these three studies included local or regional data to support the assumption that surface water nitrate and pesticide concentrations correlated with drinking water exposures to these contaminants.

Using a more refined exposure assessment than the aforementioned studies, Holtby et al. [113] conducted a case-control study of congenital anomalies in an agricultural county in Nova Scotia,

Canada. They linked maternal addresses at delivery to municipal water supply median nitrate concentrations and used kriging of monthly measurements from a network of 140 private wells to estimate drinking water nitrate concentrations in private wells. They observed no associations between drinking water nitrate and all birth defects combined for conceptions during 1987–1997. However, the prevalence of all birth defects occurring during 1998–2006 was associated with drinking water nitrate concentrations of 1–5.56 mg/L NO$_3$-N (OR 2.44, 95% CI 1.05, 5.66) and ≥5.56 mg/L (OR 2.25, 95% CI 0.92, 5.52).

None of the studies of congenital anomalies accounted for maternal consumption of bottled water or the quantity of water consumed during the first trimester, the most critical period of organ/structural morphogenesis. Attempting to overcome some of these limitations, Brender, Weyer, and colleagues [38,114] conducted a population-based, case-control study in the states of Iowa and Texas where they: (1) linked maternal addresses during the first trimester to public water utilities and respective nitrate measurements; (2) estimated nitrate intake from bottled water based on a survey of products consumed and measurement of nitrate in the major products; (3) predicted drinking water nitrate from private wells through modeling (Texas only); and (4) estimated daily nitrate ingestion from women's drinking water sources and daily consumption of water. The study populations were participants of the U.S. National Birth Defects Prevention Study [115]. Compared to the lowest tertile of nitrate ingestion from drinking water (<0.91 mg/day NO$_3$), mothers of babies with spina bifida were twice as likely (95% CI 1.3, 3.2) to ingest ≥5 mg/day NO$_3$ from drinking water than control mothers. Mothers of babies with limb deficiencies, cleft palate, and cleft lip were, respectively, 1.8 (95% CI 1.1, 3.1), 1.9 (95% CI 1.2, 3.1), and 1.8 (95% CI 1.1, 3.1) times more likely to ingest ≥5.4 mg/day of water NO$_3$ than controls. Women were also classified by their nitrosatable drug exposure during the first trimester [116] and by their daily nitrate and nitrite intake based on a food frequency questionnaire [117]. Higher ingestion of drinking water nitrate did not strengthen associations between maternal nitrosatable drug exposure and birth defects in offspring [38]. However, a pattern was observed of stronger associations between nitrosatable drug exposure and selected birth defects for women in the upper two tertiles of total nitrite ingestion that included contributions from drinking water nitrate and dietary intakes of nitrate and nitrite compared to women in the lowest tertile. Higher intake of food nitrate/nitrite was found to also modify the associations of nitrosatable drug exposure and birth defects in this study [118,119] as well as in an earlier study of neural tube defects conducted in south Texas [120]. Multiplicative interactions were observed between higher food nitrate/nitrite and nitrosatable drug exposures for conotruncal heart, limb deficiency, and oral cleft defects [118].

In summary, five out of six studies, conducted since the 1980s of drinking water nitrate and central nervous system defects, found positive associations between higher drinking water nitrate exposure during pregnancy and neural tube defects or central nervous system defects combined [38,120–123]. The sixth study, which did not find a relationship, did not include measures of association, but compared average drinking water nitrate concentrations between mothers with and without neural tube defect-affected births, which were comparable [124].

Table 1. Studies of drinking water nitrate [a] and adverse pregnancy outcomes published January 2005–March 2018.

First Author, Year, Country	Study Design Regional Description	Years of Outcome Ascertainment	Exposure Description	Pregnancy Outcome	Summary of Findings
Albouy-Llaty, 2016 France [107]	Historic cohort study Deux-Sèvres	2005–2010	Measurements of atrazine metabolites and NO_3 in community water systems (263 municipalities) were linked to birth addresses	Preterm birth	No association for >26.99 mg/L NO_3 vs. <14.13 mg/L NO_3 in community water systems with or without atrazine detections, adjusted for neighborhood deprivation
Brender, 2013 Weyer, 2014 USA [38]	Population-based case-control study Iowa and Texas	1997–2005	Maternal addresses during the first trimester linked to public water utility nitrate measurements; nitrate intake from bottled water estimated with survey and laboratory testing; nitrate from private wells predicted through modeling; nitrate ingestion (NO_3) estimated from reported water consumption	Congenital heart defects Limb deficiencies Neural tube defects Oral cleft defects	≥5 vs. <0.91 mg/day NO_3 from drinking water spina bifida OR = 2.0 (95% CI: 1.3, 3.2) ≥5.42 vs. <1.0 mg/day NO_3 from water: limb deficiencies OR = 1.8 (CI: 1.1, 3.1); cleft palate OR = 1.9 (CI: 1.2, 3.1) cleft lip OR = 1.8 (CI: 1.1, 3.1)
Holtby, 2014 Canada [113]	Population-based case-control study Kings County, Nova Scotia	1988–2006	Maternal addresses at delivery linked to municipal water supply median nitrate (NO_3-N) concentrations; nitrate in rural private wells estimated from historic sampling and kriging	Congenital malformations combined into one group	Conceptions in 1987–1997: no association with nitrate concentrations Conceptions in 1998–2006: 1–5.56 mg/L NO_3-N (vs. <1 mg/L) OR = 2.44 (CI: 1.05, 5.66); ≥5.56 mg/L OR = 2.25 (CI: 0.92, 5.52)
Joyce, 2008 Australia [109]	Record-based prevalence study Perth	2002–2004	Linked birth residences to 24 water distribution zones; computed average NO_3-N mg/L from historical measurements; independent sampling conducted for 6 zones as part of exposure validation; also evaluated trihalomethanes (THM)	Premature rupture of membranes at term (PROM) (37 weeks' gestation or later)	ORs for tertiles (vs. <0.125 mg/L NO_3-N): 0.125–0.350 mg/L OR = 1.23 (CI: 1.03, 1.52); >0.350 mg/L OR = 1.47 (CI: 1.20, 1.79) No association with THM levels
Mattix, 2007 USA [110]	Ecologic study Indiana	1990–2002	Monthly abdominal wall defect rates linked to monthly surface water nitrate and atrazine concentrations (USGS-NAWQA monitoring data [b])	Abdominal wall birth defects	No correlation observed between nitrate levels in surface water and monthly abdominal wall defects Positive correlation with atrazine levels

Table 1. *Cont.*

First Author, Year, Country	Study Design Regional Description	Years of Outcome Ascertainment	Exposure Description	Pregnancy Outcome	Summary of Findings
Migeot, 2013 France [26]	Historic cohort study Deux-Sèvres	2005–2009	Measurements of atrazine metabolites and NO_3 in community water systems (263 municipalities) were linked to birth addresses	Small-for-gestational age (SGA) births	ORs for tertiles (vs. <14.13 mg/L NO_3) in community water systems with no atrazine detections: 14–27 mg/L OR = 1.74 (CI: 1.10, 2.75); >27 mg/L OR = OR 1.51 (CI: 0.96, 2.4); no association with nitrate when atrazine was detected
Stayner, 2017 USA [108]	Ecologic study 46 counties in Indiana, Iowa, Missouri, and Ohio	2004–2008	Counties had one or more water utility in EPA's atrazine monitoring program; excluded counties with >20% of population on private wells and >300,000 population. Computed county-specific monthly weighted averages of NO_3-N in finished drinking water; exposure metric was average 9 months prior to birth	Preterm birth Low birth weight	Average nitrate not associated with low birth weight and preterm birth Very low birth weight: RR for 1 ppm increase in NO_3-N = 1.17 (CI: 1.08, 1.25); Very preterm birth RR for 1 ppm increase = 1.08 (CI: 1.02, 1.15)
Waller, 2010 USA [111]	Population-based case-control study Washington State	1987–2006	Calculated distance between maternal residence and closest stream monitoring site with concentrations >MCL for NO_3-N, NO_2-N, or atrazine in surface water (USGS-NAWQA data [b])	Gastroschisis	Gastroschisis was not associated with maternal residential proximity to surface water with elevated nitrate (>10 mg/L) or nitrite (>1 mg/L)
Winchester, 2009 USA [112]	Ecologic study USA-wide	1996–2002	Rates of combined and specific birth defects (computed by month of last menstrual period) linked to monthly surface water nitrate concentrations (USGS-NAWQA data [b]); also evaluated atrazine and other pesticides (combined)	Birth defects categorized into 22 groups	Birth defect category "other congenital anomalies": OR for continuous log nitrate = 1.15 (CI: 1.12, 1.18); adjusted for atrazine and other pesticides: OR = 1.18, CI: 1.14, 1.21); No association with other birth defects

Abbreviations: CI, 95% CI confidence interval; OR, odds ratio; RR, rate ratio; USGS-NAWQA, U. S. Geological Survey National Water Quality Assessment; [a] nitrate units are specified as reported in publications. NO_3 can be converted to NO_3-N by multiplying by 0.2258; [b] USGS-NAWQA data for 186 streams in 51 hydrological study areas; streams were not drinking water sources.

7. Cancer

Most early epidemiologic studies of cancer were ecologic studies of stomach cancer mortality that used exposure estimates concurrent with the time of death. Results were mixed, with some studies showing positive associations, many showing no association, and a few showing inverse associations. The results of ecologic studies through 1995 were reviewed by Cantor [125]. Our previous review included ecologic studies of the brain, esophagus, stomach, kidney, ovary, and non-Hodgkin lymphoma (NHL) published between 1999 and 2003 that were largely null [8]. We did not include ecologic studies or mortality case-control studies in this review due to the limitations of these study designs, especially their inability to assess individual-level exposure and dietary factors that influence the endogenous formation of NOC.

Since our review of drinking water nitrate and health in 2005 [8], eight case-control studies and eight analyses in three cohorts have evaluated historical nitrate levels in PWS in relation to several cancers. Nitrate levels were largely below 10 mg/L NO_3-N. Most of these studies evaluated potential confounders and factors affecting nitrosation. Table 2 shows the study designs and results of studies published from 2005 through 2018, including findings from periodic follow-ups of a cohort study of postmenopausal women in Iowa (USA) [31,37,126–129]. In the first analysis of drinking water nitrate in the Iowa cohort with follow-up through 1998, Weyer and colleagues [130] reported that ovarian and bladder cancers were positively associated with the long-term average PWS nitrate levels prior to enrollment (highest quartile average 1955–1988: >2.46 mg/L NO_3-N). They observed inverse associations for uterine and rectal cancer, but no associations with cancers of the breast, colon, rectum, pancreas, kidney, lung, melanoma, non-Hodgkin lymphoma (NHL), or leukemia. Analyses of PWS nitrate concentrations and cancers of the thyroid, breast, ovary, bladder, and kidney were published after additional follow-up of the cohort. The exposure assessment was improved by: (a) the computation of average nitrate levels and years of exposure at or above 5 mg/L NO_3-N, based on time in residence (vs. one long-term PWS average nitrate estimate used by Weyer and colleagues); and (b) by estimation of total trihalomethanes (TTHM) and dietary nitrite intake.

Thyroid cancer was evaluated for the first time after follow-up of the cohort through 2004. A total of 40 cases were identified [37]. Among women with >10 years on PWS with levels exceeding 5 mg/L NO_3-N for five years or more, thyroid cancer risk was 2.6 times higher than that of women whose supplies never exceeded 5 mg/L. With follow-up through 2010, the risk of ovarian cancer remained increased among women in the highest quartile of average nitrate in PWS [129]. Ovarian cancer risk among private well users was also elevated compared to the lowest PWS nitrate quartile. Associations were stronger when vitamin C intake was below median levels with a significant interaction for users of private wells. Overall, breast cancer risk was not associated with water nitrate levels with follow-up through 2008 [128]. Among women with folate intake ≥ 400 μg/day, risk was increased for those in the highest average nitrate quintile (Hazard Ratio (HR) = 1.40; 95% CI: = 1.05–1.87) and among private well users (HR = 1.38; 95% CI: = 1.05–1.82), compared to those with the lowest average nitrate quintile. There was no association with nitrate exposure among women with lower folate intake. With follow-up through 2010, there were 130 bladder cancer cases among women who had used PWS >10 years. Risk remained elevated among women with the highest average nitrate levels and was 1.6 times higher among women whose drinking water concentration exceeded 5 mg/L NO_3-N for at least four years [31]. Risk estimates were not changed by adjustment for TTHM, which are suspected bladder cancer risk factors. Smoking, but not vitamin C intake, modified the association with nitrate in water; increased risk was apparent only in current smokers (*p*-interaction <0.03). With follow-up through 2010, there were 125 kidney cancer cases among women using PWS; risk was increased among those in the 95th percentile of average nitrate (>5.0 mg/L NO_3-N) compared with the lowest quartile (HR = 2.2, 95% CI: 1.2–4.2) [127]. There was no positive trend with the average nitrate level and no increased risk for women using private wells, compared to those with low average nitrate in their public supply. An investigation of pancreatic cancer in the same population (follow-up through 2011) found no association with average water nitrate levels in public supplies and no association among women on private wells [126].

In contrast to the positive findings for bladder cancer among the cohort of Iowa women, a cohort study of men and women aged 55–69 in the Netherlands with lower nitrate levels in PWS found no association between water nitrate ingestion (median in top quintile = 2.4 mg/day NO_3-N) and bladder cancer risk [131]. Dietary intake of vitamins C and E and history of cigarette smoking did not modify the association. A hospital-based case-control study of bladder cancer in multiple areas of Spain [33] assessed lifetime water sources and usual intake of tap water. Nitrate levels in PWS were low, with almost all average levels below 2 mg/L NO_3-N. Risk of bladder cancer was not associated with the nitrate level in drinking water or with estimated nitrate ingestion from drinking water, and there was no evidence of interaction with factors affecting endogenous nitrosation.

Several case-control studies conducted in the Midwestern U.S. obtained lifetime histories of drinking water sources and estimated exposure for PWS users. In contrast to findings of an increased risk of NHL associated with nitrate levels in Nebraska PWS in an earlier study [132], there was no association with similar concentrations in public water sources in a case-control study of NHL in Iowa [35]. A study of renal cell carcinoma in Iowa [34] found no association with the level of nitrate in PWS, including the number of years that levels exceeded 5 or 10 mg/L NO_3-N. However, higher nitrate levels in PWS increased risk among subgroups who reported above the median intake of red meat intake or below the median intake of vitamin C (*p*-interaction <0.05). A small case-control study of adenocarcinoma of the stomach and esophagus among men and women in Nebraska [133] estimated nitrate levels among long-term users of PWS and found no association between average nitrate levels and risk.

A case-control study of colorectal cancer among rural women in Wisconsin estimated nitrate levels in private wells using spatial interpolation of nitrate concentrations from a 1994 water quality survey and found increased risk of proximal colon cancer among women estimated to have nitrate levels >10 mg/L NO_3-N compared to levels < 0.5 mg/L. Risk of distal colon cancer and rectal cancer were not associated with nitrate levels [134]. Water nitrate ingestion from public supplies, bottled water, and private wells and springs over the adult lifetime was estimated in analyses that pooled case-control studies of colorectal cancer in Spain and Italy [135]. Risk of colorectal cancer was increased among those with >2.3 mg/day NO_3-N (vs. <1.1 mg/day). There were no interactions with red meat, vitamins C and E, and fiber except for a borderline interaction (*p*-interaction = 0.07) for rectum cancer with fiber intake. A small hospital-based case-control study in Indonesia found that drinking water nitrate levels above the WHO standard (>11.3 mg/L as NO_3-N) was associated with colorectal cancer [136]. A national registry-based cohort study in Denmark [32] evaluated average nitrate concentrations in PWS and private wells in relation to colorectal cancer incidence among those whose 35th birthday occurred during 1978–2011. The average nitrate level was computed over residential water supplies from age 20 to 35. Increased risks for colon and rectum cancer were observed in association with average nitrate levels ≥9.25 mg/L NO_3 (≥2.1 as NO_3-N) and ≥3.87 mg/L NO_3 (>0.87 as NO_3-N), respectively, with a significant positive trend. Because the study did not interview individuals, it could not evaluate individual-level risk factors that might influence endogenous nitrosation.

A case-control study of breast cancer in Cape Cod, Massachusetts (US) [137] estimated nitrate concentrations in PWS over approximately 20 years as an historical proxy for wastewater contamination and potential exposure to endocrine disruption compounds. Average exposures >1.2 mg/L NO_3-N (vs. <0.3 mg/L) were not associated with risk. A hospital-based case-control study in Spain found no association between water nitrate ingestion and pre- and post-menopausal breast cancers [138].

Table 2. Case-control and cohort studies of drinking water nitrate and cancer (January 2004–March 2018) by cancer site.

First Author (Year) Country	Study Design, Years Regional Description	Exposure Description	Cancer Sites Included	Summary of Drinking-Water Findings [a,b]	Evaluation of Effect Modification [c]
Zeegers, 2006 Netherlands [131]	Cohort Incidence, 1986–1995 204 municipal registries across the Netherlands	1986 nitrate level in 364 pumping stations, exposure data available for 871 cases, 4359 members of the subcohort	Bladder	Highest vs. lowest quintile intake from water ($\geq$1.7 mg/day NO_3-N [median 2.4 mg/day] vs. <0.20) RR = 1.11 (CI: 0.87–1.41; p-trend = 0.14)	No interaction with vitamin C, E, smoking
Espejo-Herrera, 2015 Spain [33]	Hospital-based multi-center case-control Incidence, 1998–2001 Asturias, Alicante, Barcelona, Vallès-Bages, Tenerife provinces	Nitrate levels in PWS (1979–2010) and bottled water (measurements of brands with highest consumption based on a Spanish survey); analyses limited to those with $\geq$70% of residential history with nitrate estimate (531 cases, 556 controls)	Bladder	Highest vs. lowest quartile average level (age 18-interview) ($\geq$2.26 vs. 1.13 mg/L NO_3-N) OR = 1.04 (CI: 0.60–1.81) Years >2.15 mg/L NO_3-N (75th percentile) (>20 vs. 0 years) OR = 1.41 (CI: 0.89–2.24)	No interaction with vitamin C, E, red meat, processed meat, average THM level
Jones, 2016 USA [31]	Population-based cohort of postmenopausal women ages 55–69 Incidence, 1986–2010 Iowa	Nitrate levels in PWS (1955–1988) and private well use among women >10 years at enrollment residence with nitrate and trihalomethane estimates (20,945 women; 170 bladder cases); no measurements for private wells Adjusted for total trihalomethanes (TTHM)	Bladder	Highest vs. lowest quartile PWS average ($\geq$2.98 vs. <0.47 mg/L NO_3-N) HR = 1.47 (CI: 0.91–2.38; p-trend = 0.11) Years >5 mg/L ($\geq$4 years vs. 0) HR = 1.61 (CI: 1.05–2.47; p-trend = 0.03) Private well users (vs. <0.47 mg/L NO_3-N on PWS) HR = 1.53 (CI: 0.93–2.54)	Interaction with smoking (p-interaction = 0.03); HR = 3.67 (CI: 1.43–9.38) among current smokers/$\geq$2.98 mg/L vs. non-smokers/<0.47 mg/L NO_3-N); No interaction with vitamin C, TTHM levels
Mueller, 2004 USA, Canada, France, Italy, Spain [139]	Pooled case-control studies Incidence among children <15 years (USA <20 years) 7 regions of 5 countries	Water source during pregnancy and first year of child's life (836 cases, 1485 controls); nitrate test strip measurements of nitrate and nitrite for pregnancy home (except Italy) (283 cases, 537 controls; excluding bottled water users: 207 cases, 400 controls)	Brain, childhood	Private well use versus PWS associated with increased risk in 2 regions and decreased risk in one; No association with nitrate levels in water supplies Astrocytomas (excludes bottled water users): $\geq$1.5 vs. <0.3 mg/L NO_2-N OR = 5.7 (CI: 1.2–27.2)	Not described
Brody, 2006 USA [137]	Case-control Incidence, 1988–1995 Cape Cod, Massachusetts	Nitrate levels in public water supplies (PWS) since 1972 was used as an indicator of wastewater contamination and potential mammary carcinogens and endocrine disrupting compounds; excluded women on private wells	Breast	Average $\geq$1.2 mg/L NO_3-N vs. <0.3 OR = 1.8, (CI: 0.6–5.0); summed annual NO_3-N $\geq$10 vs. 1–<10 mg/L OR = 0.9, CI: 0.6–1.5); number of years >1 mg/L NO_3-N $\geq$8 vs. 0 years OR = 0.9 (CI: 0.5–1.5)	Not described

Table 2. *Cont.*

First Author (Year) Country	Study Design, Years Regional Description	Exposure Description	Cancer Sites Included	Summary of Drinking-Water Findings [a,b]	Evaluation of Effect Modification [c]
Inoue-Choi, 2012 USA [128]	Population-based cohort of postmenopausal women ages 55–69 Incidence, 1986–2008 Iowa	Nitrate levels in PWS (1955–1988) and private well use among women >10 years at enrollment residence (20,147 women; 1751 breast cases); no measurements for private wells	Breast	Highest vs. lowest quintile PWS average (≥3.8 vs. ≤0.32 mg/L NO_3-N) HR = 1.14 (CI: 0.95–1.36; p-trend = 0.11); Private well (vs. ≤ 0.32 mg/L NO_3-N) HR = 1.14 (CI: 0.97–1.34); Private well (vs. ≤0.32 mg/L NO_3-N on PWS) HR = 1.38 (CI: 1.05–1.82); No association among those with low folate <400 μg/day	Interaction with folate for PWS (p-interaction = 0.06). Folate ≥400 μg/d: (≥3.8 vs. ≤0.32 mg/L NO_3-N) HR = 1.40 (CI: 1.05–1.87; p-trend = 0.04)
Espejo-Herrera, 2016 Spain [138]	Hospital-based multi-center case-control Incidence, 2008–2013 Spain (8 provinces)	Nitrate levels in PWS (2004–2010), bottled water measurements and private wells and springs (2013 measurements in 21 municipalities in León, Spain, the area with highest non-PWS use) Analyses include women with ≥70% of period from age 18 to 2 years before interview (1245 cases, 1520 controls)	Breast	Water nitrate intake based on average nitrate levels (age 18 to 2 years prior to interview) and water intake (L/day). Post-menopausal women: >2.0 vs. 0.5 mg/day NO_3-N OR = 1.32 (0.93–1.86); Premenopausal women: >1.4 vs. 0.4 mg/day NO_3-N OR = 1.14 (0.67–1.94)	No interaction with red meat, processed meat, vitamin C, E, smoking for pre- and post-menopausal women
McElroy, 2008 USA [134]	Population-based case-control, women Incidence, 1990–1992 and 1999–2001 Wisconsin	Limited to women in rural areas with no public water system (475 cases, 1447 controls); nitrate levels at residence (presumed to be private wells) estimated by kriging using data from a 1994 representative sample of 289 private wells	Colorectal	All colon cancers: Private wells ≥10.0 mg/L NO_3-N vs. <0.5 OR = 1.52 (CI: 0.95–2.44); Proximal colon cancer: OR = 2.91 (CI: 1.52–5.56)	Not described
Espejo-Herrera, 2016 Spain, Italy [135]	Multi-center case-control study Incidence, 2008–2013 Spain (9 provinces) and population-based controls; Italy (two provinces) and hospital-based controls	Nitrate levels in PWS (2004–2010) for 349 water supply zones, bottled water (measured brands with highest consumption), and private wells and springs (measurements in 2013 in 21 municipalities in León, Spain, the area with highest non-PWS use) Analyses include those with nitrate estimates for ≥70% of period 30 years before interview (1869 cases, 3530 controls)	Colorectal	Water nitrate intake based on average nitrate levels (estimated 30 to 2 years prior to interview) and water intake (L/day) Highest vs. lowest exposure quintiles (≥2.3 vs. <1.1 mg NO_3-N) OR = 1.49 (CI:1.24–1.78); Colon OR = 1.52 (CI: 1.24–1.86). Rectum OR = 1.62 (CI: 1.23–2.14)	Interaction with fiber for rectum (p-interaction = 0.07); >20 g/day fiber + >1.0 mg/L NO_3-N vs. <20 g/day + ≤1.0 mg/L HR = 0.72 (CI: 0.52–1.00). No interaction with red meat, vitamin C, E

Table 2. *Cont.*

First Author (Year) Country	Study Design, Years Regional Description	Cancer Sites Included	Exposure Description	Summary of Drinking-Water Findings [a,b]	Evaluation of Effect Modification [c]
Fathmawati, 2017 Indonesia [136]	Hospital-based case-control Incidence, 2014–2016 Indonesia (3 provinces)	Colorectal	Nitrate levels in well water collected during the raining season (Feb–March 2016) and classified based on >11.3 or ≤11.3 mg/L as NO_3-N and duration of exposure >10 and ≤10 years. Analyses included participants who reported drinking well water (75 cases, 75 controls)	Water nitrate > WHO standard vs. below (>11.3 vs. ≤11.3 mg/L NO_3-N) OR = 2.82 (CI: 1.08–7.40); >10 years: 4.31 (CI: 11.32–14.10); ≤10 years: 1.41 (CI: 0.14–13.68)	Not described
Schullehner, 2018 Denmark [32]	Population-based record-linkage cohort of men and women ages 35 and older, 1978–2011 Denmark	Colorectal	Nitrate levels in PWS and private wells among 1,742,321 who met exposure assessment criteria (5944 colorectal cancer cases, including 3700 with colon and 2308 with rectal cancer)	Annual average nitrate exposure between ages 20–35 among those who lived ≥75% of study period at homes with a water sample within 1 year (61% of Danish population). Highest vs. lowest exposure quintile (≥2.1 vs. 0.16 mg/L NO_3-N); Colorectal: HR = 1.16 (CI: 1.08–1.25); colon: 1.15 (CI: 1.05–1.26); rectum: 1.17 (CI: 1.04–1.32)	No information on dietary intakes or smoking
Ward, 2007 USA [34]	Population-based case control Incidence, 1986–1989 Iowa	Kidney (renal cell carcinomas)	Nitrate levels in PWS among those with nitrate estimates for ≥70% of person-years ≥1960 (201 cases, 1244 controls)	Highest vs. lowest quartile PWS average (≥2.8 mg/L NO_3-N vs. <0.62) OR = 0.89 (CI 0.57–1.39); Years >5mg/L NO_3-N 11+ vs. 0 OR = 1.03 (CI: 0.66–1.60)	Interaction with red meat intake (p-interaction = 0.01); OR = 1.91 (CI 1.04–3.51) among 11+ years >5 mg/L NO_3-N and red meat ≥1.2 servings/day. Interaction with vitamin C showed similar pattern (p-interaction = 0.13)
Jones, 2017 USA [127]	Population-based cohort of postmenopausal women ages 55–69 Incidence, 1986–2010 Iowa	Kidney	Nitrate levels in PWS (1955–1988) and private well use among women >10 years at enrollment residence. PWS measurements for nitrate and TTHM; no measurements for private wells (20,945 women; 163 kidney cases)	Nitrate and TTHM metrics computed for duration at water source (11+ years). 95th percentile vs. lowest quartile PWS average (≥5.00 vs. <0.47 mg/L NO_3-N) HR = 2.23 (CI: 1.19–4.17; p-trend = 0.35). Years >5 mg/L (≥4 years vs. 0) HR = 1.54 (CI: 0.97–2.44; p-trend = 0.09). Private well users (vs. <0.47 mg/L NO_3-N in PWS) HR = 0.96 (CI: 0.59–1.58)	No interaction with smoking, vitamin C
Ward, 2006 USA [35]	Population-based case-control Incidence, 1998–2000 Iowa	Non-Hodgkin lymphoma	Nitrate levels in PWS among those with nitrate estimates for ≥70% of person-years ≥1960 (181 case, 142 controls); nitrate measurements for private well users at time of interviews (1998–2000; 54 cases, 44 controls)	Private wells: >5.0 mg/L NO_3-N vs. ND OR = 0.8 (CI 0.2–2.5). PWS average: ≥2.9 mg/L NO_3-N vs. <0.63 OR = 1.2 (CI 0.6–2.2). Years ≥5mg/L NO3-N: 10+ vs. 0 OR = 1.4 (CI: 0.7–2.9)	No interaction with vitamin C, smoking

Table 2. *Cont.*

First Author (Year) Country	Study Design, Years Regional Description	Exposure Description	Cancer Sites Included	Summary of Drinking-Water Findings [a,b]	Evaluation of Effect Modification [c]
Inoue-Choi, 2015 USA [129]	Population-based cohort of postmenopausal women ages 55–69 Incidence, 1986–2010 Iowa	Nitrate levels in PWS (1955–1988) and private well use among women >10 years at enrollment residence; PWS measurements for nitrate and TTHM; no measurements for private wells (17,216 women; 190 ovarian cases)	Ovary	Nitrate and TTHM metrics computed for reported duration at water source (11+ years) Highest vs. lowest quartile PWS average (≥2.98 mg/L vs. <0.47 mg/L NO_3-N) HR = 2.03 (CI = 1.22–3.38; p-trend = 0.003) Years >5 mg/L (≥4 years vs. 0) HR = 1.52 (CI: 1.00–2.31; p-trend = 0.05) Private well users (vs. <0.47 mg/L NO_3-N in PWS) HR = 1.53 (CI: 0.93–2.54)	No interaction with vitamin C, red meat intake, smoking for PWS nitrate Interaction with private well use and vitamin C intake (p-interaction = 0.01)
Quist, 2018 USA [126]	Population-based cohort of postmenopausal women ages 55–69 Incidence, 1986–2011 Iowa	Nitrate levels in PWS (1955–1988) and private well use among women >10 years at enrollment residence; nitrate and TTHM estimates for PWS (20,945 women; 189 pancreas cases); no measurements for private wells Adjusted for TTHM (1955–1988), measured levels in 1980s, prior year levels estimated by expert)	Pancreas	Nitrate and TTHM metrics computed for reported duration at water source (11+ years) 95th percentile vs. lowest quartile PWS average (≥5.69 vs. <0.47 mg/L NO_3-N) HR = 1.16 (CI: 0.51–2.64; p-trend = 0.97) Years >5 mg/L (≥4 years vs. 0) HR = 0.90 (CI: 0.55–1.48; p-trend = 0.62) Private well users (vs. <0.47 mg/L NO_3-N) HR = 0.92 (CI: 0.55–1.52)	No interaction with smoking, vitamin C
Ward, 2008 USA [133]	Population-based case control Incidence, 1988–1993 Nebraska	Controls from prior study of lymphohematopoetic cases and controls interviewed in 1992–1994; Proxy interviews for 80%, 76%, 61% of stomach, esophagus, controls, respectively. Nitrate levels (1965–1985) in PWS for ≥70% of person-years (79 distal stomach, 84, esophagus, 321 controls); Private well users sampling at interview (15 stomach, 22 esophagus, 44 controls)	Stomach and esophagus (adenocarcinomas)	Highest vs. lowest quartile PWS average (>4.32 vs. <2.45 mg/L NO_3-N): stomach OR = 1.2 (CI 0.5–2.7); esophagus OR = 1.3 (CI: 0.6–3.1); Years >10 mg/L NO_3-N (9+ vs. 0): stomach OR = 1.1 (CI: 0.5–2.3); esophagus OR = 1.2 (CI: 0.6–2.7) Private well users (>4.5 mg/L NO_3-N vs. <0.5) stomach OR = 5.1 (CI: 0.5–52; 4 cases, 13 controls); esophagus OR = 0.5 (CI: 0.1–2.9; 8 cases; 13 controls)	No interaction with vitamin C, processed meat, or red meat for either cancer
Ward, 2010 USA [37]	Population-based cohort of postmenopausal women ages 55–69 Incidence, 1986–2004 Iowa	Nitrate levels in PWS (1955–1988) and private well use among women >10 years at enrollment residence (21,977 women; 40 thyroid cases); no measurements for private wells	Thyroid	Highest vs. lowest quartile PWS average (>2.46 vs. <0.36 mg/L NO_3-N) HR = 2.18 (CI: 0.83–5.76; p-trend = 0.02) Years >5 mg/L (≥5 years vs. 0) HR = 2.59 (CI: 1.09–6.19; p-trend = 0.04); Private well (vs. <0.36 mg/L NO_3-N on PWS) HR = 1.13 (CI: 0.83–3.66) Dietary nitrate intake quartiles positively associated with risk (p-trend = 0.05)	No interaction with smoking, vitamin C, body mass index, education, residence location (farm/rural vs. urban)

ND = not detected; PWS = public water supplies; [a] nitrate or nitrite levels presented in the publications as mg/L were converted to mg/L as NO_3-N or NO_2-N; [b] Odds ratios (OR) for case-control studies, incidence rate ratios (RR) and hazard ratios (HR) for cohort studies, and 95% confidence intervals (CI); [c] Factors evaluated are noted. Interaction refers to reported $p ≤ 0.10$ from test of heterogeneity.

Animal studies demonstrate that in utero exposure to nitrosamides can cause brain tumors in the exposed offspring. Water nitrate and nitrite intake during pregnancy was estimated in a multi-center case-control study of childhood brain tumors in five countries based on the maternal residential water source [139]. Results for the California and Washington State sites were reported in our previous review [8,140]. Nitrate/nitrite levels in water supplies were measured using a nitrate test strip method in four countries including these U.S. sites; most of these measurements occurred many years after the pregnancy. Measured nitrate concentrations were not associated with risk of childhood brain tumors. However, higher nitrite levels (>1.5 mg/L NO_2-N) in the drinking water were associated with increased risk of astrocytomas.

8. Thyroid Disease

Animal studies demonstrate that ingestion of nitrate at high doses can competitively inhibit iodine uptake and induce hypertrophy of the thyroid gland [141]. An early study of women in the Netherlands consuming water with nitrate levels at or above the MCL, found increased prevalence of thyroid hypertrophy [142]. Since the last review, five studies have evaluated nitrate ingestion from drinking water (the Iowa cohort study also assessed diet) and prevalence of thyroid disease. A study of school-age children in Slovakia found increased prevalence of subclinical hypothyroidism among children in an area with high nitrate levels (51–274 mg/L NO_3) in water supplies compared with children ingesting water with nitrate ≤50 mg/L (11 mg/L NO_3-N). In Bulgarian villages with high nitrate levels (75 mg/L NO_3) and low nitrate levels (8 mg/L), clinical examinations of the thyroids of pregnant women and school children revealed an approximately four- and three-fold increased prevalence of goiter, respectively, in the high nitrate village [143,144]. The iodine status of the populations in both studies was adequate. Self-reported hypothyroidism and hyperthyroidism among a cohort of post-menopausal women in Iowa was not associated with average nitrate concentrations in PWS [37]. However, dietary nitrate, the predominant source of intake, was associated with increased prevalence of hypothyroidism but not hyperthyroidism. Modeled estimates of nitrate concentrations in private wells among a cohort of Old Order Amish in Pennsylvania (USA) were associated with increased prevalence of subclinical hypothyroidism as determined by thyroid stimulating hormone measurements, among women but not men [145].

9. Other Health Effects

Associations between nitrate in drinking water and other non-cancer health effects, including type 1 childhood diabetes (T1D), blood pressure, and acute respiratory tract infections in children were previously reviewed [8]. Since 2004, a small number of studies have contributed additional mixed evidence for these associations. Animal studies indicate that NOC may play a role in the pathology of T1D through damage to pancreatic beta cells [146]. A registry-based study in Finland [147] found a positive trend in T1D incidence with levels of nitrate in drinking water. In contrast, an ecological analysis in Italy showed an inverse correlation with water nitrate levels and T1D rates [148]. A small T1D case-control study in Canada with 57 cases showed no association between T1D and estimated intake of nitrate from drinking water (highest quartile >2.7 mg/day NO_3-N) [149]. Concentrations of nitrate in drinking water (median ~2.1 mg/L NO_3-N) were not associated with progression to T1D in a German nested case-control study of islet autoantibody-positive children, who may be at increased risk of the disease [150].

In a prospective, population-based cohort study in Wisconsin (USA), increased incidence of early and late age-related macular degeneration was positively associated with higher nitrate levels (≥5 mg/L vs. <5 mg/L NO_3-N) in rural private drinking water supplies [151]. The authors suggested several possible mechanisms, including methemoglobin-induced lipid peroxidation in the retina.

Potential benefits of nitrate ingestion include lowering of blood pressure due to production of nitric oxide in the acidic stomach and subsequent vasodilation, antithrombotic, and immunoregulatory effects [152]. Experimental studies in animals and controlled feeding studies in humans have demonstrated mixed evidence of these effects and on other cardiovascular endpoints such as vascular hypertrophy, heart failure, and myocardial infarction (e.g., [152–154]). Ingested nitrite from diet has also been associated with increased blood flow in certain parts of the brain [155]. Epidemiologic studies of these effects are limited to estimation of dietary exposures or biomarkers that integrate exposures from nitrate from diet and drinking water. Recent findings in the Framingham Offspring Study suggested that plasma nitrate was associated with increased overall risk of death that attenuated when adjusted for glomerular function (HR: 1.16, 95% CI: 1.0–1.35) but no association was observed for incident cardiovascular disease [156]. No epidemiologic studies have specifically evaluated nitrate ingested from drinking water in relation to these outcomes. Another potential beneficial effect of nitrate is protection against bacterial infections via its reduction to nitrite by enteric bacteria. In an experimental inflammatory bowel disease mouse model, nitrite in drinking water was associated with both preventive and therapeutic effects [157]. However, there is limited epidemiologic evidence for a reduced risk of gastrointestinal disease in populations with high drinking water nitrate intake. One small, cross-sectional study in Iran found no association between nitrate levels in public water supplies with mean levels of ~5.6 mg/L NO_3-N and gastrointestinal disease [158].

10. Discussion

Since our last review of studies through 2004 [8], more than 30 epidemiologic studies have evaluated drinking water nitrate and risk of cancer, adverse reproductive outcomes, or thyroid disease. However, the number of studies of any one outcome was not large and there are still too few studies to allow firm conclusions about risk. The most common endpoints studied were colorectal cancer, bladder, and breast cancer (three studies each) and thyroid disease (four studies). Considering all studies to date, the strongest evidence for a relationship between drinking water nitrate ingestion and adverse health outcomes (besides methemoglobinemia) is for colorectal cancer, thyroid disease, and neural tube defects. Four of the five published studies of colorectal cancer found evidence of an increased risk of colorectal cancer or colon cancer associated with water nitrate levels that were mostly below the respective regulatory limits [32,134,135,159]. In one of the four positive studies [159], increased risk was only observed in subgroups likely to have increased nitrosation. Four of the five studies of thyroid disease found evidence for an increased prevalence of subclinical hypothyroidism with higher ingestion of drinking water nitrate among children, pregnant women, or women only [37,144,145,160]. Positive associations with drinking water nitrate were observed at nitrate concentrations close to or above the MCL. The fifth study, a cohort of post-menopausal women in Iowa, had lower drinking water nitrate exposure but observed a positive association with dietary nitrate [37]. To date, five of six studies of neural tube defects showed increased risk with exposure to drinking water nitrate below the MCL. Thus, the evidence continues to accumulate that higher nitrate intake during the pregnancy is a risk factor for this group of birth defects.

All but one of the 17 cancer studies conducted since 2004 were in the U.S. or Europe, the majority of which were investigations of nitrate in regulated public drinking water. Thyroid cancer was studied for the first time [37] with a positive finding that should be evaluated in future studies. Bladder cancer, a site for which other drinking water contaminants (arsenic, disinfection by-products [DBPs]) are established or suspected risk factors, was not associated with drinking water nitrate in three of the four studies. Most of the cancer studies since 2004 evaluated effect modification by factors known to influence endogenous nitrosation, although few observed evidence for these effects. Several studies of adverse reproductive outcomes since 2004 have indicated a positive association between maternal prenatal exposure to nitrate concentrations below the MCL and low birth weight and small for gestational age births. However, most studies did not account for co-exposure to other water contaminants, nor did they adjust for potential risk factors. The relation between drinking water nitrate and spontaneous abortion continues to be understudied. Few cases of methemoglobinemia, the health concern that lead to the regulation of nitrate in public water supplies, have been reported in the U.S. since the 1990s. However, as described by Knobeloch et al. [96], cases may be underreported and only a small proportion of cases are thoroughly investigated and described in the literature. Based on published reports, [100] areas of the world of particular concern include several eastern European countries, Gaza, and Morocco, where high nitrate concentrations in water supplies have been linked to high levels of methemoglobin in children. Therefore, continued surveillance and education of physicians and parents will be important. Biological plausibility exists for relationships between nitrate ingestion from drinking water and a few other health outcomes including diabetes and beneficial effects on the cardiovascular system, but there have been only a limited number of epidemiologic studies.

Assessment of drinking water nitrate exposures in future studies should be improved by obtaining drinking water sources at home and at work, estimating the amount of water consumed from each source, and collecting information on water filtration systems that may impact exposure. These efforts are important for reducing misclassification of exposure. Since our last review, an additional decade of PWS monitoring data are available in the U.S. and European countries, which has allowed assessment of exposure over a substantial proportion of participants' lifetimes in recent studies. Future studies should estimate exposure to multiple water contaminants as has been done in recent cancer studies [31,33,127,129]. For instance, nitrate and atrazine frequently occur together in drinking water in agricultural areas [161] and animal studies have found this mixture to be teratogenic [162]. Regulatory monitoring data for pesticides in PWS has been available for over 20 years in the U.S.; therefore, it is now feasible to evaluate co-exposure to these contaminants. Additionally, water supplies in agricultural areas that rely on alluvial aquifers or surface water often have elevated levels of both DBPs and nitrate. Under this exposure scenario, there is the possibility of formation of the nitrogenated DBPs including the carcinogenic NDMA, especially if chloramination treatment is used for disinfection [163,164]. Studies of health effects in countries outside the U.S. and Europe are also needed.

A comprehensive assessment of nitrate and nitrite from drinking water and dietary sources as well as estimation of intakes of antioxidants and other inhibitors of endogenous nitrosation including dietary polyphenols and flavonoids is needed in future studies. Heme iron from red meat, which increases fecal NOC in human feeding studies, should also be assessed as a potential effect modifier of risk from nitrate ingestion. More research is needed on the potential interaction of nitrate ingestion and nitrosatable drugs (those with secondary and tertiary amines or amides). Evidence from several studies of birth defects [38,118–120] implicates nitrosatable drug intake during pregnancy as a risk factor for specific congenital anomalies especially in combination with nitrate. Drugs with nitrosatable groups include many over-the-counter and prescription drugs. Future studies with electronic medical records and record-linkage studies in countries like Denmark with national pharmacy data may provide opportunities for evaluation of these exposures.

Populations with the highest exposure to nitrate from their drinking water are those living in agricultural regions, especially those drinking water from shallow wells near nitrogen sources (e.g., crop fields, animal feeding operations). Estimating exposure for private well users is important because it allows assessment of risk over a greater range of nitrate exposures compared to studies focusing solely on populations using PWS. Future health studies should focus on these populations, many of which may have been exposed to elevated nitrate in drinking water from early childhood into adulthood. A major challenge in conducting studies in these regions is the high prevalence of private well use with limited nitrate measurement data for exposure assessment. Recent efforts to model nitrate concentrations in private wells have shown that it is feasible to develop predictive models where sufficient measurement data are available [41,48,49]. However, predictive models from one area are not likely to be directly translatable to other geographic regions with different aquifers, soils, and nitrogen inputs.

Controlled human feeding studies have demonstrated that endogenous nitrosation occurs after ingestion of drinking water with nitrate concentrations above the MCL of 10 mg/L NO_3-N (~44 mg/L as NO_3). However, the extent of NOC formation after ingestion of drinking water with nitrate concentrations below the MCL has not been well characterized. Increased risks of specific cancers and central nervous system birth defects in study populations consuming nitrate below the MCL is indirect evidence that nitrate ingestion at these levels may be a risk factor under some conditions. However, confounding by other exposures or risk factors can be difficult to rule out in many studies. Controlled human studies to evaluate endogenous nitrosation at levels below the MCL are needed to understand interindividual variability and factors that affect endogenous nitrosation at drinking water nitrate levels below the MCL.

A key step in the endogenous formation of NOC is the reduction of nitrate, which has been transported from the bloodstream into the saliva, to nitrite by the nitrate-reducing bacteria that are located primarily in the crypts on the back of the tongue [165–167]. Tools for measuring bacterial DNA and characterizing the oral microbiome are now available and are currently being incorporated into epidemiologic studies [168,169]. Buccal cell samples that have been collected in epidemiologic studies can be used to characterize the oral microbiome and to determine the relative abundance of the nitrate-reducing bacteria. Studies are needed to characterize the stability of the nitrate-reducing capacity of the oral microbiome over time and to determine factors that may modify this capacity such as diet, oral hygiene, and periodontal disease. Interindividual variability in the oral nitrate-reducing bacteria may play an important role in modifying endogenous NOC formation. The quantification of an individual's nitrate-reducing bacteria in future epidemiologic studies is likely to improve our ability to classify participants by their intrinsic capacity for endogenous nitrosation.

In addition to characterizing the oral microbiome, future epidemiologic studies should incorporate biomarkers of NOC (e.g., urinary or fecal NOC), markers of genetic damage, and determine genetic variability in NOC metabolism. As many NOC require α-hydroxylation by CYP2E1 for bioactivation and for formation of DNA adducts, it is important to investigate the influence of polymorphisms in the gene encoding for this enzyme. Studies are also needed among populations with medical conditions that increase nitrosation such as patients with inflammatory bowel disease and periodontal disease [8]. Because NOC exposures induce characteristic gene expression profiles [170,171], further studies linking drinking water intake to NOC excretion and gene expression responses are relevant to our understanding of health risks associated with drinking water nitrate. The field of 'Exposome-research' [172,173] generates large numbers of genomics profiles in human population studies for which dietary exposures and biobank materials are also available. These studies provide opportunities to measure urinary levels of nitrate and NOC that could be associated with molecular markers of exposure and disease risk.

Nitrate concentrations in global water supplies are likely to increase in the future due to population growth, increases in nitrogen fertilizer use, and increasing intensity and concentration of animal agriculture. Even with increased inputs, mitigation of nitrate concentrations in water resources is possible through local, national, and global efforts. Examples of the latter are the International Nitrogen Initiative [174] and the EU Nitrates Directive [17,18], which aim to quantify human effects on the nitrogen cycle and to validate and promote methods for sustainable nitrogen management. Evidence for the effectiveness of these efforts, which include the identification of vulnerable areas, establishment of codes of good agricultural practices, and national monitoring and reporting are indicated by decreasing trends in groundwater nitrate concentrations in some European countries after the implementation of the EU Nitrates Directive [19]. However, the effect of this initiative was variable across the EU. In the U.S., nitrogen applications to crop fields are not regulated and efforts to reduce nitrogen runoff are voluntary. Although strategies such as appropriate timing of fertilizer applications, diversified crop rotations, planting of cover crops, and reduced tillage can be effective [175], concentrations in U.S. ground and surface water have continued to increase in most areas [10]. Climate change is expected to affect nitrogen in aquatic ecosystems and groundwater through alterations of the hydrological cycle [176]. Climatic factors that affect nitrate in groundwater include the amount, intensity, and timing of precipitation. Increasing rainfall intensity, especially in the winter and spring, can lead to increases in nitrogen runoff from agricultural fields and leaching to groundwater.

11. Conclusions

In summary, most adverse health effects related to drinking water nitrate are likely due to a combination of high nitrate ingestion and factors that increase endogenous nitrosation. Some of the recent studies of cancer and some birth defects have been able to identify subgroups of the population likely to have greater potential for endogenous nitrosation. However, direct methods of assessing these individuals are needed. New methods for quantifying the nitrate-reducing bacteria in the oral microbiome and characterizing genetic variation in NOC metabolism hold promise for identifying high risk groups in epidemiologic studies.

To date, the number of well-designed studies of individual health outcomes is still too few to draw firm conclusions about risk from drinking water nitrate ingestion. Additional studies that incorporate improved exposure assessment for populations on PWS, measured or predicted exposure for private well users, quantification of nitrate-reducing bacteria, and estimates of dietary and other factors affecting nitrosation are needed. Studies of colorectal cancer, thyroid disease, and central nervous system birth defects, which show the most consistent associations with water nitrate ingestion, will be particularly useful for clarifying these risks. Future studies of other health effects with more limited evidence of increased risk are also needed including cancers of the thyroid, ovary, and kidney, and the adverse reproductive outcomes of spontaneous abortion, preterm birth, and small for gestational age births.

Acknowledgments: This work was partly supported by the Intramural Research Program of the National Cancer Institute, Division of Cancer Epidemiology and Genetics, Occupational and Environmental Epidemiology Branch. Two authors (TMdK, SvB) acknowledge financial support from the European Commission in the context of the integrated project PHYTOME financed under the Seventh Framework Programme for Research and Technology Development of the European Commission (EU-FP7 grant agreement no. 315683), investigating the possible replacement of nitrite in meat products by natural compounds. CMV notes that ISGlobal is a member of the CERCA Programme, Generalitat de Catalunya.

Conflicts of Interest: The authors declare no conflict of interest.

References

1. Davidson, E.A.; David, M.B.; Galloway, J.N.; Goodale, C.L.; Haeuber, R.; Harrison, J.A.; Howarth, R.W.; Jaynes, D.B.; Lowrance, R.R.; Nolan, B.T.; et al. Excess nitrogen in the U.S. environment: Trends, risks, and solutions. In *Issues in Ecology*; Ecological Society of America: Washington, DC, USA, 2012.
2. Vitousek, P.M.; Aber, J.D.; Howarth, R.W.; Likens, G.E.; Matson, P.A.; Schindler, D.W.; Schlesinger, W.H.; Tilman, D. Human alteration of the global nitrogen cycle: Sources and consequences. *Ecol. Appl.* **1997**, *7*, 737–750. [CrossRef]
3. Howarth, R.W. Coastal nitrogen pollution: A review of sources and trends globally and regionally. *Harmful Algae* **2008**, *8*, 14–20. [CrossRef]
4. USEPA. Regulated Drinking Water Contaminants: Inorganic Chemicals. Available online: https://www.epa.gov/ground-water-and-drinking-water/table-regulated-drinking-water-contaminants (accessed on 23 September 2017).
5. International Agency for Research on Cancer (IARC). *IARC Monographs on the Evaluation of Carcionogenic Risks to Humans: Ingested Nitrate and Nitrite and Cyanobacterial Peptide Toxins*; IARC: Lyon, France, 2010.
6. National Research Council (NRC). *The Health Effects of Nitrate, Nitrite, and N-Nitroso Compounds*; NRC: Washington, DC, USA, 1981.
7. Mirvish, S.S. Role of N-nitroso compounds (NOC) and N-nitrosation in etiology of gastric, esophageal, nasopharyngeal and bladder cancer and contribution to cancer of known exposures to NOC. *Cancer Lett.* **1995**, *93*, 17–48. [CrossRef]

8. Ward, M.H.; deKok, T.M.; Levallois, P.; Brender, J.; Gulis, G.; Nolan, B.T.; VanDerslice, J. Workgroup report: Drinking-water nitrate and health-recent findings and research needs. *Environ. Health Perspect.* **2005**, *113*, 1607–1614. [CrossRef] [PubMed]

9. Maupin, M.A.; Kenny, J.F.; Hutson, S.S.; Lovelace, J.K.; Barber, N.L.; Linsey, K.S. *Estimated Use of Water in the United States in 2010*; US Geological Survey: Reston, VA, USA, 2014; p. 56.

10. U.S. Geological Survey. USGS Water Data for the Nation. Available online: https://waterdata.usgs.gov/nwis (accessed on 1 January 2018).

11. Dubrovsky, N.M.; Burow, K.R.; Clark, G.M.; Gronberg, J.M.; Hamilton, P.A.; Hitt, K.J.; Mueller, D.K.; Munn, M.D.; Nolan, B.T.; Puckett, L.J.; et al. *The Quality of Our Nation's Waters—Nutrients in the Nation's Streams and Groundwater, 1992–2004*; U.S. Geological Survey: Reston, VA, USA, 2010; p. 174.

12. Lindsey, B.D.; Rupert, M.G. *Methods for Evaluating Temporal Groundwater Quality Data and Results of Decadal-Scale Changes in Chloride, Dissolved Solids, and Nitrate Concentrations in Groundwater in the United States, 1988–2010*; U.S. Geological Survey Scientific Investigations Report: 2012–5049; U.S. Geological Survey: Reston, VA, USA, 2012; p. 46.

13. Pennino, M.J.; Compton, J.E.; Leibowitz, S.G. Trends in Drinking Water Nitrate Violations across the United States. *Environ. Sci. Technol.* **2017**, *51*, 13450–13460. [CrossRef] [PubMed]

14. Van Grinsven, H.J.M.; Tiktak, A.; Rougoor, C.W. Evaluation of the Dutch implementation of the nitrates directive, the water framework directive and the national emission ceilings directive. *NJAS-Wagening. J. Life Sci.* **2016**, *78*, 69–84. [CrossRef]

15. Vock, D.C. Iowa Farmers Won a Water Pollution Lawsuit, But at What Cost? Available online: http://www.governing.com/topics/transportation-infrastructure/gov-des-moines-water-utility-lawsuit-farmers.html (accessed on 10 February 2018).

16. Des Moines Water Works. On Earth Day, Des Moines Water Works Reflects on Resources Spent to Manage Agrotoxins in Source Waters. Available online: http://www.dmww.com/about-us/news-releases/on-earth-day-des-moines-water-works-reflects-on-resources-spent-to-manage-agrotoxins-in-source-water.aspx (accessed on 10 February 2018).

17. European Commission. The Nitrates Directive. Available online: http://ec.europa.eu/environment/water/water-nitrates/index_en.html (accessed on 10 May 2018).

18. European Union (EU). *Council Directive 91/676/EEC of 12 December 1991 Concerning the Protection of Waters against Pollution Caused by Nitrates from Agricultural Sources*; European Union (EU): Brussels, Belgium, 1991.

19. Hansen, B.; Thorling, L.; Dalgaard, T.; Erlandsen, M. Trend Reversal of Nitrate in Danish Groundwater—A Reflection of Agricultural Practices and Nitrogen Surpluses since 1950. *Environ. Sci. Technol.* **2011**, *45*, 228–234. [CrossRef] [PubMed]

20. European Environment Agency (EEA). Groundwater Nitrate. Available online: https://www.eea.europa.eu/data-and-maps/daviz/groundwater-nitrate#tab-chart_1_filters=%7B%22rowFilters%22%3A%7B%7D%3B%22columnFilters%22%3A%7B%22pre_config_country%22%3A%5B%22Slovenia%22%5D%7D%7D (accessed on 10 February 2018).

21. Schullehner, J.; Hansen, B. Nitrate exposure from drinking water in Denmark over the last 35 years. *Environ. Res. Lett.* **2014**, *9*, 095001. [CrossRef]

22. Vitoria, I.; Maraver, F.; Sanchez-Valverde, F.; Armijo, F. Nitrate concentrations in tap water in Spain. *Gac. Sanit.* **2015**, *29*, 217–220. [CrossRef] [PubMed]

23. Espejo-Herrera, N.; Kogevinas, M.; Castano-Vinyals, G.; Aragones, N.; Boldo, E.; Ardanaz, E.; Azpiroz, L.; Ulibarrena, E.; Tardon, A.; Molina, A.J.; et al. Nitrate and trace elements in municipal and bottled water in Spain. *Gac. Sanit.* **2013**, *27*, 156–160. [CrossRef] [PubMed]

24. Gunnarsdottir, M.J.; Gardarsson, S.M.; Jonsson, G.S.; Bartram, J. Chemical quality and regulatory compliance of drinking water in Iceland. *Int. J. Hyg. Environ. Health* **2016**, *219*, 724–733. [CrossRef] [PubMed]

25. D'Alessandro, W.; Bellomo, S.; Parello, F.; Bonfanti, P.; Brusca, L.; Longo, M.; Maugeri, R. Nitrate, sulphate and chloride contents in public drinking water supplies in Sicily, Italy. *Environ. Monit. Assess.* **2012**, *184*, 2845–2855. [CrossRef] [PubMed]

26. Migeot, V.; Albouy-Llaty, M.; Carles, C.; Limousi, F.; Strezlec, S.; Dupuis, A.; Rabouan, S. Drinking-water exposure to a mixture of nitrate and low-dose atrazine metabolites and small-for-gestational age (SGA) babies: A historic cohort study. *Environ. Res.* **2013**, *122*, 58–64. [CrossRef] [PubMed]

27. Taneja, P.; Labhasetwar, P.; Nagarnaik, P.; Ensink, J.H.J. The risk of cancer as a result of elevated levels of nitrate in drinking water and vegetables in Central India. *J. Water Health* **2017**, *15*, 602–614. [CrossRef] [PubMed]

28. Suthar, S.; Bishnoi, P.; Singh, S.; Mutiyar, P.K.; Nema, A.K.; Patil, N.S. Nitrate contamination in groundwater of some rural areas of Rajasthan, India. *J. Hazard. Mater.* **2009**, *171*, 189–199. [CrossRef] [PubMed]

29. Gupta, I.; Salunkhe, A.; Rohra, N.; Kumar, R. Groundwater quality in Maharashtra, India: Focus on nitrate pollution. *J. Environ. Sci. Eng.* **2011**, *53*, 453–462. [PubMed]

30. Weinthal, E.; Vengosh, A.; Marei, A.; Kloppmann, W. The water crisis in the Gaza strip: Prospects for resolution. *Ground Water* **2005**, *43*, 653–660. [CrossRef] [PubMed]

31. Jones, R.R.; Weyer, P.J.; DellaValle, C.T.; Inoue-Choi, M.; Anderson, K.E.; Cantor, K.P.; Krasner, S.; Robien, K.; Freeman, L.E.B.; Silverman, D.T.; et al. Nitrate from drinking water and diet and bladder cancer among postmenopausal women in Iowa. *Environ. Health Perspect.* **2016**, *124*, 1751–1758. [CrossRef] [PubMed]

32. Schullehner, J.; Hansen, B.; Thygesen, M.; Pedersen, C.B.; Sigsgaard, T. Nitrate in drinking water and colorectal cancer risk: A nationwide population-based cohort study. *Int. J. Cancer* **2018**, *1*, 73–79. [CrossRef] [PubMed]

33. Espejo-Herrera, N.; Cantor, K.P.; Malats, N.; Silverman, D.T.; Tardon, A.; Garcia-Closas, R.; Serra, C.; Kogevinas, M.; Villanueva, C.M. Nitrate in drinking water and bladder cancer risk in Spain. *Environ. Res.* **2015**, *137*, 299–307. [CrossRef] [PubMed]

34. Ward, M.H.; Rusiecki, J.A.; Lynch, C.F.; Cantor, K.P. Nitrate in public water supplies and the risk of renal cell carcinoma. *Cancer Causes Control* **2007**, *18*, 1141–1151. [CrossRef] [PubMed]

35. Ward, M.H.; Cerhan, J.R.; Colt, J.S.; Hartge, P. Risk of non-Hodgkin lymphoma and nitrate and nitrite from drinking water and diet. *Epidemiology* **2006**, *17*, 375–382. [CrossRef] [PubMed]

36. Schullehner, J.; Stayner, L.; Hansen, B. Nitrate, Nitrite, and Ammonium Variability in Drinking Water Distribution Systems. *Int. J. Environ. Res. Public Health* **2017**, *14*, 276. [CrossRef] [PubMed]

37. Ward, M.H.; Kilfoy, B.A.; Weyer, P.J.; Anderson, K.E.; Folsom, A.R.; Cerhan, J.R. Nitrate intake and the risk of thyroid cancer and thyroid disease. *Epidemiology* **2010**, *21*, 389–395. [CrossRef] [PubMed]

38. Brender, J.D.; Weyer, P.J.; Romitti, P.A.; Mohanty, B.P.; Shinde, M.U.; Vuong, A.M.; Sharkey, J.R.; Dwivedi, D.; Horel, S.A.; Kantamneni, J.; et al. Prenatal nitrate intake from drinking water and selected birth defects in offspring of participants in the national birth defects prevention study. *Environ. Health Perspect.* **2013**, *121*, 1083–1089. [CrossRef] [PubMed]

39. Baris, D.; Waddell, R.; Beane Freeman, L.E.; Schwenn, M.; Colt, J.S.; Ayotte, J.D.; Ward, M.H.; Nuckols, J.; Schned, A.; Jackson, B.; et al. Elevated Bladder Cancer in Northern New England: The Role of Drinking Water and Arsenic. *J. Natl. Cancer Inst.* **2016**, *108*. [CrossRef] [PubMed]

40. Nolan, B.T.; Hitt, K.J. Vulnerability of shallow groundwater and drinking-water wells to nitrate in the United States. *Environ. Sci. Technol.* **2006**, *40*, 7834–7840. [CrossRef] [PubMed]

41. Messier, K.P.; Kane, E.; Bolich, R.; Serre, M.L. Nitrate variability in groundwater of North Carolina using monitoring and private well data models. *Environ. Sci. Technol.* **2014**, *48*, 10804–10812. [CrossRef] [PubMed]

42. Eckhardt, D.A.V.; Stackelberg, P.E. Relation of ground-water quality to land use on Long Island, New York. *Ground Water* **1995**, *33*, 1019–1033. [CrossRef]

43. Nolan, B.T.; Hitt, K.J.; Ruddy, B.C. Probability of nitrate contamination of recently recharged groundwaters in the conterminous United States. *Environ. Sci. Technol.* **2002**, *36*, 2138–2145. [CrossRef] [PubMed]

44. Rupert, M.G. *Probability of Detecting Atrazine/Desethyl-Atrazine and Elevated Concentrations of Nitrate in Ground Water in Colorado*; Water-Resources Investigations Report 02-4269; U.S. Geological Survey: Denver, CO, USA, 2003; p. 35.

45. Tesoriero, A.J.; Voss, F.D. Predicting the probability of elevated nitrate concentrations in the Puget Sound Basin: Implications for aquifer susceptibility and vulnerability. *Ground Water* **1997**, *35*, 1029–1039. [CrossRef]

46. Warner, K.L.; Arnold, T.L. *Relations that Affect the Probability and Prediction of Nitrate Concentration in Private Wells in the Glacial Aquifer System in the United States*; U.S. Geological Survey Scientific Investigations Report 2010–5100; U.S. Geological Survey: Reston, VA, USA, 2010; p. 55.

47. Elith, J.; Leathwick, J.R.; Hastie, T. A working guide to boosted regression trees. *J. Anim. Ecol.* **2008**, *77*, 802–813. [CrossRef] [PubMed]

48. Wheeler, D.C.; Nolan, B.T.; Flory, A.R.; DellaValle, C.T.; Ward, M.H. Modeling groundwater nitrate concentrations in private wells in Iowa. *Sci. Total Environ.* **2015**, *536*, 481–488. [CrossRef] [PubMed]

49. Ransom, K.M.; Nolan, B.T.; Traum, J.A.; Faunt, C.C.; Bell, A.M.; Gronberg, J.A.M.; Wheeler, D.C.; Rosecrans, C.Z.; Jurgens, B.; Schwarz, G.E.; et al. A hybrid machine learning model to predict and visualize nitrate concentration throughout the Central Valley aquifer, California, USA. *Sci. Total Environ.* **2017**, *601–602*, 1160–1172. [CrossRef] [PubMed]

50. Leach, S.A.; Thompson, M.; Hill, M. Bacterially catalyzed *N*-nitrosation reactions and their relative importance in the human stomach. *Carcinogenesis* **1987**, *8*, 1907–1912. [CrossRef] [PubMed]

51. Lv, J.; Neal, B.; Ehteshami, P.; Ninomiya, T.; Woodward, M.; Rodgers, A.; Wang, H.; MacMahon, S.; Turnbull, F.; Hillis, G.; et al. Effects of intensive blood pressure lowering on cardiovascular and renal outcomes: A systematic review and meta-analysis. *PLoS Med.* **2012**, *9*, e1001293. [CrossRef] [PubMed]

52. Spiegelhalder, B.; Eisenbrand, G.; Preussmann, R. Influence of dietary nitrate on nitrite content of human saliva: Possible relevance to in vivo formation of *N*-nitroso compounds. *Food Cosmet. Toxicol.* **1976**, *14*, 545–548. [CrossRef]

53. Tricker, A.R.; Kalble, T.; Preussmann, R. Increased urinary nitrosamine excretion in patients with urinary diversions. *Carcinogenesis* **1989**, *10*, 2379–2382. [CrossRef] [PubMed]

54. Eisenbrand, G.; Spiegelhalder, B.; Preussmann, R. Nitrate and nitrite in saliva. *Oncology* **1980**, *37*, 227–231. [CrossRef] [PubMed]

55. Eisenbrand, G. *The Significance of N-Nitrosation of Drugs*; Nicolai, H.V., Eisenbrand, G., Bozler, G., Eds.; Gustav Fischer Verlag, Stuttgart: New York, NY, USA, 1990; pp. 47–69.

56. Ceccatelli, S.; Lundberg, J.M.; Fahrenkrug, J.; Bredt, D.S.; Snyder, S.H.; Hokfelt, T. Evidence for involvement of nitric oxide in the regulation of hypothalamic portal blood flow. *Neuroscience* **1992**, *51*, 769–772. [CrossRef]

57. Moncada, S.; Palmer, R.M.J.; Higgs, E.A. Nitric oxide: Physiology, pathophysiology, and pharmacology. *Pharmacol. Rev.* **1991**, *43*, 109–142. [PubMed]

58. Rees, D.D.; Palmer, R.M.; Moncada, S. Role of endothelium-derived nitric oxide in the regulation of blood pressure. *Proc. Natl. Acad. Sci. USA* **1989**, *86*, 3375–3378. [CrossRef] [PubMed]

59. Palmer, R.M.; Ferrige, A.G.; Moncada, S. Nitric oxide release accounts for the biological activity of endothelium-derived relaxing factor. *Nature* **1987**, *327*, 524–526. [CrossRef] [PubMed]

60. Radomski, M.W.; Palmer, R.M.; Moncada, S. Endogenous nitric oxide inhibits human platelet adhesion to vascular endothelium. *Lancet* **1987**, *2*, 1057–1058. [CrossRef]

61. Radomski, M.W.; Palmer, R.M.J.; Moncada, S. The Anti-Aggregating Properties of Vascular Endothelium—Interactions between Prostacyclin and Nitric-Oxide. *Br. J. Pharmacol.* **1987**, *92*, 639–646. [CrossRef] [PubMed]

62. Larsen, F.J.; Schiffer, T.A.; Weitzberg, E.; Lundberg, J.O. Regulation of mitochondrial function and energetics by reactive nitrogen oxides. *Free Radic. Biol. Med.* **2012**, *53*, 1919–1928. [CrossRef] [PubMed]

63. Ceccatelli, S.; Hulting, A.L.; Zhang, X.; Gustafsson, L.; Villar, M.; Hokfelt, T. Nitric oxide synthase in the rat anterior pituitary gland and the role of nitric oxide in regulation of luteinizing hormone secretion. *Proc. Natl. Acad. Sci. USA* **1993**, *90*, 11292–11296. [CrossRef] [PubMed]

64. Green, S.J.; Scheller, L.F.; Marletta, M.A.; Seguin, M.C.; Klotz, F.W.; Slayter, M.; Nelson, B.J.; Nacy, C.A. Nitric oxide: Cytokine-regulation of nitric oxide in host resistance to intracellular pathogens. *Immunol. Lett.* **1994**, *43*, 87–94. [CrossRef]

65. Langrehr, J.M.; Hoffman, R.A.; Lancaster, J.R.; Simmons, R.L. Nitric oxide—A new endogenous immunomodulator. *Transplantation* **1993**, *55*, 1205–1212. [CrossRef] [PubMed]

66. Wei, X.Q.; Charles, I.G.; Smith, A.; Ure, J.; Feng, G.J.; Huang, F.P.; Xu, D.; Muller, W.; Moncada, S.; Liew, F.Y. Altered immune responses in mice lacking inducible nitric oxide synthase. *Nature* **1995**, *375*, 408–411. [CrossRef] [PubMed]

67. D'Ischia, M.; Napolitano, A.; Manini, P.; Panzella, L. Secondary Targets of Nitrite-Derived Reactive Nitrogen Species: Nitrosation/Nitration Pathways, Antioxidant Defense Mechanisms and Toxicological Implications. *Chem. Res. Toxicol.* **2011**, *24*, 2071–2092. [CrossRef] [PubMed]

68. Mirvish, S.S. Formation of N-nitroso compounds: Chemistry, kinetics, and in vivo occurrence. *Toxicol. Appl. Pharmacol.* **1975**, *31*, 325–351. [CrossRef]

69. Ridd, J.H. Nitrosation, diazotisation, and deamination. *Q. Rev.* **1961**, *15*, 418–441. [CrossRef]

70. Akuta, T.; Zaki, M.H.; Yoshitake, J.; Okamoto, T.; Akaike, T. Nitrative stress through formation of 8-nitroguanosine: Insights into microbial pathogenesis. *Nitric Oxide* **2006**, *14*, 101–108. [CrossRef] [PubMed]

71. Loeppky, R.N.; Bao, Y.T.; Bae, J.Y.; Yu, L.; Shevlin, G. Blocking nitrosamine formation—Understanding the chemistry of rapid nitrosation. In *Nitrosamines and Related N-Nitroso Compounds: Chemistry and Biochemistry*; Loeppky, R.N., Michejda, C.J., Eds.; American Chemical Society: Washington, DC, USA, 1994; Volume 553, pp. 52–65.

72. Qin, L.Z.; Liu, X.B.; Sun, Q.F.; Fan, Z.P.; Xia, D.S.; Ding, G.; Ong, H.L.; Adams, D.; Gahl, W.A.; Zheng, C.Y.; et al. Sialin (SLC17A5) functions as a nitrate transporter in the plasma membrane. *Proc. Natl. Acad. Sci. USA* **2012**, *109*, 13434–13439. [CrossRef] [PubMed]

73. Stich, H.F.; Dunn, B.P.; Pignatelli, B.; Ohshima, H.; Bartsch, H. *Dietary Phenolics and Betel Nut Extracts as Modifiers of n Nitrosation in Rat and Man*; IARC Scientific Publications: Lyon, France, 1984; pp. 213–222.

74. Vermeer, I.T.; Moonen, E.J.; Dallinga, J.W.; Kleinjans, J.C.; van Maanen, J.M. Effect of ascorbic acid and green tea on endogenous formation of N-nitrosodimethylamine and N-nitrosopiperidine in humans. *Mutat. Res.* **1999**, *428*, 353–361. [CrossRef]

75. Vermeer, I.T.; Pachen, D.M.; Dallinga, J.W.; Kleinjans, J.C.; van Maanen, J.M. Volatile N-nitrosamine formation after intake of nitrate at the ADI level in combination with an amine-rich diet. *Environ. Health Perspect.* **1998**, *106*, 459–463. [PubMed]

76. Chung, M.J.; Lee, S.H.; Sung, N.J. Inhibitory effect of whole strawberries, garlic juice or kale juice on endogenous formation of N-nitrosodimethylamine in humans. *Cancer Lett.* **2002**, *182*, 1–10. [CrossRef]

77. Helser, M.A.; Hotchkiss, J.H.; Roe, D.A. Influence of fruit and vegetable juices on the endogenous formation of N-nitrosoproline and N-nitrosothiazolidine-4-carboxylic acid in humans on controlled diets. *Carcinogenesis* **1992**, *13*, 2277–2280. [CrossRef] [PubMed]

78. Zeilmaker, M.J.; Bakker, M.I.; Schothorst, R.; Slob, W. Risk assessment of N-nitrosodimethylamine formed endogenously after fish-with-vegetable meals. *Toxicol. Sci.* **2010**, *116*, 323–335. [CrossRef] [PubMed]

79. Khandelwal, N.; Abraham, S.K. Intake of anthocyanidins pelargonidin and cyanidin reduces genotoxic stress in mice induced by diepoxybutane, urethane and endogenous nitrosation. *Environ. Toxicol. Pharmacol.* **2014**, *37*, 837–843. [CrossRef] [PubMed]

80. Conforti, F.; Menichini, F. Phenolic Compounds from Plants as Nitric Oxide Production Inhibitors. *Curr. Med. Chem.* **2011**, *18*, 1137–1145. [CrossRef] [PubMed]

81. Abraham, S.K.; Khandelwal, N. Ascorbic acid and dietary polyphenol combinations protect against genotoxic damage induced in mice by endogenous nitrosation. *Mutat. Res.* **2013**, *757*, 167–172. [CrossRef] [PubMed]

82. De Kok, T.M.; (Maastricht, The Netherlands). Unpublished work. 2018.

83. Haorah, J.; Zhou, L.; Wang, X.J.; Xu, G.P.; Mirvish, S.S. Determination of total N-nitroso compounds and their precursors in frankfurters, fresh meat, dried salted fish, sauces, tobacco, and tobacco smoke particulates. *J. Agric. Food Chem.* **2001**, *49*, 6068–6078. [CrossRef] [PubMed]

84. Cross, A.J.; Pollock, J.R.; Bingham, S.A. Haem, not protein or inorganic iron, is responsible for endogenous intestinal N-nitrosation arising from red meat. *Cancer Res.* **2003**, *63*, 2358–2360. [PubMed]

85. Bingham, S.A.; Pignatelli, B.; Pollock, J.R.A.; Ellul, A.; Malaveille, C.; Gross, G.; Runswick, S.; Cummings, J.H.; O'Neill, I.K. Does increased endogenous formation of N-nitroso compounds in the human colon explain the association between red meat and colon cancer? *Carcinogenesis* **1996**, *17*, 515–523. [CrossRef] [PubMed]

86. Bingham, S.A.; Hughes, R.; Cross, A.J. Effect of white versus red meat on endogenous N-nitrosation in the human colon and further evidence of a dose response. *J. Nutr.* **2002**, *132*, 3522s–3525s. [CrossRef] [PubMed]

87. Bingham, S.A. High-meat diets and cancer risk. *Proc. Nutr. Soc.* **1999**, *58*, 243–248. [CrossRef] [PubMed]

88. Bouvard, V.; Loomis, D.; Guyton, K.Z.; Grosse, Y.; Ghissassi, F.E.; Benbrahim-Tallaa, L.; Guha, N.; Mattock, H.; Straif, K. International Agency for Research on Cancer Monograph Working, G. Carcinogenicity of consumption of red and processed meat. *Lancet Oncol.* **2015**, *16*, 1599–1600. [CrossRef]

89. International Agency for Research on Cancer (IARC). *IARC Monographs on the Evaluation of Carcionogenic Risks to Humans: Red Meat and Processed Meat*; IARC: Lyon, France, 2018.

90. Phytochemicals to Reduce Nitrite in Meat Products (PHYTOME). Available online: www.phytome.eu (accessed on 3 May 2018).

91. Greer, F.R.; Shannon, M. American Academy of Pediatrics Committee on Nutrition and the Committee on Environmental Health. Infant methemoglobinemia: The role of dietary nitrate in food and water. *Pediatrics* **2005**, *116*, 784–786. [CrossRef] [PubMed]

92. Sanchez-Echaniz, J.; Benito-Fernandez, J.; Mintegui-Raso, S. Methemoglobinemia and consumption of vegetables in infants. *Pediatrics* **2001**, *107*, 1024–1028. [CrossRef] [PubMed]

93. Charmandari, E.; Meadows, N.; Patel, M.; Johnston, A.; Benjamin, N. Plasma nitrate concentrations in children with infectious and noninfectious diarrhea. *J. Pediatr. Gastroenterol. Nutr.* **2001**, *32*, 423–427. [CrossRef] [PubMed]

94. Comly, H.H. Landmark article 8 September 1945: Cyanosis in infants caused by nitrates in well-water. By Hunter H. Comly. *JAMA* **1987**, *257*, 2788–2792. [CrossRef] [PubMed]

95. Walton, G. Survey of literature relating to infant methemoglobinemia due to nitrate-contaminated water. *Am. J. Public Health Nation's Health* **1951**, *41*, 986–996. [CrossRef]

96. Knobeloch, L.; Salna, B.; Hogan, A.; Postle, J.; Anderson, H. Blue babies and nitrate-contaminated well water. *Environ. Health Perspect.* **2000**, *108*, 675–678. [CrossRef] [PubMed]

97. Johnson, C.J.; Bonrud, P.A.; Dosch, T.L.; Kilness, A.W.; Senger, K.A.; Busch, D.C.; Meyer, M.R. Fatal outcome of methemoglobinemia in an infant. *JAMA* **1987**, *257*, 2796–2797. [CrossRef] [PubMed]

98. Lutynski, R.; Steczek-Wojdyla, M.; Wojdyla, Z.; Kroch, S. The concentrations of nitrates and nitrites in food products and environment and the occurrence of acute toxic methemoglobinemias. *Prz. Lek.* **1996**, *53*, 351–355. [PubMed]

99. Ayebo, A.; Kross, B.C.; Vlad, M.; Sinca, A. Infant Methemoglobinemia in the Transylvania Region of Romania. *Int. J. Occup. Environ. Health* **1997**, *3*, 20–29. [CrossRef] [PubMed]

100. World Health Organization. *Water and Health in Europe*; World Health Organization: Geneva, Switzerland, 2002.

101. Abu Naser, A.A.; Ghbn, N.; Khoudary, R. Relation of nitrate contamination of groundwater with methaemoglobin level among infants in Gaza. *East Mediterr. Health J.* **2007**, *13*, 994–1004. [CrossRef] [PubMed]

102. Sadeq, M.; Moe, C.L.; Attarassi, B.; Cherkaoui, I.; ElAouad, R.; Idrissi, L. Drinking water nitrate and prevalence of methemoglobinemia among infants and children aged 1–7 years in Moroccan areas. *Int. J. Hyg. Environ. Health* **2008**, *211*, 546–554. [CrossRef] [PubMed]

103. Zeman, C.; Beltz, L.; Linda, M.; Maddux, J.; Depken, D.; Orr, J.; Theran, P. New Questions and Insights into Nitrate/Nitrite and Human Health Effects: A Retrospective Cohort Study of Private Well Users' Immunological and Wellness Status. *J. Environ. Health* **2011**, *74*, 8–18. [PubMed]

104. Manassaram, D.M.; Backer, L.C.; Messing, R.; Fleming, L.E.; Luke, B.; Monteilh, C.P. Nitrates in drinking water and methemoglobin levels in pregnancy: A longitudinal study. *Environ. Health* **2010**, *9*, 60. [CrossRef] [PubMed]

105. Grant, W.; Steele, G.; Isiorho, S.A. Spontaneous abortions possibly related to ingestion of nitrate-contaminated well water: LaGrange County, Indiana, 1991–1994. *Morb. Mortal. Wkly. Rep.* **1996**, *45*, 569–572.

106. Aschengrau, A.; Zierler, S.; Cohen, A. Quality of community drinking water and the occurrence of spontaneous abortion. *Arch Environ. Health* **1989**, *44*, 283–290. [CrossRef] [PubMed]

107. Albouy-Llaty, M.; Limousi, F.; Carles, C.; Dupuis, A.; Rabouan, S.; Migeot, V. Association between Exposure to Endocrine Disruptors in Drinking Water and Preterm Birth, Taking Neighborhood Deprivation into Account: A Historic Cohort Study. *Int. J. Environ. Res. Public Health* **2016**, *13*, 796. [CrossRef] [PubMed]

108. Stayner, L.T.; Almberg, K.; Jones, R.; Graber, J.; Pedersen, M.; Turyk, M. Atrazine and nitrate in drinking water and the risk of preterm delivery and low birth weight in four Midwestern states. *Environ. Res.* **2017**, *152*, 294–303. [CrossRef] [PubMed]

109. Joyce, S.J.; Cook, A.; Newnham, J.; Brenters, M.; Ferguson, C.; Weinstein, P. Water disinfection by-products and prelabor rupture of membranes. *Am. J. Epidemiol.* **2008**, *168*, 514–521. [CrossRef] [PubMed]

110. Mattix, K.D.; Winchester, P.D.; Scherer, L.R. Incidence of abdominal wait defects is related to surface water atrazine and nitrate levels. *J. Pediatr. Surg.* **2007**, *42*, 947–949. [CrossRef] [PubMed]

111. Waller, S.A.; Paul, K.; Peterson, S.E.; Hitti, J.E. Agricultural-related chemical exposures, season of conception, and risk of gastroschisis in Washington State. *Am. J. Obstet. Gynecol.* **2010**, *202*, e241–e246. [CrossRef] [PubMed]

112. Winchester, P.D.; Huskins, J.; Ying, J. Agrichemicals in surface water and birth defects in the United States. *Acta Paediatr.* **2009**, *98*, 664–669. [CrossRef] [PubMed]

113. Holtby, C.E.; Guernsey, J.R.; Allen, A.C.; VanLeeuwen, J.A.; Allen, V.M.; Gordon, R.J. A Population-Based Case-Control Study of Drinking-Water Nitrate and Congenital Anomalies Using Geographic Information Systems (GIS) to Develop Individual-Level Exposure Estimates. *Int. J. Environ. Res. Public Health* **2014**, *11*, 1803–1823. [CrossRef] [PubMed]

114. Weyer, P.J.; Brender, J.D.; Romitti, P.A.; Kantamneni, J.R.; Crawford, D.; Sharkey, J.R.; Shinde, M.; Horel, S.A.; Vuong, A.M.; Langlois, P.H. Assessing bottled water nitrate concentrations to evaluate total drinking water nitrate exposure and risk of birth defects. *J. Water Health* **2014**, *12*, 755–762. [CrossRef] [PubMed]

115. Yoon, P.W.; Rasmussen, S.A.; Lynberg, M.C.; Moore, C.A.; Anderka, M.; Carmichael, S.L.; Costa, P.; Druschel, C.; Hobbs, C.A.; Romitti, P.A.; et al. The National Birth Defects Prevention Study. *Public Health Rep.* **2001**, *116* (Suppl. 1), 32–40. [CrossRef] [PubMed]

116. Brender, J.D.; Kelley, K.E.; Werler, M.M.; Langlois, P.H.; Suarez, L.; Canfield, M.A. National Birth Defects Prevention Study. Prevalence and Patterns of Nitrosatable Drug Use among U.S. Women during Early Pregnancy. *Birth Defects Res. A* **2011**, *91*, 258–264. [CrossRef] [PubMed]

117. Griesenbeck, J.S.; Brender, J.D.; Sharkey, J.R.; Steck, M.D.; Huber, J.C., Jr.; Rene, A.A.; McDonald, T.J.; Romitti, P.A.; Canfield, M.A.; Langlois, P.H.; et al. Maternal characteristics associated with the dietary intake of nitrates, nitrites, and nitrosamines in women of child-bearing age: A cross-sectional study. *Environ. Health* **2010**, *9*, 10. [CrossRef] [PubMed]

118. Brender, J.D.; Werler, M.M.; Shinde, M.U.; Vuong, A.M.; Kelley, K.E.; Huber, J.C., Jr.; Sharkey, J.R.; Griesenbeck, J.S.; Romitti, P.A.; Malik, S.; et al. Nitrosatable drug exposure during the first trimester of pregnancy and selected congenital malformations. *Birth Defects Res. A* **2012**, *94*, 701–713. [CrossRef] [PubMed]

119. Brender, J.D.; Werler, M.M.; Kelley, K.E.; Vuong, A.M.; Shinde, M.U.; Zheng, Q.; Huber, J.C., Jr.; Sharkey, J.R.; Griesenbeck, J.S.; Romitti, P.A.; et al. Nitrosatable drug exposure during early pregnancy and neural tube defects in offspring: National Birth Defects Prevention Study. *Am. J. Epidemiol.* **2011**, *174*, 1286–1295. [CrossRef] [PubMed]

120. Brender, J.D.; Olive, J.M.; Felkner, M.; Suarez, L.; Marckwardt, W.; Hendricks, K.A. Dietary nitrites and nitrates, nitrosatable drugs, and neural tube defects. *Epidemiology* **2004**, *15*, 330–336. [CrossRef] [PubMed]

121. Dorsch, M.M.; Scragg, R.K.; McMichael, A.J.; Baghurst, P.A.; Dyer, K.F. Congenital malformations and maternal drinking water supply in rural South Australia: A case-control study. *Am. J. Epidemiol.* **1984**, *119*, 473–486. [CrossRef] [PubMed]

122. Croen, L.A.; Todoroff, K.; Shaw, G.M. Maternal exposure to nitrate from drinking water and diet and risk for neural tube defects. *Am. J. Epidemiol.* **2001**, *153*, 325–331. [CrossRef] [PubMed]

123. Arbuckle, T.E.; Sherman, G.J.; Corey, P.N.; Walters, D.; Lo, B. Water nitrates and CNS birth defects: A population-based case-control study. *Arch Environ. Health* **1988**, *43*, 162–167. [CrossRef] [PubMed]

124. Ericson, A.; Kallen, B.; Lofkvist, E. Environmental factors in the etiology of neural tube defects: A negative study. *Environ. Res.* **1988**, *45*, 38–47. [CrossRef]

125. Cantor, K.P. Drinking water and cancer. *Cancer Causes Control* **1997**, *8*, 292–308. [CrossRef] [PubMed]

126. Quist, A.J.L.; Inoue-Choi, M.; Weyer, P.J.; Anderson, K.E.; Cantor, K.P.; Krasner, S.; Freeman, L.E.B.; Ward, M.H.; Jones, R.R. Ingested nitrate and nitrite, disinfection by-products, and pancreatic cancer risk in postmenopausal women. *Int. J. Cancer* **2018**, *142*, 251–261. [CrossRef] [PubMed]

127. Jones, R.R.; Weyer, P.J.; DellaValle, C.T.; Robien, K.; Cantor, K.P.; Krasner, S.; Freeman, L.E.B.; Ward, M.H. Ingested nitrate, disinfection by-products, and kidney cancer risk in older women. *Epidemiology* **2017**, *28*, 703–711. [CrossRef] [PubMed]

128. Inoue-Choi, M.; Ward, M.H.; Cerhan, J.R.; Weyer, P.J.; Anderson, K.E.; Robien, K. Interaction of nitrate and folate on the risk of breast cancer among postmenopausal women. *Nutr. Cancer* **2012**, *64*, 685–694. [CrossRef] [PubMed]

129. Inoue-Choi, M.; Jones, R.R.; Anderson, K.E.; Cantor, K.P.; Cerhan, J.R.; Krasner, S.; Robien, K.; Weyer, P.J.; Ward, M.H. Nitrate and nitrite ingestion and risk of ovarian cancer among postmenopausal women in Iowa. *Int. J. Cancer* **2015**, *137*, 173–182. [CrossRef] [PubMed]

130. Weyer, P.J.; Cerhan, J.R.; Kross, B.C.; Hallberg, G.R.; Kantamneni, J.; Breuer, G.; Jones, M.P.; Zheng, W.; Lynch, C.F. Municipal drinking water nitrate level and cancer risk in older women: The Iowa Women's Health Study. *Epidemiology* **2001**, *12*, 327–338. [CrossRef] [PubMed]

131. Zeegers, M.P.; Selen, R.F.; Kleinjans, J.C.; Goldbohm, R.A.; van den Brandt, P.A. Nitrate intake does not influence bladder cancer risk: The Netherlands cohort study. *Environ. Health Perspect.* **2006**, *114*, 1527–1531. [CrossRef] [PubMed]

132. Ward, M.H.; Mark, S.D.; Cantor, K.P.; Weisenburger, D.D.; Correa-Villasenor, A.; Zahm, S.H. Drinking water nitrate and the risk of non-Hodgkin's lymphoma. *Epidemiology* **1996**, *7*, 465–471. [CrossRef] [PubMed]

133. Ward, M.H.; Heineman, E.F.; Markin, R.S.; Weisenburger, D.D. Adenocarcinoma of the stomach and esophagus and drinking water and dietary sources of nitrate and nitrite. *Int. J. Occup. Environ. Health* **2008**, *14*, 193–197. [CrossRef] [PubMed]

134. McElroy, J.A.; Trentham-Dietz, A.; Gangnon, R.E.; Hampton, J.M.; Bersch, A.J.; Kanarek, M.S.; Newcomb, P.A. Nitrogen-nitrate exposure from drinking water and colorectal cancer risk for rural women in Wisconsin, USA. *J. Water Health* **2008**, *6*, 399–409. [CrossRef] [PubMed]

135. Espejo-Herrera, N.; Gracia-Lavedan, E.; Boldo, E.; Aragones, N.; Perez-Gomez, B.; Pollan, M.; Molina, A.J.; Fernandez, T.; Martin, V.; La Vecchia, C.; et al. Colorectal cancer risk and nitrate exposure through drinking water and diet. *Int. J. Cancer* **2016**, *139*, 334–346. [CrossRef] [PubMed]

136. Fathmawati; Fachiroh, J.; Gravitiani, E.; Sarto; Husodo, A.H. Nitrate in drinking water and risk of colorectal cancer in Yogyakarta, Indonesia. *J. Toxicol. Environ. Health Part A* **2017**, *80*, 120–128. [CrossRef] [PubMed]

137. Brody, J.G.; Aschengrau, A.; McKelvey, W.; Swartz, C.H.; Kennedy, T.; Rudel, R.A. Breast cancer risk and drinking water contaminated by wastewater: A case control study. *Environ. Health-Glob.* **2006**, *5*, 28. [CrossRef] [PubMed]

138. Espejo-Herrera, N.; Gracia-Lavedan, E.; Pollan, M.; Aragones, N.; Boldo, E.; Perez-Gomez, B.; Altzibar, J.M.; Amiano, P.; Zabala, A.J.; Ardanaz, E.; et al. Ingested Nitrate and Breast Cancer in the Spanish Multicase-Control Study on Cancer (MCC-Spain). *Environ. Health Perspect.* **2016**, *124*, 1042–1049. [CrossRef] [PubMed]

139. Mueller, B.A.; Nielsen, S.S.; Preston-Martin, S.; Holly, E.A.; Cordier, S.; Filippini, G.; Peris-Bonet, R.; Choi, N.W. Household water source and the risk of childhood brain tumours: Results of the SEARCH International Brain Tumor Study. *Int. J. Epidemiol.* **2004**, *33*, 1209–1216. [CrossRef] [PubMed]

140. Mueller, B.A.; Newton, K.; Holly, E.A.; Preston-Martin, S. Residential water source and the risk of childhood brain tumors. *Environ. Health Perspect.* **2001**, *109*, 551–556. [CrossRef] [PubMed]

141. De Groef, B.; Decallonne, B.R.; Van der Geyten, S.; Darras, V.M.; Bouillon, R. Perchlorate versus other environmental sodium/iodide symporter inhibitors: Potential thyroid-related health effects. *Eur. J. Endocrinol.* **2006**, *155*, 17–25. [CrossRef] [PubMed]

142. Van Maanen, J.M.; Welle, I.J.; Hageman, G.; Dallinga, J.W.; Mertens, P.L.; Kleinjans, J.C. Nitrate contamination of drinking water: Relationship with HPRT variant frequency in lymphocyte DNA and urinary excretion of N-nitrosamines. *Environ. Health Perspect.* **1996**, *104*, 522–528. [CrossRef] [PubMed]

143. Radikova, Z.; Tajtakova, M.; Kocan, A.; Trnovec, T.; Sebokova, E.; Klimes, I.; Langer, P. Possible effects of environmental nitrates and toxic organochlorines on human thyroid in highly polluted areas in Slovakia. *Thyroid Off. J. Am. Thyroid Assoc.* **2008**, *18*, 353–362. [CrossRef] [PubMed]

144. Tajtakova, M.; Semanova, Z.; Tomkova, Z.; Szokeova, E.; Majoros, J.; Radikova, Z.; Sebokova, E.; Klimes, I.; Langer, P. Increased thyroid volume and frequency of thyroid disorders signs in schoolchildren from nitrate polluted area. *Chemosphere* **2006**, *62*, 559–564. [CrossRef] [PubMed]

145. Aschebrook-Kilfoy, B.; Heltshe, S.L.; Nuckols, J.R.; Sabra, M.M.; Shuldiner, A.R.; Mitchell, B.D.; Airola, M.; Holford, T.R.; Zhang, Y.; Ward, M.H. Modeled nitrate levels in well water supplies and prevalence of abnormal thyroid conditions among the Old Order Amish in Pennsylvania. *Environ. Health* **2012**, *11*, 6. [CrossRef] [PubMed]

146. Longnecker, M.P.; Daniels, J.L. Environmental contaminants as etiologic factors for diabetes. *Environ. Health Perspect.* **2001**, *109* (Suppl. 6), 871–876. [CrossRef] [PubMed]

147. Moltchanova, E.; Rytkonen, M.; Kousa, A.; Taskinen, O.; Tuomilehto, J.; Karvonen, M.; Spat Study, G. Finnish Childhood Diabetes Registry, G. Zinc and nitrate in the ground water and the incidence of Type 1 diabetes in Finland. *Diabet. Med.* **2004**, *21*, 256–261. [CrossRef] [PubMed]

148. Muntoni, S.; Cocco, P.; Muntoni, S.; Aru, G. Nitrate in community water supplies and risk of childhood type 1 diabetes in Sardinia, Italy. *Eur. J. Epidemiol.* **2006**, *21*, 245–247. [CrossRef] [PubMed]

149. Benson, V.S.; Vanleeuwen, J.A.; Taylor, J.; Somers, G.S.; McKinney, P.A.; Van Til, L. Type 1 diabetes mellitus and components in drinking water and diet: A population-based, case-control study in Prince Edward Island, Canada. *J. Am. Coll. Nutr.* **2010**, *29*, 612–624. [CrossRef] [PubMed]

150. Winkler, C.; Mollenhauer, U.; Hummel, S.; Bonifacio, E.; Ziegler, A.G. Exposure to environmental factors in drinking water: Risk of islet autoimmunity and type 1 diabetes—The BABYDIAB study. *Horm. Metab. Res.* **2008**, *40*, 566–571. [CrossRef] [PubMed]

151. Klein, B.E.K.; McElroy, J.A.; Klein, R.; Howard, K.P.; Lee, K.E. Nitrate-nitrogen levels in rural drinking water: Is there an association with age-related macular degeneration? *J. Environ. Sci. Health Part A* **2013**, *48*, 1757–1763. [CrossRef] [PubMed]
152. Ahluwalia, A.; Gladwin, M.; Coleman, G.D.; Hord, N.; Howard, G.; Kim-Shapiro, D.B.; Lajous, M.; Larsen, F.J.; Lefer, D.J.; McClure, L.A.; et al. Dietary Nitrate and the Epidemiology of Cardiovascular Disease: Report From a National Heart, Lung, and Blood Institute Workshop. *J. Am. Heart Assoc.* **2016**, *5*, e003402. [CrossRef] [PubMed]
153. Kapil, V.; Khambata, R.S.; Robertson, A.; Caulfield, M.J.; Ahluwalia, A. Dietary nitrate provides sustained blood pressure lowering in hypertensive patients: A randomized, phase 2, double-blind, placebo-controlled study. *Hypertension* **2015**, *65*, 320–327. [CrossRef] [PubMed]
154. Omar, S.A.; Webb, A.J.; Lundberg, J.O.; Weitzberg, E. Therapeutic effects of inorganic nitrate and nitrite in cardiovascular and metabolic diseases. *J. Intern. Med.* **2016**, *279*, 315–336. [CrossRef] [PubMed]
155. Presley, T.D.; Morgan, A.R.; Bechtold, E.; Clodfelter, W.; Dove, R.W.; Jennings, J.M.; Kraft, R.A.; King, S.B.; Laurienti, P.J.; Rejeski, W.J.; et al. Acute effect of a high nitrate diet on brain perfusion in older adults. *Nitric Oxide* **2011**, *24*, 34–42. [CrossRef] [PubMed]
156. Maas, R.; Schwedhelm, E.; Kahl, L.; Li, H.; Benndorf, R.; Luneburg, N.; Forstermann, U.; Boger, R.H. Simultaneous assessment of endothelial function, nitric oxide synthase activity, nitric oxide-mediated signaling, and oxidative stress in individuals with and without hypercholesterolemia. *Clin. Chem.* **2008**, *54*, 292–300. [CrossRef] [PubMed]
157. Jadert, C.; Phillipson, M.; Holm, L.; Lundberg, J.O.; Borniquel, S. Preventive and therapeutic effects of nitrite supplementation in experimental inflammatory bowel disease. *Redox Biol.* **2014**, *2*, 73–81. [CrossRef] [PubMed]
158. Khademikia, S.; Rafiee, Z.; Amin, M.M.; Poursafa, P.; Mansourian, M.; Modaberi, A. Association of nitrate, nitrite, and total organic carbon (TOC) in drinking water and gastrointestinal disease. *J. Environ. Public Health* **2013**, *2013*, 603468. [CrossRef] [PubMed]
159. De Roos, A.J.; Ward, M.H.; Lynch, C.F.; Cantor, K.P. Nitrate in public water supplies and the risk of colon and rectum cancers. *Epidemiology* **2003**, *14*, 640–649. [CrossRef] [PubMed]
160. Gatseva, P.D.; Argirova, M.D. High-nitrate levels in drinking water may be a risk factor for thyroid dysfunction in children and pregnant women living in rural Bulgarian areas. *Int. J. Hyg. Environ. Health* **2008**, *211*, 555–559. [CrossRef] [PubMed]
161. Toccalino, P.L.; Norman, J.E.; Scott, J.C. Chemical mixtures in untreated water from public-supply wells in the U.S.—Occurrence, composition, and potential toxicity. *Sci. Total Environ.* **2012**, *431*, 262–270. [CrossRef] [PubMed]
162. Joshi, N.; Rhoades, M.G.; Bennett, G.D.; Wells, S.M.; Mirvish, S.S.; Breitbach, M.J.; Shea, P.J. Developmental abnormalities in chicken embryos exposed to *N*-nitrosoatrazine. *J. Toxicol. Environ. Health Part A* **2013**, *76*, 1015–1022. [CrossRef] [PubMed]
163. Mitch, W.A.; Sharp, J.O.; Rhoades Trussell, R.; Valentine, R.L.; Alvarez-Cohen, L.; DSedlak, D.L. *N*-Nitrosodimethylamine (NDMA) as a Drinking Water Contaminant: A Review. *Environ. Eng. Sci.* **2003**, *20*, 389–404. [CrossRef]
164. Krasner, S.W. The formation and control of emerging disinfection by-products of health concern. *Philos. Trans.* **2009**, *367*, 4077–4095. [CrossRef] [PubMed]
165. Hezel, M.P.; Weitzberg, E. The oral microbiome and nitric oxide homoeostasis. *Oral Dis.* **2015**, *21*, 7–16. [CrossRef] [PubMed]
166. Hyde, E.R.; Andrade, F.; Vaksman, Z.; Parthasarathy, K.; Jiang, H.; Parthasarathy, D.K.; Torregrossa, A.C.; Tribble, G.; Kaplan, H.B.; Petrosino, J.F.; et al. Metagenomic analysis of nitrate-reducing bacteria in the oral cavity: Implications for nitric oxide homeostasis. *PLoS ONE* **2014**, *9*, e88645. [CrossRef] [PubMed]
167. Burleigh, M.C.; Liddle, L.; Monaghan, C.; Muggeridge, D.J.; Sculthorpe, N.; Butcher, J.P.; Henriquez, F.L.; Allen, J.D.; Easton, C. Salivary nitrite production is elevated in individuals with a higher abundance of oral nitrate-reducing bacteria. *Free Radic. Biol. Med.* **2018**, *120*, 80–88. [CrossRef] [PubMed]
168. Vogtmann, E.; Chen, J.; Amir, A.; Shi, J.; Abnet, C.C.; Nelson, H.; Knight, R.; Chia, N.; Sinha, R. Comparison of Collection Methods for Fecal Samples in Microbiome Studies. *Am. J. Epidemiol.* **2017**, *185*, 115–123. [CrossRef] [PubMed]

169. Sinha, R.; Abu-Ali, G.; Vogtmann, E.; Fodor, A.A.; Ren, B.; Amir, A.; Schwager, E.; Crabtree, J.; Ma, S.; The Microbiome Quality Control Project Consortium; et al. Assessment of variation in microbial community amplicon sequencing by the Microbiome Quality Control (MBQC) project consortium. *Nat. Biotechnol.* **2017**, *35*, 1077–1086. [PubMed]

170. Hebels, D.G.; Jennen, D.G.; van Herwijnen, M.H.; Moonen, E.J.; Pedersen, M.; Knudsen, L.E.; Kleinjans, J.C.; de Kok, T.M. Whole-genome gene expression modifications associated with nitrosamine exposure and micronucleus frequency in human blood cells. *Mutagenesis* **2011**, *26*, 753–761. [CrossRef] [PubMed]

171. Hebels, D.G.; Jennen, D.G.; Kleinjans, J.C.; de Kok, T.M. Molecular signatures of N-nitroso compounds in Caco-2 cells: Implications for colon carcinogenesis. *Toxicol. Sci.* **2009**, *108*, 290–300. [CrossRef] [PubMed]

172. Vineis, P.; Chadeau-Hyam, M.; Gmuender, H.; Gulliver, J.; Herceg, Z.; Kleinjans, J.; Kogevinas, M.; Kyrtopoulos, S.; Nieuwenhuijsen, M.; Phillips, D.H.; et al. The exposome in practice: Design of the EXPOsOMICS project. *Int. J. Hyg. Environ. Health* **2017**, *220*, 142–151. [CrossRef] [PubMed]

173. Hebels, D.G.; Georgiadis, P.; Keun, H.C.; Athersuch, T.J.; Vineis, P.; Vermeulen, R.; Portengen, L.; Bergdahl, I.A.; Hallmans, G.; Palli, D.; et al. Performance in omics analyses of blood samples in long-term storage: Opportunities for the exploitation of existing biobanks in environmental health research. *Environ. Health Perspect.* **2013**, *121*, 480–487. [CrossRef] [PubMed]

174. International Nitrogen Initiative. Available online: http://www.initrogen.org/ (accessed on 22 April 2018).

175. Dinnes, D.L.; Karlen, D.L.; Jaynes, D.B.; Kaspar, T.C.; Hatfield, J.L.; Colvin, T.S.; Cambardella, C.A. Nitrogen management strategies to reduce nitrate leaching in tile-drained midwestern soils. *Agron. J.* **2002**, *94*, 153–171. [CrossRef]

176. Baron, J.S.; Hall, E.K.; Nolan, B.T.; Finlay, J.C.; Bernhardt, E.S.; Harrison, J.A.; Chan, F.; Boyer, E.W. The interactive effects of excess reactive nitrogen and climate change on aquatic ecosystems and water resources of the United States. *Biogeochemistry* **2013**, *114*, 71–92. [CrossRef]

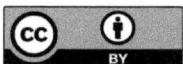

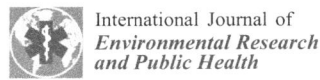

Article

Heterogeneity in the Relationship between Disinfection By-Products in Drinking Water and Cancer: A Systematic Review

Tarik Benmarhnia [1,*,†], Ianis Delpla [2,†], Lara Schwarz [1], Manuel J. Rodriguez [2] and Patrick Levallois [3,4]

1   Department of Family Medicine and Public Health & Scripps Institution of Oceanography, University of California, San Diego, CA 92093, USA; lnschwar@ucsd.edu
2   École Supérieure D'aménagement du Territoire et de Développement Régional (ESAD), Université Laval, 1624 Pavillon Savard, Québec, QC G1K-7P4, Canada; Ianis.Delpla@crad.ulaval.ca (I.D.); Manuel.Rodriguez@esad.ulaval.ca (M.J.R.)
3   Direction de la Santé Environnementale et de la Toxicologie, Institut National de Santé Publique du Québec, Québec, QC G1V 5B3, Canada; Patrick.Levallois@msp.ulaval.ca
4   Axe Santé des Populations et Pratiques Optimales en Santé, Centre de Recherche du Centre Hospitalier Universitaire (CHU) de Québec, Québec, QC G1V 2M2, Canada
*   Correspondence: tbenmarhnia@ucsd.edu
†   These authors contributed equally to this work.

Received: 28 February 2018; Accepted: 9 May 2018; Published: 14 May 2018

Abstract: The epidemiological evidence demonstrating the effect of disinfection by-products (DBPs) from drinking water on colon and rectal cancers is well documented. However, no systematic assessment has been conducted to assess the potential effect measure modification (EMM) in the relationship between DBPs and cancer. The objective of this paper is to conduct a systematic literature review to determine the extent to which EMM has been assessed in the relationship between DBPs in drinking water in past epidemiological studies. Selected articles ($n = 19$) were reviewed, and effect estimates and covariates that could have been used in an EMM assessment were gathered. Approximately half of the studies assess EMM ($n = 10$), but the majority of studies only estimate it relative to sex subgroups ($n = 6$ for bladder cancer and $n = 2$ both for rectal and colon cancers). Although EMM is rarely assessed, several variables that could have a potential modification effect are routinely collected in these studies, such as socioeconomic status or age. The role of environmental exposures through drinking water can play an important role and contribute to cancer disparities. We encourage a systematic use of subgroup analysis to understand which populations or territories are more vulnerable to the health impacts of DBPs.

Keywords: THMs; cancer; effect measure modification; drinking water

1. Introduction

Disinfection is widely used for drinking water treatment to inactivate pathogens and to prevent waterborne diseases. This process can produce disinfection by-products (DBPs), which result from a chemical reaction between disinfectants such as chlorine and organic or inorganic matter in the water [1]. Among the various DBPs (>600) [2], trihalomethanes (THMs) are the most studied due to their relatively high prevalence and concentration in drinking water.

Numerous studies assess the association between exposure to chlorinated water and diverse health outcomes. Some of them investigate the influence of chlorinated water or THMs on reproductive health, such as small for gestational age [3,4], stillbirth, and low birth rate [3,5]. However, the majority of epidemiological studies investigate the impact of such water quality exposure on cancer outcomes.

Epidemiological studies have shown that DBP exposure through drinking water is associated particularly with some types of cancer, namely, colon, rectal, and bladder [2,6–8], though contrasting results for colon and rectal cancers have been found [6]. Reviews revealing a consistent association between long-term exposure to THMs and risk of bladder cancer have been published in recent years [8–10]. Additionally, several epidemiological studies found other risk factors for colon, rectal, and bladder cancer, such as tobacco consumption [11–15], and dietary and genetic factors [13,16–21]. Other potential risk factors include urban residence [13,22] and alcohol consumption [13,16]. The duration of exposure is also associated with an increasing risk of bladder cancer [7].

In a pooled analysis published in 2004, it was observed that the effect of THMs on bladder cancer risk was more pronounced in men than women [23]. Several explanations were discussed, including residual confounding and biological plausibility such as sex differences in metabolizing DBPs. A proposed mechanism to explain this difference is the role of sex hormones in the modulation of enzymes that metabolize chlorination by-products (for chloroform and brominated THMs) into reactive metabolites. Other possible explanations are anatomic differences or variation in voiding frequency between men and women, which can influence the action of DBPs as hormone disruptors [23].

To our knowledge, besides the study described above, no systematic review has attempted to synthesize the literature that directly evaluates potential effect measure modifiers other than sex in the association between disinfection by-products in drinking water and cancer. Yet, several other potential effect measure modifiers such as socio-economic status could be particularly relevant to shaping policies that target vulnerable populations or territories and aim to reduce inequalities in cancer risks. This could help frame interventions to target specific subgroups and ensure exposure of DBPs, such as THMs and HAAs, are below harmful levels. Such assessments for populations that are unfairly treated in regard to their environmental exposures are relevant to the field of environmental justice, which has drawn recent attention with important concerns about other water contaminants such as with lead exposure in the Flint crisis [24]. In addition, these assessments can identify which populations and territories are more vulnerable to the harmful effects of exposure to THMs and inform interventions to reduce health disparities.

The literature in relation to environmental health inequalities emerged during these last two decades and distinguishes two types of environmental inequalities: (i) inequalities related to the level of exposure and (ii) inequalities related to the level of vulnerability (when the effect of an environmental exposure is modified according to different sub-groups strata of the population) [25–28].

Findings from studies investigating differential exposure have shown that deprived populations can be more exposed to contaminants in drinking water [5,24,29–35]. Among the few studies dedicated to the analysis of environmental inequalities associated with DBPs, all focus on inequalities related to the level of exposure, and show contrasting results. Briggs et al. [36] found a positive association between levels of THMs in drinking water and an index of multiple deprivation. Inversely, Delpla et al. [32] showed that municipalities with a lower material deprivation index have a lower risk of elevated THMs levels at their tap. Evans et al. [33] and Vrijheid et al. [35] found no significant relationships between individuals or community deprivation and THM concentrations in drinking water. The absence of an association could be linked to one or more of the following: geographical size of a study that could attenuate the associations when extending the studied area [36], lower participation among people of lower education, type of exposure studied, location of both the early-life and current residence of the person, and/or type of socio-economic indicator chosen [35].

This review focuses on differential vulnerability, which refers to the notion of "effect measure modification" in epidemiology. This concept of vulnerability can be defined as a "greater likelihood of an adverse outcome given a specific exposure, compared with the general population, including both host (individual) and environmental (contextual) factors" [37]. We will focus this review on socioeconomic status (SES) variables, but we will also consider potential vulnerability factors as sex/gender and health behaviors.

Differences in health opportunities and resources related to social class, race, and geographic area can lead to a lower health status for vulnerable groups [38]. For example, it has been shown in the last decade that that neighborhood SES can modify the effect of air pollutants [38,39] on mortality. Such evidence has been used to provide recommendations towards interventions aimed at specific low SES areas to reduce inequalities in mortality [40]. Understanding the effect measure modification (EMM) in the health impacts of DBPs will be useful in shaping policies to reduce cancer inequalities through proportionated interventions aimed at reducing exposure to DBPs. Yet, some drinking water distribution systems may span large geographic areas and serve large and diverse populations, so interventions on the distribution systems may be insufficient. In such a case, targeted local interventions in the infrastructure or through awareness campaigns may be relevant.

The overall objectives of this paper are to synthetize the literature studying the role of EMM in the relationship between DBPs in drinking water and cancer, and understand the extent to which it has been assessed in past epidemiological studies. If this epidemiological information is available in existing publications, this review will allow us to report the epidemiological evidence on the differential vulnerability of DBPs to cancer risk. If epidemiological information is lacking on this topic, the review will serve to highlight the knowledge gap and motivate future studies in this area. Two successive stages are performed: (i) An updated systematic review is conducted on studies measuring the association between DBPs in drinking water and colorectal and bladder cancers and (ii) The presence of EMM is evaluated according to socio-demographic characteristics and individual behaviors considered in the identified studies.

2. Materials and Methods

2.1. Search Strategy

We aim to identify all epidemiological studies investigating the effects of DBPs in drinking water on colorectal and bladder cancers published in English in scientific journals between January 1975 and August 2015. The strategy used to conduct this review, in accordance with the PRISMA guidelines [41], consisted of grouping keywords that represented (i) the exposure (namely DBPs in drinking water) and (ii) the health outcomes (namely, colon and rectal cancer (CRC) and bladder cancer). Keywords, titles, and abstracts were searched in PubMed and Elsevier Embase on the Ovid SP portal and Web of Science. There was no restriction on geographical location.

The keywords used for the literature search are as follows: (Disinfection by-products OR Disinfection-by-products OR water disinfection OR chlorination by-products OR water chlorination OR trichloromethane OR chloroform OR bromoform OR tribromomethane OR dichlorobromomethane OR dibromochloromethane OR THM OR Haloacetic acids) AND (colorectal cancer OR colorectal neoplasm OR colon cancer OR rectal cancer OR bladder cancer OR CRC).

Terms describing EMM were not included at this stage to avoid being too restrictive. Instead, we appraised the EMM assessment during the data extraction process (see below). We did not include keywords related to study design at this stage, but instead assessed this question while selecting studies (see below).

2.2. Selection of Studies

In the first stage, the first two authors of this paper read and screened the abstract of each returned article.

Papers meeting the following criteria were excluded from our review:

- Commentaries, editorials, review articles, or meta-analysis
- Studies not performed on human populations
- Studies not published in English
- Studies not including DBPs in drinking water or chlorinated water as the exposure

- Qualitative studies

When reviewers disagreed about whether a study should be excluded, the two met in person to discuss until an agreement was reached.

In a second stage, papers selected in the previous stage were fully screened and then excluded according to the following criteria:

- Studies not reporting a quantitative estimate between DBPs in drinking water or chlorinated waters and colorectal cancer or bladder cancer
- Studies not including colorectal cancer and/or bladder cancer as health outcomes
- Studies using an ecological design or only a spatial analysis

In addition, the reference section of studies identified was searched, and relevant references that were not initially identified were added.

2.3. Data Extraction

Selected articles were reviewed separately by the first two researchers, and each documented the first author, location, date of publication, sample size, study design (case-control, cohort study or case-cohort), exposure measurement, health outcomes assessed, effect size and CI (Confidence Interval), whether they included EMM assessment, and which subgroup was included in this assessment.

Finally, among studies that did not include an assessment of EMM, collected variables (i.e., those presented in the sample description used as confounders) that could potentially be used for an EMM assessment were reported. We included variables for which there is some evidence of EMM in other environmental determinants of population health and with documented mechanisms leading to a differential effect. We thus included the following variables: age [42–45], socio-economic factors [39,46], urbanization level [47,48], smoking status, and other health behaviors (alcohol consumption, diet, and physical activity) [49,50]. Sex was also included in the review. Socio-economic factors include SES variables such as education and occupation, as well as indexes that were used in the studies selected.

3. Results

3.1. Description of Studies Selected

The abstracts of 226 articles were assessed, and 26 articles were retained for in-depth review after applying the first stage of exclusion criteria. Nine articles were added after screening the references of selected papers. Finally, 19 scientific articles were retained following the second stage exclusion criteria (Figure 1).

Table 1 summarizes the studies that provide a measure of the cancer risk associated with exposure to disinfection by-products through drinking water.

Eleven studies were conducted in North America, six in Europe, and two in Asia (Taiwan). The studies were published between 1981 and 2010. The majority of studies focus on bladder cancer ($n = 14$), followed by colon cancer ($n = 4$) and rectal cancer ($n = 5$). All are case-control studies, with the exception of Wilkins and Comsock, [51] and Koivusalo et al., [52] which are cohort studies. The majority of studies use values of THMs issued from field measurements ($n = 10$) or modeling ($n = 3$) to assess the exposure. The remaining ones use presence or absence of chlorinated water ($n = 4$) or the level of mutagenicity of waters ($n = 2$) as a marker of exposure to DBPs. THMs cut-offs varied between studies, because the exposure was calculated differently. Studies use long term (>30 years), fixed [53,54], or variable duration of exposure [55,56], although the majority use fixed levels (but different values) of DBPs [57–62]. The association between exposure and health issues is almost always assessed using logistic regression, with Odds Ratios (OR) or Risks Ratios (RR) being reported.

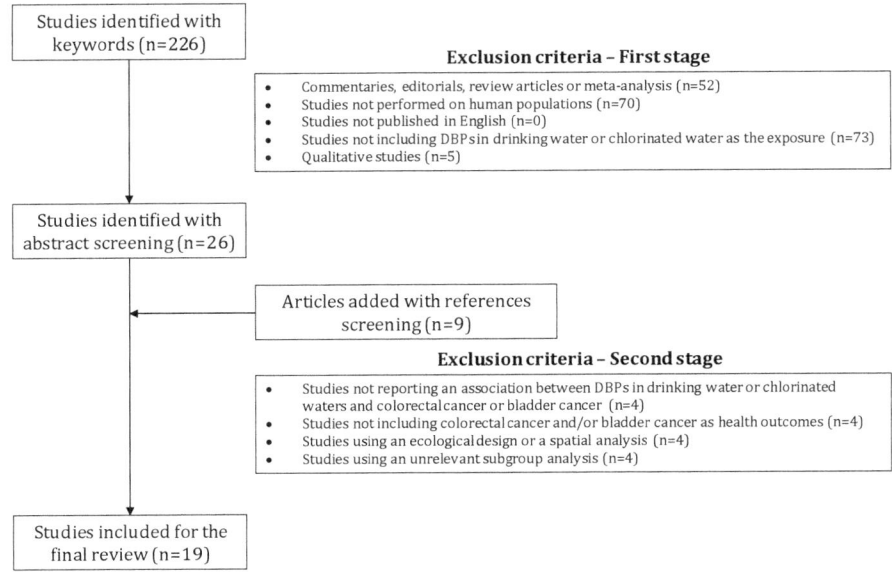

Figure 1. Flowchart of the selection of studies.

Odds Ratios in the studies selected are between 1.20 and 2.99 for bladder cancer, 0.90 and 1.66 for colon cancer, and 1.01 and 1.68 for rectal cancer (for OR calculated on the whole population under study). Fourteen studies found a significant relationship with cancer [52,53,55,57–60,62–68]. Five studies did not find a significant relationship between exposure to chlorinated water/DBPs and cancer, four of which studied bladder cancer [51,54,56,61] and one which studied colon cancer [69]. The majority of studies considered the exposure to THMs as a group of compounds without assessing the effects of the different compounds. Only the studies of Bove et al. [59,63] considered different species of THMs (chloroform, bromoform, bromodichloromethane, and chlorodibromomethane) in their analysis.

Approximately half of the studies assess EMM ($n = 10$), but the majority of them estimate it relative to different sex subgroups (total: $n = 8$, $n = 6$ for bladder cancer and $n = 2$ both for rectal and colon cancers). Generally, higher ORs and relationships that are more significant were noted for men when studying bladder and colon cancers. For example, in the study of Cantor et al. [64], an OR of 1.8 for men compared to an OR of 0.6 for women was found for bladder cancer. For rectal cancer, the results are contradictory, but the number of studies is too limited ($n = 2$) to draw any conclusion relative to sex. For women, only one study, which is also a cohort study [52], noted positive relationships for bladder and rectal cancer. Moreover, the study of Koivusalo et al. [52] is the only one that found higher risks for women than men (for the three different types of cancer). The duration of exposure was associated with an increase in bladder cancer risk for men only [7,64]. Fewer studies assessed the EMM relative to smoking status ($n = 3$). Finally, one study assessed EMM considering gene polymorphisms [62]. Generally, in all studies, the EMM assessment was conducted with stratified analyses. In the study of King et al. [57], an interaction term between exposure and sex was calculated.

Table 1. Description of studies included in the review.

(a) Bladder cancer.

Studies	Location	Year of Publication	Sample Size	Study Design	Disinfection by-Products Measurement	Subgroups Included in the Analysis	Effect Size and CI
Wilkins and Comstock [51]	Maryland, USA	1981	81 cases and 30,699 controls	Cohort	Exposure to chlorinated drinking water	Sex	All: RR = 2.2 (0.71–9.39); Men: RR = 1.80 (0.80–4.75); Women: RR = 1.60 (0.54–6.32)
Zierler et al. [55]	Massachusetts, USA	1988	614 cases and 1074 controls	Case-control	Duration of exposure to chlorinated drinking water	n.d.	All: OR = 2.7 (1.7–4.3)
McGeehin et al. [53]	Colorado, USA	1993	327 bladder cancer and 261 other-cancer controls	Case-control	Questionnaire & data for TTHM from site visit of water utilities	Smoking Status	Non-Smokers: OR = 2.9 (1.2–7.4); Smokers: OR = 2.1 (1.1–3.8)
King and Marrett [67]	Ontario, Canada	1996	696 cases and 1545 controls	Case-control	Questionnaire about source of water. Water source and chlorination status were provided directly by treatment plant surveys. TTHMs modelling	n.d.	All: OR = 1.66 (1.11–2.51)
Freedman et al. [54]	Maryland, USA	1997	294 cases and 2326 controls	Case-control	Exposure to chlorinated drinking water	Sex, smoking habits	All: OR = 1.4 (0.7–2.9); Men: OR = 2.2 (0.8–5.1); Women: OR = 0.6 (0.2–2.2)
Koivusalo et al. [52]	Finland	1997	621 431	Cohort	Questionnaires. Information on water-pipe connections, past drinking water quality, and treatment practices by waterworks was obtained from administrative registers and municipal waterworks. The level of mutagenicity was estimated by modelling	Sex	All: RR = 1.12 (0.93–1.36); Men: RR = 1.03 (0.82–1.28); Women: RR = 1.48 (1.01–2.18)
Cantor et al. [64]	Iowa, USA	1998	1123 cases and 1983 controls	Case-control	TTHMs in tap water (measures + estimations)	Sex, smoking habits	All: OR = 1.3 (0.9–2.0); Men: OR = 1.8 (1.2–2.7); Women: OR = 0.6 (0.3–1.4)
Koivusalo et al. [56]	Finland	1998	732 cases and 914 controls	Case-control	Questionnaires. Information on water-pipe connections, past drinking water quality, and treatment practices by waterworks was obtained from administrative registers and municipal waterworks. The level of mutagenicity was estimated by modelling	Sex	Men: OR = 1.17 (0.87–1.57); Women: OR = 1.14 (0.71–1.82)
Chevrier et al. [58]	France	2004	281 cases and 272 controls	Case-control	TTHMs modelling	Sex	All: OR = 2.99 (1.1–8.5); Men: OR = 3.73 (1.2–11), Women: OR = 1.55 (0.1–32)
Bove et al. [59]	New York, USA	2007	182 cases and 385 controls	Case-control	TTHM in tap water + water consumption	n.d.	THM: OR = 2.34 (1.01–3.66); CLF: OR = 2.55 (1.25–4.66); BRF: OR = 3.05 (1.51–5.69); BDCM: OR = 2.49 (1.19–4.48)
Chang et al. [60]	Taiwan	2007	403 cases and 403 controls	Case-control	TTHMs in tap water	n.d.	All: OR = 2.11 (1.43–3.11)
Michaud et al. [61]	Spain	2007	397 cases and 664 controls	Case-control	Questionnaire and records searches (including THM measurements)	n.d.	All: OR = 2.06 (0.83–5.08)
Villanueva et al. [68]	Spain	2007	1219 cases and 1271 controls	Case-control	Questionnaire and records searches (including THM measurements)	Sex	All: OR = 2.10 (1.09, 4.02); Men: OR = 2.53 (1.23, 5.20); Women: OR = 1.50 (0.26, 8.61)
Cantor et al. [62]	Spain	2010	680 cases and 714 controls	Case-control	TTHMs in tap water	Gene polymorphism	All: OR = 1.8 (0.9–3.5)

NB: n.d.: No data; OR: Odds Ratio; RR: Risk Ratio; CLF: Chloroform; BRF: Bromoform; BDCM: Bromodichloromethane; Q1: lowest THM concentrations quartile; Q4: highest THM concentrations quartile.

(b) Colon and rectal cancers.

Studies	Location	Year of Publication	Sample Size	Study Design	Exposition Measurement	Site of Cancer	Subgroups Included in the Analysis	Effect Size and CI
Gottlieb and Carr [65]	Louisiana, USA	1982	546 cases and 534 controls	Case-control	Exposure to chlorinated drinking water	Rectal	n.d.	All: OR = 1.68 (1.17–2.42)
Koivusalo et al. [52]	Finland	1997	621 431	Cohort	Questionnaires. Information on water pipe connections, past drinking water quality, and treatment practices by waterworks was obtained from administrative registers and municipal waterworks. The level of mutagenicity was estimated by modelling.	Colon and rectal	Sex	Colon: All: RR = 0.90 (0.77–1.04); Men: RR = 0.83 (0.66–1.04); Women: RR = 0.95 (0.78–1.85). Rectal: All: RR = 1.04 (0.86–1.26); Men: RR = 0.85 (0.66–1.09); Women: RR = 1.38 (1.03–1.85).
Hildesheim et al. [66]	Iowa, USA	1998	560 colon cases, 537 rectal cases, and 1983 controls	Case-control	TTHMs in tap water	Colon and rectal	n.d.	Colon: OR = 1.06 (0.7–1.6); Rectal: OR = 1.66 (1.1–2.6)
King et al. [57]	Ontario, Canada	2000	767 colon cases, 661 rectal cases, and 1545 controls	Case-control	Questionnaire about source of water. Water source and chlorination status were provided directly by treatment plant surveys. TTHMs modelling.	Colon and rectal	Sex	Colon: OR = 1.87 (1.15–3.05) for Men, OR = 0.92 (0.49–1.71) for Women. Rectal: OR = 0.98 (0.56–1.72) for Men, OR = 0.72 (0.34–1.53) for Women
Bove et al. [63]	New York State, USA	2007	128 cases and 253 controls	Case-control	TTHMs in tap water + water consumption	Rectal	n.d.	THM4: OR = 1.01 (0.98–1.03); CLF: OR = 1.00 (0.93–1.09); BRF: OR = 1.20 (1.05–1.35)
Kuo et al. [69]	Taiwan	2009	2195 cases and 2195 controls	Case-control	Questionnaire & data on TTHM levels in drinking water in study. Municipalities were collected from the Taiwan Environmental Protection Administration	Colon	n.d.	All: OR = 1.04 (0.89–1.21)

NB: n.d.: No data; OR: Odds Ratio; RR: Risk Ratio; CLF: Chloroform; BRF: Bromoform; BDCM: Bromodichloromethane.

3.2. Covariables Collected

Table 2 reports the variables collected that could be used for potential EMM assessment for each of the selected studies.

Table 2. Co-variables collected in the selected studies (candidates for a potential effect measure modification assessment).

Study	Age	Sex	Socio-Economic Factors *	Urbanization Level	Smoking	Other Health Behaviors
Wilkins and Comstock 1981 [51]	X	X	X		X	
Gottlieb and Carr 1982 [65]	X	X				
Zierler et al. 1988 [55]				X	X	
McGeehin et al. 1993 [53]					X	
King and Marrett 1996 [67]	X	X	X		X	
Freedman et al. 1997 [54]	X		X	X		
Koivusalo et al. 1997 [52]	X	X	X	X	X	
Cantor et al. 1998 [64]	X	X	X		X	
Hildesheim et al. 1998 [66]				X		X
Koivusalo et al. 1998 [56]	X	X	X	X	X	
King et al. 2000 [57]	X	X	X			X
Chevrier et al. 2004 [58]	X		X	X	X	
Bove et al. 2007 [63]	X		X			X
Bove et al. 2007 [59]	X				X	X
Chang et al. 2007 [60]	X			X		
Michaud et al. 2007 [61]	X	X	X			
Villanueva et al. 2007 [68]	X	X	X	X	X	
Kuo et al. 2009 [69]	X	X		X		
Cantor et al. 2010 [62]	X	X	X		X	

* Include education, occupation status, or SES index.

Although EMM is not assessed in the majority of the selected papers, some studies collect covariables that could be used in the future for an heterogeneity assessment. Information about age is commonly collected in selected studies ($n = 16$). Moreover, other individual data such as education and/or occupation status are collected in some of the studies ($n = 11$). Others report an SES index ($n = 12$). Information about the level of urbanization is also frequently collected ($n = 9$).

4. Discussion

The majority of studies assessing the relationship between THMs and cancer are case-control studies that focus on bladder cancer. These studies use exposure data issued from direct measurements or modelling. The majority of studies found an association between chronic exposure to THMs and bladder cancer. This review revealed that the majority of studies assessed EMM, but primarily for the effect of sex. Six studies show that the EMM of sex in the association between exposure to DBPs and bladder cancer may exist, with a higher effect for men than for women. However, only a very small number of studies have assessed this effect modification for other cancer sites such as colon and rectal cancer ($n = 2$ for both cancers), thus preventing any further conclusion about this parameter. Sex has been found as a more consistent EMM in bladder cancer, and several mechanisms have been proposed, as previously mentioned. More precisely, pharmacokinetic models in humans have shown that the activity of CYP2E1, which plays a role in chloroform metabolism, could be higher in men than in women [70,71]. The role of sex hormones in the modulation of enzymes that metabolizes DBPs has also been proposed. Brominated THMs are metabolized through a glutathione conjugation reaction and several studies have shown that glutathione transferases are regulated by thyroid and sex hormones [23].

The duration of exposure is also an important factor, as the outcomes are cancers at different sites with different latencies, and it is associated with an increase in bladder cancer risk for men [7,64]. Despite this, the exposure metrics (duration of exposure and means of exposure assessment) differ between studies selected. This could influence the results obtained in the different studies selected.

Furthermore, many epidemiological studies on DBPs collect other covariables in addition to sex, such as SES, age, urbanization level, and smoking status but without evaluating the EMM. This information could be used to conduct an EMM assessment in future studies and document the existence of vulnerability factors in the association between DBPs and risk of cancer (notably, bladder, colon, and rectal cancers). Of course, EMM assessments should be motivated and rely on a documented hypothesis. These assessments are particularly useful in targeting populations or territories that public policies should prioritize to reduce socio-demographic inequalities in cancer risks from water contaminants exposure. We thus strongly encourage further studies to assess the role of socio-demographic factors such as SES, age, or urbanization level as potential EMMs in the relationship between DBPs and cancer risk. It is also important to mention that various methods exist in the literature that assess EMM, such as the Breslow-Day test, the Wald χ^2 test, and the regression-based test of interaction [72,73].

This review is subject to a number of limitations. We included studies that measured THMs exposure in a range of different approaches. THMs exposure measurement methods have drastically evolved in the last decades, but we decided to include older studies, as they can inform one of our aims to reveal possible EMM in the association between THMs exposure and cancer risk. We added 9 studies after the screening of references of existing papers. This may be due to some missing keywords (e.g., "treated drinking water") despite the fact that we used similar keywords to other systematic reviews on this topic. Finally, some papers that have been recently published are not included in our review. For instance, a case–control study conducted in Spain and Italy by Villanueva et al. [74] assessed the impact of long-term exposure to THMs on colorectal cancer and found no association, considering the total population without including any EMM assessment.

The majority of the studies quantitatively include gender as a subgroup analysis, but very few studies focused on other potentially relevant EMMs such as SES. However, we observed that many studies included in the review collected standard details on covariates that could be, but often are not, used as stratifying variables. By doing so, we aim to highlight that EMM assessments are easily feasible in future studies using data that is already collected. We hope that this assessment will encourage future studies that will assess which populations are more vulnerable to the impacts of THMs exposure.

Studies on EMM are important to improve public health interventions and better estimate the potential benefits of an intervention (or its public health impact). For instance, within a large community/municipality that is supplied by a unique water treatment plant, inequalities in DBP exposure can be associated with the geographical location of deprived population groups within the municipality, living in neighborhoods or sectors with relatively high concentration of DBPs in drinking water (explained by variable residence time of water in the distribution network, pipe material, age and maintenance, or plumbing systems characteristics). In these cases, local interventions can reduce DBP exposure and could include two dimensions: (i) infrastructure: for instance, the renewal of distribution system pipes locally, including plumbing systems, the improving of the local hydraulic management of the system to reduce stagnation of water, or a better management of booster disinfection; and (ii) promoting awareness campaigns directed at deprived population concerning the exposure to DBPs through tap water and other domestic water uses as bath and showering (for example, the adequate use of domestic equipment to reduce DBPs, such as domestic water filtering, boiling, and refrigeration).

5. Conclusions

Inequalities in cancer incidence according to socio-demographic characteristics [75–77] or location (ex: rural areas compared to urban areas) have been highlighted in the literature. The role of environmental exposures such as drinking water contaminants can play an important role in such disparities. However, the documentation of EMM evidence is still lacking. We therefore strongly recommend greater use of subgroup analysis when possible, which will provide a greater understanding of which populations or territories are more vulnerable to the impacts of DBPs.

Author Contributions: T.B. and I.D. contributed to the study design, conducted the review, and took the lead in drafting the manuscript. L.S., M.J.R., and P.L. contributed to interpretation of data, provided critical revisions to the manuscript, and approved the final draft.

Conflicts of Interest: The authors declare no conflict of interest.

References

1. Rook, J.J. Formation of haloforms during chlorination of natural waters. *J. Water Treat. Exam* **1974**, *23*, 234–243.
2. Richardson, S.D.; Plewa, M.J.; Wagner, E.D.; Schoeny, R.; DeMarini, D.M. Occurrence, genotoxicity, and carcinogenicity of regulated and emerging disinfection by-products in drinking water: A review and roadmap for research. *Mutat. Res.* **2007**, *636*, 178–242. [CrossRef] [PubMed]
3. Grellier, J.; Bennett, J.; Patelarou, E.; Smith, R.B.; Toledano, M.B.; Rushton, L.; Briggs, D.J.; Nieuwenhuijsen, M.J. Exposure to Disinfection By-Products, Fetal Growth, and Prematurity: A Systematic Review and Meta-analysis. *Epidemiology* **2010**, *21*, 300–313. [CrossRef] [PubMed]
4. Levallois, P.; Gingras, S.; Marcoux, S.; Legay, C.; Catto, C.; Rodriguez, M.; Tardif, R. Maternal exposure to drinking-water chlorination by-products and small-for-gestational-age neonates. *Epidemiology* **2012**, *23*, 267–276. [CrossRef] [PubMed]
5. Toledano, M.B.; Nieuwenhuijsen, M.J.; Best, N.; Whitaker, H.; Hambly, P.; de Hoogh, C.; Fawell, J.; Jarup, L.; Elliott, P. Relation of trihalomethane concentrations in public water supplies to stillbirth and birth weight in three water regions in England. *Environ. Health Perspect.* **2005**, *113*, 225–232. [CrossRef] [PubMed]
6. Rahman, M.B.; Driscoll, T.; Cowie, C.; Armstrong, B.K. Disinfection by-products in drinking water and colorectal cancer: A meta-analysis. *Int. J. Epidemiol.* **2010**, *39*, 733–745. [CrossRef] [PubMed]
7. Villanueva, C.M.; Fernandez, F.; Malats, N.; Grimalt, J.O.; Kogevinas, M. Meta-analysis of studies on individual consumption of chlorinated drinking water and bladder cancer. *J. Epidemiol. Community Health* **2003**, *57*, 166–173. [CrossRef] [PubMed]
8. Villanueva, C.M.; Cordier, S.; Font-Ribera, L.; Salas, L.A.; Levallois, P. Overview of disinfection by-products and associated health effects. *Curr. Environ. Health Rep.* **2015**, *2*, 107–115. [CrossRef] [PubMed]
9. Hrudey, S.E.; Fawell, J. 40 years on: What do we know about drinking water disinfection by-products (DBPs) and human health? *Water Sci. Technol. Water Supply* **2015**, *15*, 667. [CrossRef]
10. Parbery, G.; Tivey, D.; McArthur, A. Epidemiological association between chlorinated water and overall risk of cancer: A systematic review. *JBI Database Syst. Rev. Implement. Rep.* **2012**, *10*, 1–14. [CrossRef]
11. Chyou, P.-H.; Nomura, A.M.; Stemmermann, G.N. A prospective study of colon and rectal cancer among Hawaii Japanese men. *Ann. Epidemiol.* **1996**, *6*, 276–282. [CrossRef]
12. Engel, L.S.; Taioli, E.; Pfeiffer, R.; Garcia-Closas, M.; Marcus, P.M.; Lan, Q.; Boffetta, P.; Vineis, P.; Autrup, H.; Bell, D.A. Pooled analysis and meta-analysis of glutathione S-transferase M1 and bladder cancer: A HuGE review. *Am. J. Epidemiol.* **2002**, *156*, 95–109. [CrossRef] [PubMed]
13. Haggar, F.A.; Boushey, R.P. Colorectal cancer epidemiology: Incidence, mortality, survival, and risk factors. *Clin. Colon Rectal Surg.* **2009**, *22*, 191–197. [CrossRef] [PubMed]
14. Heineman, E.F.; Zahm, S.H.; McLaughlin, J.K.; Vaught, J.B. Increased risk of colorectal cancer among smokers: Results of a 26-year follow-up of us veterans and a review. *Int. J. Cancer* **1994**, *59*, 728–738. [CrossRef] [PubMed]
15. Kälble, T. Etiopathology, risk factors, environmental influences and epidemiology of bladder cancer. *Der Urol. Ausg. A* **2001**, *40*, 447–450. [CrossRef]
16. Freudebhiem, J.; Graham, S.; Marshall, J.R.; Haughey, B.P.; Wilkinson, G. A case-control study of diet and rectal cancer in western New York. *Am. J. Epidemiol.* **1990**, *131*, 612–624. [CrossRef]
17. Kiemeney, L.A.; Schoenberg, M. Familial transitional cell carcinoma. *J. Urol.* **1996**, *156*, 867–872. [CrossRef]
18. Ross, R.K.; Jones, P.A.; Yu, M.C. Bladder cancer epidemiology and pathogenesis. *Semin. Oncol.* **1996**, *23*, 536–545. [PubMed]
19. Slattery, M.L.; Sweeney, C.; Murtaugh, M.; Ma, K.N.; Caan, B.J.; Potter, J.D.; Wolff, R. Associations between vitamin D, vitamin D receptor gene and the androgen receptor gene with colon and rectal cancer. *Int. J. Cancer* **2006**, *118*, 3140–3146. [CrossRef] [PubMed]

20. Vena, J.E.; Graham, S.; Freudenheim, J.; Marshall, J.; Zielezny, M.; Swanson, M.; Sufrin, G. Drinking water, fluid intake, and bladder cancer in western New York. *Arch. Environ. Health Int. J.* **1993**, *48*, 191–198. [CrossRef] [PubMed]
21. Woolcott, C.; King, W.; Marrett, L. Coffee and tea consumption and cancers of the bladder, colon and rectum. *Eur. J. Cancer Prev.* **2002**, *11*, 137–145. [CrossRef] [PubMed]
22. Sharp, L.; Donnelly, D.; Hegarty, A.; Carsin, A.-E.; Deady, S.; McCluskey, N.; Gavin, A.; Comber, H. Risk of several cancers is higher in urban areas after adjusting for socioeconomic status. Results from a two-country population-based study of 18 common cancers. *J. Urban Health* **2014**, *91*, 510–525. [CrossRef] [PubMed]
23. Villanueva, C.M.; Cantor, K.P.; Cordier, S.; Jaakkola, J.J.K.; King, W.D.; Lynch, C.F.; Porru, S.; Kogevinas, M. Disinfection byproducts and bladder cancer: A pooled analysis. *Epidemiology* **2004**, *15*, 357–367. [CrossRef] [PubMed]
24. Hanna-Attisha, M.; LaChance, J.; Sadler, R.C.; Champney Schnepp, A. Elevated blood lead levels in children associated with the Flint drinking water crisis: A spatial analysis of risk and public health response. *Am. J. Public Health* **2016**, *106*, 283–290. [CrossRef] [PubMed]
25. Brulle, R.J.; Pellow, D.N. Environmental justice: Human health and environmental inequalities. *Annu. Rev. Public Health* **2006**, *27*, 103–124. [CrossRef] [PubMed]
26. Evans, G.W.; Kantrowitz, E. Socioeconomic status and health: The potential role of environmental risk exposure. *Ann. Rev. Public Health* **2002**, *23*, 303–331. [CrossRef] [PubMed]
27. Pearce, J.R.; Richardson, E.A.; Mitchell, R.J.; Shortt, N.K. Environmental justice and health: The implications of the socio-spatial distribution of multiple environmental deprivation for health inequalities in the United Kingdom. *Trans. Inst. Br. Geogr.* **2010**, *35*, 522–539. [CrossRef]
28. O'Neill, M.S.; Jerrett, M.; Kawachi, I.; Levy, J.I.; Cohen, A.J.; Gouveia, N.; Wilkinson, P.; Fletcher, T.; Cifuentes, L.; Schwartz, J. Health, wealth, and air pollution: Advancing theory and methods. *Environ. Health Perspect.* **2003**, *111*, 1861–1870. [CrossRef] [PubMed]
29. Balazs, C.; Morello-Frosch, R.; Hubbard, A.; Ray, I. Social Disparities in Nitrate Contaminated Drinking Water in California's San Joaquin Valley. *Environ. Health Perspect.* **2011**, 1272–1278. [CrossRef] [PubMed]
30. Balazs, C.L.; Morello-Frosch, R.; Hubbard, A.E.; Ray, I. Environmental justice implications of arsenic contamination in California's San Joaquin Valley: A cross-sectional, cluster-design examining exposure and compliance in community drinking water systems. *Environ. Health* **2012**, *11*, 84. [CrossRef] [PubMed]
31. Balazs, C.L.; Ray, I. The drinking water disparities framework: On the origins and persistence of inequities in exposure. *Am. J. Public Health* **2014**, *104*, 603–611. [CrossRef] [PubMed]
32. Delpla, I.; Benmarhnia, T.; Lebel, A.; Levallois, P.; Rodriguez, M.J. Investigating social inequalities in exposure to drinking water contaminants in rural areas. *Environ. Pollut.* **2015**, *207*, 88–96. [CrossRef] [PubMed]
33. Evans, A.M.; Wright, J.M.; Meyer, A.; Rivera-Núñez, Z. Spatial variation of disinfection by-product concentrations: Exposure assessment implications. *Water Res.* **2013**, *47*, 6130–6140. [CrossRef] [PubMed]
34. Hales, S.; Black, W.; Skelly, C.; Salmond, C.; Weinstein, P. Social deprivation and the public health risks of community drinking water supplies in New Zealand. *J. Epidemiol. Community Health* **2003**, *57*, 581–583. [CrossRef] [PubMed]
35. Vrijheid, M.; Martinez, D.; Aguilera, I.; Ballester, F.; Basterrechea, M.; Esplugues, A.; Guxens, M.; Larrañaga, M.; Lertxundi, A.; Mendez, M.; et al. Socioeconomic status and exposure to multiple environmental pollutants during pregnancy: Evidence for environmental inequity? *J. Epidemiol. Community Health* **2012**, *66*, 106–113. [CrossRef] [PubMed]
36. Briggs, D.; Abellan, J.J.; Fecht, D. Environmental inequity in England: Small area associations between socio-economic status and environmental pollution. *Soc. Sci. Med.* **2008**, *67*, 1612–1629. [CrossRef] [PubMed]
37. Kuh, D.; Ben-Shlomo, Y.; Lynch, J.; Hallqvist, J.; Power, C. Life course epidemiology. *J. Epidemiol. Community Health* **2003**, *57*, 778–783. [CrossRef] [PubMed]
38. Barceló, M.A.; Saez, M.; Saurina, C. Spatial variability in mortality inequalities, socioeconomic deprivation, and air pollution in small areas of the Barcelona Metropolitan Region, Spain. *Sci. Total Environ.* **2009**, *407*, 5501–5523. [CrossRef] [PubMed]
39. Hajat, A.; Hsia, C.; O'Neill, M.S. Socioeconomic Disparities and Air Pollution Exposure: A Global Review. *Curr. Environ. Health Rep.* **2015**, *2*, 440–450. [CrossRef] [PubMed]

40. Benmarhnia, T.; Rey, L.; Cartier, Y.; Clary, C.M.; Deguen, S.; Brousselle, A. Addressing equity in interventions to reduce air pollution in urban areas: A systematic review. *Int. J. Public Health* **2014**, *59*, 933–944. [CrossRef] [PubMed]

41. Moher, D.; Liberati, A.; Tetzlaff, J.; Altman, D.G. Preferred reporting items for systematic reviews and meta-analyses: The PRISMA statement. *Ann. Intern. Med.* **2009**, *151*, 264–269. [CrossRef] [PubMed]

42. Bell, M.L.; Zanobetti, A.; Dominici, F. Who is more affected by ozone pollution? A systematic review and meta-analysis. *Am. J. Epidemiol.* **2014**, *180*, 15–28. [CrossRef] [PubMed]

43. Boffetta, P. Human cancer from environmental pollutants: The epidemiological evidence. *Mutat. Res.* **2006**, *608*, 157–162. [CrossRef] [PubMed]

44. Gouveia, N.; Fletcher, T. Time series analysis of air pollution and mortality: Effects by cause, age and socioeconomic status. *J. Epidemiol. Community Health* **2000**, *54*, 750–755. [CrossRef] [PubMed]

45. Gundry, S.; Wright, J.; Conroy, R. A systematic review of the health outcomes related to household water quality in developing countries. *J. Water Health* **2004**, *2*, 1–13. [PubMed]

46. Hajat, A.; Diez-Roux, A.V.; Adar, S.D.; Auchincloss, A.H.; Lovasi, G.S.; O'Neill, M.S.; Sheppard, L.; Kaufman, J.D. Air pollution and individual and neighborhood socioeconomic status: Evidence from the Multi-Ethnic Study of Atherosclerosis (MESA). *Environ. Health Perspect.* **2013**, *121*, 1325. [CrossRef] [PubMed]

47. Bertin, M.; Chevrier, C.; Serrano, T.; Monfort, C.; Rouget, F.; Cordier, S.; Viel, J.-F. Association between prenatal exposure to traffic-related air pollution and preterm birth in the PELAGIE mother–child cohort, Brittany, France. Does the urban–rural context matter? *Environ. Res.* **2015**, *142*, 17–24. [CrossRef] [PubMed]

48. Madrigano, J.; Jack, D.; Anderson, G.B.; Bell, M.L.; Kinney, P.L. Temperature, ozone, and mortality in urban and non-urban counties in the northeastern United States. *Environ. Health* **2015**, *14*, 3. [CrossRef] [PubMed]

49. Turner, M.C.; Krewski, D.; Pope, C.A., III; Chen, Y.; Gapstur, S.M.; Thun, M.J. Long-term ambient fine particulate matter air pollution and lung cancer in a large cohort of never-smokers. *Am. J. Respir. Crit. Care Med.* **2011**, *184*, 1374–1381. [CrossRef] [PubMed]

50. Sobue, T. Association of indoor air pollution and lifestyle with lung cancer in Osaka, Japan. *Int. J. Epidemiol.* **1990**, *19* (Suppl. 1), S62–S66. [CrossRef] [PubMed]

51. Wilkins, J.R.; Comstock, G.W. Source of drinking water at home and site-specific cancer incidence in Washington County, Maryland. *Am. J. Epidemiol.* **1981**, *114*, 178–190. [CrossRef] [PubMed]

52. Koivusalo, M.; Pukkala, E.; Vartiainen, T.; Jaakkola, J.J.; Hakulinen, T. Drinking water chlorination and cancer–a historical cohort study in Finland. *Cancer Cause Control* **1997**, *8*, 192–200. [CrossRef]

53. McGeehin, M.A.; Reif, J.S.; Becher, J.C.; Mangione, E.J. Case-control study of bladder cancer and water disinfection methods in Colorado. *Am. J. Epidemiol.* **1993**, *138*, 492–501. [CrossRef] [PubMed]

54. Freedman, D.M.; Cantor, K.P.; Lee, N.L.; Chen, L.-S.; Lei, H.-H.; Ruhl, C.E.; Wang, S.S. Bladder cancer and drinking water: A population-based case-control study in Washington County, Maryland (United States). *Cancer Cause Control* **1997**, *8*, 738–744. [CrossRef]

55. Zierler, S.; Feingold, L.; Danley, R.A.; Craun, G. Bladder cancer in Massachusetts related to chlorinated and chloraminated drinking water: A case-control study. *Arch. Environ. Health Int. J.* **1988**, *43*, 195–200. [CrossRef] [PubMed]

56. Koivusalo, M.; Hakulinen, T.; Vartiainen, T.; Pukkala, E.; Jaakkola, J.J.; Tuomist, J. Drinking water mutagenicity and urinary tract cancers: A population-based case-control study in Finland. *Am. J. Epidemiol.* **1998**, *148*, 704–712. [CrossRef] [PubMed]

57. King, W.D.; Marrett, L.D.; Woolcott, C.G. Case-control study of colon and rectal cancers and chlorination by-products in treated water. *Cancer Epidemiol. Biomark. Prev.* **2000**, *9*, 813–818. [PubMed]

58. Chevrier, C.; Junod, B.; Cordier, S. Does ozonation of drinking water reduce the risk of bladder cancer? *Epidemiology* **2004**, *15*, 605–614. [CrossRef] [PubMed]

59. Bove, G.E.; Rogerson, P.A.; Vena, J.E. Case-control study of the effects of trihalomethanes on urinary bladder cancer risk. *Arch. Environ. Occup. Health* **2007**, *62*, 39–47. [CrossRef] [PubMed]

60. Chang, C.-C.; Ho, S.-C.; Wang, L.-Y.; Yang, C.-Y. Bladder cancer in Taiwan: Relationship to trihalomethane concentrations present in drinking-water supplies. *J. Toxicol. Environ. Health Part A* **2007**, *70*, 1752–1757. [CrossRef] [PubMed]

61. Michaud, D.S.; Kogevinas, M.; Cantor, K.P.; Villanueva, C.M.; Garcia-Closas, M.; Rothman, N.; Malats, N.; Real, F.X.; Serra, C.; Garcia-Closas, R. Total fluid and water consumption and the joint effect of exposure to disinfection by-products on risk of bladder cancer. *Environ. Health Perspect.* **2007**, 1569–1572. [CrossRef] [PubMed]

62. Cantor, K.P.; Villanueva, C.M.; Silverman, D.T.; Figueroa, J.D.; Real, F.X.; Garcia-Closas, M.; Malats, N.; Chanock, S.; Yeager, M.; Tardon, A. Polymorphisms in GSTT1, GSTZ1, and CYP2E1, disinfection by-products, and risk of bladder cancer in Spain. *Environ. Health Perspect.* **2010**, *118*, 1545–1550. [CrossRef] [PubMed]

63. Bove, G.E.; Rogerson, P.A.; Vena, J.E. Case control study of the geographic variability of exposure to disinfectant byproducts and risk for rectal cancer. *Int. J. Health Geogr.* **2007**, *6*, 18. [CrossRef] [PubMed]

64. Cantor, K.P.; Lynch, C.F.; Hildesheim, M.; Dosemeci, M.; Lubin, J.; Alavanja, M.; Craun, G. Drinking Water Source and Chlorination Byproducts I. Risk of Bladder Cancer. *Epidemiology* **1998**, *9*, 21–28. [CrossRef] [PubMed]

65. Gottlieb, M.S.; Carr, J.K. Case-control cancer mortality study and chlorination of drinking water in Louisiana. *Environ. Health Perspect.* **1982**, *46*, 169. [CrossRef] [PubMed]

66. Hildesheim, M.E.; Cantor, K.P.; Lynch, C.F.; Dosemeci, M.; Lubin, J.; Alavanja, M.; Craun, G. Drinking Water Source and Chlorination Byproducts II. Risk of Colon and Rectal Cancers. *Epidemiology* **1998**, *9*, 29–35. [CrossRef] [PubMed]

67. King, W.D.; Marrett, L.D. Case-control study of bladder cancer and chlorination by-products in treated water (Ontario, Canada). *Cancer Cause Control* **1996**, *7*, 596–604. [CrossRef]

68. Villanueva, C.M.; Cantor, K.P.; Grimalt, J.O.; Malats, N.; Silverman, D.; Tardon, A.; Garcia-Closas, R.; Serra, C.; Carrato, A.; Castaño-Vinyals, G.; et al. Bladder cancer and exposure to water disinfection by-products through ingestion, bathing, showering, and swimming in pools. *Am. J. Epidemiol.* **2007**, *165*, 148–156. [CrossRef] [PubMed]

69. Kuo, H.-W.; Tiao, M.-M.; Wu, T.-N.; Yang, C.-Y. Trihalomethanes in drinking water and the risk of death from colon cancer in Taiwan. *J. Toxicol. Environ. Health Part A* **2009**, *72*, 1217–1222. [CrossRef] [PubMed]

70. Tanaka, E. Gender-related differences in pharmacokinetics and their clinical significance. *J. Clin. Pharmacol. Ther.* **1999**, *24*, 339–346. [CrossRef]

71. Meibohm, B.; Beierle, I.; Derendorf, H. How important are gender differences in pharmacokinetics? *Clin. Pharmacokinet.* **2002**, *41*, 329–342. [CrossRef] [PubMed]

72. Kaufman, J.S.; MacLehose, R.F. Which of these things is not like the others? *Cancer* **2013**, *119*, 4216–4222. [CrossRef] [PubMed]

73. Altman, D.G.; Bland, J.M. Interaction revisited: The difference between two estimates. *Br. Med. J.* **2003**, *326*, 219. [CrossRef]

74. Villanueva, C.M.; Gracia-Lavedan, E.; Bosetti, C.; Righi, E.; Molina, A.J.; Martín, V.; Boldo, E.; Aragonés, N.; Perez-Gomez, B.; Pollan, M.; et al. Colorectal cancer and long-term exposure to trihalomethanes in drinking water: A multicenter case–control study in Spain and Italy. *Environ. Health Perspect.* **2017**, *125*, 56–65. [CrossRef] [PubMed]

75. Askari, A.; Aziz, O.; Currie, A.; Athanasiou, T.; Faiz, O. Inequalities in Colorectal Cancer Risk and Educational Level in Developed Countries: A Systematic Review and Meta-Analysis of Observational Studies. *Br. J. Surg.* **2015**, *2015*, 187.

76. Choi, K.M. Investigation of cancer mortality inequalities between rural and urban areas in South Korea. *Aust. J. Rural Health* **2016**, *24*, 61–66. [CrossRef] [PubMed]

77. Woods, L.; Rachet, B.; Coleman, M. Origins of socio-economic inequalities in cancer survival: A review. *Ann. Oncol.* **2006**, *17*, 5–19. [CrossRef] [PubMed]

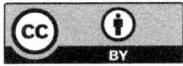

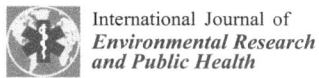

International Journal of
Environmental Research and Public Health

Article

Atrazine Contamination of Drinking Water and Adverse Birth Outcomes in Community Water Systems with Elevated Atrazine in Ohio, 2006–2008

Kirsten S. Almberg [1,*], Mary E. Turyk [2], Rachael M. Jones [1], Kristin Rankin [2], Sally Freels [2] and Leslie T. Stayner [2]

[1] Environmental and Occupational Health Sciences Division, School of Public Health,
     University of Illinois at Chicago, 1603 W. Taylor Street, Chicago, IL 60612, USA; rjones25@uic.edu
[2] Epidemiology and Biostatistics Division, School of Public Health, University of Illinois at Chicago,
     1603 W. Taylor Street, Chicago, IL 60607, USA; mturyk1@uic.edu (M.E.T.); krankin@uic.edu (K.R.);
     sallyf@uic.edu (S.F.); lstayner@uic.edu (L.T.S.)
*   Correspondence: almberg@uic.edu; Tel.: +1-312-996-9477

Received: 23 July 2018; Accepted: 28 August 2018; Published: 31 August 2018

Abstract: Atrazine, a common water contaminant in the U.S., has been associated with adverse birth outcomes in previous studies. This study aimed to determine if atrazine concentrations in drinking water are associated with adverse birth outcomes including small for gestational age (SGA), term low birth weight (term LBW), very low birth weight (VLBW), preterm birth (PTB), and very preterm birth (VPTB). This study included 14,445 live singleton births from Ohio communities served by 22 water systems enrolled in the U.S. Environmental Protection Agency's Atrazine Monitoring Program between 2006 and 2008. Mean gestational and trimester-specific atrazine concentrations were calculated. Significantly increased odds of term LBW birth was associated with atrazine exposure over the entire gestational period (OR 1.27, 95% CI 1.10, 1.45), as well as the first (OR 1.20, 95% CI 1.08, 1.34) and second trimesters (OR 1.13, 95% CI 1.07, 1.20) of pregnancy. We observed no evidence of an association between atrazine exposure via drinking water and SGA, VLBW, PTB, or VPTB. Our results suggest that atrazine exposure is associated with reduced birth weight among term infants and that exposure to atrazine in drinking water in early and mid-pregnancy may be most critical for its toxic effects on the fetus.

Keywords: atrazine; community water system; low birth weight; preterm birth; small for gestational age; water contamination; endocrine disruptor

1. Introduction

Atrazine is the second most widely used herbicide in the United States, primarily applied to corn and sorghum crops [1]. Much of the concern about atrazine arises from its persistence in soil and its transport to surface and groundwater drinking water sources [2], making it the most commonly detected pesticide in surface water sources in the United States and frequently detected in groundwater sources as well [1,3].

Atrazine is an endocrine disruptor [1,4,5], and while some aspects of the toxic mechanisms are unclear, atrazine disrupts the hypothalamic-pituitary-gonadal axis by inhibiting luteinizing hormone production, increasing aromatase production, and disrupting ovarian function [6–9]. Low ecologically relevant doses of atrazine have been shown to decrease testosterone levels, reduce spermatogenesis, and alter gonad development in amphibians, leading sometimes to complete chemical feminization of male frogs [10,11]. Exposure to atrazine induces delayed puberty, decreased testosterone and increased estradiol levels, reduced sperm counts, and altered testis architecture [8,12–15] among male rats and delayed puberty, lengthened estrous cycles, and decreased number of menstrual cycles [9,16] among females.

There is limited epidemiologic evidence of an effect of prenatal exposure to atrazine on adverse birth outcomes in humans. Winchester et al. [17] observed a temporal association between atrazine application and birth defects in an ecologic study in the U.S. Two studies of births in the Midwest have found that increased atrazine levels in drinking water sources is associated with elevated odds of small for gestational age (SGA), with one indicating that the timing of exposure is critical for understanding this association [18,19]. Exposure to atrazine through contaminated drinking water has been associated with increased risk of preterm birth in Kentucky [20] and four Midwestern states [21]. In France, Chevrier et al. [22] reported that the presence of atrazine biomarkers in maternal urine was associated with lower birth weight, length, and head circumference. A recent study found an association between atrazine and both preterm birth and very preterm births in Midwestern counties in which <10% of the population is using private well water [21]. With the exception of the one prospective cohort study in France [22], all previous epidemiological studies of atrazine and birth outcomes have relied on ecologic exposure estimates obtained retrospectively through environmental monitoring data.

The United States Environmental Protection Agency (USEPA) defines the legal limits for water contaminants and water testing schedules, as mandated in the Safe Drinking Water Act. The maximum contaminant level (MCL) for atrazine in drinking water is 3 µg/L [23]. Public water systems are required to test for atrazine quarterly, unless atrazine concentrations are consistently below the MCL, at which point testing can be reduced to once every three years. Those water systems that have atrazine or total combined triazine measurements exceeding 2.6 µg/L in finished water, or 12.5 µg/L in raw water, over a 90-day average are inducted into the Atrazine Monitoring Program (AMP) for 5 years. Community water systems (CWS) in the AMP are required to measure atrazine weekly during the season of peak atrazine use and biweekly throughout the remainder of the year [24].

The primary objective of this study was to examine the association between atrazine concentrations in drinking water and selected adverse birth outcomes among those communities receiving drinking water from community water systems that were part of USEPA's Atrazine Monitoring Program between 2006 and 2008 in the state of Ohio. This study also aimed to explore the utility of environmental and health data collected through routine monitoring by state and federal agencies for addressing epidemiologic questions, in line with the Centers for Disease Control and Prevention Environmental Public Health Tracking Program [25].

2. Materials and Methods

2.1. Study Population

This study used birth certificate data from all births occurring within the 22 Ohio communities receiving drinking water from a CWS in the USEPA's AMP between 2006 and 2008. There were 14,897 births in these cities, of which 14,445 (97%) were singleton births. This analysis was restricted to singleton births as multiple births (e.g., twins and more) have smaller birth weights and shorter gestational periods [26]. The singleton births in this analysis comprised 3.4% of births state-wide (*n* = 428,804) during this time period. Individual-level, de-identified birth certificate data for children born in Ohio were provided by the Ohio Department of Health.

2.2. Birth Outcomes

The birth outcomes of interest in this study were small for gestational age (SGA), term low birth weight (term LBW), very low birth weight (VLBW), preterm birth (PTB), and very preterm birth (VPTB). SGA was defined as the smallest 10% of infants, according to birth weight, at each gestational age in the population [26]. Small for gestational age status was calculated using sex- and gestational age-specific national birth weight references [27]. Term LBW was defined as an infant weighing <2500 g at time of delivery among term infants (≥37 weeks gestation). An infant was considered VLBW if it weighed <1500 g at time of delivery, regardless of gestational age. Preterm birth and VPTB were defined as infants delivered prior to 37 and 32 weeks gestation, respectively. Gestational age was based on the reported last normal menstrual period. If the last menstrual period was unknown or implausible, a clinical estimate of gestation was used. All birth outcomes were either reported directly on or were calculated from variables reported on the birth certificates.

2.3. Exposure Assessment

Drinking water measurements of atrazine in finished water from 2005 to 2008 were obtained from the USEPA's AMP public data portal [28] for all 22 AMP water systems in Ohio. Each of these water systems were enrolled in the AMP for all years of the study. We made the assumption that the service boundaries of each CWS in the AMP corresponded to the city limits in which the water system was located. To verify this assumption, we attempted to contact an employee at each AMP water system in Ohio. We successfully reached personnel at 70% of water systems included in this study, and our assumption regarding city and water system boundaries was verified by personnel at 10 of the 15 water systems where contact was made (Ohio Atrazine Monitoring Program Community Water Systems, 2015, personal communications). Personnel at the remaining five water systems were not able to provide this information.

Monthly mean estimates of atrazine in each AMP water system were calculated from the weekly and biweekly samples in the AMP data. Using the mean monthly estimates, we calculated the mean atrazine concentrations for the entire gestational period of the pregnancy ("gestational atrazine") as well as for each trimester of pregnancy, based on date of birth and gestational age at birth. The limit of detection for atrazine was 0.1 µg/L in 2006 and was 0.05 µg/L in 2007 and 2008 [29]. Measurements below the limit of detection (LOD) were assigned a value of the LOD/2 in this analysis. Surface water was the source for all water systems included in this analysis. Atrazine exposure measures were linked with birth records by the city code of the mother's residence, which is provided on the birth certificate, as well as the year and month of birth of the infant.

2.4. Covariates

The covariates examined in this study included infant sex, maternal age at birth, maternal race/ethnicity, maternal educational attainment, marital status, prenatal care status, socioeconomic status, parity, cigarette use, and maternal pre-pregnancy body mass index (BMI). Maternal age was categorized as <20, 20–34, and $\geq$35 years of age. Maternal race/ethnicity was defined as non-Hispanic white, non-Hispanic black, Hispanic, and other/unknown. Maternal educational attainment was categorized as less than a high school degree, high school degree, some college, and college degree or higher. Marital status was dichotomized as married or unmarried. The unmarried category includes mothers who responded single, widowed, or divorced. The Kotelchuck index was used to define the adequacy of prenatal care utilization, based on the month of entry into prenatal care and total number of prenatal care visits [30]. Women were categorized as inadequate, intermediate, adequate, or adequate plus—a category that indicates an individual has had more than the recommended amount of prenatal care. Maternal smoking was dichotomized as smoker versus non-smoker. The cigarette use data was non-specific to the window of time including pregnancy. Whether or not the mother was enrolled in the Women, Infant, and Children (WIC) supplemental nutrition program was used as a proxy for low SES. The WIC program is a federally funded nutrition and assistance program for low-income pregnant and post-partum women, infants, and children under the age of five [31]. Maternal pre-pregnancy BMI was categorized according to the Centers for Disease Control and Prevention definitions of underweight, normal, overweight, and obese [32]. Parity was categorized as having had 0, 1, 2, or $\geq$3 previous live births.

2.5. Data Analysis

This is a cross-sectional study of dichotomous birth outcomes among singleton births in Ohio cities served by AMP CWSs. Bivariate associations between atrazine concentrations, outcomes, and covariates were assessed using t-tests for continuous variables, Rao-Scott Chi-Square tests for dichotomous variables, and ANOVA test for covariates with >2 categories. Potential confounders were considered as those variables that were associated with both the exposure measures and outcome measures and were not conceptually in the causal pathway.

We developed generalized estimating equation (GEE) logistic regression models, with an exchangeable working correlation structure and robust standard errors, to estimate the association between atrazine in drinking water and each birth outcome—SGA, term LBW, VLBW, PTB, and VPTB—while accounting for clustering at the city level. Models of continuous and categorical (tertiles) atrazine exposure were tested. Maternal age, maternal race/ethnicity, and year of birth were included in all adjusted models based on a priori knowledge. We assessed confounding throughout the model building process and in an effort to maximize parsimony, we retained only those variables that had a substantial (>10%) effect on the estimate of the effect of atrazine in the models. Final adjusted models were built using the gestational atrazine exposure measure. The covariates identified as confounders in these models were applied to models of trimester-specific atrazine exposure. Third trimester models were not performed for the outcome VLBW because only two of the VLBW births in this population were delivered at full term. Linear GEE regression models of birth weight and gestation in weeks were performed controlling for those covariates identified in the logistic regression model-building procedures. Between 0.5 and 3.5% of observations were not used due to missing data on covariates, exposure, or outcome status. All analyses were performed using SAS®, Version 9.4 [33].

We performed a sensitivity analysis to further reduce exposure misclassification by restricting the analysis to only those water systems where we had confirmation from on-site representatives that the service boundaries of the water system corresponded to the city limits in which it was located and that >95% of the population was likely to be receiving their public water from the AMP water system in question (*n* = 10 water systems). Additionally, we restricted the data set to those with a gestational atrazine concentration ≤3 µg/L to evaluate the relationship between atrazine in drinking water and selected birth outcomes when exposure is below permissible levels in public drinking water.

This work was reviewed and approved by the Institutional Review Board of the University of Illinois at Chicago (#2010-0907) and the Institutional Review Board of the Ohio Department of Health (#2016-17).

3. Results

3.1. Atrazine Concentrations in Drinking Water

Monthly mean atrazine concentrations in Ohio's AMP water systems ranged from 0 to 15.7 µg/L between 2006 and 2008 (Table 1). Atrazine measurements followed a sharp seasonal pattern, peaking in the months of May and June (Figure 1). Across all years, monthly mean concentrations were missing in 2.3% of AMP water systems, with annual variation in the missing pattern between 0.5 and 5%. Overall, less than 1% of births were missing an estimate of atrazine exposure during their entire gestation or during any of their trimester estimates of exposure.

Table 1. Summary of monthly mean atrazine concentrations reported in finished drinking water by Atrazine Monitoring Program (AMP) community water systems (*n* = 22) in Ohio, 2006–2008.

Year	Geometric Mean, GSD (µg/L)	Median Concentration (µg/L)	Minimum Concentration (µg/L)	Maximum Concentration (µg/L)	Percent Missing [a] (%)
2006	0.29, 3.04	0.17	0.00	7.22	1.5
2007	0.15, 3.43	0.16	0.03	4.23	0.4
2008	0.16, 4.35	0.17	0.03	15.66	4.9

[a] Percentage of community water systems missing monthly mean atrazine concentration. GSD: geometric standard deviation.

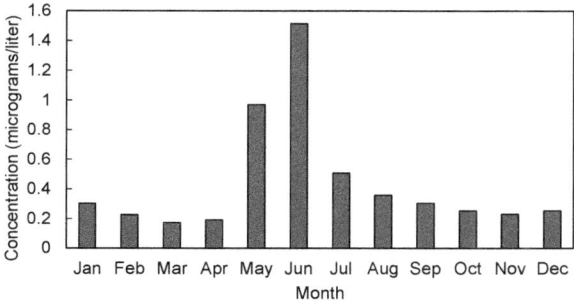

Figure 1. Seasonal variations in mean monthly atrazine concentration (μg/L) in finished water samples from 22 AMP community water systems in Ohio, 2006–2008.

3.2. Study Population

There were 14,445 live singleton births within the 22 cities which received their public drinking water supply from AMP water systems in Ohio between 2006 and 2008, of which 51% were males (Table 2). The majority of these births were born to mothers who were non-Hispanic white (86%), between 20 and 34 years old (81%), were married (54%), and parous (59%). Half of the births during this time period were born to mothers with a high school degree or less. Overall, 68% of mothers reported adequate plus, intermediate, or adequate prenatal care, but 19% had an unknown level of prenatal care. The proportion of infants born to mothers enrolled in the WIC program in our sample was higher than for the state as a whole (50% versus 42%) as was the proportion of infants born to mothers who reported smoking (35% versus 26%) (not shown). There was a high prevalence of pre-pregnancy obesity (25%) among the mothers in this population. Among live singleton births, 10.3% were SGA, 1.1% were very low birth weight, 9.9% were preterm, and 1.6% very preterm. Among singleton term births, 2.4% were term LBW. Between <1% and 3% of observations were dropped in fully covariate-adjusted models due to missing data on either outcomes, covariates, or exposure estimates.

Table 2. Distribution of demographic and economic covariates across the population of live singleton births (*n* = 14,445) and the prevalence of outcomes by covariates in Atrazine Monitoring Program communities in Ohio, 2006–2008.

Variable	*n* (%)	SGA	Term LBW	VLBW	PTB	VPTB
		%	%	%	%	%
Gender						
Male	7431 (51)	9.9	1.9	1.1	10.5	1.7
Female	7014 (49)	10.6	3.4	1.1	9.3	1.6
Race/Ethnicity						
Non-Hispanic white	12,471 (86)	9.7	2.4	1.0	9.5	1.5
Non-Hispanic black	1068 (7)	17.8	6.2	2.4	13.9	2.9
Hispanic	689 (5)	8.9	1.8	1.5	10.3	2.0
Other	217 (2)	9.7	3.2	1.4	13.4	2.3
Maternal Age at Birth						
<20	1811 (13)	15.4	4.0	1.7	13.2	2.7
20–34	11,710 (81)	9.7	2.5	1.0	9.4	1.4
35+	923 (6)	7.8	2.7	1.5	10.1	2.1
Maternal Education						
High School or less	7203 (50)	12.8	3.1	1.4	11.4	2.0
Some College/Degree	7203 (50)	7.7	2.2	0.8	8.4	1.3

Table 2. *Cont.*

Variable	n (%)	SGA	Term LBW	VLBW	PTB	VPTB
		%	%	%	%	%
Maternal Smoking						
Yes	4995 (35)	7.9	3.9	1.4	11.5	2.1
No	9449 (65)	14.7	2.0	0.9	9.1	1.4
Prenatal Care						
Inadequate	1861 (13)	13.2	3.8	1.0	11.2	1.9
Intermediate/Adequate	5970 (41)	9.7	1.6	0.3	3.0	0.4
Adequate Plus	3902 (27)	9.6	3.8	1.4	17.5	2.2
Unknown	2712 (19)	10.6	3.0	2.5	13.3	3.3
WIC use [a]						
Yes	7064 (50)	12.6	3.3	1.2	9.1	1.8
No	7108 (50)	7.9	2.0	1.0	10.6	1.4
Pre-pregnancy BMI						
Underweight	673 (8)	17.8	6.8	1.2	11.6	1.5
Normal	6664 (47)	11.2	2.8	1.1	9.9	1.7
Overweight	3170 (22)	8.8	2.0	1.0	9.2	1.4
Obese	3781 (26)	8.6	2.4	1.2	10.2	1.6
Parity						
0	5892 (41)	12.0	3.2	1.3	10.0	1.8
1	4515 (32)	8.3	2.3	0.9	9.0	1.4
2	2334 (16)	9.3	2.0	1.0	9.6	1.5
≥3	1483 (10)	11.2	2.9	0.7	12.8	1.7
Marital Status						
Married	7765 (54)	7.1	1.8	0.8	8.5	1.0
Unmarried	6680 (46)	13.9	3.8	1.5	11.6	2.3

[a] WIC use indicates participation in the Women, Infant and Children nutrition and assistance program. SGA: small for gestational age; Term LBW: term low birth weight; VLBW: very low birth weight; PTB: preterm birth; VPTB: very preterm birth.

3.3. Regression Analyses

We found weak and statistically non-significant evidence of a positive association between gestational averages of atrazine and SGA in either crude or fully covariate-adjust models (AOR 1.06, 95% CI 0.96, 1.17) (Table 3). In our examination of trimester-specific exposure windows, we similarly observed only a weak association between average atrazine exposure in the first trimesters and SGA (Table 4).

Mean gestational atrazine exposure was associated with significantly increased odds of term LBW birth in both crude and adjusted models (Table 3; AOR 1.27, 95% CI 1.10, 1.45). In our models of trimester-specific exposure windows, we observed a significant increase in odds of term LBW birth with increasing atrazine exposure during the first and second trimesters, but not in the third trimester (Table 4; Figure 2). In categorical analyses, we observed a significant increase in odds of term LBW among those in the highest tertile of mean gestational atrazine exposure compared to those in the lowest (Table 5), although odds increased across each tertile of exposure (test for trend $p = 0.0007$).

Results from linear regression analyses indicated that an increasing gestational atrazine exposure was related to decreased birth weight among term infants (-2.7 grams per $1\mu g/L$ increase, $p = 0.77$) and gestational age in weeks among all infants (-0.03 weeks per $1\ \mu g/L$ increase, $p = 0.62$), but these findings were non-significant.

We observed no evidence of an association between gestational or trimester averages of atrazine exposure with odds of VLBW, PTB, or VPTB in this population (Tables 3 and 4).

Table 3. Associations [a] between gestational mean atrazine concentrations in drinking water and SGA, term LBW, VLBW, PTB, and VPTB in AMP communities (*n* = 22) in Ohio, 2006–2008.

Outcome	Model	*n*	OR [g] (95% CI)
SGA [b]	Crude	13,942	0.99 (0.88, 1.12)
	Adjusted	13,942	1.06 (0.96, 1.17)
Term LBW [c]	Crude	12,567	1.15 (1.01, 1.31)
	Adjusted	12,567	1.27 (1.10, 1.45)
VLWB [d]	Crude	14,089	0.90 (0.50, 1.60)
	Adjusted	14,089	0.81 (0.47, 1.39)
PTB [e]	Crude	14,098	1.01 (0.89, 1.14)
	Adjusted	14,098	0.99 (0.88, 1.11)
VPTB [f]	Crude	14,349	1.15 (0.86, 1.55)
	Adjusted	14,349	1.11 (0.81, 1.51)

[a] All adjusted models included maternal race/ethnicity, maternal age, and birth year a priori. [b] Small for gestational age defined as the smallest 10% of infants, according to birth weight, at each gestational age in the population. In addition to a priori variables, the final model for SGA included maternal education, WIC status, marital status, maternal pre-pregnancy BMI. [c] Term low birth weight is defined as < 2500 g among term births (≥ 37 weeks gestation). In addition to a priori variables, the final model for term LBW included infant sex, maternal education, WIC status, marital status, maternal smoking status, and maternal pre-pregnancy BMI. [d] Very low birth weight is defined as < 1500 g at time of delivery. In addition to a priori variables, the final model for term LBW included maternal education, marital status, and parity. [e] Preterm births defined as infants delivered before 37 weeks gestation. In addition to a priori variables, the final model for PTB included maternal education, maternal smoking status, and parity. [f] Very preterm births defined as infants delivered before 32 weeks gestation. In addition to a priori variables, the final model for PTB included maternal marital status. [g] Odds ratios reflect increase in odds per 1 μg/L increase in atrazine in drinking water.

Table 4. Associations [a] between trimester-specific atrazine concentrations (μg/L) and SGA, term LBW, VLBW, PTB and VPTB among AMP communities (*n* = 22) in Ohio, 2006–2008.

Outcome	Model	*n*	OR [g] (95%CI)
First Trimester			
SGA [b]	Crude	14,022	1.02 (0.95, 1.09)
	Adjusted	14,022	1.04 (0.98, 1.11)
Term LBW [c]	Crude	12,647	1.14 (1.01, 1.28)
	Adjusted	12,647	1.20 (1.08, 1.34)
VLWB [d]	Crude	14,170	1.09 (0.86, 1.37)
	Adjusted	14,170	1.07 (0.86, 1.34)
PTB [e]	Crude	14,179	1.01 (0.90, 1.13)
	Adjusted	14,179	0.99 (0.90, 1.10)
VPTB [f]	Crude	14,432	1.11 (0.81, 1.53)
	Adjusted	14,432	1.11 (0.81, 1.53)
Second Trimester			
SGA [a]	Crude	14,002	0.97 (0.93, 1.00)
	Adjusted	14,002	0.99 (0.96, 1.02)
Term LBW	Crude	12,647	1.06 (0.98, 1.14)
	Adjusted	12,647	1.13 (1.07, 1.20)
VLWB	Crude	14,148	0.79 (0.55, 1.14)
	Adjusted	14,148	0.76 (0.51, 1.13)
PTB	Crude	14,156	0.99 (0.95, 1.04)
	Adjusted	14,156	0.99 (0.95, 1.04)

Table 4. *Cont.*

Outcome	Model	*n*	OR [g] (95%CI)
Third Trimester			
SGA [a]	Crude	12,648	0.98 (0.87, 1.10)
	Adjusted	12,648	1.00 (0.93, 1.08)
Term LBW	Crude	12,647	0.97 (0.80, 1.16)
	Adjusted	12,647	1.03 (0.87, 1.22)

[a] All adjusted models included maternal race/ethnicity, maternal age, and birth year a priori. [b] Small for gestational age defined as the smallest 10% of infants, according to birth weight, at each gestational age in the population. In addition to a priori variables, the final model for SGA included maternal education, WIC status, marital status, and maternal pre-pregnancy BMI. [c] Term low birth weight is defined as <2500 g among term births (≥37 weeks gestation). In addition to a priori variables, the final model for term LBW included infant sex, maternal education, WIC status, marital status, maternal smoking status, and maternal pre-pregnancy BMI. [d] Very low birth weight is defined as <1500 g at time of delivery. In addition to a priori variables, the final model for term LBW included maternal education, marital status, and parity. [e] Preterm births defined as infants delivered before 37 weeks' gestation. In addition to a priori variables, the final model for PTB included maternal education, maternal smoking status, and parity. [f] Very preterm births defined as infants delivered before 32 weeks' gestation. In addition to a priori variables, the final model for PTB included maternal marital status. [g] Odds ratios reflect increase in odds per 1 µg/L increase in atrazine in drinking water.

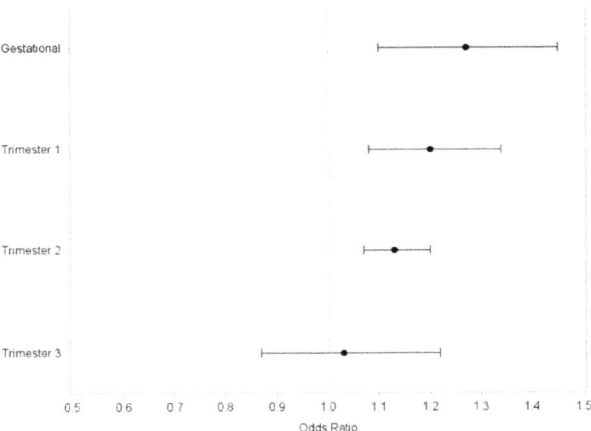

Figure 2. Association between gestational and trimester mean estimates of atrazine exposure in drinking water and term LBW in communities served by water systems enrolled in USEPA's AMP (*n* = 22) in Ohio, 2006–2008.

Table 5. Association [a] between term low birth weight births and tertiles of gestational atrazine exposure among live singleton births in AMP communities (*n* = 22) in Ohio, 2006–2008.

Tertile	Exposure Range (µg/L)	OR [a] (95% CI)
1	0–0.1537	Ref.
2	0.1538–0.4622	1.11 (0.92, 1.34)
3	0.4623–5.9337	1.26 (1.11, 1.44)
		p for trend = 0.0007

[a] Model adjusted for maternal race/ethnicity, maternal age, birth year, infant sex, maternal education, WIC status, marital status, maternal smoking status, and maternal pre-pregnancy BMI.

3.4. Sensitivity Analyses

We restricted the mean gestational and trimester-specific atrazine exposure models to include only those water systems where an on-site representative confirmed that the service boundaries corresponded to the city boundaries. There were 4488 births within these 10 AMP water systems. We observed elevated odds of term LBW per 1 μg/L increase in mean gestational atrazine in this subgroup (AOR 1.16, 95% CI 0.77, 1.74), but the association was not significant (Table 6). We observed no association between gestational atrazine concentrations and SGA or PTB. Covariate-adjusted models did not converge for VPT or VLBW, but no association between atrazine and either outcome was seen in crude models.

Table 6. Associations [a] between gestational and trimester-specific mean concentrations of atrazine in drinking water and term LBW among AMP communities with verified service boundaries (*n* = 10) in Ohio, 2006–2008.

Exposure	Model	*n*	OR [b] (95% CI)
Gestational mean	Crude	3929	1.04 (0.62, 1.72)
	Adjusted	3929	1.16 (0.77, 1.74)
First trimester	Crude	3961	1.13 (0.96, 1.33)
	Adjusted	3961	1.17 (1.03, 1.34)
Second trimester	Crude	3961	0.95 (0.77, 1.17)
	Adjusted	3961	1.01 (0.83, 1.22)
Third trimester	Crude	3961	0.96 (0.66, 1.40)
	Adjusted	3961	1.01 (0.72, 1.41)

[a] Term low birth weight is defined as <2500 g among term births (≥37 weeks' gestation). All adjusted models included maternal race/ethnicity, maternal age, birth year, infant sex, maternal education, WIC status, marital status, maternal smoking status, and maternal pre-pregnancy BMI. [b] Odds ratios reflect increase in odds per 1 μg/L increase in atrazine in drinking water.

Mean exposure to atrazine in the first trimester was significantly associated with an increase in the odds of term LBW in these restricted models (AORT1 1.17, 95% CI 1.03, 1.34) (Table 6). Atrazine exposure during the first trimester was inversely associated with the odds of PTB in crude and adjusted models. No association between atrazine exposure in the second or third trimesters and either SGA, term LBW, or PTB was observed in adjusted models. Third trimester atrazine exposure was not assessed for its relationship to PTB.

In a separate sensitivity analysis of term LBW, we restricted the data set to include only those term births with a mean gestational atrazine concentration ≤3 μg/L (*n* = 12,980), the current MCL set by the USEPA. Used as a continuous measure in the models, mean gestational atrazine exposure was associated with a significant increase in the odds of term LBW (AOR 1.33, 95% CI 1.08, 1.64). Odds of term LBW increased across tertiles of mean atrazine exposure, but only those in the highest tertile of gestational atrazine exposure were at significantly increased odds of term LBW compared to those in the lowest tertile (AOR 1.25, 95% CI 1.10, 1.43).

4. Discussion

The aim of this study was to examine the relationship between atrazine exposure during pregnancy and selected adverse birth outcomes among communities that have been served by water systems monitored by the USEPA's Atrazine Monitoring Program. Furthermore, this research was aimed at elucidating the window of exposure that is most critical for these birth outcomes. In this analysis of all live singleton births within AMP communities in Ohio between 2006 and 2008, we observed a significant increase in odds of term LBW births with increasing atrazine exposure. This association was observed within models of atrazine exposure averaged over the entire gestation of the pregnancy. Furthermore, our results suggest that atrazine exposure within the first and second trimesters of pregnancy, but not during the third trimester, are associated with term LBW, indicating that exposure to atrazine in drinking water in early and mid-pregnancy may be most critical for its toxic effects on the fetus. We observed no significant evidence of an association between atrazine exposure via drinking water and SGA, VLBW, PTB, or VPTB.

The exact mechanism through which atrazine would reduce birth weight is not well understood. Findings from rat models showing reduced pup weight after in utero exposure to atrazine lend biologic plausibility to our findings [34,35]. Our findings are consistent with previous epidemiologic research which has shown an inverse relationship between atrazine exposure and birth weight [22], but conflicts with another study which found no association between atrazine exposure via drinking water and low birth weight in a population of infants in Brittany, France [36]. While previous studies have shown evidence of an association between atrazine exposure and small for gestational age and preterm birth [21], we found no evidence of these associations in our study of singleton births occurring within communities served by AMP water systems in Ohio from 2006 to 2008.

Reduced birth weight has serious public health impacts. The risk of neonatal mortality is highest among the smallest and largest infants, as measured by birth weight. This same pattern of increased risk is seen later in life as well, with a reversed "J" shape association between birthweight and cardiovascular disease and all-cause mortality [26]. Our findings suggest that the morbidity and mortality burden from this adverse birth outcome can be lessened through reducing gestational exposures to atrazine in drinking water.

Water systems are enrolled in the AMP as a result of repeated exceedances of the 3 µg/L MCL for atrazine, but only 4% of samples from the water systems in this study exceeded the MCL. Our findings are unchanged when we remove those observations for which gestational atrazine estimates exceeded the MCL. While further epidemiologic research is needed, these results suggest that the current MCL for atrazine may not be protective against some adverse birth outcomes such as term low birth weight.

Most previous epidemiologic studies of atrazine and birth outcomes have been limited by ecologic exposure and outcome assessment. In the present study, birth outcomes and covariates were assessed at the individual level from birth certificates, providing more accurate outcome ascertainment and robust control of confounding. Atrazine exposure was estimated at the water system level in this study, which offers substantial refinement of exposure classification from the ecologic measurements that combine observations across multiple CWSs used in some of the prior studies [18,20,36]. Furthermore, the sampling frame under the USEPA's Atrazine Monitoring Program is more intensive than the frame for low-risk CWSs, which allows more robust determination of monthly atrazine concentrations and minimizes the number of months missing data in this analysis. Despite the reduction in exposure misclassification by estimating atrazine for each unique water system, we remain unable to account for personal drinking water behaviors (e.g., use of bottled water or filters), which can substantially influence an individual's exposure. We lacked data on atrazine exposure from other sources such as diet, although atrazine residue is not often detected on food products and is not considered to be a significant contributor to overall atrazine exposure in the general population [37]. Furthermore, this study assessed the relationship between exposure to one contaminant and multiple birth outcomes, which does not address the fact that drinking water contains varying levels of multiple contaminants.

We made an assumption that the service boundaries of the AMP water systems in this study corresponded to the geographic boundaries of the city in which each was located. For nearly half of these water systems, we received verbal confirmation from treatment plant operators and water system managers that this was in fact the case. We performed a sensitivity analysis by restricting the gestational atrazine models to only these confirmed water systems to attempt to further reduce exposure misclassification. In this sub-group analysis, we saw consistent magnitude and direction of association between atrazine and term low birth weight compared with the full sample, but lacked sufficient numbers to detect a significant increase in odds of this rare outcome.

Our outcome and covariate data originated from birth certificates. The reliability of birth certificate data, however, varies widely by data element. Overall, the Ohio birth certificate data contained low levels (<3%) of missing data on the key covariates used in these analyses. A notable exception is the high level of missing data on prenatal care (26%). Those who were missing data on their prenatal care status were more likely to be non-Hispanic black, "Other" race/ethnicity, and young. We chose to only use those covariates that are considered to be well-reported and highly accurate on birth certificates, such as maternal age, race/ethnicity, marital status, parity, plurality, infant gender, birth weight, and gestational age [38–45].

We lacked information on whether or not the mothers of the infants in these analyses had moved at any point during their pregnancy and assumed that the residence listed on the birth certificate was the residence throughout the entire pregnancy. Rates of pregnancy mobility are estimated between 12 and 32% [46–49], and vary by geography and demographic factors.

Our study was restricted to a small percentage of births (3%) in the state of Ohio for this analysis of AMP water systems. The population in these AMP communities differed from the state population in important ways. A much higher percentage of infants were born to mothers who were non-Hispanic white (86%) compared to the state as a whole (76%). Additionally, these AMP communities had a higher proportion of births from women enrolled in WIC (50% versus 42%) and who reported smoking (35% versus 26%). The small sample size relative to the state population and the demographic differences between the AMP communities and the state as a whole limit the generalizability of the study results. Ideally, future research on the association between atrazine in drinking water and adverse birth outcomes would include a representative sample of births to increase the generalizability of study findings.

Despite these limitations, the study had several notable strengths. The exposure estimates used in this study are highly geographically and temporally refined, which allowed specific exposure windows, such as trimesters, to be examined. The large number of births included in this study allowed the examination of two rare outcomes, very preterm birth and very low birth weight, which have not been reported previously. Furthermore, this study also benefited from individual-level data on important covariates.

Our findings suggest that additional epidemiologic research should examine the reproductive effects of exposure to atrazine in areas of relatively low contaminant exposure. Ideally, future research would employ biomarkers of exposure or individual assessment of drinking water exposures rather than relying on the ecologic exposure measures presented in these analyses. Despite the limitations in the exposure ascertainment, our findings demonstrate that linking environmental monitoring data with health outcomes data, such as vital statistics databases, holds promise for identifying potential associations, which can subsequently be investigated using with more refined exposure and outcome ascertainment.

5. Conclusions

We found an association between atrazine concentrations in drinking water and the odds of term LBW births within communities served by water systems enrolled in USEPA's Atrazine Monitoring Program in Ohio. This is the first study to show such an association for term LBW by linking maternal residence to a specific water system. Water systems are enrolled in the AMP as a result of repeated exceedances of the 3 µg/L MCL for atrazine, but only 4% of samples from the water systems in this study exceeded the MCL. We observed an increase in the odds of term LBW births among those with average gestational atrazine below the current MCL. While further epidemiologic research is needed, these results suggest that the current MCL for atrazine may not be protective against some adverse birth outcomes such as term LBW.

Author Contributions: Conceptualization, K.S.A., L.T.S., and M.E.T.; Methodology, K.S.A., R.M.J, and S.F.; Formal Analysis, K.S.A.; Investigation, K.S.A., L.T.S., and M.E.T.; Data Curation, L.T.S., M.E.T., and R.M.J; Writing–Original Draft Preparation, K.S.A.; Writing–Review and Editing, K.S.A, M.E.T, R.M.J, K.R., S.F., L.T.S.; Funding Acquisition, L.T.S., M.E.T., R.M.J.

Funding: This research was supported in part by the US Centers for Disease and Control Prevention's Environmental Public Health Tracking Program (#200-2010-37442).

Conflicts of Interest: The authors declare no conflict of interest. The founding sponsors had no role in the design of the study; in the collection, analyses, or interpretation of data; in the writing of the manuscript, and in the decision to publish the results. The contents of this document including data analysis, interpretation or conclusions are solely the responsibility of the authors and do not represent the official views of Ohio Department of Health.

References

1. United States Environmental Protection Agency (USEPA) Atrazine Chemical Summary 2007. Available online: https://archive.epa.gov/region5/teach/web/pdf/atrazine_summary.pdf (accessed on 5 July 2018).
2. Jayachandran, K.; Steinheimer, T.R.; Somasundaram, L.; Moorman, T.B.; Kanwar, R.S.; Coats, J.R. Occurrence of atrazine and degradates as contaminants of subsurface drainage and shallow groundwater. *J. Environ. Qual.* **1994**, *23*, 311–319. [CrossRef]
3. Gilliom, R.J.; Barbash, J.E.; Crawford, C.G.; Hamilton, P.A.; Martin, J.D.; Nakagaki, N.; Nowell, L.; Scott, J.C.; Stackelberg, P.E.; Thelin, G.P.; et al. *Pesticides in the Nation's Streams and Ground Water, 1992–2001*; Revised February 2007; U.S. Geological Survey: Reston, VA, USA, 2006.
4. Quignot, N.; Arnaud, M.; Robidel, F.; Lecomte, A.; Tournier, M.; Cren-Olivé, C.; Barouki, R.; Lemazurier, E. Characterization of endocrine-disrupting chemicals based on hormonal balance disruption in male and female adult rats. *Reprod. Toxicol.* **2012**, *33*, 339–352. [CrossRef] [PubMed]
5. Vandenberg, L.N.; Colborn, T.; Hayes, T.B.; Heindel, J.J.; Jacobs, D.R.; Lee, D.H.; Shioda, T.; Soto, A.M.; vom Saal, F.S.; Welshons, W.V.; et al. Hormones and endocrine-disrupting chemicals: Low-dose effects and nonmonotonic dose responses. *Endocr. Rev.* **2012**, *33*, 378–455. [CrossRef] [PubMed]
6. Cooper, R.L.; Stoker, T.E.; Goldman, J.M.; Parrish, M.B.; Tyrey, L. Effect of atrazine on ovarian function in the rat. *Reprod. Toxicol.* **1996**, *10*, 257–264. [CrossRef]
7. Cooper, R.L.; Stoker, T.E.; Tyrey, L.; Goldman, J.M.; McElroy, W.K. Atrazine disrupts the hypothalamic control of pituitary-ovarian function. *Toxicol. Sci.* **2000**, *53*, 297–307. [CrossRef] [PubMed]
8. Victor-Costa, A.B.; Bandeira, S.M.C.; Oliveira, A.G.; Mahecha, G.A.B.; Oliveira, C.A. Changes in testicular morphology and steroidogenesis in adult rats exposed to Atrazine. *Reprod. Toxicol.* **2010**, *29*, 323–331. [CrossRef] [PubMed]
9. Zorrilla, L.M.; Gibson, E.K.; Stoker, T.E. The effects of simazine, a chlorotriazine herbicide, on pubertal development in the female Wistar rat. *Reprod. Toxicol.* **2010**, *29*, 393–400. [CrossRef] [PubMed]
10. Hayes, T.B.; Collins, A.; Lee, M.; Mendoza, M.; Noriega, N.; Stuart, A.A.; Vonk, A. Hermaphroditic, demasculinized frogs after exposure to the herbicide atrazine at low ecologically relevant doses. *Proc. Natl. Acad. Sci. USA* **2002**, *99*, 5476–5480. [CrossRef] [PubMed]
11. Hayes, T.B.; Khoury, V.; Narayan, A.; Nazir, M.; Park, A.; Brown, T.; Adame, L.; Chan, E.; Buchholz, D.; Stueve, T.; et al. Atrazine induces complete feminization and chemical castration in male African clawed frogs (*Xenopus laevis*). *Proc. Natl. Acad. Sci. USA* **2010**, *107*, 4612–4617. [CrossRef] [PubMed]
12. Stoker, T.E.; Laws, S.C.; Guidici, D.L.; Cooper, R.L. The effect of atrazine on puberty in male Wistar rats: An evaluation in the protocol for the assessment of pubertal development and thyroid function. *Toxicol. Sci.* **2000**, *58*, 50–59. [CrossRef] [PubMed]
13. Friedmann, A.S. Atrazine inhibition of testosterone production in rat males following peripubertal exposure. *Reprod. Toxicol.* **2002**, *16*, 275–279. [CrossRef]
14. Belloni, V.; Dessì-Fulgheri, F.; Zaccaroni, M.; Di Consiglio, E.; De Angelis, G.; Testai, E.; Santochirico, M.; Alleva, E.; Santucci, D. Early exposure to low doses of atrazine affects behavior in juvenile and adult CD1 mice. *Toxicology* **2011**, *279*, 19–26. [CrossRef] [PubMed]
15. Jin, Y.; Wang, L.; Fu, Z. Oral exposure to atrazine modulates hormone synthesis and the transcription of steroidogenic genes in male peripubertal mice. *Gen. Comp. Endocrinol.* **2013**, *184*, 120–127. [CrossRef] [PubMed]
16. Wetzel, L.T.; Luempert, L.G.; Breckenridge, C.B.; Tisdel, M.O.; Stevens, J.T.; Thakur, A.K.; Extrom, P.J.; Eldridge, J.C. Chronic effects of atrazine on estrus and mammary tumor formation in female Sprague-Dawley and Fischer 344 rats. *J. Toxicol. Environ. Health* **1994**, *43*, 169–182. [CrossRef] [PubMed]
17. Winchester, P.D.; Huskins, J.; Ying, J. Agrichemicals in surface water and birth defects in the United States. *Acta. Paediatr.* **2009**, *98*, 664–669. [CrossRef] [PubMed]

18. Munger, R.; Isacson, P.; Hu, S.; Burns, T.; Hanson, J.; Lynch, C.F.; Cherryholmes, K.; Van Dorpe, P.; Hausler, W.J. Intrauterine growth retardation in Iowa communities with herbicide-contaminated drinking water supplies. *Environ. Health Perspect.* **1997**, *105*, 308–314. [CrossRef] [PubMed]

19. Ochoa-Acuña, H.; Frankenberger, J.; Hahn, L.; Carbajo, C. Drinking-water herbicide exposure in Indiana and prevalence of small-for-gestational-age and preterm delivery. *Environ. Health Perspect.* **2009**, *117*, 1619–1624. [CrossRef] [PubMed]

20. Rinsky, J.L.; Hopenhayn, C.; Golla, V.; Browning, S.; Bush, H.M. Atrazine exposure in public drinking water and preterm birth. *Public Health Rep.* **2012**, *127*, 72–80. [CrossRef] [PubMed]

21. Stayner, L.T.; Almberg, K.; Jones, R.; Graber, J.; Pedersen, M.; Turyk, M. Atrazine and nitrate in drinking water and the risk of preterm delivery and low birth weight in four Midwestern states. *Environ. Res.* **2017**, *152*, 294–303. [CrossRef] [PubMed]

22. Chevrier, C.; Limon, G.; Monfort, C.; Rouget, F.; Garlantézec, R.; Petit, C.; Durand, G.; Cordier, S. Urinary biomarkers of prenatal atrazine exposure and adverse birth outcomes in the PELAGIE birth cohort. *Environ. Health Perspect.* **2011**, *119*, 1034–1041. [CrossRef] [PubMed]

23. 40 CFR 141.61-Maximum Contaminant Levels for Organic Contaminants. Available online: https://www.gpo.gov/fdsys/granule/CFR-2012-title40-vol24/CFR-2012-title40-vol24-sec141-61 (accessed on 5 July 2018).

24. United States Environmental Protection Agency (USEPA) Atrazine-Background and Updates. Available online: https://www.epa.gov/ingredients-used-pesticide-products/atrazine-background-and-updates#drinking-water (accessed on 5 July 2018).

25. Balluz, L.S. CDC's environmental public health tracking network: an innovative dynamic surveillance system for you. *J. Environ. Health* **2014**, *76*, 48–50. [PubMed]

26. Wilcox, A.J. *Fertility and Pregnancy: An. Epidemiologic Perspective*, 1st ed.; Oxford University Press: New York, NY, USA, 2010.

27. Duryea, E.L.; Hawkins, J.S.; McIntire, D.D.; Casey, B.M.; Leveno, K.J. A revised birth weight reference for the United States. *Obstet. Gynecol.* **2014**, *124*, 16–22. [CrossRef] [PubMed]

28. United States Environmental Protection Agency Atrazine Monitoring Program Data and Results. Available online: https://www.epa.gov/ingredients-used-pesticide-products/atrazine-monitoring-program-data-and-results (accessed on 5 July 2018).

29. Jones, R.M.; Stayner, L.T.; Demirtas, H. Multiple imputation for assessment of exposures to drinking water contaminants: Evaluation with the Atrazine Monitoring Program. *Environ. Res.* **2014**, *134*, 466–473. [CrossRef] [PubMed]

30. Kotelchuck, M. The adequacy of prenatal care utilization index: Its US distribution and association with low birthweight. *Am. J. Public Health* **1994**, *84*, 1486–1489. [CrossRef] [PubMed]

31. United States Department of Agriculture the Special Supplemental Nutrition Program for Women, Infants and Children (WIC Program) 2018. Available online: https://fns-prod.azureedge.net/sites/default/files/wic/wic-fact-sheet.pdf (accessed on 16 August 2018).

32. Centers for Disease Control and Prevention about Adult BMI | Healthy Weight | CDC. Available online: https://www.cdc.gov/healthyweight/assessing/bmi/adult_bmi/index.html (accessed on 5 July 2018).

33. *SAS*, version 9.4; SAS Institute: Cary, NC, USA, 2002.

34. Rayner, J.L.; Enoch, R.R.; Fenton, S.E. Adverse effects of prenatal exposure to atrazine during a critical period of mammary gland growth. *Toxicol. Sci.* **2005**, *87*, 255–266. [CrossRef] [PubMed]

35. Rayner, J.L.; Wood, C.; Fenton, S.E. Exposure parameters necessary for delayed puberty and mammary gland development in Long-Evans rats exposed in utero to atrazine. *Toxicol. Appl. Pharmacol.* **2004**, *195*, 23–34. [CrossRef] [PubMed]

36. Villanueva, C.M.; Durand, G.; Coutté, M.B.; Chevrier, C.; Cordier, S. Atrazine in municipal drinking water and risk of low birth weight, preterm delivery, and small-for-gestational-age status. *Occup. Environ. Med.* **2005**, *62*, 400–405. [CrossRef] [PubMed]

37. Agency for Toxic Substances and Disease Registry Toxicological Profile for Atrazine. Available online: https://www.atsdr.cdc.gov/toxprofiles/tp.asp?id=338&tid=59 (accessed on 27 August 2018).

38. Querec, L.J. Comparability of reporting between the birth certificate and the National Natality Survey. *Vital Health Stat. Ser. 2* **1980**, *83*, 1–44.

39. Schoendorf, K.C.; Parker, J.D.; Batkhan, L.Z.; Kiely, J.L. Comparability of the birth certificate and 1988 Maternal and Infant Health Survey. *Vital Health Stat. Ser. 2* **1993**, *116*, 1–19.

40. Green, D.C.; Moore, J.M.; Adams, M.M.; Berg, C.J.; Wilcox, L.S.; McCarthy, B.J. Are we underestimating rates of vaginal birth after previous cesarean birth? The validity of delivery methods from birth certificates. *Am. J. Epidemiol.* **1998**, *147*, 581–586. [CrossRef] [PubMed]

41. Reichman, N.E.; Hade, E.M. Validation of birth certificate data. A study of women in New Jersey's Health Start program. *Ann. Epidemiol.* **2001**, *11*, 186–193. [CrossRef]

42. DiGiuseppe, D.L.; Aron, D.C.; Ranbom, L.; Harper, D.L.; Rosenthal, G.E. Reliability of birth certificate data: A multi-hospital comparison to medical records information. *Matern. Child Health J.* **2002**, *6*, 169–179. [CrossRef] [PubMed]

43. Roohan, P.J.; Josberger, R.E.; Acar, J.; Dabir, P.; Feder, H.M.; Gagliano, P.J. Validation of birth certificate data in New York State. *J. Community Health* **2003**, *28*, 335–346. [CrossRef] [PubMed]

44. Northam, S.; Knapp, T.R. The reliability and validity of birth certificates. *J. Obstet. Gynecol. Neonatal Nurs.* **2006**, *35*, 3–12. [CrossRef] [PubMed]

45. Zollinger, T.W.; Przybylski, M.J.; Gamache, R.E. Reliability of Indiana birth certificate data compared to medical records. *Ann. Epidemiol.* **2006**, *16*, 1–10. [CrossRef] [PubMed]

46. Fell, D.B.; Dodds, L.; King, W.D. Residential mobility during pregnancy. *Paediatr. Perinat. Epidemiol.* **2004**, *18*, 408–414. [CrossRef] [PubMed]

47. Canfield, M.A.; Ramadhani, T.A.; Langlois, P.H.; Waller, D.K. Residential mobility patterns and exposure misclassification in epidemiologic studies of birth defects. *J. Expo. Sci. Environ. Epidemiol.* **2006**, *16*, 538–543. [CrossRef] [PubMed]

48. Miller, A.; Siffel, C.; Correa, A. Residential mobility during pregnancy: Patterns and correlates. *Matern. Child Health J.* **2010**, *14*, 625–634. [CrossRef] [PubMed]

49. Zender, R.; Bachand, A.M.; Reif, J.S. Exposure to tap water during pregnancy. *J. Expo. Anal. Environ. Epidemiol.* **2001**, *11*, 224–230. [CrossRef] [PubMed]

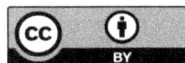

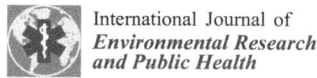

International Journal of
Environmental Research and Public Health

Article

Associations between Water Quality Measures and Chronic Kidney Disease Prevalence in Taiwan

Kuan Y. Chang [1,†], I-Wen Wu [2,†], Bo-Ruei Huang [1], Jih-Gau Juang [3], Jia-Chyi Wu [3], Su-Wei Chang [4,5] and Chung Cheng Chang [6,*]

[1] Department of Computer Science and Engineering, National Taiwan Ocean University, Keelung 202, Taiwan; kchang@ntou.edu.tw (K.Y.C.); rrayhhuang@gmail.com (B.-R.H.)
[2] Division of Nephrology, Keelung Chang Gung Memorial Hospital, Keelung 204, Taiwan; fliawu@yahoo.com
[3] Department of Communications, Navigation and Control Engineering, National Taiwan Ocean University, Keelung 202, Taiwan; jgjuang@mail.ntou.edu.tw (J.-G.J.); jcwu@mail.ntou.edu.tw (J.-C.W.)
[4] Clinical Informatics and Medical Statistics Research Center, College of Medicine, Chang Gung University, Taoyuan 333, Taiwan; shwchang@mail.cgu.edu.tw
[5] Division of Allergy, Asthma, and Rheumatology, Department of Pediatrics, Chang Gung Memorial Hospital at Linkou, Taoyuan 333, Taiwan
[6] Department of Electrical Engineering, National Taiwan Ocean University, Keelung 202, Taiwan
* Correspondence: ccchang@mail.ntou.edu.tw; Tel.: +886-2-2462-2192 (ext. 6350)
† These authors contributed equally to this work.

Received: 16 October 2018; Accepted: 28 November 2018; Published: 3 December 2018

Abstract: To determine the relationships between exposure to environmental contaminants in water and chronic kidney disease (CKD), we investigated the associations of 61 water attributes with the prevalence of CKD and End-Stage Renal Disease (ESRD) using data from 2005 to 2011 from all 22 counties and cities in the main island of Taiwan. We acquired patient information from the Taiwan Longitudinal Health Insurance Database to calculate the age-standardized CKD and ESRD prevalence rates and linked the patients' residences to the water quality monitoring data, which were sampled periodically for a total of over 45,000 observations obtained from the Taiwan Environmental Water Quality Information Database. The association analysis adjusting for gender, age, and annual effects showed that the zinc (Zn), ammonia, chemical oxygen demand (COD), and dissolved oxygen in rivers were weakly correlated with CKD ($\tau = 0.268/0.250/0.238/-0.267$, $p = 6.01 \times 10^{-6}/2.52 \times 10^{-5}/6.05 \times 10^{-5}/3.30 \times 10^{-5}$, respectively), but none for ESRD. The importances of Zn and COD in rivers were also demonstrated in a CKD regression model. Moreover, an unusually high CKD prevalence was related to arsenic contamination in groundwater. A further prospective cohort study would improve our understanding of what level of environmental water with risky properties could affect the development of CKD.

Keywords: chronic kidney disease; end-stage renal disease; water contaminants; zinc; ammonia; chemical oxygen demand; dissolved oxygen; arsenic

1. Introduction

Understanding risk factors is key to preventing and controlling the development of chronic kidney disease (CKD). The known risk factors for developing CKD can be put into four categories. First, demographic conditions. People at risk are, for example, female [1], over 75 years old [2], non-Hispanic blacks [3], receiving only primary education or no education [4,5], and having a family history of chronic renal diseases [6]. Second, comorbidities include diabetes [1,7], hypertension [1,8], metabolic syndrome [9], heart failure [10], hepatitis B [11], hepatitis C [12], glomerulonephritis [13], hyperuricemia [14], hyperlipidemia [1], anemia [15], and systemic lupus erythematosus [16]. Third, lifestyles, including smoking for more than five pack-years [17], drinking alcohol heavily with 30 g/day [18], betel nut chewing [19], exercising lightly with <30 min of bicycling per day or an equal amount of activities [20], and having a low water intake of <2.0 L/day [21]. The last category is environmental and physiological conditions, including having cadmium in one's blood and/or urine [22], lead in the blood [23], and organophosphorus herbicides in water [24]. A recent study even suggested that dehydration resulted from climate change may also be a risk factor for developing CKD [25]. Among all of these factors, diabetes and hypertension are highly recognized to associated with CKD [8,26].

Taiwan, infamous for the highest prevalence rate of end-stage renal disease (ESRD) in the world [27,28], has suffered the prevalence of CKD. CKD is also a global health problem. Approximately 13.4% of the world's population has CKD [29]. The CKD prevalence rate in Taiwan was approximately 11.9%, estimated by a large-scale study of 462,293 Taiwanese adults in 2006 [27]. In other words, approximately 2.03 million Taiwanese people had CKD [27]. CKD, which can be divided into five stages of increasing severity, is becoming an increasingly serious health problem worldwide. Until 2015, Taiwan had the highest prevalence of ESRD in the world (3317 cases per million people) [28]. A total of 77,920 Taiwanese patients received an ESRD diagnosis in 2015 [28]. ESRD is not only life-threatening and inconvenient for patients' daily living, but also a burden on the society's medical resources. Therefore, the early diagnosis and prevention of CKD are critical objectives in maintaining a healthy public.

Unprocessed raw water can affect one's health. Not only can unprocessed water be a source of drinking water, but it can also influence agricultural soils, plants, and animals, subsequently affecting our health. In Taiwan, three categories of water resources (reservoirs, rivers, and groundwater) dominate the sources of drinking water. About three-fourths drinking water is tap water [30]. More than half of tap water comes from reservoirs, about one third from surface water like rivers, and about ten percent from groundwater [31]. Raw water before drinking undergoes a series of water treatment processes, which involve physical, chemical, and biological processes in order to remove contaminants such as pesticides, organic pollutants, and volatile organics. Yet, the remaining contaminants may still be delivered into human bodies.

Although water is essential for kidney function, a full-scale investigation into the environment's exposure to water contaminants in the development of CKD/ERSD has yet to be conducted in Taiwan in order to identify any potential water-related risk factors for CKD/ESRD. This study aimed to investigate the associations between the 61 water attributes of the three water resources and the CKD/ESRD prevalence rates in Taiwan from 2005 to 2011. To our knowledge, this is the first study to assess the relationships between CKD/ESRD and a wide range of water properties in the environment.

2. Materials and Methods

To evaluate the relationships between large-scale water attributes and CKD/ESRD, an ecological study using longitudinal data was performed. The examined longitudinal data involved aggregated de-identified health records and water monitoring data in Taiwanese counties and cities from 2005 to 2011. The unit of observation was either a county or a city in a specific year. To detect a significant relationship, both the annual average water quality values and age-standardized CKD/ESRD prevalence rates of the subjects were utilized. An annual average water quality was derived from the data from all monitoring stations within a particular county or city in a year, where each sample was given an equal weight. Finally, to lower the Type I error, the significances of the 61 relationships were determined using partial correlation with a Bonferroni–Holm correction [32] at an α level of 0.01.

2.1. Study Area

Taiwan is a narrow and long island with a north-to-south orientation. The total area of the island is approximately 36,193 km². It is located southeast of the Asian continent and is part of the East Asian island arcs in the west bank of the Pacific Ocean. Located in the subtropical climate zone (23° N,

120° E), Taiwan neighbors the archipelagos of Japan and Ryukyu to the north, the Philippines to the south, and mainland China to the west. The two-thirds island area is dominated by rugged mountains that are covered by forests and the rest of the island consists of rolling hills, plateaus, coastal plains, and basins. There are a total of 22 counties and cities in Taiwan (Figure 1).

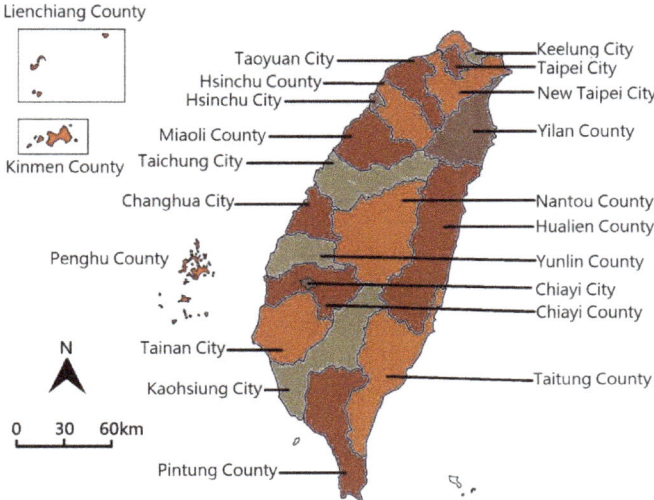

Figure 1. The 22 counties and cities in Taiwan. The map colors have no special meanings.

2.2. Water-Quality Monitoring Data

The water-monitoring data were acquired from the Environmental Water Quality Information Database maintained by the Environmental Protection Administration of Taiwan [33]. The monitoring data are divided into five categories according to the source of water resources: reservoirs, groundwater, rivers, beaches, and coastal oceans. Because water resources in Taiwan are distributed unevenly, the number of monitoring stations and observations in each county or city vary. Of all the 1096 water monitoring stations in Taiwan, 448 stations were for groundwater, 319 for rivers, 121 for reservoirs, 105 for coastal oceans, and 103 for beaches. Between 2005 and 2011, these stations collected a total of 51,037 water-monitoring observations, comprising 9345 observations of groundwater, 31,791 of rivers, 4710 of reservoirs, 2662 of oceans, and 2529 of beaches. We selected groundwater, rivers, and reservoirs to be examined because they are closely related to tap water.

There were 61 water quality measures that we examined: 23 for groundwater, 15 for reservoirs, and 23 for rivers. Each water resource monitored a different subset of 36 water quality items. A total of 20 of the 36 monitored items were specific metal or inorganic substances in water and the rest (16 items) belonged to the physicochemical and biological properties of water. Tables S1–S3 for groundwater, reservoirs, and rivers show the levels of water attributes in the study area.

2.3. CKD/ESRD Prevalence Rates

The age-adjusted standardized CKD/ESRD prevalence rates standardized by the World Health Organization (WHO) 2000–2025 standard population were used. This study adhered to the Declaration of Helsinki and was approved by the ethics committee of the Institutional Review Board of Chang Gung Memorial Hospital (IRB No. 100-4385A3 and 102-2508B). This study employed de-identified secondary data from the National Health Insurance Database (NHID) and thus was exempted from informed consent. The original prevalence data were retrieved from NHID, which covered almost 99%

of the entire population of Taiwan [34]. The prevalent CKD patients were defined by the presence of the several diagnostic codes (ICD-9-CM codes: 250.4, 274.1, 283.11, 403.1, 404.2, 404.3, 440.1, 442.1, 447.3, 572.3, 580–588, 593, 642.1, 646.2, and 753.1) in at least three ambulatory claims or one inpatient claim between 2005 and 2011. The prevalent ESRD patients were identified if the patient had both an ICD-9-CM code of 585 and an inclusion in the Registry for Catastrophic Illness [1,35–37], a rigorous requisite for the NHI payment of dialysis therapies. The details of ICD-9 codes for CKD and ESRD are listed at Tables A1 and A2. Those excluded were patients who died, who lacked IDs, who were less than 18 years old, and those who exited the insurance program or underwent renal transplantation. The township of cases was identified by the location of the medical setting of the patient with CKD. Briefly, the standardized prevalence rates were age-adjusted to the WHO 2000–2025 standard population using 18 age groups (0–4, 5–9, . . . , 80–84, 85+). The standardized CKD/ESRD prevalence rates of this study are consistent with those of previous studies [38–40].

Like the prevalence rates, the gender ratios—one of the controlling factors—were also standardized with age adjustment. The other demographic variables including the national population estimates, the townships' population densities, and the townships' population median ages were obtained from Taiwan's socio-economic database (http://segis.moi.gov.tw/STAT/). Out of the 25.56 million individuals enrolled in NHID, about 1,000,000 enrolled beneficiaries were randomly sampled in 2005 and were followed up with until 2011. Table 1 describes the baseline characteristics of the study population from 2005 to 2011.

Table 1. The baseline characteristics of the study population.

Year	2005	2006	2007	2008	2009	2010	2011
Total population, *n*	1,075,535	1,074,803	1,070,511	1,065,938	1,061,195	1,056,549	1,051,921
Age (mean ± SD)	36.4 ± 23.3	37.3 ± 23.4	38.2 ± 23.4	39.2 ± 23.4	40.1 ± 23.5	41.0 ± 23.5	41.9 ± 23.5
Age group							
<40	59.53%	58.30%	56.95%	55.58%	54.20%	52.77%	51.39%
40–49	15.84%	15.94%	16.12%	16.31%	16.42%	16.57%	16.67%
50–59	11.05%	11.89%	12.59%	13.17%	13.75%	14.29%	14.65%
60–69	6.66%	6.61%	6.73%	6.98%	7.30%	7.63%	8.17%
70–79	4.69%	4.80%	4.93%	5.03%	5.15%	5.29%	5.43%
>80	2.24%	2.46%	2.69%	2.93%	3.18%	3.45%	3.69%
Male	48.60%	48.53%	48.45%	48.37%	48.29%	48.21%	48.11%
CKD prevalence	4.00%	4.24%	4.49%	4.73%	4.97%	5.21%	5.53%
ESRD prevalence	0.20%	0.21%	0.23%	0.24%	0.26%	0.27%	0.28%
Comorbidity							
Diabetes	6.40%	7.00%	7.20%	8.20%	8.90%	9.60%	10.30%
Hypertension	11.70%	12.70%	13.80%	14.80%	15.80%	16.80%	17.80%
Hyperlipidemia	7.50%	8.50%	9.61%	10.70%	11.81%	12.90%	14.00%

CKD: chronic kidney disease; ESRD: end-stage renal disease.

2.4. Correlation between Water Quality and CKD/ESRD

To assess the relationship between the average water quality and the CKD/ESRD prevalence rates, partial Kendall correlations [41] were applied. Partial correlation $\tau_{yx \cdot z}$ calculates the correlation between X and Y by controlling Z or, more literally, by removing the effects of Z. Its formula is as follows:

$$\tau_{yx \cdot z} = \frac{\tau_{yx} - (\tau_{yz})(\tau_{xz})}{\sqrt{1 - \tau_{yz}^2}\sqrt{1 - \tau_{xz}^2}} \tag{1}$$

where τ_{yx}, τ_{zx}, and τ_{yz} are Kendall's correlations [42] between Y and X, Z and X, and Y and Z, respectively. The correlation magnitude was classified into four levels: strong ($1.0 \geq \tau \geq 0.7$), moderate ($0.7 > \tau \geq 0.4$), weak ($0.4 > \tau \geq 0.1$), and negligible ($0.1 > \tau \geq 0$). When the difference between $\tau_{yx \cdot z}$ and

τ_{yx} was negligible, Z had no effect on the relationship between Y and X, suggesting that Y and X may have a direct relationship. When $\tau_{yx \cdot z} < \tau_{yx}$, it meant that Y and X may have a spurious relationship or that Z may be a common cause or an intermediate factor between Y and X. When $\tau_{yx \cdot z} > \tau_{yx}$, the suggestion is that the effect of X on Y might be independent of that of Z on Y. In other words, X and Z have no correlation but, by removing the covariates between Y and Z, the correlation between Y and X improves. In our case, we aimed to control the confounding factors such as gender, age, annul, or time-dependent bias. That is, X, Y, and Z are water quality, the prevalence of CKD/ESRD, and control variables (population gender ratio, population median age, and sampling year), respectively. The "ppcor" package in R was used to perform the partial Kendall's correlation.

2.5. CKD Regression Analysis Using Selected Water Attributes

We built a CKD prevalence prediction model using nonparametric generalized additive models (GAMs) [43]. GAMs were used to associate the regional CKD prevalence rates as the dependent variable and the corresponding regional water attributes as the independent variables. In this study, multiple GAMs were constructed and the optimal model was determined using the Akaike Information Criterion [44]. A GAM adjusting for confounding sex, age, and year can be expressed as follows:

$$E(Y) = B_0 + s(Sex) + s(Age) + s(Year) + s_1(X_1) + s_2(X_2) + \cdots + s_n(X_n) \tag{2}$$

where $E(Y)$ refers to the expected regional CKD prevalence rate during the year, $s(\ )$ are the smoothing functions by splines, and X_i are the selected river quality attributes such as Zn, COD, DO, and NH_3. The "mgcv" package in R was applied to build the GAMs.

3. Results

3.1. Associations between Water Attributes and CKD in Taiwan

Table 2 presents the partial correlations adjusted for region-wise population, gender, age, and time-dependent annual effects between the water attributes and the CKD prevalence rates. Only four out of the 61 water attributes that passed the Bonferroni–Holm test displayed significant associations: the CKD prevalence rate was significantly correlated with the magnitude of Zn, ammonia (NH_3-N), and the chemical oxygen demand (COD) of rivers ($\tau = 0.268/0.250/0.238$, $p = 6.01 \times 10^{-6}/2.52 \times 10^{-5}/6.05 \times 10^{-5}$, respectively) and it was inversely correlated with the magnitude of the dissolved oxygen (DO) of rivers ($\tau = -0.267$, $p = 3.30 \times 10^{-5}$). The results indicated that a region with a higher CKD prevalence rate may be associated with a larger amount of Zn, ammonia, or COD of rivers, as well as a lower magnitude of DO of rivers.

3.2. Associations between Water Attributes and ESRD in Taiwan

Table 3 presents the partial correlations adjusted for region-wise population, gender, age, and time-dependent annual effects between the water attributes and the ESRD prevalence rates. None of the 61 water attributes displayed a significant association with the ESRD prevalence rates because they all failed the Bonferroni–Holm correction test.

3.3. Influential Observations Found in the Scatter Plots

Figure 2 illustrates the influential observations between arsenic in groundwater and CKD/ESRD. Seven highly influential observations that were far away from the other observations on the X axis were identified on the top right corner of Figure 2. We realized that all these high influencers came from the same region, Chiayi city. A clear trend was revealed in that the arsenic in the groundwater accompanying the CKD/ESRD prevalence in Chiayi city increased with time. The Z-score bar chart of all the monitored substances of Chiayi city (Figure S1) indicates that Chiayi city was like the other places in Taiwan except that it had an unusual high level of arsenic in the groundwater, with a Z-score was 3.85. In other words, the concentration of arsenic in the groundwater in Chiayi city was over 75 μg/L, a value that was exceptionally higher than those of the other regions in Taiwan.

Table 2. The correlation between water attribute and age-standardized CKD prevalence rate, adjusting for gender, age, and annual effects (2005–2011).

Substance	Groundwater		Reservoir		River	
	τ	*p*-Value	τ	*p*-Value	τ	*p*-Value
Metal and Inorganics						
Ag	-		-		−0.088	0.139
As	0.140	0.018	-		0.074	0.213
Ca	0.007	0.902	-		-	
Cd	0.089	0.132	-		−0.038	0.520
Cl	−0.007	0.912	-		-	
Cr	−0.072	0.227	-		−0.009	0.873
Cu	−0.057	0.335	-		0.022	0.714
Fe	−0.091	0.126	-		-	
Hg	-		-		−0.017	0.779
K	0.005	0.933	-		-	
Mg	0.044	0.457	-		-	
Mn	−0.028	0.636	-		0.032	0.594
Na	0.070	0.236	-		-	
NH_3-N	0.030	0.613	−0.077	0.282	0.250 **	2.52×10^{-5} **
NO_2-N	-		−0.073	0.363	0.211 *	3.79×10^{-4} *
NO_3-N	−0.180	0.002	0.078	0.272	0.191	0.001
Pb	−0.034	0.568	-		0.059	0.318
Se	-		-		−0.061	0.383
SO_4^{2-}	−0.010	0.869	-		-	
Zn	−0.047	0.426	-		0.268 **	6.01×10^{-6} **
Physicochemical and biological properties						
Alk	0.090	0.128	0.266 *	1.89×10^{-4} *	-	
BOD	-		-		0.222 *	1.84×10^{-4} *
Chl-A	-		0.021	0.773	-	
COD	-		0.032	0.648	0.238 **	6.05×10^{-5} **
Coliform	-		-		0.148	0.013
DO	-		0.031	0.687	−0.267 **	3.30×10^{-5} **
EC	0.062	0.292	0.159	0.026	−0.048	0.416
pH	0.125	0.035	0.015	0.833	−0.194	0.001
SD	-		−0.088	0.276	-	
SS	-		0.197	0.006	0.022	0.706
TB	-		0.167	0.019	-	
TDS	0.051	0.389	-		-	
TH	0.019	0.745	0.174	0.014	-	
TKN	-		-		0.235	0.044
TOC	0.031	0.597	0.035	0.627	0.181	0.002
WT	0.130	0.028	0.036	0.618	0.143	0.016

Significance levels of the Bonferroni–Holm test: ** $\leq$ 0.01, * $\leq$ 0.05. Abbreviations: Alk: Alkalinity; BOD: Biochemical Oxygen Demand; Chl-A: Chlorophyll-A; COD: Chemical Oxygen Demand; DO: Dissolved Oxygen; EC: Electrical conductivity; SD: Secchi Depth (Transparency); SS: Suspended Solids; TB: Turbidity; TDS: Total Dissolved Solids; TH: Total Hardness; TKN: Total Kjeldahl nitrogen; TOC: Total Organic Carbon; WT: Water Temperature.

Table 3. The correlation between water attribute and age-standardized ESRD prevalence rate adjusting for gender, age, and annual effects (2005–2011).

Substance	Groundwater		Reservoir		River	
	τ	*p*-Value	τ	*p*-Value	τ	*p*-Value
Metal and Inorganics						
Ag	-		-		−0.034	0.568
As	0.106	0.073	-		−0.017	0.777
Ca	0.007	0.900	-		-	
Cd	0.165	0.005	-		0.021	0.718
Cl	−0.058	0.379	-		-	
Cr	−0.043	0.472	-		−0.009	0.878
Cu	−0.061	0.300	-		0.004	0.949
Fe	−0.079	0.182	-		-	
Hg	-		-		−0.080	0.179
K	−0.112	0.058	-		-	
Mg	−0.097	0.100	-		-	
Mn	−0.016	0.793	-		0.074	0.214
Na	−0.059	0.319	-		-	
NH_3-N	0.018	0.764	−0.176	0.013	0.094	0.111
NO_2-N	-		−0.064	0.426	0.109	0.067
NO_3-N	−0.113	0.057	0.055	0.441	0.086	0.149
Pb	0.030	0.616	-		0.046	0.438
Se	-		-		−0.012	0.867
SO_4^{2-}	−0.103	0.084	-		-	
Zn	−0.135	0.023	-		0.167	0.005
Physicochemical and biological properties						
Alk	0.005	0.932	−0.008	0.914	-	
BOD	-		-		0.073	0.215
Chl-A	-		−0.017	0.807	-	
COD	-		−0.056	0.429	0.138	0.020
Coliform	-		-		0.018	0.762
DO	-		0.052	0.501	−0.056	0.388
EC	−0.033	0.577	−0.096	0.178	−0.081	0.172
pH	0.100	0.090	−0.134	0.060	−0.132	0.026
SD	-		0.047	0.560	-	
SS	-		−0.021	0.768	−0.044	0.459
TB	-		0.002	0.973	-	
TDS	−0.021	0.728	-		-	
TH	−0.018	0.766	−0.088	0.218	-	
TKN	-		-		−0.047	0.685
TOC	−0.046	0.439	−0.050	0.486	0.077	0.077
WT	0.010	0.865	0.014	0.845	0.054	0.364

None passed the Bonferroni–Holm test. Abbreviations: Alk: Alkalinity; BOD: Biochemical Oxygen Demand; Chl-A: Chlorophyll-A; COD: Chemical Oxygen Demand; DO: Dissolved Oxygen; EC: Electrical conductivity; SD: Secchi Depth (Transparency); SS: Suspended Solids; TB: Turbidity; TDS: Total Dissolved Solids; TH: Total Hardness; TKN: Total Kjeldahl nitrogen; TOC: Total Organic Carbon; WT: Water Temperature.

We performed an additional analysis by excluding Chiayi city because we suspected that the arsenic in the groundwater of Chiayi city could dominate the association of the CKD/ESRD prevalence. However, albeit with some differences, the associations were rather stable.

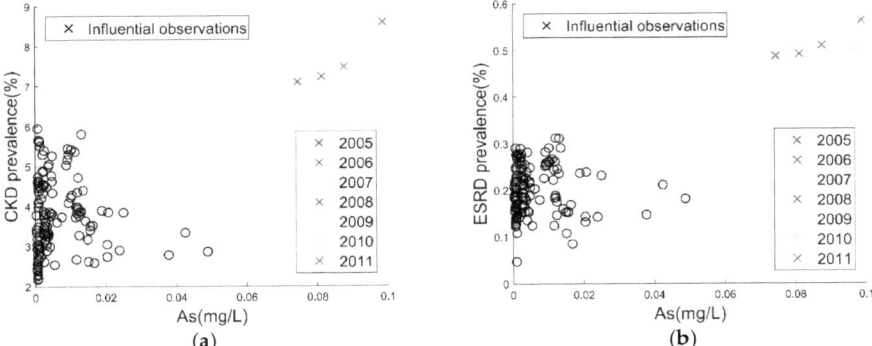

Figure 2. The relationship between arsenic in groundwater and age-standardized chronic kidney disease (CKD)/ end-stage renal disease (ESRD) prevalence rates (2005–2011): (**a**) the CKD prevalence rate in groundwater and (**b**) the ESRD prevalence rate in groundwater. The influential observations are labeled by the color-coded year symbols '×'.

3.4. Optimal CKD Regression Model Using Selected River Attributes

Table 4 indicates that the GAM built by Zn and the COD of rivers with confounding covariates (sex, age, and year) was the optimal model with the minimum AIC value (−987.6). The larger model with one additional parameter (NH_3) and the smaller model that considered only Zn had similar AIC performance values to the optimal model, differing by AIC values of 1.3 and 2.4, respectively.

Table 4. The generalized additive models (GAMs) of CKD prevalence in Taiwan using selected river attributes.

Model	AIC	ΔAIC	R^2	DE (%)
sex + age + year	−955.0	32.6	0.742	70.7
sex + age + year + COD	−972.2	15.4	0.769	75.0
sex + age + year + DO	−844.2	143.4	0.788	77.2
sex + age + year + NH_3	−973.0	14.6	0.772	75.6
sex + age + year + Zn	−985.2	2.4	0.821	78.2
sex + age + year + Zn + COD	−987.6	0	0.820	78.8
sex + age + year + Zn + DO	−846.5	141.1	0.805	78.2
sex + age + year + Zn + NH_3	−983.9	3.7	0.817	78.5
sex + age + year + Zn + COD + NH_3	−986.3	1.3	0.818	78.9
sex + age + year + Zn + COD + DO + NH_3	−850.3	137.3	0.809	80.1

$\Delta AIC_i = AIC_i - AIC_{min}$; Abbreviations: AlC: Akaike Information Criterion; COD: Chemical Oxygen Demand; DE: Deviance explained; DO: Dissolved Oxygen.

4. Discussion

To our knowledge, this is the first ecological study with seven years of monitoring to associate the CKD and ESRD prevalence rates with a wide range of water attributes of the environment. We found that Zn, ammonia, COD, and DO of rivers were weakly correlated with the CKD prevalence rates, but none of them were linked to ESRD under the stringent Bonferroni–Holm test.

The GAM with the Zn and COD of rivers was the best model for the given data (Table 4). Although including additional NH_3 or omitting COD in the model led to a similar AIC performance when compared to the best model, the results did not support the inclusion of one more parameter (NH_3). However, the necessity of the inclusion of COD in the model was unclear. The differences in AIC did not support the notion that the Zn only model was substantially inferior to the best model.

Zn in the environment has been linked to CKD. In fact, both our correlation and regression results supported that Zn was a relatively stronger indicator of CKD prevalence than the three other river attributes. A recent study that indicated that Zn in residential soil was a risk factor for CKD progression also supports our findings [45]. We suspect that a Zn contaminated river, which can pollute soil, may reach CKD patients in the same way that Zn contaminated soil does. On the other hand, Zn homeostasis is important for kidney function. A Zn deficiency is present in CKD patients [46]. Although oxidized Zn particles which interfere with Zn homeostasis in rats are toxic [47], further investigations are needed to confirm whether exposure to environmental Zn could cause the development of CKD in humans.

To our knowledge, this is also the first report to link environmental water quality indicators to CKD in humans. Ammonia, COD, and DO all are indicative measures of water quality. They are interrelated in some way. For example, ammonia can acidify water, consume oxygen, and raise the COD. Ammonia can be a key indicator to determine whether water resources are undergoing anthropogenic pollution. Excessive anthropogenic pollutants—which mainly come from unprocessed livestock wastewater, domestic sewage, and industrial manufacturing—are enriched with ammonia. Elevated levels of ammonia in the water have been demonstrated to degenerate the kidneys of Nile tilapia [48]. However, further studies are needed to verify its role in humans.

Like a high level of ammonia in water, a low DO may mean a poor water quality. A low DO may be caused by overfertilization, causing water plants to overgrow and dead plants to draw a lot of bacteria, which, in turn, depletes the DO level. A river with a lower DO can support less aquatic organisms, implying that the environment's water is more toxic. A region with a lower DO may mean that its environment is more toxic, thus linking it to CKD patients. Besides, hypoxia, a condition defined by the body being deprived of oxygen, is known to accelerate CKD progression [49]. An adequate oxygen supply is important for the functioning of the kidneys. However, it is unclear whether oxygen-deprived water would reduce the oxygen levels in the kidneys.

A high COD, which indicates more oxidizable pollutants, also suggest that the environment is more toxic in our findings. However, there is a lack of direct evidence that a high COD in water would lead to the development of CKD.

Our results linked arsenic in groundwater to higher CKD prevalence. In fact, the relationship between arsenic and CKD has been extensively studied. Previous animal research on mice and dogs confirmed that exposure to arsenic may damage kidney function [50,51]. A recent systematic review of studies on exposure to arsenic and kidney disease mortality in humans over the past 30 years found evidence that generally supported a positive association between the arsenic and CKD [52]. Our study strengthens their finding through the prevalence rate of kidney disease, not the mortality rate, suggesting that exposure to arsenic in groundwater may relate to the development of CKD/ESRD in Taiwan.

The alarmingly high arsenic concentration in groundwater concurrent with the high prevalence rate of CKD/ESRD in Chiayi city might be the best example to demonstrate a plausible link between exposure to arsenic and CKD/ESRD. Low-dose arsenic levels did not exhibit a clear correlation, suggesting that arsenic in groundwater may need to pass a certain threshold to be associated with CKD/ESRD. Because arsenic exists in the natural environment, such as in the soil, air, water, and food, it may enter human bodies through breathing, drinking, or eating. Chiayi is infamous for its 1950s Blackfoot disease endemic [53], which resulted from the exposure to arsenic in drinking water from artesian wells, consequently impairing the blood vessels of the lower limbs of patients and causing them to develop gangrene. Based on the 1962 groundwater data, two ecological studies linked arsenic to the increased mortality of kidney disease in Chiayi [54,55]. They also indicated the exposure to arsenic in locals had since ceased [54,55]. Instead, we used contemporary water monitoring data to associate arsenic with the prevalence of kidney disease. The results led us to speculate the possible long latent effects of arsenic or the recurrent arsenic contamination in Chiayi in its drinking water, crops, or farmed seafood. A recent study reported that arsenic in drinking water in Taiwan was linked to the progression of CKD [56]. However, further investigations are needed to verify our speculation.

Because this was a longitudinal study, patients enrolled in this ecological population-based study were aging. Some died and the population declined each year. The mean age of our patients may be older than the national estimate because only those older than 18 years were included in our analysis. Younger patients were excluded from the study to avoid possible confounding effects in renal diseases that are genetic disorders. However, the aging and shrinking populations should not affect our results as the age factor was controlled and the prevalence rates were applied in our analyses.

The reason why CKD and ESRD did not share the same correlation magnitude with water attributes may either be due to random fluctuations or may involve a complex progression of kidney disease. To determine the reason, more information is required.

Limitations and Strengths

This study has some limitations. First, this is an observational study at the city or county level so we cannot account for cases smaller than a city or county (e.g., a town or village). Second, although we already adjusted for the gender, age, and annual effects, we still cannot eliminate the possibility that the associations may result from other confounding factors that we did not adjust for. Third, we did not have direct quality measures of drinking water. We instead examined three related water resources. Thus, oral exposure may not necessarily be the same as the environmental exposure studied here. Fourth, unlike incidence cases, prevalence may not capture the full risks of abruptly developing diseases. However, to manifest a renal disease, a long-term exposure may be needed. The exact date at which the exposure started is unknown and to follow up from the first exposure is unfeasible due to the burden of the disease [57,58]. We thus preferred using prevalence data instead of incident cases to measure the burden of the disease during a seven-year time lapse in the Taiwanese population in this ecological study.

However, the use of nationwide health data; the extensive coverage of inorganic, physicochemical, and biological properties of water quality data; and computational analyses adjusted for important covariates, have strengthened the conjecture of this study. Although unmeasured confounders may be still present, we adjusted our data to all the possible covariates whose data were available to us. Needless to say, environmental raw water is important not only because it can be a source of drinking water but also because it is connected to our health through the food chain via agriculture and animals. Although the three water resources were only an approximate to drinking water, they—representing the majority of drinking water sources in Taiwan—were the best ones with a massive amount of information available for this study. Overall, we examined a total of 45,846 water-monitoring observations between 2005 and 2011 to address the issue of the temporality of association. Consequently, the monitored water attributes were found to correlate with the national cohort of patients since 2005 and to 2011 in the development of CKD or ESRD. The seven years of data should be reliable enough to establish meaningful associations in a clinical setting.

In fact, this study has several implications. First, the poor water quality in the environment may be linked to renal disease. Second, regulatory water monitoring of these suspicious contaminants should be strictly done from a public health perspective. Third, water with highly suspicious contaminants should be re-treated or drunk with caution. Fourth, water quality management could be imperative for current public health policymaking. Finally, further clinical trials should be warranted to assure the exact roles of the implicated environmental contaminants, such as Zn in rivers, in renal disease mechanisms.

5. Conclusions

Environmental exposure to water containments such as heavy metal Zn is weakly but significantly associated with CKD. Out of the 61 water attributes, only the rivers' Zn, ammonia, and COD, as well as DO, were found to be weakly correlated with the CKD prevalence rates. Moreover, arsenic contamination in groundwater may be linked to an unusually high CKD prevalence. To confirm our findings, further investigation of individual exposure to the exact amount of water containments should be conducted. Reducing water pollution and better managing the water quality may benefit public health and CKD patients.

Supplementary Materials: Supplementary materials can be found at http://www.mdpi.com/1660-4601/15/12/2726/s1, Figure S1: The Z-score bar chart of monitoring water attributes of Chiayi City, Taiwan. Table S1: Descriptive statistics for groundwater in Taiwan. Table S2: Descriptive statistics for reservoirs in Taiwan. Table S3: Descriptive statistics for rivers in Taiwan.

Author Contributions: K.Y.C., J.-G.J., J.-C.W. and C.C.C. conceived and designed the experiments; K.Y.C. and B.-R.H. performed the experiments; K.Y.C., I. -W.W., B.-R.H. and S.-W.C. analyzed the data; K.Y.C. and I.-W.W. contributed reagents/materials/analysis tools; K.Y.C. and I.-W.W. wrote the paper.

Acknowledgments: The authors thank Andy Liu, Tim Li, and Tien-Ling Tsai for technical support and Shwu-Jing Chang for the helpful discussion in the early stage of this study. The work was supported by National Taiwan Ocean University (NTOU-106-012) and the Chang Gung Memorial Hospital Research Projects (CMRPG2C0093 and CLRPG2C0021). This work was based in part on data from the NHIRD-TW provided by the National Health Insurance Administration, Ministry of Health and Welfare and managed by the National Health Research Institutes (registration number: NHIRD-102-238). The interpretations and conclusions contained herein do not represent those of the National Health Insurance Administration, Ministry of Health and Welfare or National Health Research Institutes.

Conflicts of Interest: The authors declare no conflict of interest. The founding sponsors had no role in the design of the study; in the collection, analyses, or interpretation of data; in the writing of the manuscript, and in the decision to publish the results.

Abbreviations

The following abbreviations are used in this manuscript:

Alk	Alkalinity
BOD	Biochemical Oxygen Demand
Chl-A	Chlorophyll-A
CKD	Chronic Kidney Disease
COD	Chemical Oxygen Demand
DO	Dissolved Oxygen
EC	Electrical conductivity
ESRD	End Stage Renal Disease
SD	Secchi Depth (Transparency)
SS	Suspended Solids
TB	Turbidity
TDS	Total Dissolved Solids
TH	Total Hardness
TKN	Total Kjeldahl nitrogen
TOC	Total Organic Carbon
WHO	World Health Organization
WT	Water Temperature

Appendix A

Table A1. ICD-9 codes for CKD and ESRD.

Disease	ICD-9 Codes
CKD	250.4, 274.1, 283.11, 403.1, 404.2, 404.3, 440.1, 442.1, 447.3, 572.3, 580–588, 593, 642.1, 646.2, 753.1
ESRD	585 and associates

Table A2. Description of ICD-9 codes.

ICD-9 Codes	Disease Description
250.4	Diabetic Nephropathy
274.1	Gouty Nephropathy
283.11	Hemolytic Uremic Syndrome
403.1	Hypertensive Nephropathy
404.2	Malignant hypertension with renal and cardiac complication
404.2	Malignant hypertension with renal and cardiac failure
440.1	Renovascular atherosclerotic disease
442.1	Aneurysm of renovascular system
447.3	Renovascular hyperplasia
572.3	Renovascular hypertension
580	Acute glomerulonephritis
581	Nephrotic syndrome
582	Chronic glomerulonephritis
583	Nephritis and renal disease
584	Acute kidney failure
585	Chronic kidney failure
586	Kidney failure
587	Renal sclerosis
588	Disease complicated by renal failure
593	Renal and ureter disease
642.1	Gestational, pregnancy related renal disease
646.2	Gestational, pregnancy related renal disease
753.1	Polycystic kidney disease

References

1. Kuo, H.W.; Tsai, S.S.; Tiao, M.M.; Yang, C.Y. Epidemiological features of CKD in Taiwan. *Am. J. Kidney Dis.* **2007**, *49*, 46–55. [CrossRef] [PubMed]
2. Yamagata, K.; Ishida, K.; Sairenchi, T.; Takahashi, H.; Ohba, S.; Shiigai, T.; Narita, M.; Koyama, A. Risk factors for chronic kidney disease in a community-based population: A 10-year follow-up study. *Kidney Int.* **2007**, *71*, 159–166. [CrossRef] [PubMed]
3. Sarathy, H.; Henriquez, G.; Abramowitz, M.K.; Kramer, H.; Rosas, S.E.; Johns, T.; Kumar, J.; Skversky, A.; Kaskel, F.; Melamed, M.L. Abdominal obesity, race and chronic kidney disease in young adults: Results from NHANES 1999–2010. *PLoS ONE* **2016**, *11*, e0153588. [CrossRef] [PubMed]
4. Tsai, S.Y.; Tseng, H.F.; Tan, H.F.; Chien, Y.S.; Chang, C.C. End-stage renal disease in Taiwan: A case-control study. *J. Epidemiol.* **2009**, *19*, 169–176. [CrossRef]
5. Vart, P.; Gansevoort, R.T.; Crews, D.C.; Reijneveld, S.A.; Bultmann, U. Mediators of the association between low socioeconomic status and chronic kidney disease in the United States. *Am. J. Epidemiol.* **2015**, *181*, 385–396. [CrossRef]
6. Wanigasuriya, K.P.; Peiris-John, R.J.; Wickremasinghe, R.; Hittarage, A. Chronic renal failure in north central province of Sri Lanka: An environmentally induced disease. *Trans. R. Soc. Trop. Med. Hyg.* **2007**, *101*, 1013–1017. [CrossRef]
7. Lin, M.Y.; Chiu, Y.W.; Lee, C.H.; Yu, H.Y.; Chen, H.C.; Wu, M.T.; Hwang, S.J. Factors associated with CKD in the elderly and nonelderly population. *Clin. J. Am. Soc. Nephrol.* **2013**, *8*, 33–40. [CrossRef]
8. Bang, H.; Vupputuri, S.; Shoham, D.A.; Klemmer, P.J.; Falk, R.J.; Mazumdar, M.; Gipson, D.; Colindres, R.E.; Kshirsagar, A.V. Screening for occult renal disease (scored): A simple prediction model for chronic kidney disease. *Arch. Intern. Med.* **2007**, *167*, 374–381. [CrossRef]
9. Singh, A.K.; Kari, J.A. Metabolic syndrome and chronic kidney disease. *Curr. Opin. Nephrol. Hypertens.* **2013**, *22*, 198–203. [CrossRef]
10. Liu, M.; Li, X.C.; Lu, L.; Cao, Y.; Sun, R.R.; Chen, S.; Zhang, P.Y. Cardiovascular disease and its relationship with chronic kidney disease. *Eur. Rev. Med. Pharmacol. Sci.* **2014**, *18*, 2918–2926.
11. Ayodele, O.E.; Salako, B.L.; Kadiri, S.; Arije, A.; Alebiosu, C.O. Hepatitis b virus infection: Implications in chronic kidney disease, dialysis and transplantation. *Afr. J. Med. Med. Sci.* **2006**, *35*, 111–119. [PubMed]

12. Chen, Y.C.; Lin, H.Y.; Li, C.Y.; Lee, M.S.; Su, Y.C. A nationwide cohort study suggests that hepatitis c virus infection is associated with increased risk of chronic kidney disease. *Kidney Int.* **2014**, *85*, 1200–1207. [CrossRef] [PubMed]

13. Warady, B.A.; Abraham, A.G.; Schwartz, G.J.; Wong, C.S.; Munoz, A.; Betoko, A.; Mitsnefes, M.; Kaskel, F.; Greenbaum, L.A.; Mak, R.H.; et al. Predictors of rapid progression of glomerular and nonglomerular kidney disease in children and adolescents: The chronic kidney disease in children (CKID) cohort. *Am. J. Kidney Dis.* **2015**, *65*, 878–888. [CrossRef] [PubMed]

14. Johnson, R.J.; Nakagawa, T.; Jalal, D.; Sanchez-Lozada, L.G.; Kang, D.H.; Ritz, E. Uric acid and chronic kidney disease: Which is chasing which? *Nephrol. Dial. Transplant.* **2013**, *28*, 2221–2228. [CrossRef] [PubMed]

15. Stauffer, M.E.; Fan, T. Prevalence of anemia in chronic kidney disease in the United States. *PLoS ONE* **2014**, *9*, e84943. [CrossRef] [PubMed]

16. Pokroy-Shapira, E.; Gelernter, I.; Molad, Y. Evolution of chronic kidney disease in patients with systemic lupus erythematosus over a long-period follow-up: A single-center inception cohort study. *Clin. Rheumatol.* **2014**, *33*, 649–657. [CrossRef] [PubMed]

17. Orth, S.R.; Ogata, H.; Ritz, E. Smoking and the kidney. *Nephrol. Dial. Transplant.* **2000**, *15*, 1509–1511. [CrossRef] [PubMed]

18. White, S.L.; Polkinghorne, K.R.; Cass, A.; Shaw, J.E.; Atkins, R.C.; Chadban, S.J. Alcohol consumption and 5-year onset of chronic kidney disease: The AUSDIAB study. *Nephrol. Dial. Transplant.* **2009**, *24*, 2464–2472. [CrossRef]

19. Kang, I.M.; Chou, C.Y.; Tseng, Y.H.; Huang, C.C.; Ho, W.Y.; Shih, C.M.; Chen, W. Association between betelnut chewing and chronic kidney disease in adults. *J. Occup. Environ. Med.* **2007**, *49*, 776–779. [CrossRef]

20. Eidemak, I.; Haaber, A.B.; Feldt-Rasmussen, B.; Kanstrup, I.L.; Strandgaard, S. Exercise training and the progression of chronic renal failure. *Nephron* **1997**, *75*, 36–40. [CrossRef]

21. Sontrop, J.M.; Dixon, S.N.; Garg, A.X.; Buendia-Jimenez, I.; Dohein, O.; Huang, S.-H.S.; Clark, W.F. Association between water intake, chronic kidney disease, and cardiovascular disease: A cross-sectional analysis of NHANES data. *Am. J. Nephrol.* **2013**, *37*, 434–442. [CrossRef] [PubMed]

22. Ferraro, P.M.; Costanzi, S.; Naticchia, A.; Sturniolo, A.; Gambaro, G. Low level exposure to cadmium increases the risk of chronic kidney disease: Analysis of the NHANES 1999–2006. *BMC Public Health* **2010**, *10*, 304. [CrossRef]

23. Muntner, P.; He, J.; Vupputuri, S.; Coresh, J.; Batuman, V. Blood lead and chronic kidney disease in the general United States population: Results from NHANES III. *Kidney Int.* **2003**, *63*, 1044–1050. [CrossRef]

24. Jayasumana, C.; Gunatilake, S.; Senanayake, P. Glyphosate, hard water and nephrotoxic metals: Are they the culprits behind the epidemic of chronic kidney disease of unknown etiology in Sri Lanka? *Int. J. Environ. Res. Public health* **2014**, *11*, 2125–2147. [CrossRef]

25. Glaser, J.; Lemery, J.; Rajagopalan, B.; Diaz, H.F.; Garcia-Trabanino, R.; Taduri, G.; Madero, M.; Amarasinghe, M.; Abraham, G.; Anutrakulchai, S.; et al. Climate change and the emergent epidemic of CKD from heat stress in rural communities: The case for heat stress nephropathy. *Clin. J. Am. Soc. Nephrol.* **2016**, *11*, 1472–1483. [CrossRef]

26. Plummer, M.; Franceschi, S.; Vignat, J.; Forman, D.; de Martel, C. Global burden of gastric cancer attributable to helicobacter pylori. *Int. J. Cancer* **2015**, *136*, 487–490. [CrossRef]

27. Wen, C.P.; Cheng, T.Y.; Tsai, M.K.; Chang, Y.C.; Chan, H.T.; Tsai, S.P.; Chiang, P.H.; Hsu, C.C.; Sung, P.K.; Hsu, Y.H.; et al. All-cause mortality attributable to chronic kidney disease: A prospective cohort study based on 462 293 adults in Taiwan. *Lancet* **2008**, *371*, 2173–2182. [CrossRef]

28. Saran, R.; Robinson, B.; Abbott, K.C.; Agodoa, L.Y.C.; Bhave, N.; Bragg-Gresham, J.; Balkrishnan, R.; Dietrich, X.; Eckard, A.; Eggers, P.W.; et al. Us renal data system 2017 annual data report: Epidemiology of kidney disease in the United States. *Am. J. Kidney Dis.* **2018**, *71*, A7. [CrossRef] [PubMed]

29. Hill, N.R.; Fatoba, S.T.; Oke, J.L.; Hirst, J.A.; O'Callaghan, C.A.; Lasserson, D.S.; Hobbs, F.D. Global prevalence of chronic kidney disease—A systematic review and meta-analysis. *PLoS ONE* **2016**, *11*, e0158765. [CrossRef] [PubMed]

30. Environmental Protection Administration. *Investigation on Household Drinking Water in Taiwan (Translation)*; Environmental Protection Administration: Taipei, Taiwan, 2014.

31. Taiwan Water Corporation. *2017 Annual Report on Taiwan Tap Water (Translation)*; Taiwan Water Corporation: Taipei, Taiwan, 2017; Volume 40.

32. Holm, S. A simple sequentially rejective multiple test procedure. *Scand. J. Stat.* **1979**, *6*, 65–70.

33. Taiwan Environmental Water Quality Information Database. Available online: http://wq.epa.gov.tw/Code/ ?Languages=en (accessed on 17 February 2017).

34. Morrison, D.S.; Parr, C.L.; Lam, T.H.; Ueshima, H.; Kim, H.C.; Jee, S.H.; Murakami, Y.; Giles, G.; Fang, X.; Barzi, F.; et al. Behavioural and metabolic risk factors for mortality from colon and rectum cancer: Analysis of data from the Asia-Pacific cohort studies collaboration. *Asian Pac. J. Cancer Prev.* **2013**, *14*, 1083–1087. [CrossRef]

35. Quan, H.; Sundararajan, V.; Halfon, P.; Fong, A.; Burnand, B.; Luthi, J.C.; Saunders, L.D.; Beck, C.A.; Feasby, T.E.; Ghali, W.A. Coding algorithms for defining comorbidities in ICD-9-cm and ICD-10 administrative data. *Med. Care* **2005**, *43*, 1130–1139. [CrossRef]

36. Navaneethan, S.D.; Jolly, S.E.; Schold, J.D.; Arrigain, S.; Saupe, W.; Sharp, J.; Lyons, J.; Simon, J.F.; Schreiber, M.J., Jr.; Jain, A.; et al. Development and validation of an electronic health record-based chronic kidney disease registry. *Clin. J. Am. Soc. Nephrol.* **2011**, *6*, 40–49. [CrossRef]

37. Winkelmayer, W.C.; Schneeweiss, S.; Mogun, H.; Patrick, A.R.; Avorn, J.; Solomon, D.H. Identification of individuals with CKD from medicare claims data: A validation study. *Am. J. Kidney Dis.* **2005**, *46*, 225–232. [CrossRef]

38. Chan, T.C.; Fan, I.C.; Liu, M.S.; Su, M.D.; Chiang, P.H. Addressing health disparities in chronic kidney disease. *Int. J. Environ. Res. Public Health* **2014**, *11*, 12848–12865. [CrossRef]

39. Lin, Y.-C.; Hsu, C.-Y.; Kao, C.-C.; Chen, T.-W.; Chen, H.-H.; Hsu, C.-C.; Wu, M.-S. Incidence and prevalence of ESRD in Taiwan renal registry data system (TWRDS): 2005–2012. *Acta Nephrol.* **2014**, *28*, 65–68.

40. Wu, M.-S.; Wu, I.-W.; Shih, C.-P.; Hsu, K.-H. Establishing a platform for battling end-stage renal disease and continuing quality improvement in dialysis therapy in Taiwan-Taiwan renal registry data system (TWRDS). *Acta Nephrol.* **2011**, *25*, 148–153.

41. Guilford, J.P. *Fundamental Statistics in Psychology and Education*; McGraw-Hill: New York, NY, USA, 1942.

42. Kendall, M.G. A new measure of rank correlation. *Biometrika* **1938**, *30*, 81–93. [CrossRef]

43. Hastie, T.J.; Tibshirani, R.J. *Generalized Additive Models*; Chapman & Hall/CRC: London, UK, 1990.

44. Akaike, H. A new look at the statistical model identification. *IEEE Trans. Autom. Control* **1974**, *19*, 716–723. [CrossRef]

45. Tsai, C.C.; Wu, C.L.; Kor, C.T.; Lian, I.B.; Chang, C.H.; Chang, T.H.; Chang, C.C.; Chiu, P.F. Prospective associations between environmental heavy metal exposure and renal outcomes in adults with chronic kidney disease. *Nephrology (Carlton)* **2017**, *23*, 830–836. [CrossRef]

46. McGregor, D.O.; Dellow, W.J.; Lever, M.; George, P.M.; Robson, R.A.; Chambers, S.T. Dimethylglycine accumulates in uremia and predicts elevated plasma homocysteine concentrations. *Kidney Int.* **2001**, *59*, 2267–2272. [CrossRef]

47. Kao, Y.Y.; Chen, Y.C.; Cheng, T.J.; Chiung, Y.M.; Liu, P.S. Zinc oxide nanoparticles interfere with zinc ion homeostasis to cause cytotoxicity. *Toxicol. Sci.* **2012**, *125*, 462–472. [CrossRef]

48. Benli, A.C.; Koksal, G.; Ozkul, A. Sublethal ammonia exposure of Nile tilapia (Oreochromis niloticus l.): Effects on gill, liver and kidney histology. *Chemosphere* **2008**, *72*, 1355–1358. [CrossRef]

49. Fu, Q.; Colgan, S.P.; Shelley, C.S. Hypoxia: The force that drives chronic kidney disease. *Clin. Med. Res.* **2016**, *14*, 15–39. [CrossRef]

50. Tsukamoto, H.; Parker, H.R.; Gribble, D.H.; Mariassy, A.; Peoples, S.A. Nephrotoxicity of sodium arsenate in dogs. *Am. J. Vet. Res.* **1983**, *44*, 2324–2330.

51. Liu, J.; Liu, Y.; Habeebu, S.M.; Waalkes, M.P.; Klaassen, C.D. Chronic combined exposure to cadmium and arsenic exacerbates nephrotoxicity, particularly in metallothionein-i/ii null mice. *Toxicology* **2000**, *147*, 157–166. [CrossRef]

52. Zheng, L.; Kuo, C.C.; Fadrowski, J.; Agnew, J.; Weaver, V.M.; Navas-Acien, A. Arsenic and chronic kidney disease: A systematic review. *Curr. Environ. Health Rep.* **2014**, *1*, 192–207. [CrossRef]

53. Tseng, C.H. Blackfoot disease and arsenic: A never-ending story. *J. Environ. Sci. Health C Environ. Carcinog. Ecotoxicol. Rev.* **2005**, *23*, 55–74. [CrossRef]

54. Tsai, S.M.; Wang, T.N.; Ko, Y.C. Mortality for certain diseases in areas with high levels of arsenic in drinking water. *Arch. Environ. Health* **1999**, *54*, 186–193. [CrossRef]

55. Chiu, H.F.; Yang, C.Y. Decreasing trend in renal disease mortality after cessation from arsenic exposure in a previous arseniasis-endemic area in southwestern Taiwan. *J. Toxicol. Environ. Health A* **2005**, *68*, 319–327. [CrossRef]
56. Cheng, Y.Y.; Huang, N.C.; Chang, Y.T.; Sung, J.M.; Shen, K.H.; Tsai, C.C.; Guo, H.R. Associations between arsenic in drinking water and the progression of chronic kidney disease: A nationwide study in Taiwan. *J. Hazard. Mater.* **2017**, *321*, 432–439. [CrossRef] [PubMed]
57. Pearce, N. Classification of epidemiological study designs. *Int. J. Epidemiol.* **2012**, *41*, 393–397. [CrossRef] [PubMed]
58. Noordzij, M.; Dekker, F.W.; Zoccali, C.; Jager, K.J. Measures of disease frequency: Prevalence and incidence. *Nephron Clin. Pract.* **2010**, *115*, c17–c20. [CrossRef] [PubMed]

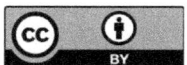

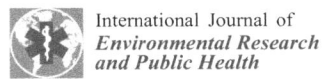

Article

Deriving A Drinking Water Guideline for A Non-Carcinogenic Contaminant: The Case of Manganese

Mathieu Valcke [1,2], Marie-Hélène Bourgault [1], Sami Haddad [2], Michèle Bouchard [2], Denis Gauvin [1] and Patrick Levallois [1,3,*]

1   Direction de la Santé Environnementale et de la Toxicologie, Institut National de Santé Publique du Québec, 945 Avenue Wolfe, Québec, QC G1V 5B3, Canada; mathieu.valcke@inspq.qc.ca (M.V.); marie-helene.bourgault@inspq.qc.ca (M.-H.B.); denis.gauvin@inspq.qc.ca (D.G.)

2   Department of Environmental and Occupational health, École de Santé Publique, C.P. 6128, Succursale Centre-Ville, Montréal, QC H3C 3J7, Canada; sami.haddad@umontreal.ca (S.H.); michele.bouchard@umontreal.ca (M.B.)

3   Department of Social and Preventive Medicine, Faculté de Médecine, Pavillon Ferdinand-Vandry, 1050 Avenue de la Médecine Local 00241, Université Laval, Québec, QC G1V 0A6, Canada

*   Correspondence: patrick.levallois@msp.ulaval.ca; Tel.: +1-418-650-5115 (ext. 5216)

Received: 19 May 2018; Accepted: 16 June 2018; Published: 20 June 2018

Abstract: Manganese is a natural contaminant of water sources. It is an essential oligo-element, which may exert toxicity at high doses, particularly via inhalation. Its toxicity by the oral route is less known, but epidemiological and experimental studies tend to support its neurodevelopmental toxicity in infants and children. This paper describes the method used by a middle-size public health institution to derive a Drinking Water Guideline (DWG) for manganese. After reviewing the work done by major public health institutions, authors confirmed the use of experimental data to derive a point-of-departure (POD) of 25 mg of manganese/kg/day, based on neurodevelopmental effects on pup rats. Then, a total uncertainty factor of 450 was applied to calculate a Toxicological Reference Value (TRV) of 55 µg/kg/day. The final DWG proposed for manganese is 60 µg/L and is based on a relative source contribution (RSC) of water of 20% and an infant drinking scenario of 182 mL/kg of body weight (BW) of water (95th percentile of the ingestion rate distribution for 0–6 months). Despite its limitations, e.g., starting with the work done by other agencies, such an approach demonstrates in a transparent way the rationale and challenging choices made by regulators when deriving a DWG.

Keywords: drinking water; inorganic manganese; health-based guideline; infants

1. Introduction

Manganese is a metal mostly occurring naturally in the environment. Food is the main source of exposure for humans, but water may sometimes become a significant source. In particular, high levels of manganese may be found in surface or groundwater, occurring in aerobic or low oxidation conditions [1]. Inorganic manganese is considered an essential element for human beings, despite few reported cases of clinical deficiency [2]. It has a well-known toxicity in workers exposed by inhalation, leading to neurotoxic effects and Parkinson-like symptoms, sometimes called manganism [3]. However, its toxicity by the oral route has long been considered low, particularly due to homeostasis control of its excretion.

Very few epidemiological studies were conducted on manganese exposure from drinking water in adults. They had limited designs and gave mixed results [4,5]. However, several studies with better designs have since then reported possible negative impact on the neurodevelopment of infants and young children [6–9]. Infants might be particularly vulnerable to overexposure due to their greater gastrointestinal absorption and immaturity of their homeostatic control of bile excretion [2,10]. Therefore, growing concerns with regard to manganese neurotoxicity are being expressed [10,11].

Until now, few jurisdictions have proposed a drinking water quality criteria for manganese based on health effects. The last version of the WHO guidelines did not report any formal guideline for manganese, due to the fact aesthetic acceptability problems usually occur before health concerns [1]. The USEPA has proposed a lifetime health advisory of 300 μg/L based on a dietary daily intake of 10 mg for adults and 20% contribution for drinking water [12]. The same value was also recommended for infants younger than 6 months for an acute exposure of 10 days, contrary to 1 mg/L for older children and adults, because of concerns of possible overexposure of infants [12]. More recently, the Minnesota Department of Health has proposed a short term Health-Based Value of 100 μg/L [13]. In doing so, the possible higher risk for the neurodevelopment of infants bottle fed with plain tap water or given reconstituted formula is specifically targeted. Indeed, this guideline is based on cognitive and behavioral effects found in newborn rats exposed to manganese in water [14] and accounts for infant-specific body weight-adjusted drinking water ingestion rate.

Such a guideline brings out the growing concerns of public health institutions with regard to the particular susceptibility of young infants to manganese, not only from the perspective of the health effect but also of the increase exposure, also highlighted by Goeden [15] (in this *IJERPH* special issue). Given the presence of manganese in several groundwater sources in Quebec [16,17] and the absence of any official health based standard for this parameter in Quebec and Canada, the Institut de santé publique du Québec (INSPQ, Québec, QC, Canada) was asked by the Quebec Ministry of Healh and Social Services to propose a health-based guideline value for manganese in drinking water. The objective of this paper is to describe a systematic method applied by the INSPQ to derive a Drinking Water Guideline (DWG) for the non-carcinogenic contaminant that is manganese.

2. Methodology

We present here the method used by the INSPQ to derive its health-based drinking water guideline for manganese in Quebec [18]. It relies mainly on the critical use of assessments already made available by public health institutions around the world for manganese. The approach includes four mains steps, namely: (1) identification of the existing relevant toxicological reference values (TRV) derived by these institutions in order to select the most appropriate point of departure (POD); (2) determination of the required uncertainty factors (UF) based on available data rather than default values if possible; (3) application of the required UF to divide the POD determined in step 1 and (4) consideration of the relative source contribution and drinking water ingestion rate in order to compute the final numerical value of the DWG.

2.1. Inventory of Available TRVs for Selection of the Most Appropriate POD

TRVs for manganese were searched among the following sources: Health Canada's Drinking Water Documents [19], US EPA's IRIS and Drinking Water Health advisoires [12,20], CalEPA's Public Health Goals [21], the Human Health-Based Water Guidances from the Minnesota Department of Health (MDH, St. Paul, MN, USA) [22], WHO's Drinking Water Guidelines [1], ATSDR's Minimum Risk Levels (MRL)s [23], and the Advices for Drinking Water Quality from the French Agency for Food, Environment and Occupational Health & Safety (ANSES, Maisons-Alfort, France) [24]. These represent the most commonly cited public health institutions with regard to the determination of populationnal TRVs for environmental contaminants. Not only official positions are retained at this step, but also provisional guidelines and draft documents when they are publicly available.

The POD that could be identified for manganese from these institution reviews were critically analyzed based on the following criteria: (1) the relevance of the exposure route to the targeted guideline; (2) the robustness of the original dose-response curve that have lead to the determination of the POD; (3) the correspondence with the most sensitive adverse health effect.

Precisely, given that the DWG purpose is to limit exposure resulting from the ingestion of drinking water, TRV for the oral route are to be focused on. In the case of animal studies, administration via drinking water rather than food or gavage is to be privileged, but epidemiological data are prioritized over animal data when both types are considered of equivalent quality and robustness. With regard specifically to the POD, benchmark doses are to be prioritized over NOAELs, as they include all the available information provided by the dose-response curve, contrary to a single experimental point, such as the NOAEL [25]. If none of these critical doses are available, LOAELs can be used. Finally, should several PODs appear relevant based on the preceding criteria, the one corresponding to the most sensitive effect, that is the lowest, is chosen.

2.2. Review and Application of The Required Uncertainty Factors

The application of uncertainty factors (UF) follows the general principles edicted by the US EPA [26]. Such factors are applied to compensate for the uncertainty resulting from the use of a POD that has been determined in conditions that differ from the conditions to which the targeted TRV applies [27–29]. Thus, UF for animal-to-human extrapolation (UF_A), interhuman variability (UF_H), subchronic-to-chronic extrapolation (UF_S), LOAEL-to-NOAEL extrapolation (UF_L) are considered. All these UFs are usually attributed a 10 default value. Additionally, the available studies, among which the one used for the determination of the POD is included, must comprise at least two chronic toxicity studies and two developmental toxicity studies by the relevant exposure route, in a rodent and non-rodent mammal species, as well as a multigenerational reproduction study. Otherwise, an additional factor is applied to account for the deficiency in the database (UF_D) [27–29]. The approach considered here implies that the value attributed to UF_D is either 3, if one or two of the aforementioned studies is missing, or 10 if more than two these studies are missing, or if the pattern of the dose-response curve is unclear, if suspected evidences of epigenetic carcinogenicity are present or any other justification that cannot be covered by the above-mentioned UFs. Once all the required UFs are identified, a so-called "customized" TRV can be calculated, as the POD divided by the product of each selected UF.

In accordance with the WHO/IPCS and US EPA guidances on the application of chemical-specific or data-derived extrapolation adjustment factors [30–32], it is recommended to consider the possible replacement of the 10-fold default value generally applied UF_A and UF_H by numerical values that are computed from data relevant to the chemical of interest. This is proposed under the premise that the default 10-fold value in fact corresponds to two components, one for toxicodynamic (TD) and one for toxicokinetic (TK) variability.

In the case of manganese, available data only allow this replacement for UF_H, for which the default TK and TD component values are being attributed the value of square root of 10, that is 3.16 [30–32]. First, the comparison between average and sensitive individuals in both species was based on available experimental data in rats and population biomonitoring data in humans [33–36]. This allowed to evaluate whether or not the interindividual TK variability is greater in humans than in rats. Such evaluation was necessary given that the POD retained results from a study conducted in neonate rats (see Results), thus suggesting that the presumed increased sensitivity of newborn individuals, as compared to adults, is intrinsically accounted for by this POD selection. The magnitude of the interindividual TK variability that is possibly not accounted for by this POD selection was then evaluated. Indeed, it cannot be excluded that some TK variability remains within the sensitive human subpopulation itself, while it is apparently virtually limited in rats [33]. Thus, total blood Mn concentrations measured in several human subpopulations presumed more sensitive to the effect of Mn were taken from the literature, and the magnitude of the TK variability computed as prescribed by the WHO/IPCS [30] and US EPA [31], and total UF_H was calculated by multiplying resulting TK and TD component accordingly.

2.3. Caclulation of the Drinking Water Health-Based Guideline

The drinking water health-based guideline for manganese is calculated based on the oral TRV determined above following the state-of-the-art approach for non-carcinogenic effects [1,37–39], given that the critical effect of manganese is of neurotoxic nature [3,11,40]. Precisely, equation 1 show that the relative source contribution (RSC), the body weight (BW) and the drinking water ingestion rate (IR) are factored in for the guideline calculation:

$$DWG = (TRV \times RSC \times BW)/IR \qquad (1)$$

where, DWG is in mg/L, TRV is in mg/kg/day, RSC is unitless, BW is in kg, and IR is in L/day.

The relative source contribution (RSC) of drinking water corresponds to a fraction of the TRV to which the exposure resulting from the use of drinking water can contribute. Indeed, it is necessary from a public health perspective to ensure that this contribution does not result into exceeding the TRV if summed to the exposure resulting from the non-drinking water potential sources [1,41–44]. Given the default assumption that total exposure to an environmental contaminant may come from 5 medias (drinking water, air, soil, food and household products; [1,41]), it is considered that up to one fifth of this total exposure can be attributed to drinking water, thus triggering a default 20% RSC value for all age groups. In certain circumstances, for which further details are provided in Supplemental materials, an RSC value that differ from this 20% default can be chosen. That is, a RSC greater than 20% is justifiable when drinking water is believed to be the main or the only source of exposure, while an RSC lower than 20% can be attributed when it is estimated that the other exposure sources than drinking water, notably food, may contribute in total, to more than 80% of the TRV [1,41–44]. Manganese being an essential element and given that its main exposure source is in fact food, its RSC was herein validated based on data of its concentrations found in cow or soya milk formula, which constitutes the main manganese dietary exposure source for non-breast-fed neonates.

The choice of the values that are used in Equation (1) for BW and IR is driven by three considerations, namely (1) the period of life during which the exposure that has allowed the determination of the POD has occurred; (2) the concern for protecting the most sensitive individuals; and (3) making sure that the DWG is adequately protective for the high-end consumers of drinking water. The specific values chosen in the case of manganese are detailed and justified in Results, hereafter.

3. Results

3.1. Available Oral TRV for Manganese

The oral TRVs adopted for manganese by the various institutions investigated are detailed in Table 1. They originate either from human or animal data. With the exception of MDH, every reviewed institution have determined an oral TRV that applies to chronic exposure of the general population. In the case of MDH, two TRV were determined, namely one for the chronic exposure of the general population, which in fact is the same as the US EPA's, and another one for exposure occuring in the first year of life (short-term TRV). Oral TRV chosen by the US EPA, WHO and ATSDR are based on human data, whereas the short-term TRV derived by MDH is based on animal data.

In addition to the institutions indicated in Table 1, Health Canada has also recently proposed, as part of a public consultation, an oral TRV of 25 µg/kg BW/day based on a LOAEL of 25 mg/kg/day divided by a composite UF of 1000 [19]. This value has not been officialy adopted to date, but is still considered for the purpose of the present work, as it counts among the most recent documents published on manganese by a recognized public health organization.

Table 1. Oral TRV recommended by various public health institutions.

Institution	POD (mg/kg/day)	Type of POD	Composite UF	Oral TRV (µg/kg/day)
TRV based on human data				
US EPA and MDH [12,20,45]	0.140 [1]	NOAEL	1 or 3 [2]	140 or 47 [2]
WHO [1]	0.183 [3]	NOAEL	3	61
ATSDR [3]	0.160	NOAEL	1	160 [4]
TRV based on animal data				
MDH [13]	25	LOAEL	300	83 [5]

[1] Rounded value, based on a NOAEL of 10 mg/day for a 70 kg adult; [2] Uncertainty factor that applies only to non-dietary manganese exposure, including drinking water, for individuals older than 1 year-old. [3] WHO has selected a NOAEL of 11 mg/day for a 60 kg adult. [4] Interim guideline. [5] This TRV only applies to infants younger than 1 year old.

3.2. Determination of the Most Relevant POD

The TRV derived by the US EPA, WHO and ATSDR are all based on the upper bound estimated daily dietary intake of manganese in the average vegetarian adult, determined as safe by various authors after further analyses [2,46–50]. However, this TRV is not determined based on a toxicological evaluation [10]. Moreover, either no data related to dietary manganese exposure are presented in the cited sources, either these sources refer to other studies with limited data and for which there was no focus on health outcome. Also noteworthy, these studies have been published back to at least the 80's, and as early as the 60's. For these reasons, the human data-derived POD from the US EPA, WHO and ATSDR is not retained here for the DWG derivation for manganese.

Conversely, considering the increasing weight-of-evidence towards infant neurotoxicity of manganese in drinking water as the critical effect of interest, MDH and Health Canada have evaluated the possibility to determine such guideline based on corresponding epidemiological data [13,19]. However, due to important limitations of available studies in this regard, both organizations have considered that animal data are to be privileged. The INSPQ agrees with this evaluation. Thus, a POD corresponding to a LOAEL of 25 mg/kg/day for neurobehavioral, motor and cognitive effects obtained in juvenile rats exposed on post-natal days 1–21 (*per os*), or longer (via drinking water) to doses of 0, 25 or 50 mg/kg/day of manganese under the form of manganese chloride (MnCl$_2$·4H$_2$O), was retained by both institutions [13,19]. This POD results from a series of three studies conducted by the same research team [14,51,52]. In each one of these studies, at least one adverse effect occurred at exposure doses of 25 mg/kg/day on post-natal days 1–21 [14,51] or during the entire 54 weeks following birth [52], thus corresponding to a LOAEL (Table 2).

Table 2. Summary of the neurological effects observed in rats exposed orally to Mn following birth, at doses of 0 (control group), 25 and 50 mg/kg/day.

Study	Postnatal Exposure Days	Postnatal Effect Days [1]	Critical Observed Effect	LOAEL or NOAEL (mg/kg/day) [2]
Kern et al., 2010 [14]	1–21	33-46	Decreased learning capacity (increase use of stereotyped response strategy) [3]	25 (LOAEL)
Kern et al., 2011 [51]	1–21	24 [4]	Increased expression of glial acid protein in the prefrontal cortex [5]	25 (LOAEL)
Beaudin et al., 2013 [52]	1–21 1–400	120–150 [6]	Decreased fine sensorimotor function [7]	25 (NOAEL) 25 (LOAEL)

[1] Lifestage where the observed effect has been measured. [2] n = 20 rats per dose. [3] This strategy consisted in finding food hidden at extremities of an 8-arms labyrinth by systematically moving from one adjacent arm to the other. [4] n = 16 to 24 rats per dose. [5] Results in an astrocytes activation, which constitutes a sign of neurological inflammation. [6] n = 11 or 12 rats per dose. [7] Consist into seasing and eating food granules during the staircase test.

Given the good quality of all three studies listed in Table 2 (precise experimental protocols, control of confounding's, justification of the chosen exposure doses), this neurodevelopmental LOAEL of 25 mg of manganese/kg/day was chosen as a POD for the current DWG derivation. Although other LOAEL lower than those POD have been proposed in some studies (reviewed by Health Canada [19], see Supplemental materials), important limitations preclude their use in the present context. In particular, these studies often included a single experimental dose or involved controls that were not readily comparable to the exposed group, which equals to testing a single experimental dose.

3.3. Application of Uncertainty Factors

3.3.1. Default 10-Fold Value or not Applied (UF = 1) Uncertainty Factors

Given that no available data suggest a value that differs from the default 10-fold uncertainty factor for animal-to-human extrapolation (UF_A), it was retained for the current assessment.

The POD retained reflects an exposure that has occurred over a short period of time during the first three weeks of life of the experimental pup rats, and to which are associated neurodevelopmental effects occurring up to three months later. But prolonged exposure throughout lifetime did not result in a different LOAEL [52]. Likely, this brings out the evidence of a mechanism of toxicity that involves a window of susceptibility, and that the adverse effect that may occur following exposure during this period is in fact the most sensitive one. Therefore, even though exposure may persist for longer duration, it will likely not trigger another adverse effect than the one associated to that specific window of susceptibility. This is further evidenced by the fact that LOAELs observed in chronic animal studies for other adverse effect than the one considered here almost always exceeded 25 mg/kg/day [3]. Two exceptions are the studies of Gupta et al. [53] and Ishizuka et al. [54] which however the number of individuals exposed was very low (4 rhesus monkeys and 2 mice, respectively), providing evidences of very limited robustness. Thus, no subchronic-to-chronic uncertainty (UF_S) factor was applied here.

3.3.2. Uncertainty Factors Different from the Default 10-Fold Value

Uncertainty factors that were applied and exhibit a magnitude that differ from the default 10-fold value include those for human variability (UF_H), for LOAEL-to-NOAEL extrapolation (UF_L) and for the incomplete database (UF_D).

Human Variability

Experimental kinetic data on manganese in rats suggest that more than 80% of an administered dose in neonate rats is retained as body burden [33] whereas this fraction is only about 5% in pup rats and stays around this level until adulthood [34], suggesting a 16-fold variations between identified sensitive and average rat. This is attributable to a reduce homeostatic capacity in the first few weeks of life [33,34]. In humans, Japanese data were available with regard to measures specifically conducted in newborns. Indeed, Mizogushi et al. [35] reported an arithmetic mean ($\pm$ standard deviation (SD)) total blood concentration of manganese of 56.4 ± 16.4 µg/L in this subpopulation ($n = 14$), based on which a 95th percentile value of 83.4 µg/L can be computed as [mean value + ($1.64 \times$ SD)], assuming lognormal distribution. In comparison, the mean concentration in subjects aged 1–11 years ($n = 36$) was 14.8 µg/L. Considering the expected difference between an arithmetic mean and a geometric mean in a population distribution, this latter value compares rather well with the geometric mean concentration observed in children aged 6–11 from the Canadian Health Measure Survey (CHMS), that is 11 µg/L [36]. Besides, mean total blood manganese levels barely vary through lifetime according to CHMS, as values between 9.1 and 10 µg/L were obtained in the participants aged from 12 to 79 years old. From these elements, it can be suggested that the magnitude of the variability of manganese levels is comparable between Japanese and Canadian populations. Therefore, using the Canadian mean adult value of 9.8 µg/L for 6 to 79 years old [36], and under the WHO/IPCS approach for the calculation of chemical-specific adjustment factor [30], the magnitude of TK variability for manganese in humans can be approximated as the ratio between the 95th percentile in sensitive individuals, here newborn japanese over the median in adults, that is the Canadian value, yielding $83.4/9.8 \approx 9$. This ratio appears rather conservative, as the corresponding ratio between newborn and older Japanese children would have yield a value of ≈ 5.6 ($84.5/14.8$). Ratio values of 3 or less were observed by Park et al. [55] as well as Alarcon et al. [56] in respectively Korean and Venezuelan infants. Even when considering reported manganese levels in pregnant women, umbilical cord and neonates, including in 12 comparison studies detailed by Huang et al. [57], such ratio remains below 10 [57,58].

All in all, from the data mentioned in the preceding paragraph suggest that the magnitude of the interindividual TK variability in rats is comparable, or even slightly greater, than that calculated from human data. Although this assertion is made based on a quite limited number of measures (11–24 per dose in rats depending on the study and 14 in humans), which limits their generalizability to entire animal or human populations, it appears reasonable to propose that a major part of interindividual TK variability is presumably accounted for by the use of a POD determined in neonate rats, and the TK component of UF_H can be diminished below its default 3.16 value. Also, literature data on manganese TK variability within several presumably sensitive human subpopulations are presented in Table S1. It can be seen that following the WHO/IPCS approach, [30], the computed interindividual variability in toxicokinetics corresponds to a 1.7-fold magnitude in average, within the most sensitive human individuals. This thus replaces the 3.16 default value for interindividual TK variability factor and multiplies the other 3.16 default value for interindividual TD, yielding a resulting rounded UF_H value of 5.

LOAEL-to-NOAEL Extrapolation

Based on ATSDR's compilation, both LOAEL and NOAEL values can be identified among several of the reviewed experimental studies in neonate rodents, which covered a wide array of such effects [14,51,52,59–62]. In each one of these studies, the NOAEL is at the most 3 times lower than the LOAEL; therefore, a 3-fold LOAEL-to-NOAEL UF_L is chosen here.

Database Deficiencies

The available relevant studies on manganese detailed by Health Canada [19] include all of the required studies as per the state-of-the art determination of TRV (see Methods) [26–29]. Therefore, no UF_D would be needed under this aspect. However, some of the studies that were not retained here due to the weaknesses mentioned in 3.2, still suggest a neurodevelopmental LOAEL that could be lower than the 25 mg/kg/day value used herein (See Supplemental Materials). In particular, the studies from Dorman et al. [61] and Brennemann et al. [60] suggest LOAEL values of 11 and 22 mg/kg/day, but the toxicological significance of the adverse effects considered in these studies (increased reaction to an acoustic stimulus, and increased motor skills, respectively) is unclear. Still, a 3-fold UF_D is added in the current analysis at this step to compensate for the uncertainty added by the existence of lower LOAEL values that were not retained for the purpose of the current assessment.

3.4. Determination of a Customized TRV

Based on the POD retained in 3.2 (LOAEL of 25 mg/kg/day) and the product of every uncertainty factors applied as justified in Section 3.3 ($UF_H \times UF_A \times UF_{SC} \times UF_L \times UF_{DB} = 5 \times 10 \times 1 \times 3 \times 3 = 450$), the TRV calculated in this assessment is $25/450 = 55$ µg/kg/day.

3.5. Consideration of the Relative Source Contribution and Drinking Water Ingestion Rate

3.5.1. Relative Source Contribution

Elevated manganese concentrations, up to the range of 300 à 400 µg/L, had been found in milk formula, in particular based on soya milk [10,63]. A Canadian study has examined manganese concentrations in various drinks destinated to neonates and infants [64]. Despite limited sample size, a mean manganese concentration of 100 ± 50 µg/L was measured in a cow milk-based formula. Corresponding value for soya milk-based formula was 340 ± 110 µg/L.

Although present at roughly 3.4 times greater concentrations, manganese in soya milk-based formula is up to 8 times less bioavailable than in cow milk-based formula; this is attributed in part to the presence in soya milk of other chemicals (e.g., phitic acid) that compete with manganese for GI absorption [65]. Overall, it appears reasonable to state that cow milk-based formula represents a potential for greater internal manganese dose. Therefore, based on a 95th percentile manganese concentration of 182 µg/L in cow milk-based formula computed under the same default statistical considerations as those described in 3.3.2., an exposure dose of 33 µg/kg/day can be calculated. This figure corresponds to 60% of the TRV determined above (55 µg/kg/day) and leaves a margin of 40% of the TRV to every non-dietary sources of manganese exposure, drinking water being only one of them. Else, the available data do not suggest that dietary and other non-drinking water sources contribute to more than 80% of the total exposure. Overall then, under the premise of parting equally the above-mentioned 40% contribution between drinking water on the one hand, and every other non-dietary sources on the other hand, the default value of 20% can be retained here for DWG derivation.

3.5.2. Body Weight (BW) and Drinking Water Ingestion Rate (ING)

Given that the TRV determined above for manganese is based on a POD determined under the consideration of a specific period of susceptibility, the values considered to the parameters related to the drinking water contact rate are deemed to reflect this specific time period. Therefore, the mean BW and 95th percentile value of ING for the infants aged ≤ 6 months for the Quebec population, described elsewhere [66], are being used for the DWG calculation. This corresponds to 6.7 kg and 1.22 L/day respectively, for a BW-adjusted equivalent ingestion rate of 0.182 L/kg/day. Other elements considered by the present authors with regard to the choice of the appropriate BW-adjusted DW ingestion rate are presented in Supplemental materials.

3.6. Calculation of the Drinking Water Guideline

Applying Equation (1) above to the TRV calculated in 3.4, the DWG for manganese is 61 µg/L, rounded to 60 µg/L and based on a 20% RSC, a BW of 6.7 kg and a drinking water ingestion rate of 1.22 L/day. This guideline is more stringent than similar guidelines proposed by other public health institutions around the world, as shown by Table 3.

Table 3. Comparison of drinking water guidelines proposed by various public health institutions, including the one derived by the INSPQ.

Characteristics	Public Health Institution				
	Health Canada [19]	US EPA [12]	WHO [1]	MDH [13]	INSPQ [18]
Year of publication	2016	2004	2017	2012	2017
Critical studies, (specie)	[14,51,52], (rats)	[46,47,67], (human)	[2], (human)	[14], (rats)	[14,51,52], (rats)
POD, mg/kg/day (Type)	25 (LOAEL)	0.14 (NOAEL)	0.183 (NOAEL)	25 (LOAEL)	25 (LOAEL)
Composite UF, (detailed) [2]	1000, $(10 \times 10 \times 1 \times 10 \times 1)$	3, $(3 \times 1 \times 1 \times 1 \times 1)$	3, $(3 \times 1 \times 1 \times 1 \times 1)$	300, $(10 \times 10 \times 1 \times 3 \times 1)$	450, $(5 \times 10 \times 1 \times 3 \times 3)$
TRV, µg/kg/day	25	47	61	83	55
BW, kg	7	70	60	-	6.7
RSC, %	50	20	20	50	20
ING, L/kgBW/day [3]	0.107	0.029	0.033	0.29	0.182
Guideline value, mg/L	100	300	400	100 [1]	60

Abreviations: BW, body weight; ING, daily ingestion rate; POD, point of departure; RSC, relative source contribution; TRV, toxicological reference value; UF, uncertainty factor. [1] DWG applied to infants less than one year old. [2] $UF_H \times UF_A \times UF_{SC} \times UF_L \times UF_{DB}$, see text for meaning. [3] The body-weight adjusted ingestion rates are obtained by dividing the ingestion rate, in L/day, by the BW, in Kg, that are chosen by each institutions in the calculation of their respective drinking water guideline.

4. Discussion

The objective of this work was to derive a health-base DWG for manganese and provide a demonstration of the procedure used by a public health agency of a midsize jurisdiction such as the province of Quebec, that is INSPQ, for such activity. The work is mainly based on a systematic analysis of already existing guidelines determined by other public health institutions, with a focus on the rationale and critical points determined by these institutions to justify their methodological choices. Such an approach presents the advantage in that by building on existing work, it allows efficient process of guideline derivation while optimizing often limited time and human resources in middle size public health institutions. The DWG obtained here for manganese is 61 µg/L, rounded to 60 µg/L, and was derived by focusing specifically on the concern of protecting the most vulnerable population, that is children aged < 1 year old, not only by selecting the lowest relevant POD available and applying the required UF, but also by considering a BW and drinking water ingestion rate that corresponds specifically to this age group. Thus, the resulting guideline accounts for the greater drinking water ingestion rate in neonates as compared to adults, on a BW basis. It therefore addresses the concerns raised by Goeden [15].

Despite the fact that there are lower guidelines for manganese in drinking water based on esthetical considerations, that is 50 µg/L and currently projected to be lowered to 20 µg/L [19,68,69], the present health-based guideline is more stringent than corresponding health guidelines around the world, as the next most severe guideline is MDH's Risk Assessment Advice of 100 µg/L. Reasons for such discrepancy can be identified from the values taken by the different variables entering in the guideline calculation, which are detailed in Table 3.

The main source of greater conservatism in the current assessment as compared to the US EPA and WHO mainly stems from the choice of the POD, an animal one that triggers the application of several UFs, rather than the epidemiological POD with almost no UF applied. Indeed, the former appears more justifiable given that in the latter case, the human data that were not evaluated from the toxicological point of view, but rather the nutritional one [10].

The choice made here of the neurodevelopmental animal LOAEL of 25 mg/kg/day is also justified based on the following four elements:

(1) Neurotoxic effects of ingested manganese are the most sensitive ones based on the array of the toxicological tests listed in Table 2. Besides, this effect was observed in pup rodents at BW-adjusted exposure doses that are lower than those observed in other rodent groups (post weaning or adult animals) exposed chronically or subchronically to manganese [3]. Such sensitivity in rodent pups appears related to the immaturity of their homeostatic regulation system, with the consequent maximal absorption and minimal, if not absent, excretion during the first 15 to 18 postnatal days [33,70–72].

(2) Because of the uncertainties associated with the characterization of exposure and the role of confounders in epidemiological studies, corresponding data with regard to cognitive, motor and behavioral effects [19,73] are difficult to use for quantitative risk assessment such as the derivation of a health-based drinking water guideline.

(3) Although non-human primates would constitute the most appropriate toxicological model in order to characterize the toxicity of ingested manganese in humans [74,75], the available data do not appear sufficiently robust to do so. Indeed, such data result from experimental designs that either involve a single tested dose or a manganese exposure occurring via the intravenous route, or lacks comparable control experimental groups [53,75–82].

(4) The mechanism of action of manganese neurotoxicity through the oral exposure route is not fully elucidated. It is likely multi-process, including perturbation of dopamine transmission [40]. Given that such perturbation has been observed in both rodents and primates exposed to manganese [74], using a rat-based LOAEL to determine a DWG in humans appears relevant.

Once the choice of relying on animal data rather than human data has been made, differences in the application of UF contribute to derive a different guideline than MDH and Health Canada. However, at the end and as shown in Table 3, the composite UF of 450 positions itself in between Health Canada composite UF (1000) and MDH one (300). As a result, the TRV obtained (55 µg/kg/day) also lies midway between these two institution values (25 and 83 µg/kg/day). These numbers can be analyzed in light of the essential nature of manganese by comparison with the minimum recommended intakes of the Institute of Medicine (IOM). The TRV obtained here is significantly greater than the minimum intake recommended for neonates aged $\leq$ 6 months ($\approx$0.5 µg/kg/day) but may be lower than, or equivalent to, this recommendation for other age groups, in particular children aged 1–3 years (80 µg/kg/day) and 4–8 years (55 µg/kg/day) [2]. However, IOM recommended intakes are based on real exposure data that are deemed corresponding to the minimum intakes required. Possibly, the true required intake is much lower.

A source of greater conservatism herein is the application of 3-fold UF_{DB} to account for the fact that some lower LOAEL values—although apparently less robust than the POD selected here—could have been used (See Supplemental Materials). This factor is not applied by any other public health institution. Conversely, in some instances, less severe UF values were used. This is the case for UF_H, as a 5-fold factor was applied here contrary to the default 10-fold value applied by both MDH and Health Canada. As clearly demonstrated in Section 3.3.2, available data support the application of a less-than-ten-fold factor for UF_H. In fact, MDH and Health Canada both argue that a significant variability is observed in manganese metabolism in rats and thus such variability need to be accounted for when extrapolating to animals (personnal communication with Health Canada and MDH). However, it is the current authors position that this variability either leans towards greater variability in rats than humans, or that the toxicokinetically more sensitive individuals were accounted for by the experimental design leading to the selected animal POD. In such situation, it can be argued that only the toxicodynamic component of the UF_H, that is 3.16, need to be accounted for. Since some residual uncertainty still resides in assessing human variability from animal variability data, it appears reasonable that such situation triggers an UF_H no lower than 4, and the data-derived approach used here is coherent with this argument.

In support of the current assessment, both MDH and Health Canada have applied the default 10-fold animal-to-human extrapolation factor while neither institution applied any UF for the use of a less-than-chronic POD in guideline derivation. While MDH guideline specifically targets short-term exposure [13], this position appears well justified. Health Canada, for its part, argues that the consideration of a POD triggered by an exposure occurring during a restrained window of susceptibility, as can be concluded from the experimental design detailed in Table 2, suggests that the measured effect is likely more sensitive than any other (chronic) effect that may result from long-term exposure to manganese in drinking water and that as a result, no UF for subchronic to chronic extrapolation is required. Other coherent UF values include the 3-fold UF_L applied here like MDH and differently than the 10-fold default applied by Health Canada. This 3-fold value was also based on the review of the magnitude of the LOAEL/NOAEL ratios for a same given adverse effect, detailed by ATSDR (see also Supplemental Material). However, MDH argument differs in that it qualifies as subtle the neurological adverse effect and thus does not require a 10-fold factor.

The attribution of a RSC of 20% rather than 50% contributes significantly to the derivation of a lower guideline than MDH and Health Canada. Both institutions have justified this 50% value by the fact that neonates are mainly exposed to manganese from two sources, namely drinking water and food, each of which 50% of the overall contribution is attributed. Although this is based on some rationale, the careful analysis of the available quantitative data suggests otherwise with regard to the magnitude of this factor, as the 50% value retained by these institutions appear too high. Indeed, if 50% of the TRV of 55 µg/kg/day calculated in Section 3.4 was attributed to drinking water, the potential is real for some infants to be exposed to a total dose exceeding it. Given the 33 µg/kg figure calculated in Section 3.5.1, this corresponds to 60% of the TRV as resulting from ingestion of milk formula, leaving at the most a RSC for drinking water that should not be greater than 40%.

In this regard, it is noteworthy that Krishnan and Carrier [20] describe the US EPA methodology for deriving values that depart from default for this factor, based on available data on the presence of the contaminant of interest in the various environmental medias. Thus, an RSC lower than 20% can be required if it is estimated that the other exposure sources than drinking water may contribute, at the total, to more than 80% of the TRV [1,31], as allowing as much as 20% of RSC to drinking water in this case would undesirably translate into a total exposure that theoretically exceeds the threshold of potential effect. Conversely, an RSC greater than 20% can be envisaged when it is known that drinking water is likely the sole (e.g., up to 80%) or at least the main (e.g., at 50%) contributor to the total human exposure [1,26,28,30,31], for instance because a chemical is added for water treatment purposes (e.g., trihalomethanes, trihaloacetic acids). However, the data-derived approach implies that for a situation in which the drinking water is more contaminated than the other medium, its RSC can be greater than 20% and as a result, the guideline more permissible for more contaminated media than for less contaminated ones. Although this can be justifiable from a risk management perspective, it is more hardly so when reasoning strictly from the point of view of protecting human health. Besides, the IOM stated that, for infants, the sole source of manganese as essential element should come from dietary sources [2], therefore excluding any presence in drinking water. Obviously, this recommendation was made at a time where not many toxicological data on manganese were available. But the default 20% value was still retained here, and the data-derived approach proved to be useful in demonstrating that the 50% figure appears too permissive.

One uncertainty that is worth mentionning with regard to the DWG determined here relates to the fact that manganese speciation is sensitive to environmental conditions and drinking water sources may vary considerably with regard to their physicochemical environment. Thus it cannot be excluded that the population, for which the DWG aims at regulating its manganese exposure, in fact is exposed to chemical forms of manganese that are different than the one that was used in the study from which originates the POD used herein. Likewise, the dose-response relationship could be different. However, the manganese chloride that was used in the chosen POD study is very soluble and is ionized as Mn^{2+} in water, which happened also to be the vehicle of administration in this study. Besides, epidemiological studies that brought out concerns for the neurodevelopmental toxicity of manganese (see Introduction) have been conducted on population fed by groundwaters and it is therefore reasonable to assume that most manganese was also present as Mn^{2+}. Overall then, the impact of the uncertainty associated with the possible variations of the dose-response relationship according to the chemical form of manganese appears low with regard to the adequacy of the DWG proposed herein.

A limitation of the method presented here that needs to be acknowledged is that a complete literature review of all toxicological and epidemiological data available on manganese toxicity was not performed, but rather a critical analysis of previous work done by other Agencies was done [12,13,19]. In particular, the POD for this risk assessment was based on a critical analysis of papers, which were already selected and reviewed by those agencies. This approach was chosen in response to limited resources but still appears appropriate in view of the credibility of these agencies and the fact that, at least for the MDH [13,45] and Health Canada [19], their reviews of the literature were quite recent. Should there have been no recent review available by credible agencies, a complete literature review would have been required, but only for the time period not covered by the previous reviews. Despite the fact that such an approach has some limitations (no replication of the original literature reviews), it allows middle-size agencies to do such work with limited resources and time constraints, which is not a negligible advantage from a public health perspective.

Finally, this DWG for manganese is based on a risk assessment conducted on the most vulnerable population to this contaminant: infants fed with formula reconstituted with drinking water. Normally, for convenience and simplicity of the communication message, it might be justified to propose such a guideline for the entire population exposed to excessive concentration of manganese in drinking water. However, because the homeostatis control for oral exposure is more developed in older children and adults, and cost of measures to be applied to reduce exposure (water treatment, changing the source of water., etc.), some juridictions will prefer to use a different DWG for older populations. This is the case of MDH who has recommended to use the USEPA Health advisory of 300 µg/L for older population (>1 year old) [13]. Water treatment technologies, both at the community and individual levels are available, but their implementation may represent additional financial costs and significant challenges for drinking water system managers. However, given the organoleptic inconveniences caused by the presence of manganese for exposed population, in particular staining of laundry and plumbing fixtures, and eventually taste problems, it might be justified to implement measures to reduce the presence of manganese in drinking water for the entire population. Thus, the organoleptic recommendation of 50 µg/L, as currently proposed by US-EPA [38] and WHO [68], or a lower one as the one proposed recently by Health Canada [19], might therefore be considered as a target to be achieved for the entire population. Our proposed DWG is not very different from these esthetical guidelines.

5. Conclusions

Deriving DWG is an important activity to protect public health [1]. However, the procedures used to derive a guideline are sometimes very technical and not available in current literature. A simple method used by a middle size institution (INSPQ, Québec, QC, Canada) using the critical review of work done by other institutions as its first input was thus presented here, following a step by step method to derive a guideline for non carcinogenic contaminants.

The proposed health based guideline proposed for manganese is based on the same animal POD as the one chosen by other institutions [13,19] but its numerical value differs by using different uncertainty factors, RSC of water to the TRV and water consumption. Globally, the proposed guidelines of 60 µg/L is still higher than the usual esthetical guidelines values for manganese (50 µg/L, projected to be lowered at 20 µg/L, [1,19]) but lower that other health based values [12,13,19]. The rationale applied to the choices made herein were exposed and compared to the choices of other institutions. This might help to open a transparent debate on the issues relative to deriving health based guidelines for drinking water.

Supplementary Materials: The following are available online at http://www.mdpi.com/1660-4601/15/6/1293/s1, Table S1. Total blood concentrations (mean, standard derivation and 95th percentiles) of Mn measured in presumably sensitive human subpopulations as reported in other studies. I. Consideration regarding the application of 3-fold UF_{DB} to account for the fact that some LOAEL values lower than the POD retained in the current assessment are available in the literature. II.Considerations with regard to the choice of the appropriate BW-adjusted drinking water ingestion rate.

Author Contributions: P.L. coordinated the study and wrote part of the manuscript. M.V. and M.-H.B. designed the study, did the literature review and wrote most of the manuscript; S.H., M.B. and D.G. participated actively to the discussion and decisions about this study. All the authors did a critical review of a previous version of the manuscript and did approve its final version.

Acknowledgments: This work was not funded by external source. It was conducted by the Groupe scientifique sur l'eau (GSE) and the Comité d'experts sur les risques chimiques de l'eau (CERCeau) of the INSPQ. Authors want to thank other members of the CERCeau who also participated to the discussion and approved the content of the INSPQ report on this guidance value: Benoît Barbeau of École Polytechnique de Montréal (in particular for its inputs on issues with manganese speciation in water), Manuel Rodriguez from Université Laval of Québec city, Michel Savard from the Public health department of Laurentides region, and Cathy Vaillancourt of INRS-Institut Armand Frappier, Quebec, Canada.

Conflicts of Interest: The authors declare no conflict of interest.

References

1. WHO. *Guidelines for Drinking-Water Quality: Fourth Edition Incorporating the First Addendum*; WHO Guidelines Approved by the Guidelines Review Committee; World Health Organization: Geneva, Switzerland, 2017; ISBN 978-92-4-154995-0.

2. Institute of Medicine (IOM). *Dietary Reference Intakes for Vitamin A, Vitamin K, Arsenic, Boron, Chromium, Copper, Iodine, Iron, Manganese, Molybdenum, Nickel, Silicon, Vanadium, and Zinc*; National Academy Press: Washington, DC, USA, 2001; ISBN 978-0-309-07279-3.

3. ATSDR Toxicological Profile: Manganese. Available online: https://www.atsdr.cdc.gov/ToxProfiles/tp.asp?id=102&tid=23 (accessed on 20 September 2017).

4. Kondakis, X.G.; Makris, N.; Leotsinidis, M.; Prinou, M.; Papapetropoulos, T. Possible health effects of high manganese concentration in drinking water. *Arch. Environ. Health* **1989**, *44*, 175–178. [CrossRef] [PubMed]

5. Vieregge, P.; Heinzow, B.; Korf, G.; Teichert, H.M.; Schleifenbaum, P.; Mösinger, H.U. Long term exposure to manganese in rural well water has no neurological effects. *Can. J. Neurol. Sci. J. Can. Sci. Neurol.* **1995**, *22*, 286–289. [CrossRef]

6. Bjørklund, G.; Chartrand, M.S.; Aaseth, J. Manganese exposure and neurotoxic effects in children. *Environ. Res.* **2017**, *155*, 380–384. [CrossRef] [PubMed]

7. Sanders, A.P.; Claus Henn, B.; Wright, R.O. Perinatal and Childhood Exposure to Cadmium, Manganese, and Metal Mixtures and Effects on Cognition and Behavior: A Review of Recent Literature. *Curr. Environ. Health Rep.* **2015**, *2*, 284–294. [CrossRef] [PubMed]

8. Rahman, S.M.; Kippler, M.; Tofail, F.; Bölte, S.; Hamadani, J.D.; Vahter, M. Manganese in Drinking Water and Cognitive Abilities and Behavior at 10 Years of Age: A Prospective Cohort Study. *Environ. Health Perspect.* **2017**, *125*, 057003. [CrossRef] [PubMed]

9. Dion, L.-A.; Saint-Amour, D.; Sauvé, S.; Barbeau, B.; Mergler, D.; Bouchard, M.F. Changes in water manganese levels and longitudinal assessment of intellectual function in children exposed through drinking water. *Neurotoxicology* **2017**. [CrossRef] [PubMed]

10. Ljung, K.; Vahter, M. Time to re-evaluate the guideline value for manganese in drinking water? *Environ. Health Perspect.* **2007**, *115*, 1533–1538. [CrossRef] [PubMed]

11. Lucchini, R.; Placidi, D.; Cagna, G.; Fedrighi, C.; Oppini, M.; Peli, M.; Zoni, S. Manganese and Developmental Neurotoxicity. *Adv. Neurobiol.* **2017**, *18*, 13–34. [CrossRef] [PubMed]

12. U.S. EPA. *Drinking Water Health Advisory for Manganese*; U.S. Environmental Protection Agency: Washington, DC, USA, 2004.

13. MDH. *Toxicological Summary for: Manganese. Health Based Guidance for Water*; Minnesota Department of Health: St. Paul, MN, USA, 2018.

14. Kern, C.H.; Stanwood, G.D.; Smith, D.R. Preweaning manganese exposure causes hyperactivity, disinhibition, and spatial learning and memory deficits associated with altered dopamine receptor and transporter levels. *Synapse* **2010**, *64*, 363–378. [CrossRef] [PubMed]

15. Goeden, H. Focus on Chronic Exposure for Deriving Drinking Water Guidance Underestimates Potential Risk to Infants. *Int. J. Environ. Res. Public. Health* **2018**, *15*, 512. [CrossRef] [PubMed]

16. Barbeau, B.; Carrière, A.; Bouchard, M.F. Spatial and temporal variations of manganese concentrations in drinking water. *J. Environ. Sci. Health Part A* **2011**, *46*, 608–616. [CrossRef] [PubMed]

17. MDDELCC. *Bilan de la Qualité de L'eau Potable au Québec 2010–2014*; Ministère du Développement Durable, de l'Environnement et de la Lutte Contre les Changements Climatiques: Québec, QC, Canada, 2016; p. 80.

18. Groupe scientifique sur l'eau. *Valeur Guide Sanitaire pour le Manganèse dans l'eau Potable—Avis au Ministère de la Santé et des Services Sociaux*; Institut National de Santé Publique du Québec: Québec, QC, Canada, 2017; p. 28.

19. Health Canada. *Manganese in Drinking Water. Document for Public Consultation Prepared by the Federal-Provincial-Territorial Committee on Drinking Water Consultation period ends August 5, 2016*; Health Canada: Ottawa, ON, Canada, 2016.

20. U.S. EPA. *Integrated Risk Information System (IRIS) Chemical Assessment Summary Manganese*; CASRN 7439-96-5; U.S. Environmental Protection Agency: Washington, DC, USA, 1996.

21. OEHHA Public Health Goals (PHGs). Available online: https://oehha.ca.gov/water/public-health-goals-phgs (accessed on 3 May 2018).

22. MDH Health-Based Values and Risk Assessment Advice for Water—EH: Minnesota Department of Health. Available online: http://www.health.state.mn.us/divs/eh/risk/guidance/hbvraawater.html (accessed on 18 May 2018).

23. ATSDR ATSDR—Minimal Risk Levels for Hazardous Substances (MRLs). Available online: https://www.atsdr.cdc.gov/mrls/index.asp (accessed on 18 May 2018).

24. ANSES L'Anses, Acteur de la Qualité des eaux | Anses—Agence Nationale de Sécurité Sanitaire de L'alimentation, de L'environnement et du Travail. Available online: https://www.anses.fr/fr/content/l%E2%80%99anses-acteur-de-la-qualit%C3%A9-des-eaux (accessed on 3 May 2018).

25. U.S. EPA. *Benchmark Dose Technical Guidance*; U.S. Environmental Protection Agency: Washington, DC, USA, 2012.

26. U.S. EPA. *A Review of the Reference Dose and Reference Concentration Processes*; U.S. Environmental Protection Agency: Washington, DC, USA, 2002.

27. Dourson, M.L.; Stara, J.F. Regulatory history and experimental support of uncertainty (safety) factors. *Regul. Toxicol. Pharmacol.* **1983**, *3*, 224–238. [CrossRef]

28. Dourson, M.L.; Felter, S.P.; Robinson, D. Evolution of science-based uncertainty factors in noncancer risk assessment. *Regul. Toxicol. Pharmacol.* **1996**, *24*, 108–120. [CrossRef] [PubMed]

29. Ritter, L.; Totman, C.; Krishnan, K.; Carrier, R.; Vézina, A.; Morisset, V. Deriving uncertainty factors for threshold chemical contaminants in drinking water. *J. Toxicol. Environ. Health B Crit. Rev.* **2007**, *10*, 527–557. [CrossRef] [PubMed]

30. WHO. *Chemical-Specific Adjustment Factors for Interspecies Differences and Human Variability: Guidance Document for Use of Data in Dose/Concentration-Response Assessment*; Harmonization Project Document No. 2; World Health Organization: Geneva, Switzerland, 2005.

31. U.S. EPA. *Guidance for Applying Quantitative Data to Develop Data-Derived Extrapolation Factors for Interspecies and Intraspecies Extrapolation*; U.S. Environmental Protection Agency: Washington, DC, USA, 2014.

32. Bhat, V.S.; Meek, M.E.B.; Valcke, M.; English, C.; Boobis, A.; Brown, R. Evolution of chemical-specific adjustment factors (CSAF) based on recent international experience; increasing utility and facilitating regulatory acceptance. *Crit. Rev. Toxicol.* **2017**, *47*, 729–749. [CrossRef] [PubMed]

33. Keen, C.L.; Bell, J.G.; Lönnerdal, B. The effect of age on manganese uptake and retention from milk and infant formulas in rats. *J. Nutr.* **1986**, *116*, 395–402. [CrossRef] [PubMed]

34. Davis, C.D.; Zech, L.; Greger, J.L. Manganese metabolism in rats: An improved methodology for assessing gut endogenous losses. *Proc. Soc. Exp. Biol. Med. Soc. Exp. Biol. Med.* **1993**, *202*, 103–108. [CrossRef]

35. Mizoguchi, N.; Nishimura, Y.; Ono, H.; Sakura, N. Manganese elevations in blood of children with congenital portosystemic shunts. *Eur. J. Pediatr.* **2001**, *160*, 247–250. [CrossRef] [PubMed]

36. Health Canada Second Report on Human Biomonitoring of Environmental Chemicals in Canada. Available online: https://www.canada.ca/en/health-canada/services/environmental-workplace-health/reports-publications/environmental-contaminants/second-report-human-biomonitoring-environmental-chemicals-canada-health-canada-2013.html (accessed on 19 April 2018).

37. Sidhu, K.S. Standard setting processes and regulations for environmental contaminants in drinking water: State versus federal needs and viewpoints. *Regul. Toxicol. Pharmacol.* **1991**, *13*, 293–308. [CrossRef]

38. U.S. EPA. *2012 Edition of the Drinking Water Standards and Health Advisories*; U.S. Environmental Protection Agency: Washigton, DC, USA, 2012.

39. Tobin, R.S.; Wood, G.C.; Giddings, M.J. Development of drinking water guidelines for public health protection. *Can. Water Resour. J.* **1991**, *16*, 433–437. [CrossRef]

40. Peres, T.V.; Schettinger, M.R.C.; Chen, P.; Carvalho, F.; Avila, D.S.; Bowman, A.B.; Aschner, M. Manganese-induced neurotoxicity: A review of its behavioral consequences and neuroprotective strategies. *BMC Pharmacol. Toxicol.* **2016**, *17*, 57. [CrossRef] [PubMed]

41. Krishnan, K.; Carrier, R. The use of exposure source allocation factor in the risk assessment of drinking-water contaminants. *J. Toxicol. Environ. Health B Crit. Rev.* **2013**, *16*, 39–51. [CrossRef] [PubMed]

42. MDH. *Statement of Need and Reasonableness Proposed Amendments to the Rules on Health Risk Limits for Groundwater (Minnesota Rules, Chapter 4717, Parts 7500, 7850, and 7860)*; Minnesota Department of Health: St. Paul, MN, USA, 2015.

43. U.S. EPA. *Methodology for Deriving Ambient Water Quality Criteria for the Protection of Human Health*; U.S. Environmental Protection Agency: Washigton, DC, USA, 2000.

44. Howd, R.A.; Brown, J.P.; Fan, A.M. Risk Assessment for Chemicals in Drinking Water: Estimation of Relative Source Contribution. In Proceedings of the 43rd Annual Meeting of the Society of Toxicology, Baltimore, MD, USA, 21–25 March 2004; Volume 78.

45. MDH. *2012 Health Based Guidance for Groundwater. Manganese (Mn)*; Minnesota Department of Health: St. Paul, MN, USA, 2012.

46. WHO. *Trace Elements in Human Nutrition: Manganese*; Report of a WHO expert committee; World Health Organization: Geneva, Switzerland, 1973; pp. 34–36.

47. Schroeder, H.A.; Balassa, J.J.; Tipton, I.H. Essential trace metals in man: Manganese. A study in homeostasis. *J. Chronic Dis.* **1966**, *19*, 545–571. [CrossRef]

48. National Research Council (US) Subcommittee on Reproductive and Neurodevelopmental Toxicology. *Biologic Markers in Reproductive Toxicology*; National Academies Press (US): Washington, DC, USA, 1989; ISBN 978-0-309-03930-7.

49. NRC. *Recommended Dietary Allowances: 10th Edition*; National Academies Press (National Research Council): Washington, DC, USA, 1989.

50. Greger, J.L. Nutrition versus toxicology of manganese in humans: Evaluation of potential biomarkers. *Neurotoxicology* **1999**, *20*, 205–212. [PubMed]

51. Kern, C.H.; Smith, D.R. Preweaning Mn exposure leads to prolonged astrocyte activation and lasting effects on the dopaminergic system in adult male rats. *Synapse* **2011**, *65*, 532–544. [CrossRef] [PubMed]

52. Beaudin, S.A.; Nisam, S.; Smith, D.R. Early life versus lifelong oral manganese exposure differently impairs skilled forelimb performance in adult rats. *Neurotoxicol. Teratol.* **2013**, *38*, 36–45. [CrossRef] [PubMed]

53. Gupta, S.K.; Murthy, R.C.; Chandra, S.V. Neuromelanin in manganese-exposed primates. *Toxicol. Lett.* **1980**, *6*, 17–20. [CrossRef]

54. Ishizuka, H.; Nishida, M.; Kawada, J. Changes in stainability observed by light microscopy in the brains of ataxial mice subjected to three generations of manganese administration. *Biochem. Int.* **1991**, *25*, 677–687. [PubMed]

55. Park, S.; Sim, C.-S.; Lee, H.; Kim, Y. Blood Manganese Concentration is Elevated in Infants with Iron Deficiency. *Biol. Trace Elem. Res.* **2013**, *155*, 184–189. [CrossRef] [PubMed]

56. Alarcón, O.M.; Reinosa-Fuller, J.A.; Silva, T.; Ramirez De Fernandez, M.; Gamboa, J. Manganese Levels in Serum of Healthy Venezuelan Infants Living in Mérida. *J. Trace Elem. Med. Biol.* **1996**, *10*, 210–213. [CrossRef]

57. Huang, S.-H.; Weng, K.-P.; Lin, C.-C.; Wang, C.-C.; Lee, C.T.-C.; Ger, L.-P.; Wu, M.-T. Maternal and umbilical cord blood levels of mercury, manganese, iron, and copper in southern Taiwan: A cross-sectional study. *J. Chin. Med. Assoc.* **2017**, *80*, 442–451. [CrossRef] [PubMed]

58. Spencer, A. Whole blood manganese levels in pregnancy and the neonate. *Nutrition* **1999**, *15*, 731–734. [CrossRef]

59. Beaudin, S.A.; Strupp, B.J.; Strawderman, M.; Smith, D.R. Early Postnatal Manganese Exposure Causes Lasting Impairment of Selective and Focused Attention and Arousal Regulation in Adult Rats. *Environ. Health Perspect.* **2017**, *125*, 230–237. [CrossRef] [PubMed]

60. Brenneman, K.A.; Cattley, R.C.; Ali, S.F.; Dorman, D.C. Manganese-induced developmental neurotoxicity in the CD rat: Is oxidative damage a mechanism of action? *Neurotoxicology* **1999**, *20*, 477–487. [PubMed]

61. Dorman, D.C.; Struve, M.F.; Vitarella, D.; Byerly, F.L.; Goetz, J.; Miller, R. Neurotoxicity of manganese chloride in neonatal and adult CD rats following subchronic (21-day) high-dose oral exposure. *J. Appl. Toxicol.* **2000**, *20*, 179–187. [CrossRef]

62. Reichel, C.M.; Wacan, J.J.; Farley, C.M.; Stanley, B.J.; Crawford, C.A.; McDougall, S.A. Postnatal manganese exposure attenuates cocaine-induced locomotor activity and reduces dopamine transporters in adult male rats. *Neurotoxicol. Teratol.* **2006**, *28*, 323–332. [CrossRef] [PubMed]

63. Erikson, K.M.; Thompson, K.; Aschner, J.; Aschner, M. Manganese neurotoxicity: A focus on the neonate. *Pharmacol. Ther.* **2007**, *113*, 369–377. [CrossRef] [PubMed]

64. Cockell, K.A.; Bonacci, G.; Belonje, B. Manganese content of soy or rice beverages is high in comparison to infant formulas. *J. Am. Coll. Nutr.* **2004**, *23*, 124–130. [CrossRef] [PubMed]

65. Davidsson, L.; Cederblad, A.; Lönnerdal, B.; Sandström, B. Manganese absorption from human milk, cow's milk, and infant formulas in humans. *Am. J. Dis. Child.* **1989**, *143*, 823–827. [CrossRef] [PubMed]

66. INSPQ. *Lignes Directrices pour la Réalisation des Évaluations du Risque Toxicologique D'origine Environnementale au Québec*; Institut National de Santé Publique du Québec: Québec, QC, Canada, 2012.

67. NRC. *Biologic Markers in Reproductive Toxicology*; National Academies Press (US): Washington, DC, USA, 1989; ISBN 978-0-309-03930-7.

68. OMS. *Manganese in Drinking-Water. Background Document for Development of WHO Guidelines for Drinking-Water Quality*; Organisation Mondiale de la Santé: Genève, Switzerland, 2011.

69. U.S. EPA. Secondary Drinking Water Standards: Guidance for Nuisance Chemicals. Available online: https://www.epa.gov/dwstandardsregulations/secondary-drinking-water-standards-guidance-nuisance-chemicals (accessed on 13 June 2016).

70. Aschner, M.; Erikson, K.M.; Dorman, D.C. Manganese dosimetry: Species differences and implications for neurotoxicity. *Crit. Rev. Toxicol.* **2005**, *35*, 1–32. [CrossRef] [PubMed]

71. Tran, T.T.; Chowanadisai, W.; Crinella, F.M.; Chicz-DeMet, A.; Lönnerdal, B. Effect of high dietary manganese intake of neonatal rats on tissue mineral accumulation, striatal dopamine levels, and neurodevelopmental status. *Neurotoxicology* **2002**, *23*, 635–643. [CrossRef]

72. Miller, S.T.; Cotzias, G.C.; Evert, H.A. Control of tissue manganese: Initial absence and sudden emergence of excretion in the neonatal mouse. *Am. J. Physiol.* **1975**, *229*, 1080–1084. [CrossRef] [PubMed]

73. Zoni, S.; Lucchini, R.G. Manganese exposure: Cognitive, motor and behavioral effects on children: A review of recent findings. *Curr. Opin. Pediatr.* **2013**, *25*, 255–260. [CrossRef] [PubMed]

74. Neal, A.P.; Guilarte, T.R. Mechanisms of lead and manganese neurotoxicity. *Toxicol. Res.* **2013**, *2*, 99–114. [CrossRef] [PubMed]

75. Golub, M.S.; Hogrefe, C.E.; Germann, S.L.; Tran, T.T.; Beard, J.L.; Crinella, F.M.; Lonnerdal, B. Neurobehavioral evaluation of rhesus monkey infants fed cow's milk formula, soy formula, or soy formula with added manganese. *Neurotoxicol. Teratol.* **2005**, *27*, 615–627. [CrossRef] [PubMed]

76. Chandra, S.V.; Srivastava, R.S.; Shukla, G.S. Regional distribution of metals and biogenic amines in the brain of monkeys exposed to manganese. *Toxicol. Lett.* **1979**, *4*, 189–192. [CrossRef]

77. Guilarte, T.R.; Chen, M.-K.; McGlothan, J.L.; Verina, T.; Wong, D.F.; Zhou, Y.; Alexander, M.; Rohde, C.A.; Syversen, T.; Decamp, E.; et al. Nigrostriatal dopamine system dysfunction and subtle motor deficits in manganese-exposed non-human primates. *Exp. Neurol.* **2006**, *202*, 381–390. [CrossRef] [PubMed]

78. Schneider, J.S.; Decamp, E.; Clark, K.; Bouquio, C.; Syversen, T.; Guilarte, T.R. Effects of Chronic Manganese Exposure on Working Memory in Non-Human Primates. *Brain Res.* **2009**, *1258*, 86–95. [CrossRef] [PubMed]

79. Schneider, J.S.; Williams, C.; Ault, M.; Guilarte, T.R. Chronic Manganese Exposure Impairs Visuospatial Associative Learning in Non-Human Primates. *Toxicol. Lett.* **2013**, *221*, 146–151. [CrossRef] [PubMed]

80. Schneider, J.S.; Williams, C.; Ault, M.; Guilarte, T.R. Effects of Chronic Manganese Exposure on Attention and Working Memory in Non-Human Primates. *Neurotoxicology* **2015**, *48*, 217–222. [CrossRef] [PubMed]

81. Verina, T.; Kiihl, S.F.; Schneider, J.S.; Guilarte, T.R. Manganese exposure induces microglia activation and dystrophy in the substantia nigra of non-human primates. *Neurotoxicology* **2011**, *32*, 215–226. [CrossRef] [PubMed]

82. Schneider, J.S.; Decamp, E.; Koser, A.J.; Fritz, S.; Gonczi, H.; Syversen, T.; Guilarte, T.R. Effects of chronic manganese exposure on cognitive and motor functioning in non-human primates. *Brain Res.* **2006**, *1118*, 222–231. [CrossRef] [PubMed]

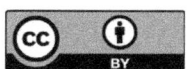

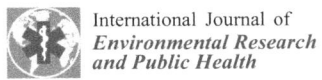

International Journal of
Environmental Research and Public Health

Article

A Method for Developing Rapid Screening Values for Active Pharmaceutical Ingredients (APIs) in Water and Results of Initial Application for 119 APIs

Ashley Suchomel *, Helen Goeden and Julia Dady

Minnesota Department of Health, Saint Paul, MN 55164, USA
* Correspondence: ashley.suchomel@state.mn.us; Tel.: +1-651-201-4512

Received: 23 May 2018; Accepted: 17 June 2018; Published: 22 June 2018

Abstract: Americans fill upward of four billion prescriptions for pharmaceuticals each year, and many of those pharmaceuticals eventually make their way into the environment. Hundreds of different active pharmaceutical ingredients (APIs) are detected in ambient waters and source water used for drinking water in the U.S. Very few of these drugs have health-based guidance values that suggest a safe level for individuals exposed in the ambient environment through drinking water. The Minnesota Department of Health (MDH) has developed a novel method to derive screening-level human health guidance values for APIs. This method was designed for rapid evaluation and relies on Food and Drug Administration (FDA)-approved drug labels and limited additional public data resources for necessary information. MDH developed an analytical framework using traditional and novel uncertainty and adjustment factors specific to the information available for APIs. This framework, along with an estimated lowest therapeutic dose (LTD), was used to derive screening reference dose (sRfD) values. Water screening values (WSV) were then derived using the sRfD, a relative source contribution factor (RSC), and a water intake rate for infants to represent a highly exposed population. MDH used this new method to derive water screening values for 119 APIs that are commonly prescribed and/or commonly monitored in Minnesota waters, including antibiotics, antidepressants, steroids, and other classes of drugs. The derived WSVs can be used to provide context to environmental detections, prioritize APIs for further health-based guidance development, prioritize APIs for future environmental monitoring studies, and inform the development or refinement of analytical methods.

Keywords: pharmaceuticals; human health; environment; drug labels; screening method; LTD; uncertainty factors; risk assessment; risk context

1. Introduction

In the past twenty-five years, the portion of the United States population that uses at least one prescription pharmaceutical has risen approximately ten percent. From 2011–2014, nearly half of all Americans used at least one prescription medication, and nearly a quarter used three or more [1]. In 2017, upward of four billion prescriptions, or 12.6 prescriptions per capita, were filled by Americans [2]. Trends show that that percentage will continue to grow in the coming years.

The rapid growth in pharmaceutical use has contributed to increased detection of pharmaceuticals in the environment [3–6]. Many pharmaceuticals are commonly detected in potential drinking water sources and treated drinking water, yet very few of these drugs have established water guidance values that inform the probability of certain health risks associated with large populations consuming water containing prescription drugs [7]. Pharmaceuticals enter the environment through a variety of pathways, including improper disposal down household drains and toilets, disposal into landfills, runoff from manure in agricultural areas after use in animals, industrial releases, and human excretion. While detected environmental concentrations may be lower than other types of contaminants, these compounds are designed to be biologically active and potent at low concentrations, warranting special scrutiny to assess potential human health risk.

Despite the widespread presence of pharmaceuticals in water, these contaminants of emerging concern are not currently regulated for drinking water and wastewater purposes. A number of methodologies have been described in the literature for screening and prioritizing the hazard and risk to human health from pharmaceuticals in the environment [8–11]. These approaches use various techniques for calculating toxicity values and mainly rely on published data in the literature for derivation of toxicity points of departure and adverse effects. The method developed by the Minnesota Department of Health (MDH) builds on many of these approaches, adding assessment factors that may be of specific concern for pharmaceuticals (e.g., endocrine activity), in addition to incorporating many elements of MDH's established risk assessment methods to derive water guidance values [12]. A key aspect of the rapid assessment method is a reliance on easily accessible data obtained from the US Food and Drug Administration (FDA) drug labels to provide the majority of the information needed. Pharmaceuticals typically have sufficient safety data as required by FDA; however, much of the data relevant for risk assessment are not available in published literature and drug studies are often considered proprietary. The data source allows for the rapid assessment of a large variety and number of pharmaceuticals that could be present in potential drinking water sources.

The objectives pursued by MDH were: (1) to create a rapid assessment framework for deriving screening reference doses (sRfDs) for orally administered pharmaceuticals using readily available information (e.g., FDA approved drug labels); and (2) to use the sRfDs to derive water screening level values for an initial set of commonly prescribed and detected pharmaceuticals. The developed values can be used for a variety of purposes, including, providing human health context to environmental detections, guiding future monitoring efforts, prioritization of development or refinement of analytical methods, and prioritization the development of health-based standards.

2. Methods

2.1. Selecting the Most Relevant Pharmaceuticals for Value Development

MDH initially planned to focus on the pharmaceuticals most relevant in Minnesota. However, prescription usage information was not available on a state-specific basis in 2013, when method development was initiated. Information on the top 200 pharmaceuticals most commonly prescribed and used in the United States from 2011–2012 [13,14] was considered representative of pharmaceutical use in Minnesota. This list, which is updated each year, provided an approximation of what may be entering the Minnesota environment, but not necessarily what is actually being found and in what amounts. In addition to the top 200 pharmaceuticals from the national lists, other pharmaceuticals were added if they were included in monitoring efforts relevant to Minnesota and were on common analyte lists from national/federal laboratories. The active pharmaceutical ingredient (API) for each pharmaceutical was identified using information from drug label information found on the National Library of Medicine drug information website DailyMed [15]. Duplicate APIs were removed from the list.

The developed framework provides a method to rapidly derive sRfDs for a large number of APIs based on information from the FDA drug label. The sRfDs are appropriate for most orally administered APIs, with a few exceptions (Table 1). The framework is not designed to address APIs with non-oral routes of administration, genotoxic effects, lack of appropriate FDA labels, and those that are only used for purposes that do not require a prescription for human use. These characteristics were used to establish exclusion criteria. Approximately one-third of the unique APIs were excluded based on the exclusion criteria.

Table 1. Exclusion Criteria for Applicable APIs.

Exclusion Criteria	Description
Non-oral route of administration	The bioavailability of an API given orally differs from that of an API given via another route of administration. Route to route modifications would be necessary to adjust for a non-oral route. The MDH method was designed to rapidly derive water screening values (WSV) related to oral ingestion, only. APIs designed to be administered vaginally, dermally, sublingually, via suppository, via injection (intraperitoneally, subcutaneously, or intravenously), and via inhalation are not appropriate for this method.
Nutritional supplement	The acceptable daily intake (ADI) values and dietary reference intake (DRI) levels for nutrients found in food and pharmaceuticals are available and more appropriate for to deriving human-health based guidance values than the calculated lowest therapeutic doses (LTD) used in this method [16].
Over-the-Counter (OTC) medication only	Labels for OTC drugs do not provide the necessary information to use the developed method.
Illicit Substance	Most illicit substances do not have an FDA-approved label. Some illicit substances may be used for therapeutic purposes with a prescription; however, the potential adverse effects may not be appropriate for analysis with this method.
Discontinued or Not Approved in US	Many discontinued products no longer have active FDA-approved labels that contain the necessary information to use the developed method. If the drug is not approved for use in the US, then it is not likely to be found in US waters in significant quantities.
Registered for Veterinary Purposes only	Labels for veterinary use APIs are not always required to provide the same level of detail as labels with APIs intended for human use.
Genotoxic or Non-Threshold Carcinogen	The developed method may not be adequate to derive an appropriately conservative screening reference doses (sRfD) or WSVs for genotoxic or non-threshold carcinogens.

If an appropriate FDA-approved label was found for an API, the description section of the label was searched for possible exclusion criteria. Exclusions based on genotoxic or non-threshold carcinogenicity were generally determined during review of the label and selection of uncertainty and adjustment factors. An unsuccessful search for an applicable FDA-approved label and supporting information usually indicated that one or more of the exclusion criteria applied.

2.2. API Data Used for Rapid Assessment

Information for each API was obtained from the most current and appropriate FDA approved label. Labels were accessed via DailyMed [15] and the most recently approved label available for oral administration of the API was selected. Additionally, MDH selected a label for a drug containing the API from an original packager, when available. If a suitable label could not be found for the API in the DailyMed database, the FDA Drugs Database [17] was searched for an applicable label. When information was not available from the drug label, or when additional data was needed to further confirm or support information from the drug label, data was gathered from other sources such as the National Toxicology Program (NTP), FDA New Drug Application (NDA) Data, International Agency for Research on Cancer (IARC), and Hazardous Substances Data Bank (HSDB) [18–20].

2.3. Lowest Therapeutic Dose Calculation

The lowest therapeutic dose (LTD), the lowest amount of an API that is necessary to produce a clinically effective outcome, was selected as the point of departure (POD) for deriving the sRfDs. The lower end of an API's therapeutic dosing range can be considered a lower threshold for biological activity, approximating a lowest adverse effect level (LOAEL). The LTD was considered an appropriate POD for the framework because API-related biological effects in the general population were considered undesirable. LTDs based on special dosing for individuals with certain physiological conditions or existing disease (e.g., renal or hepatic impairment), requiring a lower, titrated, or limited dosing, were considered not relevant for the general population and excluded from consideration. Doses on FDA labels were typically expressed as milligram per day (mg/day). In some cases, label instructions indicated dosing was required multiple times per day over various time increments to attain a minimum therapeutic level. In these cases, the LTD included the full amount per an entire 24-h day and not the minimum amount per tablet/capsule (e.g., a 10 mg tablet taken 4 times per day resulted in LTD of 40 mg/day). MDH subsequently calculated the final LTD by converting the selected dose from mg/day to mg/kg-day (Equation (1)):

$$LTD \ (mg/kg\text{-}day) = Dose \ of \ API \ (mg/kg)/BW \ based \ on \ age \ (kg) \tag{1}$$

An appropriate body weight (BW) in kilograms was selected from the US Environmental Protection Agency (EPA) Exposure Factors Handbook [21,22]. Mean weights by age, as shown in Table 2, that corresponded to the appropriate dosing recommendations from the label were used to calculate the dosage in units of mg/kg-d. If a specific age or body weight range was described on the FDA label (e.g., 12–17 years of age), the LTD calculations were performed on each age group separately (e.g., 12–13, 13–14, etc.) to determine age-group specific LTDs. In these instances, however, the age group with the highest mean weight usually produced the lowest LTD. If doses on the label were already reported in mg/kg-day, no further calculations or adjustments were made.

Table 2. Mean Weights by Age Used in Lowest Therapeutic Dose Calculations.

Age (Years)	Mean Weight (kg) [1]
6–7 [1]	22.5
7–8	27.4
8–9	31.3
9–10	36.2
10–11	39.5
11–12	44.6
12–13	50.3
13–14	56.9
14–15	61.5
15–16	65.9
16–17	68.0
17–18	66.6
≥18 [2]	80

Selected mean weights were based on the dosing age range presented on the drug label. [1] Dosing for ages under 6 years of age normally reported as mg/kg with no need for further calculation. [2] The mean weight (kg) for adults 18+ years of age is from EPA Exposure Factors Handbook 2011 Edition Table 8-1, comprising 1999–2006 data [22]. Increased weight reflects the higher average weight of a United States adult and adds to conservativeness of calculations.

2.4. Uncertainty and Adjustment Factors

Uncertainty factors (UF) and adjustment factors (AF) were used to account for a range of considerations in calculating appropriately conservative sRfDs. While the majority of the UFs applied were based on standard chemical risk assessment methods, modifications to decision criteria for application were developed to better fit specific considerations regarding APIs and the available data from FDA approved labels. Additional AFs were applied to account for special considerations and concerns related to the selected pharmaceuticals, including nonlinear (i.e., threshold) cancer potential and endocrine activity. Unlike MDH's methodology for developing health-based water guidance following in-depth review, which uses the standard RfD derivation process for nonlinear carcinogens, the MDH rapid assessment methodology for pharmaceuticals addressed carcinogenicity potential with an additional AF for cancer. In total, six potential UF or AFs, represented as UF/AF, may be applied to account for various areas of uncertainty.

A Decision Tree was established to facilitate the selection of UFs and AFs (Figure 1). Definitions and guidelines were incorporated into the Decision Tree to ensure consistency in defining and applying the UFs and AFs. Each UF or AF could be assigned a value of 1, 3, or 10. The UF/AF designation was based on the FDA-approved label data for the API or a representative API for the therapeutic class, along with additional sources as needed. A value of 1 was assigned to indicate that the particular UF or AF was not needed for the API. The minimum overall UF/AF possible (product of all six UF/AFs) was 30 (default application of an intraspecies UF of 10 and at minimum a LOAEL UF of 3) and the maximum UF/AF possible was 100,000 (a product of 10,000 for all UFs and 10 for either the AF for endocrine activity or for cancer potential). The rationale for application of specific UFs and AFs is detailed in Sections 2.4.1–2.4.6. Decision criteria for the application of each UF or AF were designed to avoid overlap application of UF/AFs based on the same information. Therefore, application of the maximum total UF/AF of 100,000 was not used in the current assessment and is highly unlikely to occur in future assessments.

Consistent with MDH and EPA risk assessment methodology [12], individual UF/AFs of 3 and 10 were expressed as 30 (3×10^1), whereas individual UF/AFs of 3 and 3 were expressed as 10 ($10^{0.5} \times 10^{0.5} = 10^1$). For the APIs evaluated, the overall UF/AF was usually at least 100. Each UF and AF is described in more detail in the following subsections and in the Decision Tree (Figure 1).

2.4.1. Cancer Adjustment Factor (AF$_C$)

MDH accounted for the risk of potential cancer of an API by applying an AF based on the available information from the FDA label. If the API was determined to be a threshold carcinogen, i.e., a carcinogen for which there is sufficient evidence that a level of exposure exists below which there is no cancer risk, the appropriate Cancer AF (AF$_C$) was determined. The FDA labels did not directly state whether or not an API had a threshold or non-threshold mode of action (MOA). Additional literature sources were consulted and professional judgement was required to make determinations. Non-threshold, i.e., linear, carcinogens were not appropriate for this method and were excluded from the evaluation. Application of UFs/AFs to a POD is not appropriate for linear carcinogens. Assessment of linear carcinogens requires access to appropriate cancer study data in order to derive a cancer slope factor rather than deriving an RfD based on a no observable adverse effect level (NOAEL) or LOAEL. For most APIs, appropriately detailed dose-response cancer data were not reported on FDA-approved labels and were not publically available because the studies were considered proprietary. Therefore, application of a rapid assessment method was not possible for linear carcinogens.

For traditional non-linear (threshold) carcinogen risk assessments, MDH evaluates the data to ensure an RfD based on non-cancer effects will also be protective for cancer. A separate cancer-based value using UFs is not typically derived for non-linear carcinogens. In contrast, the rapid screening method was used to derive a sRfD, protective of non-linear cancer effects, by using a cancer adjustment factor (AF$_C$). In many cases, drugs tested for carcinogenicity were only found to cause cancer in animals at human equivalent doses (HED) far above the maximum recommended human dose (MRHD). An HED is the human dose estimated to be equivalent to the dose administered to the test animal, based on allometric scaling. For pharmaceuticals, allometric scaling is based on relative body surface area between animals and humans. The carcinogenicity sections on the FDA labels provided the HEDs and comparisons with MRHDs necessary to make a determination about AF$_c$. An AF$_c$ of 10 was applied when the HED associated with tumors was near or below the MRHD or LTD. If the HED was far above the MRHD or LTD, an AF$_c$ was not needed. An AF$_c$ was also not applied in cases where the particular type of cancer reported in animals was not relevant to humans (rodent thyroid and liver tumors), or if the cancer was localized at the site of administration and not relevant to oral administration (carcinogenic effects only seen in studies with administration via subcutaneous or intraperitoneal injection and effects not deactivated via first pass metabolism).

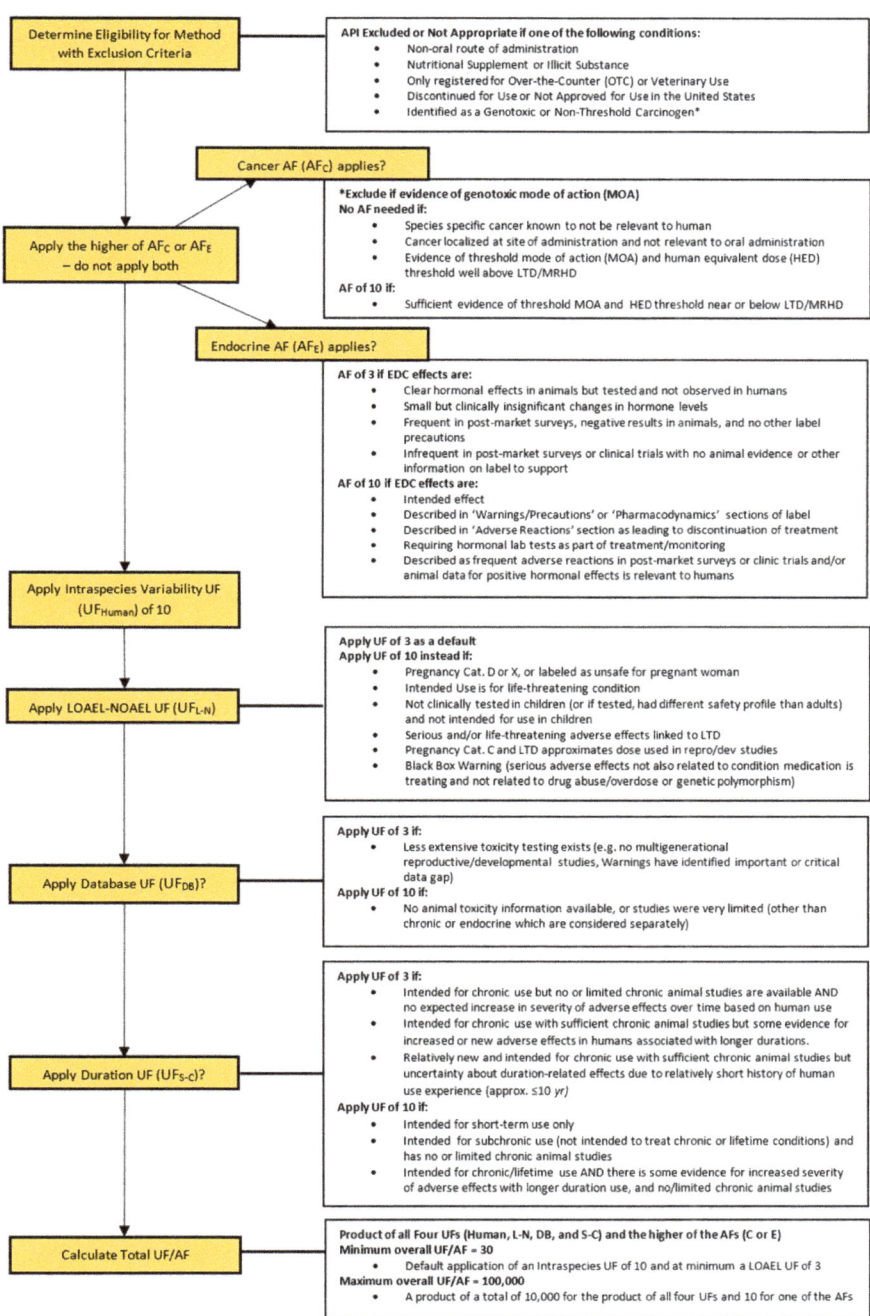

Figure 1. The decision tree provides a summary and guide for the decisions made in regards to application of Adjustment Factors (AFs), Uncertainty Factors (UFs), and calculation of Total UF/AF for use in derivation of a screening reference dose (sRfD).

2.4.2. Endocrine Activity Adjustment Factor (AF$_E$)

MDH accounted for potential adverse effects relating to endocrine activity by applying an Endocrine Activity AF (AF$_E$). The AF$_E$ was applied when endocrine activity was either the intended effect or a reported side effect of the API. Concerns that the application of the LOAEL-NOAEL UF (UF$_{L-N}$) of 10, discussed in Section 2.4.4, was not adequate to be protective of the very low-level potencies of potential endocrine active APIs warranted the use of this additional AF. MDH considered endocrine activity to include effects related to the female reproductive system, male reproductive system, pituitary gland, adrenal gland, changes in hormones (including estrogen, testosterone, and androgen), and hormonal changes related to the nervous system, blood sugar changes, and metabolism [23]. For endocrine effects aggravated by, but not caused by, the API (e.g., aggravation of diabetes symptoms in diabetic patients), an (AF$_E$) was not applied unless an endocrine mode-of-action was identified from the label. Additionally, an AF$_E$ was not applied if endocrine effects were described as rare adverse effects on the label, or the API masked signs of endocrine disease by controlling symptoms (e.g., controlled arrhythmias caused by hyperthyroidism). If the AF$_C$ was already applied, the AF$_E$ was still noted but not additionally applied. This decision was based both in part on the results of other assessment methodologies [10,24] for APIs and to avoid overlapping conservatism in the application of UF/AFs. An Endocrine Activity AF (AF$_E$) of 3 was applied when at least one of the following conditions was present on the FDA label or supporting information:

- Clear hormonal effects in animals were observed, but testing in humans was performed and no effects were observed.
- Small but clinically insignificant changes in hormone levels were seen in animal studies.
- Endocrine effects were frequent in post market surveillance in humans but negative endocrine effects were reported in animal studies, and no other precautions for endocrine effects were provided on the label.
- Infrequent endocrine effects in post market surveillance or clinical trials in humans were noted but there were no animal studies available on the label to support the observed endocrine effects.

An Endocrine Activity AF (AF$_E$) of 10 was applied when at least one of the following conditions was present on the FDA label or supporting information:

- The endocrine effects observed were the intended therapeutic effects of the API.
- The endocrine effects were described in the 'Warnings/Precautions' or 'Pharmacodynamics' section of the FDA label.
- The endocrine effects were described in the 'Adverse Reactions' section of the FDA label as leading to discontinuation of treatment.
- There were hormonal lab tests that were required or recommended as part of the treatment, or for monitoring individuals taking the API.
- The endocrine effects were described as frequent adverse reactions in post-marketing surveillance or clinical trials and/or there are animal data indicating positive hormonal effects relevant to humans.

2.4.3. Intraspecies Variability Uncertainty Factor (UF$_{Human}$)

MDH accounted for the variation in how human individuals may respond to APIs by applying an Intraspecies Variability UF of 10 to every API. This is consistent with EPA and MDH risk assessment methods for deriving health-based guidance [12,25].

2.4.4. LOAEL-NOAEL (Dosing) Uncertainty Factor (UF$_{L-N}$)

Although APIs are designed to exert a beneficial therapeutic effect on an individual, this effect may be undesirable for the general population. Adverse side effects may also occur at the LTD and drug safety studies may not report or test for effects that occur at doses lower than the LTD. As a result, the LTD was considered to be analogous to a LOAEL and could not be considered as a NOAEL. Therefore, the LOAEL-NOAEL UF (UF_{L-N}) was applied.

A LOAEL-NOAEL UF (UF_{L-N}) of 3 was applied as a default. The LOAEL-NOAEL UF (UF_{L-N}) was increased to 10 if the FDA label or supporting information indicated that the API met any of the following criteria:

- The API was labeled as Pregnancy Category D or X, or labeled as unsafe for pregnant women. FDA pregnancy categories D and X indicate that there could be side effects that may affect sensitive populations at the LTD. Category D is assigned when risks to the fetus were observed in humans, but the benefits may outweigh the risks. Category X indicates studies in animals or humans have shown fetal abnormalities or other risks to the fetus and the risks outweigh the benefits. These two category classifications warrant the use of a more protective UF. In comparison, Categories A and B indicate that adequate information in humans exist that demonstrate no substantial effect to the fetus or that studies failed to demonstrate effects to the fetus and there have been no well-controlled studies in pregnant women. Category C indicates that animal studies have shown adverse effects to the fetus and that there are no adequate studies in humans, but the potential benefits may outweigh the risks.
- The API was labeled as Pregnancy Category C and the LTD approximated the dose used in reproductive or developmental studies that was indicated on the FDA label.
- The API was intended for life threatening conditions. APIs used to treat many serious conditions often have severe side effects that can occur at the level of the LTD. The potential benefits of these APIs may outweigh the risks for those seeking the therapeutic benefit, but the side effects may not be acceptable to the general population.
- The API was not clinically tested in children or, if it was tested in children, it had a different safety profile than adults and the LTD applied only to adults. This extra level of protectiveness was warranted because children are often more sensitive to the effects of APIs.
- The LTD for the API was linked to serious and/or life threatening adverse effects.
- The FDA label for the API contained a black box warning. Certain serious warnings, particularly those that may lead to death or serious injury, are often required to be presented as a black box warning on the label with bold text marked 'Warning' [26]. Warnings for which a UF of 10 was applied included serious, life threatening effects not related to the condition or illness that the API was treating. Examples of effects where a UF of 10 was applied include statements concerning drug abuse or overdose, increased suicide from antidepressants, and those related to specific polymorphisms. Potential vulnerability due to genetic polymorphisms is addressed by the Intraspecies UF.

2.4.5. Database Uncertainty Factor (UF_{DB})

A Database UF (UF_{DB}) was applied to account for APIs with less extensive toxicity testing, especially if the data gap may be relevant to sensitive populations. A UF_{DB} of 3 was applied to APIs that may have extensive toxicity testing, but an important study appeared to be missing from the drug label. The lack of multigenerational reproductive/developmental studies was a common cause for setting this UF to 3. A UF_{DB} of 10 was applied to APIs that had no animal studies or studies with very limited endpoint testing as described on the available FDA label or other readily available sources (e.g., NTP, HSDB). Additional information may have been available in the published scientific literature, but an extensive literature search and subsequent in-depth analysis and critical review was outside the scope bounds for conducting a rapid assessment because it is very time and resource intensive.

2.4.6. Duration (of Administration) Uncertainty Factor (UF$_{SC-C}$)

A Duration UF (UF$_{SC-C}$) was applied to account for uncertainty based on the length of API use or administration, to account for limited chronic testing, or to account for the potential for increased severity of potential effects over time during the course of taking an API. A Duration UF (UF$_{SC-C}$) of 3 was applied when at least one of the following conditions applied based on the available FDA label or supporting information:

- The API was intended for chronic use (months to years) with no expected increase in severity of adverse effects over time based on extensive time of human use, but had no or limited accessible chronic animal studies.
- The API was intended for chronic use and had sufficient chronic studies in animals, but had some evidence of increased or new risk of adverse effects in humans associated with longer durations of use, including increased risk of dependence on the API.
- The API was intended for chronic use and had sufficient chronic studies in animals, but was relatively new to market, and uncertainty about possible duration-related effects due to a relatively short history of human use remains.

A Duration UF (UF$_{SC-C}$) of 10 was applied when at least one of the following conditions applied based on the available FDA label or supporting information:

- The API was intended for short-term use only (days to weeks)
- The API was intended for subchronic use (months) and had limited or no chronic testing in animals. This includes APIs not intended to treat chronic or lifetime conditions.
- The API was intended for chronic and/or lifetime use with no or limited chronic testing in animals, and there is evidence for increased severity of adverse effects with increasing and longer durations of use.

2.5. Screening Reference Dose (sRfD) Calculation

The calculated LTDs, along with the UF/AF assignments, were used in the derivation of sRfDs for each API. The sRfD is calculated in a similar manner to a traditional reference dose (RfD), a daily oral dose that is not likely to have appreciable risk or adverse effects [25,27]. MDH calculated the sRfD by dividing the LTD by the total UF/AF (Equation (2)):

$$\text{sRfD (mg/kg-d)} = \text{LTD (mg/kg-d)}/[(\text{AF}_C \text{ or } \text{AF}_E) \times \text{UF}_{Human} \times \text{UF}_{L-N} \times \text{UF}_{DB} \times \text{UF}_{S-C}] \quad (2)$$

2.6. Water Screening Value (WSV) Calculation

The WSV was derived using the calculated sRfD, a relative source contribution factor (RSC), a unit conversion factor, and a drinking water intake rate (Equation (3)). The WSV calculation is based on the MDH standard non-cancer assessment algorithm for calculating short-term water guidance values [12]:

$$\text{WSV (µg/L)} = (\text{sRfD (mg/kg-d)} \times \text{RSC} \times \text{Conversion Factor (µg/mg)})/\text{Water Intake (L/kg-d)}$$
$$\text{WSV (µg/L)} = (\text{sRfD (mg/kg-d)} \times 0.8 \times 1000 \text{ (µg/mg)})/0.289 \text{ (L/kg-d)}$$
$$(3)$$

Water intake may be only one of several pathways by which an individual may be exposed to a contaminant. An RSC is used to account for exposure other than ingestion of water (e.g., inhalation of volatilized chemicals, dermal absorption) as well as exposure from other media (e.g., diet) to ensure that the cumulative exposure does not exceed the RfD, in this case the sRfD [25]. MDH used the EPA Exposure Decision Tree [25,28] to identify the appropriate RSC value [28]. Within the EPA Decision Tree framework, RSCs can range from 0.2 up to 0.8. The EPA methodology uses a ceiling of 0.8 (80%) and minimum of 0.2 (20%) so that no more than 80% nor less than 20% of the RfD can be accounted for from ingestion of water at the developed guidance value [28]. WSVs were calculated using an RSC of 0.8 for the majority of APIs, based on the assumption that individuals not taking a prescription medication could receive the majority of their exposure through drinking water. An RSC of 0.2 was applied to a very limited number of APIs that have prescription as well as numerous over-the-counter uses, due to concerns regarding the frequency of unintended overdoses [29,30]. An example would be acetaminophen or ibuprofen, which are widely used in infants and children cough, cold and pain medications.

The intake rate used to calculate the WSV is 0.289 L/kg-d, which represents the 95th percentile human infant intake for ages 1–3 months [12]. This is consistent with MDH methodology for completing pesticide rapid assessments and with MDH risk assessment methodology for developing water guidance values [12,31,32]. The use of this intake rate is protective for infants and special susceptible populations, and was considered appropriately conservative for development of screening-level values.

3. Results

MDH identified 121 unique APIs from the 200 most prescribed pharmaceuticals in the United States from the 2011 and 2012 Pharmacy Times lists [13,14]. Forty of the 121 unique APIs were excluded from further analysis based on the exclusion criteria outlined in Table 1. Thirty-eight additional unique APIs were identified from monitoring efforts in Minnesota waters. This resulted in a total of 119 APIs for evaluation, 81 from analysis of the top 200 prescribed pharmaceuticals in the United States and 38 additional APIs that were commonly being monitored in Minnesota. Five APIs were included in the assessment even though they did not have current FDA-approved labels or were discontinued for use, despite the general exclusion criteria. These five included: lomefloxacin, norfloxacin, oxytetracycline, propoxyphene, and sulfamethizole. Labels were identified in DailyMed [15] for these five drugs, but it was discovered during the assessment that the API was either recently discontinued for use or the label was too outdated to provide all of the necessary information needed for assessment. In these cases, additional data sources [17,19,20] were relied upon to provide the needed information to derive a sRfD and WSV.

MDH calculated LTDs for each of the 119 APIs. A large majority (106 or 89%) of calculated LTDs used adult (i.e., ≥18 years of age) dosing, based on recommendations from the label. The remaining 13 (or 11%) used child or adolescent dosing and body weights (BW) from the label to serve as the basis of the LTD (Figure 2). The calculated LTDs ranged from 0.0013 to 25 mg/kg-d, spanning four orders of magnitude.

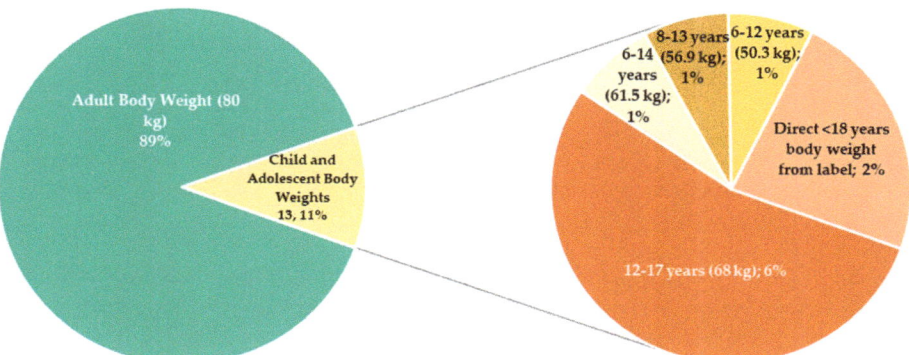

Figure 2. Breakdown of Dosing Basis for Lowest Therapeutic Dose Calculations for the 119 APIs Evaluated. The child and adolescent body weights are based on averages for the ranges [21,22] presented in Table 2.

The LTDs were then used to generate sRfDs for 119 APIs. The total UF/AF adjustment applied to the 119 APIs ranged from 100 to 30,000. The Intraspecies UF (UF_{Human}) of 10 was applied to all APIs. The LOAEL-NOAEL UF (UF_{L-N}) of 3 or 10 was applied to all APIs as well. A breakdown of the frequency of application for each UF and AF is shown in Figure 3.

A UF_{L-N} of 10 was applied to the majority of APIs (102 out of 119 or 86%) and a UF_{L-N} of 3 was applied to the remaining 17 APIs (14%) as a default UF. Often, multiple decision points for application of a UF_{L-N} of 10 applied to each API, such as a black box warning being present on the label and the API not being intended for use in children. These instances were recorded, but only one UF_{L-N} was applied in these instances. Relevant black box warnings or pregnancy category D or X statements were found on labels for 42% of APIs meeting the criteria for application of a UF_{L-N}. The label for 24% of APIs specifically indicated that the API was not intended for use in children, meeting the criteria for application of a UF_{L-N}. Serious adverse effects occurring at the LTD were noted on the label for 15% of APIs and 14% were labeled with a Pregnancy Category C classification with an LTD that approximated doses used in reproductive studies, both cases also meeting the criteria for application of a UF_{L-N} of 10.

The UF_{S-C} was applied to 92 of 119 (77%) of APIs. The UF_{S-C} of 3 was applied slightly more often (50 out of 92 or 54%) than the UF_{S-C} of 10 (42 out of 92 or 46%). The UF_{S-C} of 3 was typically applied to account for intended chronic use of an API that had sufficient testing apparent on the label or supporting information, but there was evidence of an increase in incidence or severity of effects with increased duration of use. The UF_{S-C} of 10 was most often applied to account for APIs intended for short-term use (e.g., antibiotics, pain relievers, and sedatives).

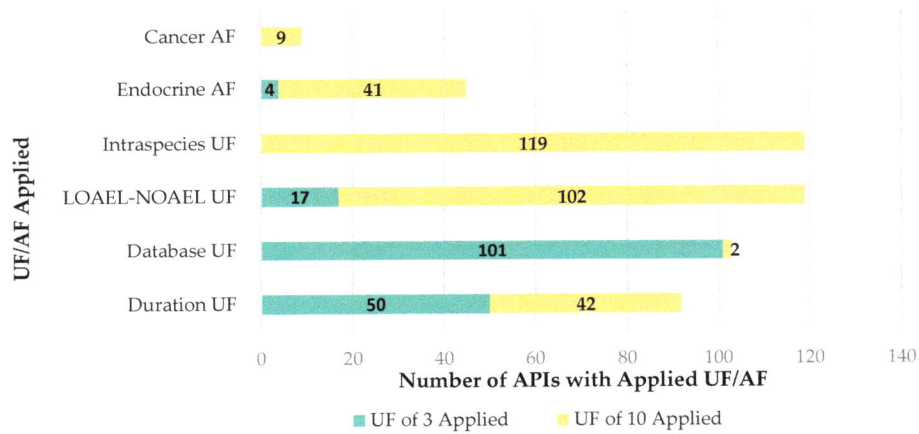

Figure 3. Frequency of Uncertainty (UF) and Adjustment (AF) Factors (described in Section 2.4) Application During Derivation of API sRfD including application of UF/AF of 3 or 10 applied for the Cancer AF (AF_C), Endocrine AF (AF_E), Intraspecies UF (UF_{Human}), LOAEL-NOAEL UF (UF_{L-N}), Database UF (UF_{DB}), and the Duration UF (UF_{S-C}).

A UF_{DB} of 3 or 10 was applied to 103 of 119 (87%) of APIs. The $UF_{DB \, of}$ 3 was most often applied (101 out of 103 or 98%) to account for a lack of multigenerational study to appropriately qualify reproductive and developmental risks. The $UF_{DB \, of}$ 10 was applied to two APIs (2%), benztropine and digoxin, to account for a lack of animal studies, most notably for reproductive and developmental endpoints, being described on the label or supporting information.

The framework for deriving sRfDs included two novel adjustment factors: Cancer AF (AF_C) and Endocrine (AF_E). These adjustment factors were applied to less than half of the 119 APIs. In cases where both factors were deemed appropriate only the higher of the two AFs was applied in deriving the sRfD. The AF_C of 10 was applied to nine APIs (digoxin, drospirenone, fenofibrate, gemofibrozil, olanzapine, pioglitazone, primidone, quetiapine, and risperidone) to account for evidence of a threshold carcinogenic mode of action with the threshold near or below the LTD or MRHD. The cancer endpoints identified for these nine APIs included liver carcinomas and tumors, mammary gland and interstitial testes tumors, bladder tumors, thyroid cancers, and adrenal gland tumors.

The AF_E was applied to 45 APIs, with the application of a AF_E of 10 being the most frequently applied value (41 out of 45). The AF_E of 10 was usually applied for one of two reasons: (1) for 61% (25 out of 41) it was based on endocrine side-effects (e.g., antidiuretic hormone effects, increased hormone levels, goitrogenic effects, gynecomastia) described in the warnings and precautions, pharmacodynamics, and adverse reactions sections of the label; or (2) for the remaining 39% (16 of 41) it was based on endocrine effects that were the intended therapeutic effect (e.g., insulin stimulation, regulation of thyroid activity) for APIs that were glucocorticoids, antidepressants, hormones, or lipid lowering drugs. The AF_E of 3, on the other hand, was usually applied to account for infrequent endocrine effects (hormone level changes) being reported in humans with no animal data to support these observed effects.

Some individual APIs lacked data to adequately evaluate carcinogenic potential or endocrine activity. During the assessment it was determined that APIs within the same class could be used to address these data gaps. Three classes of APIs (i.e., statins, sulfonamides, and tetracyclines) were assessed as a group for determining the appropriate application of the Cancer AF and/or Endocrine Activity AF. A group assessment was considered appropriate since the general modes-of-action are similar within each class.

Statins, including atorvastatin, lovastatin, pravastatin, rosuvastatin, and simvastatin, were each assigned an AF_E of 10 based on clear indications for endocrine effects on the 'Warnings and Precautions' section of the label. Sulfonamides, including sulfadiazine, sulfamethizole, and sulfamethoxazole, were each assigned an AF_E of 10 to account for known drug class effects on the thyroid. The tetracycline drug class, including demeclocycline, doxycycline, minocycline, oxytetracycline, and tetracycline, were reviewed together to determine Cancer and Endocrine AFs. The tetracycline class evaluation was based on the label for minocycline and supporting information on labels for others in the group. Tetracyclines were assigned an AF_E of 10 for thyroid effects including thyroid hyperplasia and the potential of thyroid related cancers. An AF_C of 1 was assigned to the five tetracyclines based on the lack of information provided on labels to determine relative dosing related to human doses for cancer studies, and due to the likely cancer mechanism, if present, being related to endocrine mechanisms, which was more appropriately covered with the application of the AF_E.

The sRfDs were calculated using the LTD and overall UF (Equation (2)). Each sRfD along with an RSC and an infant water intake rate were used to generate the WSV (Equation (3)). An RSC of 0.8 was used for the majority of the 119 APIs. However, an RSC of 0.2 was used for one API, ibuprofen, because it is included in multiple over-the-counter (OTC) formulations intended for children in addition to prescription pharmaceuticals. The derived sRfDs ranged from 0.00000016 mg/kg-d to 0.12 mg/kg-d, spanning six orders of magnitude. The final derived water screening values (Table 3) also spanned six orders of magnitude with values ranging from 0.0004 μg/L to 400 μg/L. A detailed breakdown of the calculation for each of the 119 APIs (i.e., LTD, sRfD, WSV, UF/AF application, and reference label sources) is provided in Table S1. Pharmaceutical Water Screening Values Table (see supplementary information).

Table 3. Derived Water Screening Values (WSV), Screening Reference Doses (sRfD), Uncertainty and Adjustment Factor (UF/AF) application, and calculated Lowest Therapeutic Doses (LTD) for 119 APIs [1].

API	CASRN	LTD (mg/kg)	Total UF/AF	sRfD (mg/kg-d)	WSV (µg/L)
Albuterol	18559-94-9	0.075	100	0.00075	2
Alendronate	66376-36-1	0.063	300	0.00021	0.6
Allopurinol	315-30-0	2.50	100	0.025	70
Alprazolam	28981-97-7	0.0094	1000	0.0000094	0.03
Amitriptyline	50-48-6	0.74	10000	0.000074	0.2
Amlodipine	88150-42-9	0.037	100	0.00037	1
Amoxicillin	26787-78-0	12.5	1000	0.013	40
Amphetamine salts	-	0.039	3000	0.000013	0.04
Ampicillin	69-53-4	12.5	3000	0.0042	10
Atenolol	29122-68-7	0.63	1000	0.00063	2
Atorvastatin	134523-00-5	0.13	3000	0.000043	0.1
Azithromycin	83905-01-5	3.13	3000	0.001	3
Benztropine	86-13-5	0.013	3000	0.0000043	0.01
Betaxolol	63659-18-7	0.13	1000	0.00013	0.4
Bisoprolol	66722-44-9	0.6	1000	0.0006	2
Carisoprodol	78-44-4	9.38	1000	0.0094	30
Carvedilol	72956-09-3	0.313	300	0.001	3
Celecoxib	169590-42-5	2.50	1000	0.0025	7
Cephalexin	15686-71-2	12.5	1000	0.013	40
Cimetidine	51481-61-9	10	1000	0.01	30
Ciprofloxacin	85721-33-1	6.25	3000	0.0021	6
Clarithromycin	81103-11-9	6.25	3000	0.0021	6
Clavulanate	58001-44-8	3.13	1000	0.0031	9
Clindamycin	18323-44-9	7.50	3000	0.0025	7
Clonazepam	1622-61-3	0.013	3000	0.0000043	0.01
Clonidine	4205-90-7	0.0025	300	0.0000083	0.02
Clopidogrel	113665-84-2	0.94	300	0.0031	9
Codeine	76-57-3	0.19	1000	0.00019	0.5
Cyclobenzaprine	303-53-7	0.19	10000	0.000019	0.05
Demeclocycline	127-33-3	7	30000	0.00023	0.6
Diazepam	439-14-5	0.044	300	0.00015	0.4
Diclofenac	15307-86-5	1.25	300	0.0042	10
Digoxin	20830-75-5	0.0016	10000	0.00000016	0.0004
Diltiazem	42399-41-7	1.5	1000	0.0015	4
Doxepin	1668-19-5	0.94	3000	0.00032	0.9
Doxycycline	564-25-0	0.91	30000	0.000030	0.08
Drospirenone	67392-87-4	0.038	10000	0.0000038	0.01
Duloxetine	116539-59-4	0.50	1000	0.0005	1
Enalapril	75847-73-3	0.063	300	0.00021	0.6
Erythromycin	114-07-8	12.5	1000	0.013	40
Escitalopram	128196-01-0	0.13	3000	0.000043	0.1
Ezetimibe	163222-33-1	0.125	300	0.00042	1
Fenofibrate	49562-28-9	0.60	3000	0.0002	0.6
Fenoprofen	31879-05-7	2.5	3000	0.00083	2
Fluconazole	86386-73-4	1.25	10000	0.00013	0.4
Fluoxetine	54910-89-3	0.25	3000	0.000083	0.2
Furosemide	54-31-9	0.25	300	0.00083	2
Gabapentin	60142-96-3	11.3	100	0.11	300
Gemfibrozil	25812-30-0	15	3000	0.005	10
Glipizide	29094-61-9	0.19	10000	0.000019	0.05
Glyburide	10238-21-8	0.016	10000	0.0000016	0.004
Hydrochlorothiazide	58-93-5	0.16	10000	0.000016	0.04
Hydrocodone	125-29-1	0.25	10000	0.000025	0.07
Hydrocortisone	50-23-7	0.25	30000	0.0000083	0.02
Ibuprofen	15687-27-1	20	3000	0.0067	5[i]
Imipramine	50-49-7	0.37	10000	0.000037	0.1
Indomethacin	53-86-1	0.63	300	0.0021	6
Ketoprofen	22071-15-4	0.94	1000	0.00094	3
Lamotrigine	84057-84-1	2.81	300	0.0094	30
Levothyroxine	51-48-9	0.0013	300	0.0000043	0.01

Table 3. *Cont.*

API	CASRN	LTD (mg/kg)	Total UF/AF	sRfD (mg/kg-d)	WSV (µg/L)
Lisdexamfetamine	608137-32-2	0.38	3000	0.00013	0.4
Lisinopril	76547-98-3	0.063	3000	0.000021	0.06
Lomefloxacin	98079-51-7	20	3000	0.0067	20
Lorazepam	846-49-1	0.025	3000	0.0000083	0.02
Losartan	114798-26-4	0.63	300	0.0021	6
Lovastatin	75330-75-5	0.13	10000	0.000013	0.04
Mefenamic acid	61-68-7	12.5	3000	0.0042	10
Meloxicam	71125-38-7	0.094	1000	0.000094	0.3
Memantine	19982-08-2	0.25	1000	0.00025	0.7
Meprobamate	57-53-4	3.98	1000	0.004	10
Metformin	657-24-9	14.7	10000	0.0015	4
Methylphenidate	113-45-1	0.25	1000	0.00025	0.7
Methylprednisolone	83-43-2	0.05	30000	0.0000017	0.005
Metoprolol	51384-51-1	0.31	300	0.001	3
Minocycline	10118-90-8	2.5	30000	0.000083	0.2
Montelukast	158966-92-8	0.081	100	0.00081	2
Naproxen	22204-53-1	6.25	1000	0.0063	20
Nebivolol	118457-14-0	0.031	1000	0.000031	0.09
Nifedipine	21829-25-4	0.38	1000	0.00038	1
Norfloxacin	70458-96-7	10	3000	0.0033	10
Ofloxacin	82419-36-1	5	3000	0.0017	5
Olanzapine	132539-06-1	0.037	10000	0.0000037	0.01
Olmesartan medoxomil	144689-63-4	0.25	300	0.00083	2
Oxycodone	76-42-6	0.25	30000	0.0000083	0.02
Oxytetracycline	79-57-2	6.25	30000	0.00021	0.6
Penicillin V	87-08-1	9.38	3000	0.0031	9
Pentoxyifylline	6493-05-6	5	300	0.017	50
Pioglitazone	111025-46-8	0.19	10000	0.000019	0.05
Pravastatin	81093-37-0	0.35	10000	0.000035	0.1
Prednisolone	50-24-8	0.06	30000	0.000002	0.006
Prednisone	53-03-2	0.063	30000	0.0000021	0.006
Pregabalin	148553-50-8	1.88	300	0.0063	20
Primidone	125-33-7	9.38	3000	0.0031	9
Progesterone	57-83-0	2.5	30000	0.000083	0.2
Promethazine	60-87-7	0.23	3000	0.000077	0.2
Propranolol	525-66-6	0.38	3000	0.00013	0.4
Propoxyphene	469-62-5	4.88	3000	0.0016	4
Quetiapine	111974-69-7	0.63	10000	0.000063	0.2
Ranitidine	66357-35-5	2	100	0.02	60
Risperidone	106266-06-2	0.0074	3000	0.0000025	0.007
Rosuvastatin	287714-41-4	0.063	10000	0.0000063	0.02
Sertraline	79617-96-2	0.31	3000	0.0001	0.3
Sildenafil	139755-83-2	0.13	1000	0.00013	0.4
Simvastatin	79902-63-9	0.063	10000	0.0000063	0.02
Sitagliptin	486460-32-6	1.25	10000	0.00013	0.4
Sulfadiazine	68-35-9	25	10000	0.0025	7
Sulfamethizole	144-82-1	12.5	30000	0.00042	1
Tadalafil	171596-29-5	0.031	300	0.0001	0.3
Tamsulosin	106133-20-4	0.005	3000	0.0000017	0.005
Temazepam	846-50-4	0.09	3000	0.00003	0.08
Tetracycline	60-54-8	18.8	30000	0.00063	2
Tramadol	27203-92-5	2.50	1000	0.0025	7
Trazodone	19794-93-5	1.88	10000	0.00019	0.5
Triamterene	396-01-0	0.47	300	0.0016	4
Trimethoprim	738-70-5	4.57	3000	0.0015	4
Valsartan	137862-53-4	1	300	0.0033	9
Verapamil	52-53-9	2.25	1000	0.0023	6
Warfarin	81-81-2	0.025	1000	0.000025	0.07
Zolpidem	82626-48-0	0.063	3000	0.000021	0.06

[1] Derived values are based on data and drug labels accessed in 2014 from DailyMed [15] and the FDA Drug Database [17].

4. Discussion

MDH developed a novel method to rapidly derive screening level values for APIs that have the potential to be found in the environment. As described in Section 2, this method relied upon established MDH risk assessment practices as well as pharmaceutical specific data to derive appropriately conservative water screening values in a rapid manner.

4.1. Data Sources

The selection of an appropriate FDA label was key to deriving a WSV for each API. As previously mentioned, it was important to find the most current and active FDA label available for oral administration of the API. Labels from the original packager and brand names, that were no more than three years old, were used to derive the screening values in 2014. When original labels were not available, repackagers and generic labels were used. When labels in DailyMed [15] were older than two years, the FDA Drugs Database [17] was consulted to confirm that it was the most up-to-date available label.

The available FDA-approved labels can change over time due to new FDA labeling requirements or availability of new safety data. Changes to labeling requirements could affect where relevant information is found on the label and could change how the available data is interpreted. During development of the 119 screening values, the FDA finalized a new Pregnancy and Lactation Labeling Rule (PLLR) that changed how pregnancy and lactation data were presented on the label [33]. The new rule removed the use of pregnancy letter categories (A, B, C, D, and X) and replaced it with three subsections labeled 'Pregnancy', 'Lactation', and 'Females and Males of Reproductive Potential'. This new rule gradually phased in the new requirements for existing products and immediately impacted newly registered products. These changes do not impact the values already derived; however, the evaluation of new products will have to be slightly altered to fit the new label presentation. The developed methodology is still useful when evaluating these new products, as the description of effects will still be available. However, the pregnancy letter categories which made the LOAEL-NOAEL UF designation easy to apply, will not be present.

Additional changes to other label sections may occur if additional rule changes are made by the FDA. Changes to labels may also occur as new safety data are added. When there is updated safety information, the FDA [34] generally directs that relevant labels be updated to reflect those changes. MDH, however, found that labels in DailyMed [15] were not always updated. Changes to labels can also be due to changes in manufacturer or packager of the API, as well as formulations being acquired by different companies as a product becomes generic. DailyMed [15] did not have an archive process for these labels when a new label was issued under the same manufacturer at the time of the MDH assessment. For these reasons, labels for assessment were chosen carefully and were identified during value derivation (Table S1). With this knowledge, MDH relied heavily on the FDA-approved label, but other sources were consulted to verify information and fill in data gaps.

The data sources used for this rapid assessment method placed constraints on the types of APIs that could be evaluated. Over-the-counter drugs (OTC), genotoxic or non-threshold carcinogens, and those with non-oral routes of administration cannot be adequately assessed using this method, even though they are often detected in the environment. The Decision Tree in Figure 1 could be easily adapted for OTC drugs; however, different sources of relevant information would need to be identified to facilitate consistent and rapid reviews since OTC labels do not contain the same level of detail as prescription labels. Appropriate risk assessments of genotoxic and non-linear carcinogens require development of cancer slope factors. However, cancer slope factors are not available on FDA-approved labels and cannot be developed without access to data that are currently not publicly available. Drugs with non-oral routes of administration need to be assessed using route-to-route extrapolation. While there are various methods available to conduct route-to-route extrapolation, there are currently no methods developed to facilitate a rapid screening assessment for non-orally administered APIs.

Additional or different methods, decision criteria data, and data sources would need be needed to address these groups of APIs.

4.2. Appropriately Conservative Methodology

The rapid assessment method was designed to derive appropriately protective sRfDs and WSVs. The method is designed to be more conservative than values generated using the established MDH methodology for in-depth chemical reviews. The level of protectiveness is appropriate for a screening value meant to protect the general population, including sensitive or highly exposed populations, based on limited data or time for assessment. To ensure that the sRfDs and WSVs were sufficiently protective, appropriately conservative selections were made for a variety of parameters used to derive sRfDs and WSVs.

An adult body weight of 80 kg was used in the LTD calculations. As seen in Figure 2, the most common body weight used in the development of the LTDs was the 80 kg adult body weight. In most risk assessment methodologies, 70 kg is the standard adult body weight. According to the EPA, the average adult body weight has increased in recent years, making the 80 kg estimate more appropriate for the current general US adult population [22]. Use of the higher adult body weight results in lower LTDs and sRfD.

The Decision Tree (Figure 1) for application of UF/AFs based on drug label and supporting information was designed to ensure that the resulting sRfD, which was based on limited data and level of evaluation, would be protective of the most sensitive members of the general population. MDH risk assessment methodology for conducting in-depth chemical reviews, uses a maximum UF of 3000 when deriving an RfDs [12]. A chemical with a UF over 3000 is deemed to have insufficient information to derive an appropriate health-based value. The rapid assessment methodology resulted in the application of overall UFs ranging from 100 to 30,000, with 33 (28%) having values greater than 3000. The majority of APIs with a total UF greater than 3000 were either endocrine-active or had a LOAEL-NOAEL UF (UF_{L-N}) of 10 (Table S1). The common application of an UF_{L-N} of 10 is not unexpected given that APIs are designed to be biologically active at low doses.

Uncertainty factors for intraspecies variability (UF_{HUMAN}), LOAEL-NOAEL extrapolation (UF_{L-N}), database deficiencies (UF_{DB}), and duration (UF_{S-to-C}) are commonly applied in established risk assessment practices for industrial and commercial product environmental contaminants. Unlike APIs, these environmental contaminants are not usually designed to be biologically active in humans. To account for this intended biological activity, MDH included additional adjustment factors for cancer (AF_C) and endocrine activity potential (AF_E) in the rapid assessment framework for pharmaceuticals. The use of additional factors for cancer and endocrine activity has precedence based on other methods and approaches described in the published literature [10,24]. The Australian government (AU) has published guidelines for water recycling that include development of surrogate acceptable daily intakes for pharmaceuticals [24]. The AU describes use of a 10-fold safety factor for hormonally active steroids because normal hormone function and fertility could be adversely affected in those not taking the medication for therapeutic benefits [24]. This hormonally-based safety factor used by the AU is similar to the endocrine activity AF applied in MDH's rapid assessment methodology. The WateReuse Foundation also identified hormonally active compounds and genotoxic carcinogens to be of particular concern and incorporated a UF of 10 in their assessment [10]. These additional AFs provided an extra degree of protection for effects that were not necessarily captured by the other UFs, and may be related to the intended biological effect of the API. The maximum LOAEL-NOAEL UF of 10 may not be adequately protective for APIs designed to effect endocrine targets or for potential carcinogens.

The use of a water intake rate based on bottle-fed infants of 0.289 L/kg-d also added to the conservative nature of the derived screening values. Bottle-fed infants have a higher intake of water on a per body weight basis than individuals at any other life-stage, and are more likely to ingest a higher dose than adults [12,32]. The high infant intake rate is protective of formula-fed infants as well as other sensitive populations. The same intake rate and rationale has been applied by MDH for deriving rapid assessment values for pesticides [31] and is recommended for screening level values [32].

Comparison of WSVs with MDH Derived Health-Based Guidance (HBG)

To test the developed method, MDH compared the WSVs derived using the rapid assessment methodology with health-based guidance values (HBGs) derived from traditional in-depth reviews for five APIs [35]). The five APIs were acetaminophen [36], carbamazepine [37], 17a-ethinylestradiol [38], sulfamethoxazole [39], and venlafaxine [40]. The HBGs are based on an in-depth evaluation of potential health risk and are preferred over WSVs when available.

The WSVs derived using the rapid assessment methodology were 2 to 250 times lower, or more conservative, than HBGs derived using established MDH in-depth review methods (Table 4). For four of the five (acetaminophen, carbamazepine, sulfamethoxazole, and venlafaxine) APIs the same RSC (0.2 for acetaminophen and 0.8 for the others) and intake rate (0.289 L/kg-d) were used to derive both the WSV and the HBG. When these inputs were the same, the resulting WSVs were lower than HBGs due, in part, to use of the LTD as the point of departure (POD) instead of a LOAEL or NOAEL, as well as of the additional UFs and AFs. Total UF/AFs for WSVs were higher than those used for HBGs. This was expected because full in-depth reviews required for HBG development were more refined and involved critical examination of much larger datasets, which reduced the degree of uncertainty.

For the remaining API, 17a-ethinylestradiol, the RSC used to derive the WSV and HBG was 0.8, but the intake rates differed. The HBG derived from a full in-depth review supported use of a lower, sub-chronic water intake rate (0.070 L/kg-d) rather than the infant intake rate (0.289 L/kg-d) used in deriving the WSV. The lower intake rate in the HBG calculation and the higher overall UF applied in the WSV calculation resulted in a nearly identical values. This indicated that even for hormonal active compounds that mimic endogenous chemicals, the derived WSVs are near or lower than values derived with traditional methods.

The two WSVs for acetaminophen represented the recommended daily dose ranges for different therapeutic purposes. For example, a simple headache might be treated effectively with only one tablet but more severe pain or chronic conditions such as arthritis might require the maximum recommended daily dosing of six tablets (i.e., 1 tablet every 4 h). The lower LTD of 3.75 mg/kg-d and WSV of 9 µg/L were based on one tablet per day while the higher LTD of 22.5 mg/kg-d and WSV of 50 µg/L were based on six tablets per day.

The limited comparison of rapid assessment-based WSVs and HBGs, which are based on an in-depth review, demonstrates a reasonable level of conservatism. Therefore, WSVs were considered appropriate for screening and prioritization purposes and were not likely to underestimate risk.

Table 4. Comparison of Inputs and Values for the Pharmaceutical Rapid Assessment Method for Deriving WSVs and MDH established traditional method for deriving Health-Based Guidance Values (HBG).

API	WSV (µg/L)	MDH HBG (µg/L)	Level of Protection	Pharmaceutical Rapid Assessment Method Inputs	MDH Guidance Value Inputs [1]
Acetaminophen [2]	9 50	200	4–22x	LTD1—3.75 LTD2—22.5 mg/kg-d UF_{HUMAN}—10 UF_{L-N}—10 UF_{DB}—3 UF_{S-C}—10 Overall UF/AF—3000	POD—7.4 mg/kg-d UF_H—10 UF_{DB}—3 Total UF—300
Carbamazepine	0.9	40	44x	LTD—1 mg/kg-d AF_C—10 UF_{HUMAN}—10 UF_{L-N}—10 UF_{S-C}—3 Overall UF/AF—3000	POD—3.8 mg/kg-d UF_H—10 UF_{L-N}—10 UF_{DB}—3 Total UF—300
17a-Ethinylestradiol	0.0001	0.0002	2x	LTD—0.00044 mg/kg-d AF_E—10 UF_{HUMAN}—10 UF_{L-N}—10 UF_{DB}—3 UF_{S-C}—3 Overall UF/AF—3000	POD—4.2×10^{-7} mg/kg-d UF_H—10 UF_A—3 Total UF—30
Sulfamethoxazole	0.4	100	250x	LTD—4.57 mg/kg-d AF_E—10 UF_{HUMAN}—10 UF_{L-N}—10 UF_{DB}—3 UF_{S-C}—10 Overall UF/AF—30,000	POD—1.2 mg/kg-d UF_H—10 UF_A—3 Overall UF—30
Venlafaxine	0.3	10	33x	LTD—25 mg/kg-d UF_{HUMAN}—10 UF_{L-N}—10 UF_{DB}—3 UF_{S-C}—10 Overall UF/AF—3000	POD—0.54 mg/kg-d UF_H—10 UF_{L-N}—10 Total UF—100

[1] Points-of-departure (POD) for derving MDH Health-Based Guidance (HBG) are NOAELS or LOAELS. Uncertainty factors (UF) used in deriving HBGs include Intraspecies UF (UF_H), Interspecies UF (UF_A), LOAEL-NOAEL UF (UF_{L-N}), and a Database UF (UF_{DB}). [2] The lower LTD of 3.75 mg/kg-d (LTD_1) and WSV of 9 µg/L were based on one tablet per day for acetaminophen, while the higher LTD of 22.5 mg/kg-d (LTD_2) and WSV of 50 µg/L were based on six tablets per day for acetaminophen. Both dosing regimens are therapeutically relevant and therefore were both included as comparison values.

4.3. Applications of the Values and Use of the Method

The WSV derived by MDH using the rapid assessment methodology are most appropriate for prioritization and screening purposes. MDH recommends using WSVs as a first tier assessment for detections of APIs in a variety of water environments, including surface water, groundwater, and treated drinking water. Ingestion of water is unlikely to pose a threat to human health when API water concentrations are below the WSV. WSVs can also be used for: (1) setting priorities for deriving new health-based guidance based on in-depth reviews; (2) setting priorities for developing new or improved laboratory analytical methods; (3) selecting APIs to be included in future monitoring projects; and (4) assisting in the evaluation of water quality. Situations in which water detections exceed the WSV, may benefit from completing a more thorough risk assessment for the API. Many APIs may not have any available analytical methods, making it impossible or difficult for them to be included in environmental monitoring programs. The WSVs may help to identify APIs that warrant development of new or improved analytical methods. The water screening values are not designed to be used as definitive estimates of risk. A more refined assessment, including detailed toxicity and exposure evaluations, should be done before specific risk management decisions are made.

To date, MDH has used the derived values to provide context to environmental detections of various monitoring studies of surface water and groundwater in Minnesota. The majority of detections have been below developed WSVs. Only two APIs, hydrochlorothiazide (WSV of 0.04 ug/L) and methylprednisolone (WSV of 0.005 ug/L), have been detected in Minnesota surface water at concentrations exceeding the WSV (0.0571 ug/L and 0.006, respectively) [41,42]. No concentrations for APIs in Minnesota groundwater have exceeded a WSV. Gabapentin, an anticonvulsant is detected frequently and at relatively high concentrations compared to other APIs in Minnesota surface waters, sometimes at concentrations over 1 ug/L [42]. While these concentrations appear of concern in contrast to concentrations of other APIs, the concentrations are well below the developed WSV of 300 ug/L indicating that gabapentin detections are not likely to pose a human health concern at detected concentrations. It should be noted that WSVs may not be protective of ecological receptors.

Although, concentrations did not exceed the WSV for most APIs in Minnesota, that does not indicate that concentrations of APIs in other areas and states are not of potential concern. The WSVs can be used to provide context to environmental detections in waters throughout the country to similarly prioritize monitoring efforts and determine potential health risk posed by detected concentrations.

Additionally, MDH compared the WSVs to available maximum detection limits (MDL) and maximum reporting limits (MRL) for analytical schedules from EPA (Methods 1694, 1698) [43,44], USGS (Methods 2434, 2440, and 2080) [45–47], and SGS Axys Analytical pharmaceutical methods [48], all of which are commonly used to analyze Minnesota monitoring samples. The MDL or MRL exceeded the WSV for eight APIs, including benztropine, digoxin, glyburide, hydrocortisone, methylprednisolone, oxycodone, prednisolone, and prednisone, indicating that efforts to improve (lower) detection limits of existing analytical methods may be warranted.

MDH was also unable to find evidence of monitoring capability for nearly 22% (18 of 81) of the most commonly prescribed APIs. Given the potential for environmental release development of analytical capabilities should be a research priority.

5. Conclusions

MDH has developed a rapid assessment method for deriving WSVs for APIs. This approach is rooted in traditional risk assessment practices and builds upon related methods created by other organizations. This method can be applied for most orally administered human prescription drugs. Screening level values were developed relatively quickly using data from FDA-approved drug labels. MDH used the rapid assessment method to derive sRfDs and WSVs for 119 unique APIs that are commonly prescribed and/or monitored in the environment. The use of FDA-approved labels and limited additional sources allowed for the derivation of consistent and appropriately conservative screening level values. These screening values filled existing data gaps in the available guidance for many of these APIs.

Over four billion pharmaceutical prescriptions were filled last year in the United States, and this estimate is expected to increase in coming years. Continually increasing trends in prescription usage means that APIs have an ever-growing presence in the natural environment. Pharmaceuticals are nearly ubiquitous in most environmental media as a result of improper disposal and normal human excretion. Growing concerns about widespread prevalence of APIs in the environment led to the realization that a rapid method for developing values to provide context for the occurrence of APIs in the environment was required. The rapid assessment method and screening values developed by MDH provide information that can be used to respond to current detections and allow risk managers opportunities to be proactive in setting future priorities. Some future priorities include continued monitoring for pharmaceuticals in environmental media, setting priorities for more detailed and impactful pharmaceutical risk assessments, and identifying the need for new or modified analytical methods.

Supplementary Materials: The following are available online at http://www.mdpi.com/1660-4601/15/7/1308/s1, Table S1: Active Pharmaceutical Ingredient (API) Rapid Assessment Method Inputs, Decisions, Values, and Supporting Information.

Author Contributions: Conceptualization, H.G.; Data curation, A.S.; Formal analysis, A.S. and J.D.; Investigation, A.S., H.G. and J.D.; Methodology, A.S., H.G. and J.D.; Project administration, A.S.; Validation, A.S., H.G. and J.D.; Writing—original draft, A.S.; Writing—review & editing, H.G. and J.D.

Funding: This work was conducted by the Minnesota Department of Health's Contaminants of Emerging Concern (CEC) Program with funds from the Clean Water Fund of the Clean Water, Land, and Legacy Amendment of Minnesota.

Acknowledgments: The authors would like to thank Chris Greene, Kris Klos, James Jacobus, Sarah Johnson, James Kelly, and Katie Nyquist for their efforts in reviewing this paper.

Conflicts of Interest: The authors declare no conflict of interest.

References

1. Centers for Disease Control and Prevention—National Center for Health Statistics. Health, United States. 2016. Available online: https://www.cdc.gov/nchs/data/hus/hus16.pdf#079 (accessed on 4 April 2018).
2. Kaiser Family Foundation. Retail Prescription Drugs Filled at Pharmacies (Annual Per Capita) and Total Number of Retail Prescription Drugs Filled at Pharmacies. Available online: https://www.kff.org/state-category/health-costs-budgets/prescription-drugs/ (accessed on 10 April 2018).
3. Daughton, C. Pharmaceutical ingredients in drinking water: Overview of occurence and significance of human exposure. In *Contaminants of Emerging Concern in the Environment: Ecological and Human Health Considerations*; American Chemical Society: Washington, DC, USA, 2010; Chapter 2; Volume 1048, pp. 9–68.
4. Fram, M.; Belitz, K. Occurence and concentrations of pharmaceutical compounds in groundwater used for public drinking water supply in California. *Sci. Total Environ.* **2011**, *409*, 3409–3417. [CrossRef] [PubMed]
5. Kolpin, D.; Furlong, E.T.; Meyer, M.T.; Thurman, E.M.; Zaugg, S.D.; Barber, L.B.; Buxton, H.T. Pharmaceuticals, hormones, and other organic wastewater contaminants in US streams, 1999–2000. A national reconnaissance. *Environ. Sci. Technol.* **2002**, *36*, 1202–1211. [CrossRef] [PubMed]
6. Lee, K.; Langer, S.; Barber, L.; Writer, J.; Ferrey, M.; Schoenfuss, H.; Furlong, E.; Foreman, W.; Gray, J.; ReVello, R.; et al. Endocrine Active Chemicals, Pharmaceuticals, and Other Chemicals of Concern in Surface Water, Wastewater-Treatment Plant Effluent, Bed Sediment, and Biological Characteristics in Selected Streams, Minnesota—Design, Methods, Data, Data Series 575. 2009. Available online: https://pubs.usgs.gov/ds/575/pdf/ds575.pdf (accessed on 4 April 2018).
7. Furlong, E.; Batt, A.L.; Glassmeyer, S.T.; Noriega, M.C.; Kolpin, D.W.; Mash, H.; Schench, K.M. Nationwide reconnaissance of contamiants of emerging concern in source and treated drinking waters of the United States: Pharmaceuticals. *Sci. Total Environ.* **2017**, *579*, 1629–1642. [CrossRef] [PubMed]
8. Schwab, B.; Hayes, E.P.; Fiori, J.M.; Mastrocco, F.J.; Roden, N.M.; Cragin, D.; Meyerhoff, R.D.; D'Aco, V.J.; Anderson, P.D. Human pharmaceuticals in US surface waters: A human health risk assessment. *Regul. Toxicol. Pharmacol.* **2005**, *42*, 296–312. [CrossRef] [PubMed]
9. US Environmental Protection Agency. Approaches to Screening for Risk from Pharmaceuticals in Drinking Water and Prioritization for Further Evaluation (Contract No. C-07-021, wa -b-02, Tasks 6 Under the Supervision of Dr. O. Conerly). Available online: https://www.acs.org/content/dam/acsorg/policy/acsonthehill/briefings/pharmaceuticalsinwater/epa-approaches-to-screening-pharmaceuticals-in-water.pdf (accessed on 4 April 2018).
10. WateReuse Research Foundation. Identifying Hormonally Active Compounds, Pharmaceuticals, and Personal Care Product Ingredients of Health Concern from Potential Presence in Water Intended for Indirect Potable Use. Available online: https://watereuse.org/watereuse-research/05-05-identifying-hormonally-active-compounds-pharmaceuticals-and-personal-care-product-ingredients-of-health-concern-from-potential-presence-in-water-intended-for-indirect-potable-reuse/ (accessed on 4 April 2018).
11. Watts and Crane Associates. Drinking Water Inspectorate: Desk Based Review of Current Knowledge on Pharmaceuticals in Drinking Water and Estimation of Potential Levels. Available online: http://dwi.defra.gov.uk/research/completed-research/reports/dwi70-2-213.pdf (accessed on 4 April 2018).
12. Minnesota Department of Health. Statement of Need and Reasonableness 11 July 2008. Available online: http://www.health.state.mn.us/divs/eh/risk/rules/water/hrlsonar08.pdf (accessed on 4 April 2018).
13. PharmacyTimes. Top 200 Drugs of 2011. Available online: www.pharmacytimes.com/publications/issue/2012/July2012/Top-200-Drugs-of-2011 (accessed on 4 April 2018).
14. PharmacyTimes. Top 200 Drugs of 2012. Available online: www.pharmacytimes.com/publications/issue/2013/July2013/Top-200-Drugs-of-2012 (accessed on 4 April 2018).

15. US National Library of Medicine. Dailymed. Available online: https://dailymed.nlm.nih.gov/dailymed/ (accessed on 4 April 2018).
16. Institute of Medicine—Food and Nutrition Board. Dietary Reference Intakes: A Risk Assessment Model for Establishing Upper Intake Levels for Nutrients. Available online: https://www.ncbi.nlm.nih.gov/books/NBK45189/ (accessed on 9 September 2015).
17. US Food and Drug Administration. US FDA Drugs Database. Available online: https://www.fda.gov/Drugs/InformationOnDrugs/ucm135821.htm (accessed on 4 April 2018).
18. International Agency for Research on Cancer (IARC). IARC Monographs on the Evaluation of Carcinogenic Risk to Humans. Available online: http://monographs.iarc.fr/ENG/Classification/index.php (accessed on 4 April 2018).
19. National Toxicology Program (NTP). Data and Resources. Available online: https://ntp.niehs.nih.gov/results/dbsearch/index.html (accessed on 4 April 2018).
20. US National Library of Medicine. Toxicology Data Network—Hazardous Substances Data Bank (HSDB). Available online: https://toxnet.nlm.nih.gov/cgi-bin/sis/htmlgen?HSDB (accessed on 4 April 2018).
21. US Environmental Protection Agency. Child Specific Exposure Factors Handbook. Available online: https://cfpub.epa.gov/ncea/risk/recordisplay.cfm?deid=199243 (accessed on 4 April 2018).
22. US Environmental Protection Agency. Exposure Factors Handbook: 2011 Edition. Available online: https://cfpub.epa.gov/ncea/risk/recordisplay.cfm?deid=236252 (accessed on 4 April 2018).
23. US Environmental Protection Agency. Endocrine Disruption Home—What is the Endocrine System? Available online: https://www.epa.gov/endocrine-disruption (accessed on 4 April 2018).
24. Australian Environmental Protection and Heritage Council; National Health and Medical Research Council; Natural Resource Management Ministerial Council. Australian Guidelines for Water Recycling—Augmentation of Drinking Water Supplies. Available online: https://www.nhmrc.gov.au/_files_nhmrc/file/publications/nhmrc_adwg_6_version_3.4_final.pdf (accessed on 4 April 2018).
25. US Environmental Protection Agency. Methodology for Deriving Ambient Water Quality Criteria for the Protection of Human Health. Available online: https://nepis.epa.gov/Exe/ZyPDF.cgi/20003D2R.PDF?Dockey=20003D2R.PDF (accessed on 4 April 2018).
26. US Food and Drug Administration. Code of Federal Regulations Title 21: Chapter 1—Food and Drug Administration Department of Health and Human Services Subchapter c—Drugs: General. Available online: https://www.accessdata.fda.gov/scripts/cdrh/cfdocs/cfcfr/cfrsearch.cfm?fr=201.57&utm_campaign=google2&utm_source=fdasearch&utm_medium=website&utm_term=21cfr201.57&utm_content=3 (accessed on 4 April 2018).
27. US Environmental Protection Agency. Risk Assessment: Conducting a Human Health Risk Assessment. Available online: https://www.epa.gov/risk/conducting-human-health-risk-assessment (accessed on 4 April 2018).
28. Krishnan, K.; Carrier, R. The use of exposure source allocation factor in the risk assessment of drinking-water contaminants. *J. Toxicol. Environ. Health B Crit. Rev.* **2013**, *16*, 39–51. [CrossRef] [PubMed]
29. Ryan, T.; Brewer, M.; Small, L. Over-the-counter cough and cold medication use in young children. *Pediatr. Nurs.* **2008**, *34*, 174–180. [PubMed]
30. Schille, S.; Shehab, N.; Thomas, K.E.; Budnitz, D.S. Medication overdoses leading to emergency department visits among children. *Am. J. Prev. Med.* **2009**, *37*, 181–187. [CrossRef] [PubMed]
31. Minnesota Department of Health. Report on Pesticide Rapid Assessments. Available online: http://www.health.state.mn.us/divs/eh/risk/guidance/dwec/rapidpest.html (accessed on 4 April 2018).
32. Goeden, H. Focus on chronic exposure for deriving drinking water guidance underestimates potential risk to infants. *Int. J. Environ. Res. Public Health* **2018**, *15*, 512. [CrossRef] [PubMed]
33. US Food and Drug Administration. Pregnancy and Lactation Labeling Final Rule. Available online: https://www.fda.gov/Drugs/DevelopmentApprovalProcess/DevelopmentResources/Labeling/ucm093307.htm (accessed on 4 April 2018).
34. US Food and Drug Administration. Medical Product Safety Information. Available online: https://www.fda.gov/Safety/MedWatch/SafetyInformation/default.htm (accessed on 4 April 2018).
35. Minnesota Department of Health. Human Health-Based Water Guidance Table. Available online: http://www.health.state.mn.us/divs/eh/risk/guidance/gw/table.html (accessed on 4 April 2018).

36. Minnesota Department of Health. Toxicological Summary for Acetaminophen. Available online: http://www.health.state.mn.us/divs/eh/risk/guidance/dwec/sumacetamin.pdf (accessed on 10 April 2018).

37. Minnesota Department of Health. Toxicological Summary Sheet for Carbamazepine. Available online: http://www.health.state.mn.us/divs/eh/risk/guidance/gw/carbamazepine.pdf (accessed on 10 April 2018).

38. Minnesota Department of Health. Toxicological Summary for 17a-Ethinylestradiol. Available online: http://www.health.state.mn.us/divs/eh/risk/guidance/gw/ethinylestsumm.pdf (accessed on 10 April 2018).

39. Minnesota Department of Health. Toxicological Summary for Sulfamethoxazole. Available online: http://www.health.state.mn.us/divs/eh/risk/guidance/gw/sulfamethoxsum.pdf (accessed on 10 April 2018).

40. Minnesota Department of Health. Toxicological Summary for Venlafaxine. Available online: http://www.health.state.mn.us/divs/eh/risk/guidance/gw/vanlafaxsumm.pdf (accessed on 10 April 2018).

41. Ferrey, M. Pharmaceuticals, Personal Care Products, and Endocrine Active Chemical Monitoring in Lakes and Rivers: 2013. Available online: https://www.pca.state.mn.us/sites/default/files/tdr-g1-18.pdf (accessed on 10 April 2018).

42. VanderMeulen, D. Screening for Contaminants of Emerging Concern in Surface Waters of the Great Lakes Network Parks. *Res. Gate* **2015**. [CrossRef]

43. US Environmental Protection Agency. *Method 1694: Pharmaceuticals and Personal Care Products in Water, Soil, Sediment, and Biosolids by HPLC/MS/MS*; EPA-821-R-08-002; EPA: Washington, DC, USA, 2007.

44. US Environmental Protection Agency. *Method 1698: Steroid and Hormones in Water, Soil, Sediment, and Biosolids by HRGC/HRMS*; EPA-821-R-08-003; EPA: Washington, DC, USA, 2007.

45. Furlong, E.; Werner, S.L.; Anderson, B.D.; Cahill, J.D. *Determination of Human-Health Pharmaceuticals in Filtered Water by Chemicallly Modified Styrene-Divinylbenzene Resin-Based Solid Phase Extraction and High-Performance Liquid Chromatography/Mass Spectrometry*; U.S. Geological Survey Techniques and Methods: Reston, VA, USA, 2008; Book 5, Section B, Chapter B5; p. 56.

46. Furlong, E.T.; Noriega, M.C.; Kanagy, C.J.; Kanagy, L.K.; Coffey, L.J.; Burkhardt, M.R. *Determination of Human-Use Pharmaceuticals in Filtered Water by Direct Aqueous Injection–High-Performance Liquid Chromatography/Tandem Mass Spectrometry*; U.S. Geological Survey Techniques and Methods: Reston, VA, USA, 2014; Book 5, Chapter B10; p. 49.

47. Foreman, W.T.; Gray, J.L.; ReVello, R.C.; Lindley, C.E.; Losche, S.A.; Barber, L.B. *Determination of Steroid Hormones and Related Compounds in Filtered and unfiltered Water by Solid-Phase Extraction, Derivatization, and Gas Chromatography with Tandem Mass Spectrometry*; U.S. Geological Survey Techniques and Methods: Reston, VA, USA, 2012; Book 5, Chapter B9; p. 118.

48. Axys Analytical Labs. Pharmaceuticals and Personal Care Products. Available online: https://www.axysanalytical.com/axys-enviro/analyses-enviro/ppcp/ (accessed on 4 April 2018).

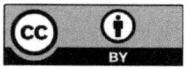

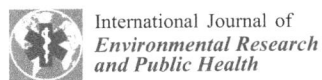

International Journal of
*Environmental Research
and Public Health*

Article

Focus on Chronic Exposure for Deriving Drinking Water Guidance Underestimates Potential Risk to Infants

Helen Goeden

Minnesota Department of Health, St. Paul, MN 55164-0975, USA; helen.goeden@state.mn.us;
Tel.: +01-651-201-4904

Received: 20 February 2018; Accepted: 11 March 2018; Published: 14 March 2018

Abstract: In 2007, the Minnesota Department of Health (MDH) developed new risk assessment methods for deriving human health-based water guidance (HBG) that incorporated the assessment of multiple exposure durations and life stages. The methodology is based on US Environmental Protection Agency recommendations for protecting children's health (US EPA 2002). Over the last 10 years, the MDH has derived multiple duration (e.g., short-term, subchronic, and chronic) water guidance for over 60 chemicals. This effort involved derivation of multiple duration reference doses (RfDs) and selection of corresponding water intake rates (e.g., infant, child, and lifetime). As expected, RfDs typically decreased with increasing exposure duration. However, the corresponding HBG frequently did not decrease with increasing duration. For more than half of the chemicals, the shorter duration HBG was lower than chronic HBG value. Conventional wisdom has been that chronic-based values will be the most conservative and will therefore be protective of less than chronic exposures. However, the MDH's experience highlights the importance of evaluating short-term exposures. For many chemicals, elevated intake rates early in life, coupled with short-term RfDs, resulted in the lowest HBG. Drinking water criteria based on chronic assessments may not be protective of short-term exposures in highly exposed populations such as formula-fed infants.

Keywords: drinking water guidance; infant exposure; chemical risk assessment; duration extrapolation

1. Introduction

Guidance values produced by human health risk assessments most often use animal experiments of different durations and key endpoints of consideration to derive a quantitative guidance value for the matrix of concern (water, air, soil, etc.). Chronic duration studies have been the preferred source of toxicity information, as these longer duration studies provide ample time for toxic effects to manifest from the exposure protocol. In recent years, a realization has been building that elevated sensitivity or exposures during the developmental time period may provide data that drive a risk assessment to a lower guidance value compared to use of longer duration chronic studies. In 1993, the National Academy of Science (NAS) [1] recommended changes to regulatory practice in order to ensure proper characterization of risks to infants and children. The specific recommendations included consideration of greater physiological sensitivity of infants and children, using exposure estimates representative of infants and children, and accounting for nondietary as well as dietary sources of exposure. The NAS report prompted passage of the Food Quality and Protection Act and amendments to the Safe Drinking Water Act related to children's health protection. The US Environmental Protection Agency (US EPA) subsequently established the reference dose/reference concentration (RfD/RfC) Technical Panel early in 1999 to evaluate the RfD/RfC derivation process with respect to how well children and other potentially sensitive subpopulations are protected. As a result of this review, the RfD/RfC Technical Panel recommended derivation of RfD/RfCs for multiple exposure durations as well as enhanced or additional testing protocols to improve children's health protection as part of the noncancer assessment process [2].

In 2007, the Minnesota Department of Health (MDH) began implementing exposure duration-specific methods that were adopted into state rule in 2009 [3]. For the derivation of noncancer health-based guidance, the MDH relied heavily upon the RfD/RfC Technical Panel recommendations [2] and additional duration- and life-stage specific US EPA guidance [4,5]. In addition, changes to MDH practice were mandated in Minnesota's 2001 Health Standards Statute, which required that safe drinking water standards include "a reasonable margin of safety to adequately protect the health of infants, children, and adults … " [6]. This statute was based on concerns regarding children's susceptibility to environmental contaminants. In response, the MDH's approach to multiple-duration guidance included consideration of "windows of sensitivity" to toxicants as well as periods of high exposures.

The MDH derives human health-based guidance (HBG) to evaluate potential health risks of environmental exposures. The focus of this manuscript are HBGs developed in response to concerns over contaminated water. MDH guidance is used by state programs as regulatory tools for groundwater protection, the prevention of exposure, remediation of contaminated sites, and to provide context for risk management. The MDH also uses HBG to advise households about chemical contamination in private wells. An HBG represents a water concentration (expressed as micrograms of chemical per liter of water, µg/L) that can be consumed with no appreciable risk to human health. HBGs are based on chemical toxicity (the dose that results in adverse effects), the duration of exposure (the time period of exposure that results in adverse effects), and the amount of water individuals drink during the exposure period.

Until 2007, the MDH used methods for deriving HBG that were similar to those used by the US EPA Office of Water for calculating chronic (lifetime) health advisories [7]. The US EPA methods for assessing noncancer health effects from lifetime exposure generally combine an adult water intake rate (2 L per day for a person weighing 70 kg, 2 L/70 kg b.w./day) with a chronic reference dose (RfD) and a relative source contribution factor (RSC) of 0.2. The RSC factor represents the maximum amount of the RfD "apportioned" to drinking water [8]. US EPA also derives 1- and 10-day health advisories using a child water intake rate (1 L per day for a child weighing 10 kg, 1 L/10 kg b.w./day) and no RSC (allowing 100% of the RfD to be from consumption of water). This approach typically results in short-term health advisory values that are greater than longer-term lifetime health advisory values. In contrast, the MDH's implementation of exposure duration-specific methods has resulted in HBGs that have been more frequently driven by less-than-chronic exposure scenarios.

As of December 2017, the MDH has utilized the multiduration methodology discussed above to derive HBG for 85 chemicals or chemical groups. A wide range of chemicals have been evaluated, including, solvents, pesticides, consumer product/personal care-related chemicals, pharmaceuticals, and perfluorinated compounds. This publication is a retrospective evaluation of the MDH's decade long experience of incorporating multiple duration evaluations into their process for deriving HBGs for water. The specific objectives of the evaluation are to: (1) evaluate the significance of incorporating multiple duration assessment methodology for deriving HBG intended for the general population (rather than the traditional single chronic duration) and (2) determine the overall utility of conducting multiple duration assessments for public health protection.

2. Materials and Methods

To derive HBG, the MDH followed the standard US EPA four-step risk assessment process: hazard identification; dose–response/toxicity evaluation; exposure assessment; and risk characterization [9]. Hazard identification is a determination of the type of adverse effects posed by a chemical or substance. Dose–response or toxicity evaluation describes the quantitative relationship between the amount of exposure (i.e., dose) to a substance and the extent of toxic injury or disease. Exposure assessment typically includes the magnitude, frequency, duration, and route of exposure. Finally, when applied to developing standards or guidance, risk characterization integrates all three previously mentioned steps to derive a level of exposure that is unlikely to pose a health risk to the population of interest.

2.1. Hazard Assessment and Dose–Response

The chemicals chosen for review were identified by state agencies and the public as chemicals known or anticipated to be groundwater or surface water contaminants in Minnesota. For each chemical, government reports and peer-reviewed literature were searched for toxicity study information that encompassed various life stages and durations. The MDH adopted the duration definitions as recommended by the US EPA [2], as shown in Table 1.

Table 1. Defined study exposure duration [2].

Duration	Definition
Short-term	Repeated exposure for more than 24 h, up to 30 days.
Subchronic	Repeated exposure for more than 30 days, up to approximately 10 percent of a lifetime (approximately 90 days in typical laboratory rodent studies)
Chronic	Repeated exposure for more than approximately 10 percent of a lifespan (more than 90 days, to 2 years in typical laboratory rodent studies)

For each chemical assessment and each toxicity bioassay, the MDH evaluated information regarding the specific periods of time (e.g., life stage most susceptible to a toxic effect) and durations of exposure necessary to elicit an adverse effect. The MDH found that data were often not available for all dose–response time points or all life stages of potential interest, such as fetal or neonatal life stages. In addition, the time-point or exposure duration associated with effects was often not clear, since many parameters (e.g., histopathology) were assessed only at study termination. Studies that did include exposure during development (e.g., gestation, birth, and nursing) typically did not report the dose to the fetus or neonate. In these cases, the MDH used the maternal dose as a surrogate.

Studies that did not include developmental exposure were useful for assessing shorter-duration dose–response for non-developmental health endpoints. Unless data to the contrary were available, these non-developmental endpoints (e.g., hepatotoxicity) were assumed to be relevant to any age group, including infants and children, when matched to the appropriate exposure duration.

Reference Dose Derivation and Selection

Using the systematic approach recommended by the US EPA [2], the MDH derived an RfD for each duration for which sufficient toxicity data were available. An appropriate point of departure (e.g., no observable adverse effect level (NOAEL), lower confidence limit of a benchmark dose (BMDL), or lowest observable adverse effect level (LOAEL)) was identified and adjusted by applicable human equivalent dose conversion [10], uncertainty, and variability factors [3].

Since the RfD for each duration should be protective of all health endpoints that could occur within the given duration of exposure [2,3], the MDH considered and compared the short-term, subchronic, and chronic duration-based RfDs for a chemical prior to final RfD determination. Standard short-term, subchronic, and chronic toxicity bioassays typically do not encompass all life stages or may not assess all sensitive endpoints. In cases where the shorter-duration RfD was lower (more protective) than a longer-duration RfD due to life stage sensitivity or health effect assessed in the shorter duration study but not assessed in the longer-duration studies, the shorter-duration RfD was used as the longer-duration RfD as well. For example, a short-term RfD, based on developmental effects, may be lower than the chronic RfD based on evaluation of adult animals only. Since assessment of early life stages was not included in the chronic studies, the final chronic RfD would be set at the lower short-term RfD to ensure that short-term exposures that occur within a chronic durations are adequately protected. Shorter duration RfDs that were lower because of differences in study dose selection were not used as RfDs for longer durations. For example, wider dose spacing in the subchronic study could result in a lower subchronic RfD because the subchronic NOAEL was lower than the chronic NOAEL. The differences in the RfDs is due to the different dose levels selected alone and not due to the lack of life stage or endpoint assessment. This approach is consistent with US EPA recommendations [2] and recent US EPA practice [11]. Specific case where these decisions were made are described in Section 3.1.

The duration specific RfD and its basis for each chemical is available on the MDH's website (http://www.health.state.mn.us/divs/eh/risk/guidance/gw/table.html) in the form of chemical-specific toxicity summaries. Links to the chemical specific summaries are also provided in Table S1 of the Supplemental Information.

2.2. Exposure Assessment—Drinking Water Intake Rates and the RSC

Estimation of human doses from drinking water exposures requires a drinking water intake rate for assessing exposure in the context of the RfD. An HBG is derived by incorporating a drinking water intake rate, which is the quantity of water consumed per kilogram of body weight per day (L/kg per day). In 2007, the MDH used the US EPA's report, "Estimated Per Capita Water Ingestion and Body Weight in the United States—An Update" [12] as a source of intake rates for the general population and subpopulations (e.g., children, pregnant women). As recommended by the US EPA Science Advisory Board (SAB) [13], the MDH used estimates of intake based on data for individuals who drank at least some tap water (i.e., consumer-only). The US EPA has since updated the Exposure Factors Handbook [14], which now serves as the source of water intake rates for the MDH's HBG (see Table 2).

Table 2. Age group water ingestion rates (Tables 3-1 and 3-3, consumers only [14]).

Age Group	Mean (L/kg-Day)	Ratio to All Ages	95th Percentile (L/kg-Day)	Ratio to All Ages
Birth to <1 month	0.137	8.6	0.238	5.4
1 to <3 months	0.119	7.4	0.285	6.5
3 to <6 months	0.080	5.0	0.173	3.9
6 to <12 months	0.053	3.3	0.129	2.9
1 to <2 years	0.027	1.7	0.075	1.7
2 to <3 years	0.026	1.6	0.062	1.4
3 to <6 years	0.021	1.3	0.052	1.2
6 to <11 years	0.017	1.1	0.047	1.1
11 to <16 years	0.012	0.8	0.035	0.8
16 to <18 years	0.010	0.6	0.030	0.7
18 to <21 years	0.011	0.7	0.036	0.8
≥21 years	0.016	1.0	0.042	1.0
All ages (lifetime)	0.016		0.044	
Pregnant women	0.014	0.9	0.043	1.0
Lactating women	0.026	1.6	0.055	1.3

Infancy and early childhood are clearly periods during which exposure to water is the greatest, as demonstrated by the much larger water intake rates on a per body weight (L/kg per day) basis. Intake rates drop sharply with age, approximating adult rates on a per body weight basis by 6 to 11 years of age. The MDH selected the 95th percentile intake rates for HBG derivation. This ensured that the HBG was protective of individuals who consume most of their water from a single source, such as a private well.

For deriving short-term duration HBG, the MDH selected the 1 to <3 months old infant intake rate of 0.285 L/kg per day. For longer-durations, the MDH calculated time-weighted averages (TWA) starting at birth. The resulting subchronic (birth to approximately 8 years) and chronic (birth to approximately 70 years) duration TWA intake rates were 0.070 and 0.044 L/kg per day, respectively. These intake rates represent default values. Other exposure values were used if sufficient chemical-specific information indicated that a different duration or intake rate was more appropriate. For example, if a developmental effect was identified as the most sensitive effect and the susceptible period was limited to *in utero* development for the health effect of concern (e.g., cardiac malformations), the intake rate for pregnant women was used to calculate the HBG value.

Another aspect of exposure is the relative contribution that ingestion of water adds to the total exposure to a chemical. Water intake may constitute only one of several exposure pathways. A relative source contribution (RSC) factor is used to account for non-water ingestion related exposures (e.g., inhalation of volatilized chemicals, dermal absorption) as well as exposures via other media (e.g., consumer products, food, air, and soil) to ensure that the cumulative exposure does not exceed the RfD.

The use of an RSC is mandated by Minnesota state statute [15] and is based on the US EPA's historic use of the RSC to derive drinking water health advisories and ambient water quality criteria. US EPA guidance for the latter includes an exposure decision tree for selecting RSC values [8]. The decision tree consists of a series of decision points at which the availability and quality of chemical and exposure data are evaluated. In general, a lack of statistically significant exposure data will steer the process towards a lower, more protective, RSC value. Higher RSC values may result if situation-specific data indicate that alternate exposures may not be as significant as water ingestion. US EPA [8] recommends that RSC values stay within the range of 0.2 to 0.8; the lower end of the range protects against other routes of exposure when uncertainty is high, and the upper end of the range allows for unknown exposures when uncertainty is low. Because the HBG are derived for exposure to the general public rather than a site-specific situation the application of the decision tree results in an RSC of 0.2 for most chemicals, which means that ingestion of water accounts for 20 percent of the RfD, with the remaining 80 percent coming from other pathways or sources of exposure.

A default RSC of 0.2 was used for the multiple duration HBG developed for most of the 85 chemicals studied, with some exceptions. The narrower range of environments encountered by an infant during the first few months of life justified the use of an RSC of 0.5 for short-term (infant) exposures to most chemicals found in drinking water. The MDH used an RSC of 0.2 for all durations (including short-term based on infants) for chemicals that were classified as highly volatile, because inhalation is likely to be a significant exposure pathway for all durations. For pharmaceuticals available only through prescription, the MDH used an RSC of 0.8 for all durations because exposure from non-water sources, apart from prescription use, is unlikely. The MDH's derivation of the default RSC values using US EPA's decision tree process is documented in Appendix K of the MDH's technical support document [3].

2.3. Risk Characterization

Understanding the relationship between timing and duration of exposure to a chemical and the subsequent adverse effects was essential in completing the characterization of risk. Calculation of each HBG combines a duration-specific RfD with the corresponding intake rate and a relative source contribution factor (RSC)

$$nHBG_{duration} = \frac{RfD_{duration} \times RSC \times 1000 \ \mu g/mg}{IR_{duration}} \quad (1)$$

where:

$nHBG_{duration}$ = the noncancer health-based guidance value, for a given duration (see Table 1), expressed in units of micrograms of chemical per liter of water ($\mu g/L$).

$RfD_{duration}$ = the reference dose, for a given duration (see Table 1), expressed in units of milligrams of the chemical per kilogram of body weight per day (mg/kg per day).

RSC = the relative source contribution factor, as described above.

$IR_{duration}$ = the intake rate of water ingested for a given duration, as described above.

Departures from the HBG algorithm and parameter values discussed above were made if sufficient, appropriate chemical-specific information was available. The MDH rounded the HBG value to one significant figure, which was the least precise parameter used in the calculation.

Final Selection of Health-Based Guidance (HBG)

Similar to the decision process used for selection of RfDs, the MDH compared the longer-duration HBG with the corresponding shorter-duration HBG prior to determining the final health-protective HBG value. If the shorter-duration HBG value was lower than a longer-duration value, the shorter-duration HBG value was selected as guidance for the longer-duration exposure. This ensures that shorter-duration exposures that could occur within the longer-duration exposure period are protected.

A detailed description of the MDH's methodology for deriving drinking water HBG was published in a technical support document [3]. The MDH's application of this methodology, in the form of chemical-specific toxicological summaries, is publically available on the MDH website (http://www.health.state.mn.us/divs/eh/risk/guidance/gw/table.html).

3. Results and Discussion

Of the 85 chemical assessments conducted between 2007 and 2017, the MDH was able to derive short-term, subchronic and chronic RfDs and HBG in 63 (~74%) of the assessments. Subchronic and chronic (but not short-term RfDs) and HBG were derived for an additional 15 chemicals, for a total of 78 (92%) of the 85 assessments. For the remaining seven chemicals, only a single value could be derived (e.g., anatoxin-a, dichloromethane, 2-methylnaphthalene, NDMA, PFOA, PFOS, and triclocarban).

The retrospective evaluation focused on the comparison of short-term, subchronic, and chronic duration values and was therefore limited to the 63 assessments containing values for all three durations. The duration-specific RfDs and HBG for these 63 assessments are presented in Tables S1 and S2 (see Supplemental Information).

3.1. Comparison of Duration-Specific Reference Doses

As expected, based on established toxicological trends, the MDH found that, in general RfDs decreased with increasing duration (short-term > subchronic > chronic), as shown in Figure 1.

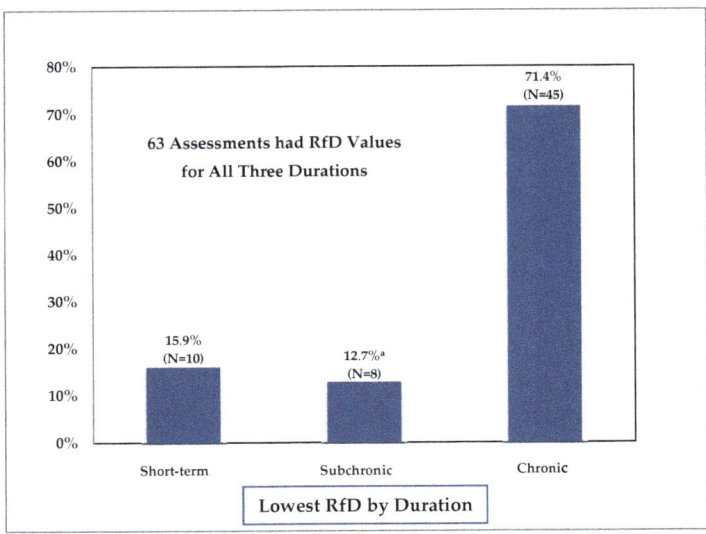

Figure 1. Comparison of reference doses (RfDs) across durations. [a] Includes four assessments in which RfD was slightly lower than the chronic RfD due to dose selection.

In 45 of the 63 (71.4%) multiple duration assessments, the calculated chronic RfD was equal to or lower than the selected short-term RfD. For 10 of the 63 (15.9%) assessments, the short-term RfD was the lowest RfD. In 6 of the 10 cases, adverse developmental effects were the basis of the short-term RfD. The six chemicals were benzo[*a*]pyrene, boron, butyl benzyl phthalate, dibutyl phthalate, di-2-ethylhexyl phthalate, and ethylene glycol. Two of the remaining four chemicals were cholinesterase inhibitors (chlorpyrifos and chlorpyrifos oxon). The final remaining two were pharmaceuticals (desvenlafaxine and venlafaxine), where the RfD was based on a minimal therapeutic dose level. The chronic studies upon which the chronic RfD was based did not assess the most sensitive life stages or physiological state (e.g., pregnancy). The chronic RfD must be protective of health effects that could result from less than chronic exposures, therefore the final chronic RfD was set to the lower short-term RfD.

In 8 of the 63 (12.7%) multiple duration assessments the subchronic RfD was the lowest calculated RfD value. In one case, trichloroethylene (TCE), the lower subchronic RfD was based on developmental immune effects observed in a subchronic duration study. For three chemicals (17α-ethinylestradiol, mestranol, and thiamethoxam), the RfD was based on male reproductive system effects observed in a subchronic duration study. In these instances, the subchronic RfD was used as the final RfD for the chronic duration as well to ensure that the chronic RfD was protective of subchronic exposures that could occur within a chronic exposure.

For the remaining four chemical assessments (*N,N*-diethyl-meta-toluamide (DEET), sulfamethozine/sulfamethoxazole, triclosan, and xylenes) the subchronic RfD was only slightly lower than the chronic RfD and was due to the different dose levels selected for the subchronic and chronic studies. For example, the NOAEL for the subchronic DEET study was lower than the NOAEL for the chronic study. Benchmark dose estimates, which might have corrected for the difference in dose selection, were not available. Another example is triclosan, in which the lowest dose tested for the subchronic study was a LOAEL whereas the point of departure for the chronic study was a NOAEL. Application of a LOAEL-to-NOAEL uncertainty factor, not differences in toxicological sensitivity, produced a lower subchronic RfD. In these four instances, the calculated chronic RfD rather than the slightly lower subchronic RfD was used as the RfD for the chronic duration.

Although the RfDs, in general, decreased with increasing duration (short-term > subchronic > chronic), the shorter duration RfDs were often not much higher than the longer duration RfDs. This is demonstrated by a geometric mean ratio of 3.5 ± 2.8 for comparison of short-term to chronic RfDs and 1.9 ± 2.0 for comparison of subchronic to chronic RfDs when all 63 assessments are considered. The 95th percentile ratios for short-term to chronic and subchronic to chronic were 24.1 and 5.4, respectively, See Table 3.

Table 3. Descriptive statistical summary analysis comparing measures of oral toxicity across exposure durations.

Study	Comparison Parameter [a]	Number of Chemicals	Geometric Mean ± GSD	95th Percentile
Short-term to Chronic				
Current Analysis	RfD	63	3.5 ± 2.8	24.1
	RfD [b]	18	2.9 ± 2.4	17.1
Batke et al. [16]	NOAEL	14	3.4 ± 3.7	29.2
Zarn et al. [17]	NOAEL (rat)	107	4.3 ± 4.7	53.2
	NOAEL (mouse)	56	3.4 ± 3.6	23.7
Malkiewicz et al. [18]	NOAEL	26	3.1 ± 2.1	
Groeneveld et al. [19]	NOAEL	35	4.9 ± 3.5	38.6
Kramer et al. [20]	NOAEL	71	4.1 ± 4.4	46
Subchronic to Chronic				
Current Analysis	RfD	63	1.9 ± 2.0	5.4
	RfD [b]	18	1.6 ± 2.0	4.6
Batke et al. [16]	NOAEL	58	1.4 ± 2.1	4.7
Zarn et al. [17]	NOAEL (rat)	222	2.5 ± 3.4	17.4
	NOAEL (mouse)	99	2.2 ± 3.9	21.4
Malkiewicz et al. [18]	NOAEL	32	2.3 ± 2.0	
Bokkers and Slob [21]	NOAEL	68	1.5 ± 5.3	22.7
	benchmark dose	189	1.7 ± 2.9	9.9
Groeneveld et al. [19]	NOAEL	70	2.3 ± 3.6	18.4
Pieters et al. [22]	NOAEL	149	1.7 ± 5.6	29

GSD—geometric standard deviation; [a] Comparison parameter: no observable adverse effect level (NOAEL); lowest observable adverse effect level (LOAEL); and oral reference dose (RfD); [b] Limited to chemical assessments in which comparison is across laboratory animal studies and the chronic RfD is based on a chronic study.

The application of duration-based uncertainty factors, as well as study design factors (e.g., dose selection), can directly influence the comparison of chronic to shorter duration RfDs. The MDH used the standard practice of applying a subchronic-to-chronic uncertainty factor if the study used as the basis of the chronic RfD was less than chronic in duration. The maximum MDH subchronic to chronic RfD ratio was 10, reflecting this practice. However, a factor of 10 was not always applied when a less than chronic study was used. The MDH evaluated the entire data set for each chemical to assess the evidence of increasing progression with increasing duration as a basis for an uncertainty factor of 1, 3, or 10. Of the 63 chronic RfDs, 44 (69.8%) were based on subchronic duration studies. Of these, four incorporated a subchronic-to-chronic uncertainty factor of 10; 20 incorporated a factor of 3; 10 incorporated a factor of 1; and 10 were set to short-term RfD values.

Limiting the comparison of RfDs across durations to the subset of chemical assessments in which the chronic RfD was based on a chronic animal study produced smaller RfD ratios. The geometric mean and 95th percentile short-term to chronic RfD ratio decrease from 3.4 to 2.9 and 24.1 to 17.1, respectively.

Likewise, the geometric mean and 95th percentile subchronic to chronic RfD ratio decrease from 1.9 to 1.6 and 5.4 to 4.6 (see Table 3).

Unlike a comparison of RfDs, the direct comparison of potential points of departure (e.g., NOAELs, LOAELs) across durations is not influenced by the application of uncertainty factors. Several investigators have compared potential points of departure across study durations ([16–22]) reporting geometric mean ratios of similar magnitude to the current analysis of RfD ratios (see Table 3).

3.2. Comparison of Duration-Specific Health-Based Guidance (HBG) Values

The short-term, subchronic, and chronic HBG for the 63 chemicals evaluated in this manuscript are presented in Table S2 (see Supplemental Information). By design and intent, the MDH selected a final HBG from the calculated values to ensure that the final chronic HBG value was protective for all life stages and exposure durations.

In testing the presumption that HBG would decrease with increasing duration (short-term > subchronic > chronic) the MDH found chronic HBG values to be the lowest (or equal to the lowest shorter duration value) calculated HBG value in only 23 of 63 (36.5%) assessments. See Figure 2. For 31 of the 63 (49.2%) assessments, the short-term HBG was the lowest HBG value. Fifty percent of the short-term to calculated chronic HBG ratios were 0.8 or less and 30 percent of the ratios were 0.5 or less. In the nine remaining assessments, the subchronic HBG was the lowest (or equal to the lowest shorter duration value). The 50th percentile subchronic to calculated chronic HBG ratio was 1.0 and 10 percent of the ratios were 0.5 or less.

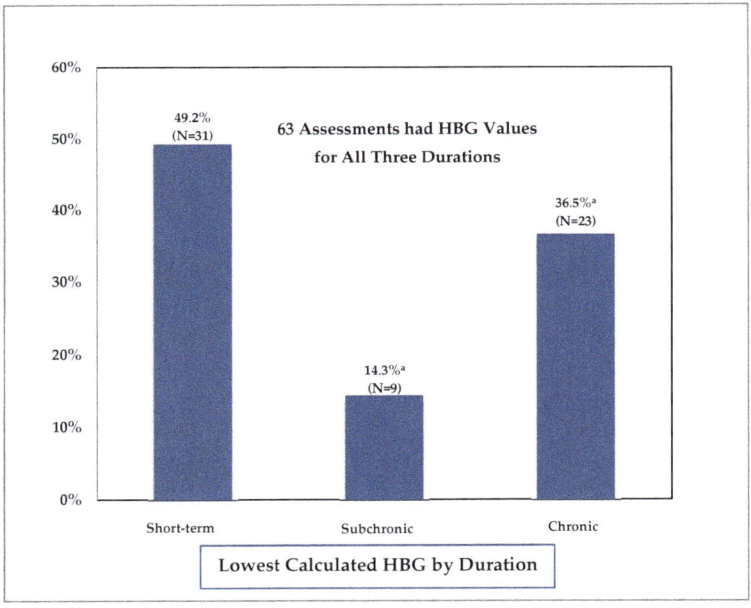

Figure 2. Comparison of health-based guidance (HBG) across durations. [a] Includes values that are equal to the lowest value (e.g., calculated subchronic HBG same as short-term HBG or calculated chronic HBG same as short-term or subchronic HBG).

High intake rates from early life exposure are a key contributing factor in these findings. As shown in Table 2, short-term duration intake rates can be six to nine times higher than chronic intake rates. The difference between the 95th percentile based short-term (0.285 L/kg per day) and chronic

(0.044 L/kg per day) water intake rates used by the MDH is 6.5-fold. When shorter- and longer-duration RfDs are similar in magnitude, the high intake rate from the shorter-duration resulted in a lower shorter-duration HBG value relative to the longer-duration HBG value. Thus, in order to ensure that the longer-duration HBG value, which encompasses all life stages, is protective for higher shorter-term exposure that occurs within its defined time span, the longer-duration HBG value must be set equal to the lower, shorter-duration HBG.

The choice of RSC can also impact the magnitude of each duration-specific HBG. The purpose of the RSC is to account for multiple sources of exposure. As noted in the introduction, the US EPA Office of Water typically does not apply an RSC factor to exposure durations that are less than chronic in duration. However, accounting for both dietary and nondietary (e.g., water ingestion) exposures was among the specific changes recommended by NAS [1].

The narrower range of environments encountered by an infant during the first few month of life justified the use of an RSC of 0.5 for short-term (infant) exposures for chemicals not considered highly volatile. For pharmaceuticals available only through prescription, the MDH used an RSC of 0.8 because exposure from non-water sources, apart from prescription use, is unlikely (see Appendix K of [3] for further explanation). Shorter duration HBG values for non-highly volatile chemicals were lower than the calculated chronic duration HBGs in 19 of 51 (37%) assessments.

For the derivation of HBG values for highly volatile chemicals, the MDH used a default RSC factor of 0.2 across all durations since the principal route of exposure is expected to be inhalation for all ages. Eight of the 12 (67%) assessments for highly volatile chemicals had a calculated shorter duration (short-term or subchronic) HBG value that was lower than the calculated chronic HBG value (see Supplemental Table S2). Therefore, when RSC is set equal across all durations, it becomes more likely that the short-term duration HBG will be lower than the chronic HBG.

As mentioned above, the US EPA Office of Water typically does not apply an RSC factor to exposure durations that are less than chronic in duration. If no RSC factor was used to derive shorter duration HBG and a default RSC factor of 0.2 was always used in deriving chronic HBG, 12 of the 63 (19%) chronic HBG values would exceed the short-term HBG values (see Supplemental Table S3). If an RSC of 0.8, US EPA's the recommended ceiling value [8], is used for all short-term HBG and an RSC of 0.2, the recommended floor value, is used for all chronic HBG the number of chronic HBG values exceeding the short-term value increases to 16 (25%).

4. Conclusions

The present study of multiple duration guidance derived by the MDH over the past 10 years clearly demonstrates the importance of incorporating shorter duration toxicity information and exposure parameters when deriving public health protective water guidance.

Twenty years ago, NAS recommended changes to regulatory practice in order to better characterize risk to infants and children. In response to these recommendations the US EPA issued their policy on evaluating risks to children, which stated that the US EPA will consistently and explicitly consider risks to infants and children as part of risk assessment and standard setting [23]. In 2013, this policy was reaffirmed by the US EPA [24]. The World Health Organization has also recently acknowledged the need to identify the most vulnerable, based on windows of sensitivity or high exposure, and to incorporate this information into risk assessment [25]. While there is consensus regarding the importance of characterizing risks to infants and children, methods to characterize these risk have generally not been widely implemented.

In 2007, the MDH implemented a multiple-duration approach which included consideration of "windows of sensitivity" to toxicants as well as periods of high exposures. As expected, RfDs typically decreased as exposure duration increased. Exceptions were developmental toxicants and fast acting neurological agents (e.g., cholinesterase inhibitors). The difference in magnitude of the RfDs, however, was often relatively small, with the majority of chronic RfDs less than four-fold lower when compared to the corresponding short-term RfD. This observation is consistent with those made by other investigators who have compared the magnitude of more direct measures of toxicity (e.g., NOAELs) across exposure durations.

Combining the short-term RfD with the high, short-term infant water intake yielded short-term duration guidance that was lower (more protective) than chronic guidance for a majority of chemicals evaluated. The main reason for this phenomenon was the high water intake rate in young infants, which is nearly seven-fold higher than in older children and adults. Derivation of short-term duration guidance may be necessary to ensure protection for all periods of susceptibility in the general population, including periods of high water intake and early-life stages.

As acknowledged by the US EPA Technical Panel [2], derivation of RfDs and RfCs has historically focused on the chronic duration. Short-term and subchronic reference values are typically not derived. Derivation of additional RfD and RfC values is resource intensive, one likely significant factor undercutting the implementation of risk assessments that focus on multiple durations.

In situations where shorter duration reference values are needed to assess risk, the panel identified the use of the chronic reference value to assess shorter duration exposures as one possible option. Based on the relatively small differential between shorter and chronic duration toxicity values for many chemicals (Table 3), utilization of a chronic RfD value, when shorter duration RfDs are not available, appears to be a reasonable screening level approach to assessing whether shorter duration exposures may be of potential concern. The MDH has incorporated the use of chronic RfDs into derivation of rapid assessments (e.g., screening values) for nearly 160 pesticides [26] and 120 pharmaceuticals [27] in water to assist in identifying situations in which potential risks from short duration exposures warrant closer scrutiny.

The MDH's HBG work, which incorporates US EPA guidance, underscores the importance of evaluating shorter duration periods of high exposure in order to afford susceptible populations such as infants and children, the same level of protection as adults. This retrospective analysis clearly demonstrates the importance of deriving shorter-duration RfDs, whether based on adult or early-life (developmental) toxicity studies, and characterizing risk for high, short-term exposure durations.

Supplementary Materials: The following are available online at: www.mdpi.com/1660-4601/15/3/512/s1, Table S1: reference dose derivation information for 63 MDH chemical assessments with short-term, subchronic, and chronic values, Table S2: health-based guidance derivation information, Table S3: health-based guidance derivation information—RSC removed from less than chronic values.

Acknowledgments: The author would like to acknowledge and thank MDH staff who conducted chemical assessments and provided helpful comments on draft versions of this manuscript. In particular, Nancy Rice and Ashley Suchomel who verified the individual RfD and HBG values in the Supplemental Tables. The author would also like to thank management at the MDH for supporting multiple duration method development and implementation. The findings and conclusions in this publication are those of the author and do not necessarily represent an official position of the MDH.

Conflicts of Interest: The author declares no conflict of interest.

References

1.   National Academy of Sciences. *Pesticides in the Diets of Infants and Children*; National Academies Press: Washington, DC, USA, 1993; Available online: https://www.nap.edu/catalog/2126/pesticides-in-the-diets-of-infants-and-children (accessed on 13 March 2018).

2.   U.S. Environmental Protection Agency (EPA). *A Review of the Reference Dose and Reference Concentration Processes*; EPA: Washington, DC, USA, 2002. Available online: https://www.epa.gov/osa/review-reference-dose-and-reference-concentration-processes (accessed on 13 March 2018).

3.   Minnesota Department of Health (MDH). *Statement of Need and Reasonableness (SONAR), July 11, 2008. Support Document Relating to Health Risk Limits for Groundwater Rules*; MDH: St Paul, MN, USA, 2008; Available online: http://www.health.state.mn.us/divs/eh/risk/rules/water/hrlsonar08.pdf (accessed on 13 March 2018).

4. U.S. Environmental Protection Agency (EPA). *Guidance on Selecting Age Groups for Monitoring and Assessing Childhood Exposures to Environmental Contaminants*; EPA: Washington, DC, USA, 2005. Available online: https: //www.epa.gov/sites/production/files/2013-09/documents/agegroups.pdf (accessed on 13 March 2018).

5. U.S. Environmental Protection Agency (EPA). *A Framework for Assessing Health Risks of Environmental Exposures to Children*; EPA: Washington, DC, USA, 2006. Available online: https://cfpub.epa.gov/ncea/risk/ recordisplay.cfm?deid=158363 (accessed on 13 March 2018).

6. Minnesota Statutes. 144.0751 Health Standards. Available online: https://www.revisor.mn.gov/statutes? id=144.0751&year=2001&keyword_type=all&keyword=144.0751 (accessed on 13 March 2018).

7. U.S. Environmental Protection Agency (EPA). *Office of Water. 2012 Edition of the Drinking Water Standards and Health Advisories*; EPA: Washington, DC, USA, 2012. Available online: https://www.epa.gov/sites/ production/files/2015-09/documents/dwstandards2012.pdf (accessed on 13 March 2018).

8. U.S. Environmental Protection Agency (EPA). *Methodology for Deriving Ambient Water Quality Criteria for the Protection of Human Health*; EPA-822-B-00-004; EPA: Washington, DC, USA, 2000. Available online: https://nepis.epa.gov/Exe/ZyPDF.cgi/20003D2R.PDF?Dockey=20003D2R.PDF (accessed on 13 March 2018).

9. U.S. Environmental Protection Agency (EPA). *Human Health Risk Assessment*; EPA: Washington, DC, USA. Available online: https://www.epa.gov/risk/human-health-risk-assessment (accessed on 13 March 2018).

10. Minnesota Department of Health (MDH). *MDH Health Risk Assessment Methods to Incorporate Human Equivalent Dose Calculations into Derivation of Oral Reference Doses*; MDH: St Paul, MN, USA, 2011; (revised 2017); Available online: http://www.health.state.mn.us/divs/eh/risk/guidance/hedrefguide.pdf (accessed on 13 March 2018).

11. U.S. Environmental Protection Agency (EPA). *Toxicological Review of Benzo[a]pyrene*; EPA: Washington, DC, USA, 2017. Available online: https://cfpub.epa.gov/ncea/iris/iris_documents/documents/toxreviews/0136tr.pdf (accessed on 13 March 2018).

12. U.S. Environmental Protection Agency (EPA). *Estimated Per Capita Water Ingestion and Body Weight in the United States—An Update. Based on Data Collected by the United States Department of Agriculture's 1994–1996 and 1998 Continuing Survey of Food Intakes by Individuals*; EPA: Washington, DC, USA, 2004.

13. U.S. Environmental Protection Agency (EPA). *An SAB Report on EPA's Per Capita Water Ingestion in the United States*; EPA-SAB-EC-00-003; EPA: Washington, DC, USA, 1999.

14. U.S. Environmental Protection Agency (EPA). Exposure Factors Handbook. Available online: https://cfpub. epa.gov/ncea/risk/recordisplay.cfm?deid=236252 (accessed on 13 March 2018).

15. Minnesota Statutes. 103H.201 Health Risk Limits; 1989. Available online: https://www.revisor.mn.gov/ statutes?id=103H&year=1989#search:"103H.201" (accessed on 13 March 2018).

16. Batke, M.; Escher, S.; Hoffmann-Doerr, S.; Melber, C.; Messinger, H.; Mangelsdorf, I. Evaluation of time extrapolation factors based on the database RepDose. *Toxicol. Lett.* **2011**, *205*, 122–129. [CrossRef] [PubMed]

17. Zarn, H.; Engeli, B.E.; Schlatter, J.R. Study parameters influencing NOAEL and LOAEL in toxicity feeding studies for pesticides: Exposure duration versus dose decrement, dose spacing, group size and chemical class. *Regul. Toxicol. Pharmacol.* **2011**, *61*, 243–250. [CrossRef] [PubMed]

18. Malkiewicz, K.; Hansson, S.O.; Ruden, C. Assessment factors for extrapolation from short-time to chronic exposure—Are the REACH guidelines adequate? *Toxicol. Lett.* **2009**, *190*, 16–22. [CrossRef] [PubMed]

19. Groenveld, C.; Hakkert, B.C.; Bos, P.M.J.; de Herr, C. Extrapolation exposure duration in Oral Toxicity: A quantitative analysis of historical Toxicity Data. *Hum. Ecol. Risk Assess.* **2004**, *10*, 709–716. [CrossRef]

20. Kramer, H.; van den Ham, W.A.; Slob, W.; Pieters, M.N. Conversion Factors estimating Indicative Chronic No-Observed-Adverse-Effect levels from short-term Toxicity Data. *Regul. Toxicol. Pharmacol.* **1996**, *23*, 249–255. [CrossRef] [PubMed]

21. Bokkers, B.; Slob, W. A comparison of ratio distributions based on the NOAEL and the Benchmark Approach for Subchronic-to-Chronic Extrapolation. *Toxicol. Sci.* **2005**, *85*, 1033–1040. [CrossRef] [PubMed]

22. Pieters, M.; Kramer, H.J.; Slob, W. Evalution of the uncertainty factor for Subchronic-to-Chronic Extrapolation: Statistical analysis of Toxicity Data. *Regul. Toxicol. Pharmacol.* **1998**, *27*, 108–111. [CrossRef] [PubMed]

23. U.S. Environmental Protection Agency (EPA). *Memorandum: New Policy on Evaluating Health Risks to Children*; EPA: Washington, DC, USA, 1995. Available online: https://www.epa.gov/sites/production/files/2014-05/ documents/1995_childrens_health_policy_statement.pdf (accessed on 13 March 2018).

24. U.S. Environmental Protection Agency (EPA). *Memorandum: Reaffirmation of the U.S. Environmental Protection Agency's 1995 Policy on Evaluating Health Risks to Children*; EPA: Washington, DC, USA, 2013. Available online: https://www.epa.gov/sites/production/files/2014-05/documents/reaffirmation_memorandum.pdf (accessed on 13 March 2018).

25. Cohen Hubal, E.; de Wet, T.; Toit, L.D.; Firestone, M.P.; Ruchirawat, M.; van Englen, J.; Vickers, C. Identifying important life stages for monitoring and assessing risks from exposures to environmental contaminants: Results of a World Health Organization review. *Regul. Toxicol. Pharmacol.* **2014**, *69*, 113–124. [CrossRef] [PubMed]

26. Minnesota Department of Health (MDH). *Report on Pesticide Rapid Assessments*; MDH: St Paul, MN, USA, 2014; Available online: http://www.health.state.mn.us/divs/eh/risk/guidance/dwec/rapidpest.html (accessed on 13 March 2018).

27. Minnesota Department of Health (MDH). *Pharmaceutical Water Screening Values Report*; MDH: St Paul, MN, USA, 2015; Available online: http://www.health.state.mn.us/divs/eh/risk/guidance/dwec/pharmproj.html (accessed on 13 March 2018).

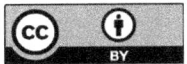

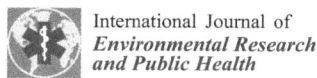

International Journal of
Environmental Research
and Public Health

MDPI

Article

Health Risk of Polonium 210 Ingestion via Drinking Water: An Experience of Malaysia

Minhaz Farid Ahmed [1], Lubna Alam [1,*], Che Abd Rahim Mohamed [2], Mazlin Bin Mokhtar [1] and Goh Choo Ta [1]

[1] Institute for Environment and Development (LESTARI), Universiti Kebangsaan Malaysia (UKM), UKM Bangi 43600, Selangor, Malaysia; minhazhmd@yahoo.com (M.F.A.); mazlin@ukm.edu.my (M.B.M.); gohchoota@ukm.edu.my (G.C.T.)

[2] School of Environmental and Natural Resource Sciences, Universiti Kebangsaan Malaysia (UKM), UKM Bangi 43600, Selangor, Malaysia; carmohd@ukm.edu.my

* Correspondence: lubna762120@gmail.com or lubna@ukm.edu.my; Tel.: +60-389-217-656

Received: 10 July 2018; Accepted: 30 August 2018; Published: 20 September 2018

Abstract: The presence of toxic polonium-210 (Po-210) in the environment is due to the decay of primordial uranium-238. Meanwhile, several studies have reported elevated Po-210 radioactivity in the rivers around the world due to both natural and anthropogenic factors. However, the primary source of Po-210 in Langat River, Malaysia might be the natural weathering of granite rock along with mining, agriculture and industrial activities. Hence, this is the first study to determine the Po-210 activity in the drinking water supply chain in the Langat River Basin to simultaneously predict the human health risks of Po-210 ingestion. Therefore, water samples were collected in 2015–2016 from the four stages of the water supply chain to analyze by Alpha Spectrometry. Determined Po-210 activity, along with the influence of environmental parameters such as time-series rainfall, flood incidents and water flow data (2005–2015), was well within the maximum limit for drinking water quality standard proposed by the Ministry of Health Malaysia and World Health Organization. Moreover, the annual effective dose of Po-210 ingestion via drinking water supply chain indicates an acceptable carcinogenic risk for the populations in the Langat Basin at 95% confidence level; however, the estimated annual effective dose at the basin is higher than in many countries. Although several studies assume the carcinogenic risk of Po-210 ingestion to humans for a long time even at low activity, however, there is no significant causal study which links Po-210 ingestion via drinking water and cancer risk of the human. Since the conventional coagulation method is unable to remove Po-210 entirely from the treated water, introducing a two-layer water filtration system at the basin can be useful to achieve SDG target 6.1 of achieving safe drinking water supplies well before 2030, which might also be significant for other countries.

Keywords: drinking water; radioactivity; annual effective dose; carcinogenic

1. Introduction

Po-210, a decay element of U-238, is a naturally occurring radionuclide mostly found in water, soil and food. The significant sources of terrestrial radiation are primordial radionuclides, namely U-238, Th-232, and K-40, which are dispersed around the Earth's crust and widely reported in Peninsular Malaysia [1]. In the Langat River, Po-210 is mainly due the natural weathering of the minerals, uraninite UO_2 (pitchblend), carnotite, and autunite of the acid intrusive granitic rock [2–4]. Therefore, human beings are at risk of ingestion of Po-210 through drinking water and exposure to annual effective doses for a long time. Moreover, Po-210 is considered as one of the primary sources of alpha exposure [5] to human beings through ingestion via drinking water [6–8]. Alam and Mohamed [5] also reported

Po-210 is about 250,000 times more toxic than hydrogen cyanide; therefore, it could be carcinogenic if ingested through drinking water [9–13].

Natural sources contribute about 80% to the radionuclides generated in Malaysia, the other sources being anthropogenic ones such as industrial activities as well as mining of natural resources along with gas and petroleum exploration [14]. Many studies in Peninsular Malaysia have investigated the existence of radioactivity from Ra-226, Ra-228, Pb-210, Cs-137, Th-232, K-40 and Rn-222 in water bodies [15–18] and it was reported that about 80 to 87% of the human exposure to radioactivity in Peninsular Malaysia results mainly from natural sources such as primordial radionuclides, cosmogenic radionuclides, etc. [14,16]. The atmospheric source is also considered as one of the sources of Po-210 in water because of the decay of Rn-222 gas and the decay of naturally occurring U-238 [15,19].

Malaysia has seriously focused on industrial expansion to achieve developed country status by 2020 [20,21]. As a result, the rivers in Malaysia have been found to be severely contaminated with heavy metals [22] as well as radioactive elements [17,23,24]. Rapid mineralization of tin ore from the Main Range Granite is the prime source of the high radioactivity associated with soil in the western region of Peninsular Malaysia [2]. In Selangor state, the maximum activity of U-238, Ra-226, Th-232, and K-40 recorded in sediments from the tin recycling ponds are higher than the rest of Malaysia and is the world's highest natural activity [25]. The DOE [26] reported that the industrial sector and quarries are responsible for the source points of pollution in the Langat River, quantified at 8.14% and 0.24%, respectively. Therefore, significant sources of primordial radionuclides in the Langat River Basin are sand and gravel extraction 56.21%, and earth material extraction 28.10%, along with granite quarries 13.73% [27].

In Malaysia, the naturally occurring radionuclides are usually generated from the mining and mineral processing industries. For instance, in Selangor, more than 30 illegal sand mining sites, mainly in the Hulu Selangor, Sepang, and Kuala Langat districts have been identified in the last 20 years, while the government has given permits to only 46 sites for sand mining in private lands [28]. In the Langat, Lui, and Semenyih River Sub-basins, the mining area is about 3.28, 10.55, and 4.63 km^2, respectively, and the mining area trend is increasing [29]. However, the Malaysian government—based on the Atomic Energy Licensing (Radioactive Waste Management) Regulations 2011—allows industries to run if the generation of natural radionuclides remains below 1 Bq/g [30,31]. Similarly, the Ministry of Health Malaysia recommends that the gross alpha (α) and gross beta (β) levels of both in the river and drinking water should not exceed 0.1 Bq/L and 1.0 Bq/L, respectively, as set by the National Standard for Drinking Water Quality [32].

Langat River in Selangor state is not only one of the primary local sources of drinking water [33,34], but rivers are in general the primary sources of drinking water in all Malaysia. Studies on natural radionuclides in the Langat River have reported that the radioactivity of some radionuclides in the river such as U-238 (3.85 Bq/L), Th-232 (1.14 Bq/L), K-40 (145.67 Bq/L) [23], and Ra-226 (0.26 Bq/L) [35] has exceeded the limit of both the gross alpha 0.1 Bq/L and gross beta 1.0 Bq/L emitters set by the Malaysian standard for raw water quality [32]. Similarly, are only a few studies on the radioactivity of radionuclides in the drinking water of Malaysia, which were reported safe through ingestion [36]. However, in some places of Malaysia the activity of Ra-226, i.e., 0.30 Bq/L in drinking water was recorded above the standard set by the United States Environmental Protection Agency. Moreover, the range of annual effective doses from radionuclides in some places of Malaysia was determined to be 0.02 mSv/year to 0.06 mSv/year [19,37].

As there is no significant study on Po-210 in the drinking water supply chain of Malaysia, there is an urgency to study the Po-210 activity in drinking water because of its high radiotoxicity. Since the Langat River is situated on the acid intrusive granite rock belt that is the prime source of U-238 including Po-210, determining the Po-210 activity in the drinking water and its annual effective dose to humans through ingestion is very important concerning human health carcinogenicity risks. Therefore, this study investigated the Po-210 activity in the drinking water of Langat River Basin and the annual effective dose through ingestion via drinking water.

2. Materials and Methods

2.1. Water Sample Collection

There are a total nine water treatment plants (WTPs) in the Langat River Basin that provide drinking water to one-third of the population in Selangor State of Malaysia [33] through the water distributor Syarikat Bekalan Air Selangor Sdn Bhd (SYABAS). Although each WTP has been designed to supply treated water in the specific areas of the basin, however, during water shortages treated water from one plant may be channeled to the areas of other plants using the same pipeline. Therefore, twenty liter water samples were collected in polyethylene containers from the Langat River precisely from where the WTPs are located, except the Semenyih WTP were we could not collect samples of raw water for treatment purposes in 2015 (Figure 1) during the rainy days. Similarly, twenty liter treated water samples were collected from the outlets of the WTPs on the same day of the raw water collection. Twenty liters of tap water from five households in the basin as well as three liters of water after filtration were also collected from the same households based on five types of household water filtration systems commonly used in the basin during the same period. Moreover, the collected water samples were analyzed before the end of the half-life of Po-210 i.e., 138 days. Overall, no special measures have been taken to analyze the samples.

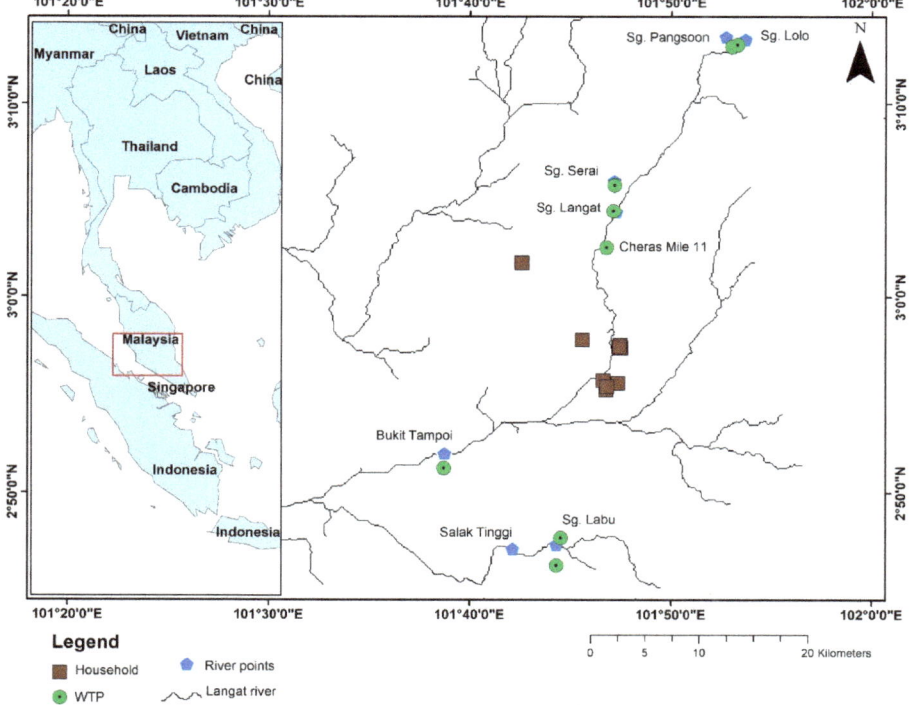

Figure 1. Water sampling points at Langat River Basin, Malaysia.

2.2. Analysis of Po-210

Water samples were filtered with the ADVANTEC membrane filter (pore size: 0.45 μm) and acidified with concentrated HNO_3 immediately after collection in order to maintain pH ≤ 2 and to avoid contamination. Then the water samples were analyzed for Po-210 following the modified

International Atomic Energy Agency (IAEA) method of $FeOH_2$ precipitation (Figure 2) [38,39]. Similarly, the activity concentrations of Po-210 in water samples were determined by a CANBERRA Apex Alpha Spectrometer (Canberra Industries, Meriden, CT, USA) with a minimum detectable activity (MDA) of less than 0.2 mBq for a counting efficiency of 12.79%.

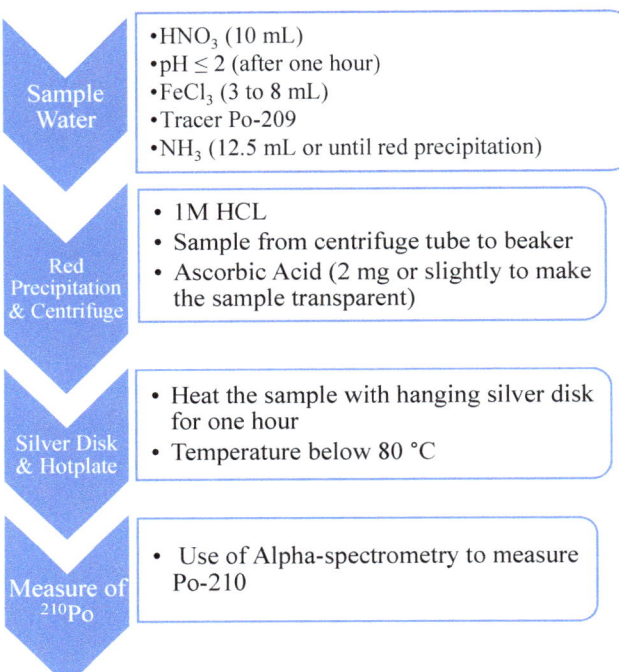

Figure 2. Steps of chemical analysis of Po-210 for fresh water sample [38].

A Po-210 tracer has been used in this study to calculate the recovery though using Equation (1) [40].

Po-209 Recovery (%) = [{cpm (tracer)/Counting Efficiency}/Spiked tracer Po-209 (dpm)] × 100   (1)

Therefore, the following amounts of tracer Po-209 have been spiked for each sample (Table 1).

Table 1. Amount of Spiked Po-209 Tracer.

Sample	Spiked Weight of Po-209 (g)	Stock Tracer Po-209 (dpm/g)	Spiked Tracer Po-209 (dpm)
Pangsoon River	0.2893	12.17	3.52
Pangsoon WTP	0.4296	1.43	0.61
Lolo River	0.2957	12.17	3.60
Lolo WTP	0.3036	12.17	3.69
Serai River	0.4987	12.17	6.07
Serai WTP	0.3506	1.43	0.50
Langat River	0.2643	12.17	3.22
Langat WTP	0.4629	12.17	5.63
Cheras River	0.4695	12.17	5.71
Cheras WTP	0.4711	12.17	5.73
Bukit River	0.3597	12.17	4.38

Table 1. *Cont.*

Sample	Spiked Weight of Po-209 (g)	Stock Tracer Po-209 (dpm/g)	Spiked Tracer Po-209 (dpm)
Bukit WTP	0.4844	12.17	5.90
Salak River	0.2297	12.17	2.80
Salak WTP	0.4430	12.17	5.39
Labu River	0.2030	1.43	0.29
Labu WTP	0.4896	12.17	5.96
Carbon Supply Hentian Kajang	0.2768	12.17	3.37
Carbon Filter Hentian Kajang	0.2186	12.17	2.66
Distilled Supply UKM	0.2090	1.43	0.30
Distilled Filter UKM	0.1940	12.17	2.36
RO Supply Hentian Kajang	0.3646	12.00	4.38
RO Filter Hentian Kajang	0.2097	12.00	2.52
Alkaline Supply Serdand	0.3289	12.17	4.00
Alkaline Filter Serdand	0.3251	12.17	3.96
UV Supply UKM	0.1880	12.17	2.29
UV Filter UKM	0.3090	12.17	3.76

2.3. Calculating Po-210 Activity

Equation (2) [40] has been used to calculate the activity of Po-210 in the water sampling date (Table 2):

$$A_0 = \frac{A}{e^{-\lambda t}} \tag{2}$$

where A_0 = Po-210 activity during sampling date, A = Po-210 activity during counting date in alpha-spectrometry, λ = Coefficient value of Po-210 is 0.005 per year, t = Half-life of Po-210 is 138 days

Table 2. Tracer Po-209 recovery (%) in drinking water supply chain samples in the Langat Basin.

Location	Water (L)	Recovery Po-209 (%)	Sampling Date	Test Date
Pangsoon River	20	19.68	6/8/2015	22/12/2015
Pangsoon WTP	20	26.43	6/8/2015	22/12/2015
Lolo River	20	19.27	6/8/2015	22/12/2015
Lolo WTP	20	33.36	6/8/2015	22/12/2015
Serai River	20	15.92	20/8/2015	2/1/2016
Serai WTP	20	58.84	20/8/2015	28/12/2015
Langat River	20	25.96	11/8/2015	22/12/2015
Langat WTP	20	20.13	11/8/2015	22/12/2015
Cheras River	20	28.70	12/8/2015	26/12/2015
Cheras WTP	20	12.87	12/8/2015	24/12/2015
Bukit River	20	16.84	13/8/2015	26/12/2015
Bukit WTP	20	25.23	13/8/2015	22/12/2015
Salak River	20	14.38	14/8/2015	23/1/2016
Salak WTP	20	11.37	14/8/2015	22/12/2015
Labu River	20	19.70	20/8/2015	2/1/2016
Labu WTP	20	20.62	20/8/2015	2/1/2016
Carbon Supply Hentian Kajang	3	44.09	20/11/2015	28/12/2015
Carbon Filter Hentian Kajang	3	18.81	20/11/2015	28/12/2015
Distilled Supply UKM	3	30.22	20/11/2015	26/12/2015
Distilled Filter UKM	3	23.83	5/5/2016	22/6/2016
RO Supply Hentian Kajang	3	40.20	18/11/2015	24/12/2015
RO Filter Hentian Kajang	3	31.94	18/11/2015	24/12/2015
Alkaline Supply Serdang	3	23.43	15/11/2015	30/1/2016
Alkaline Filter Serdang	3	26.78	15/11/2015	30/1/2016
UV Supply UKM	3	13.38	15/11/2015	30/1/2016
Carbon Supply Hentin Kajang	3	44.09	20/11/2015	28/12/2015
Carbon Filter Hentian Kajang	3	18.81	20/11/2015	28/12/2015

Note: WTP = Water Treatment Plant.

Equation (3) [38] has been used to calculate the Po-210 activity in the counting date of samples by Alpha-spectrometry:

$$A = \{cpm\ (sample)/cpm\ (tracer)\} \times [\{Spiked\ tracer\ Po\text{-}209\ (dpm)\} \times \{1/Volume\ of\ sample\ (L)\}] \quad (3)$$

where, cpm = Counts per minute; Spiked trace Po-209 (dpm) = {Spiked weight of tracer Po-209 (g) × Stock of trace Po-209 (dpm/g)}; dpm = Disintegrations per minute.

2.4. Calculating Annual Effective Dose of Po-210

The annual effective dose of Po-210 to an individual due to ingestion through drinking water was estimated using Equation (4) [24,36]:

$$D_w = C_w \times CR_w \times Dc_w \quad (4)$$

where D_w = Annual effective dose (mSv/year), C_w = Activity of Po-210 in the ingested water (Bq/L), CR_w = Annual intake of drinking water (i.e., average 1.996 L/Day by an individual in the Langat Basin through questionnaire survey, so 728.54 L/year) and Dc_w = Ingested dose conversion factor for Po-210, which is 1.2×10^{-3} mSv/Bq based on the report of International Commission on Radiological Protection (ICRP) 1996 [41,42].

2.5. Household Questionnaire Survey

According to the latest population census by the Department of Statistic Malaysia, the total number of households [43] in the Langat River Basin (Malaysia) is 1,494,865. Therefore, 402 household questionnaire surveys were conducted in the basin using Equation (5) [44,45] to get the average daily drinking water intake by the population at the basin to calculate the annual effective dose of Po-210 ingestion through drinking water (Equation (4)).

$$n = \frac{N}{1 + N(e)^2} \quad (5)$$

where n = sample size; N = population size; e = level of precision, i.e., 0.05 at 95% confidence level.

2.6. Time-Series Environmental Data

Flood Incidents data (2005–2016) for the Langat River Basin and water flow data (2005–2015) in the Langat River are obtained from the Dept. of Drainage and Irrigation Malaysia. Similarly, rainfall data (2006–2015) for the basin was collected from the Malaysian Meteorological Department. These data are plotted in the graphs below to show their trends and influences on the Po-210 activity in the Langat River Basin.

3. Results and Discussion

3.1. Po-210 Status in Raw and Treated Water

Po-210 activity ranges in the river 0.63 ± 0.29 mBq/L to 14.98 ± 1.18 mBq/L and treated water 0.34 ± 0.10 mBq/L to 6.80 ± 0.71 mBq/L (Table 3) of water treatment plants (WTPs) were within the maximum limit of raw and drinking water quality guideline of the Ministry of Health Malaysia [32] and the World Health Organization [41] i.e., 0.1×10^3 mBq/L. Although Po-210 status in raw ($t = 3.22$, $p = 0.015$) and treated water ($t = 2.924$, $p = 0.022$) was significantly safe at 95% confidence level (i.e., t statistic) through drinking water, however, the overall efficiency of all the WTPs in the basin was about 59% which might be due to an inability to remove Po-210 from treated water by the conventional method used at the plants as well as the small number of water samples. The Serai and Langat WTPs have the higher Po-210 removal efficiencies from treated water, about 93% and 81%, respectively, might be because of lower iron concentration (175 µg/L) in the upstream region of the Langat River than the downstream (264 µg/L) [46] along with higher manganese and total dissolved solids at the downstream [47,48], although all the WTPs in the basin follow a conventional coagulation method.

Table 3. Po-210 activity (mBq/L) in raw and treated water at the Langat River Basin.

Location	River	WTP	Efficiency WTP (%)	Weighted [1] Efficiency
Pangsoon	2.99 ± 0.33	1.22 ± 0.49	59	3.72
Lolo	2.54 ± 0.31	1.83 ± 0.20	28	1.49
Serai	5.02 ± 0.47	0.34 ± 0.10	93	9.83
Langat	14.98 ± 1.18	2.86 ± 0.31	81	25.49
Cheras	12.40 ± 0.84	6.80 ± 0.71	45	11.77
Bukit	7.14 ± 0.69	5.18 ± 0.42	27	4.12
Salak	1.86 ± 0.45	0.84 ± 0.20	55	2.14
Labu	0.63 ± 0.29	0.51 ± 0.11	20	0.26
Mean	5.95 ± 5.22	2.45 ± 2.37	59	58.83 (Total)
t value	3.220	2.924		
p value	0.015 *	0.022 *		
MOH (2010)	<0.1 × 10³ mBq/L			
WOH (2017)	<0.1 × 10³ mBq/L			

Note: Reported Po-210 activity is in the sampling date (A_o) and the standard deviation calculation are based on the radiochemistry method, not on the replicates [49]. [1] Sum of the river Po-210 activity of the eight sampling points has been taken as the basis of weighted average for each WTP. * Significant at 95% confidence level.

Sources of Po-210 in the Langat River

The Langat River originates at the hilly areas of Hulu Langat, Selangor, Malaysia that are an extension of the Titiwangsa Mountain Range at the north of Selangor. Hence the river drains towards west via the highly urbanized areas of Malaysia until it flows into the Strait of Malacca. Granite rock, extended from the granite batholith of Peninsular Thailand, is widespread underneath central Peninsular Malaysia, especially the entire Selangor state that is situated on two types of lithology based on intrusive rock, i.e., the formation is mainly from gabbro >500 million years ago [2,3]. Therefore, the mean dose rate of soil in Selangor is 183 ± 84 nGy/h with the range of 17.4 nGy/h to 500 nGy/h and the mean value is two times higher than the rest of Malaysia as well as the world average (i.e., 92 nGy/h) [3]. Moreover, a higher dose rate of 500 nGy/h has been recorded in Hulu Gombak because of its location in the acid intrusive granite rock in the Titiwangsa Mountain Range of East Selangor (Figure 3). Hence, through several steps such as weathering, erosion, etc. of granite, quartz rocks [4], these natural radionuclides usually migrate into the Langat River and increase the activity of radionuclides.

However, the higher Po-210 activity in the midstream of Langat River than the upstream might be due to the aerial inputs of the radionuclide, accumulation of radionuclide-rich silt and organic matter, and increased biological production [50] as well as agricultural, industrial and urban waste discharge in the river [51]; since dissolved oxygen (DO) along with a declining trend (Table 4) and conductivity shows a strongly significant inverse correlation ($r = -0.811$) at 99% confidence level (Table 5).

Table 4. Results of the Linear Regression-based Trend line of Po-210, Physiochemical and Environmental Parameters.

Parameters	Constant	River Point Coefficient	R-Square	F-Stat
Po-210	6.81 (1.56)	−0.09 (−0.22)	0.01	0.05 (0.832)
DO	10.66 (17.43)	−0.95 (−7.63)	0.91	58.21 (0.0003)
Salinity	0.001 (0.61)	0.85 (4.01)	0.73	16.09 (0.007)
Water Flow	−6.99 (−1.09)	0.89 (4.72)	0.79	22.28 (0.003)
Rainfall	3079.94 (22.62)	−0.81 (−3.43)	0.66	11.79 (0.014)
Flood Incidents	13.24 (10.56)	−0.74 (−2.70)	0.55	7.27 (0.036)

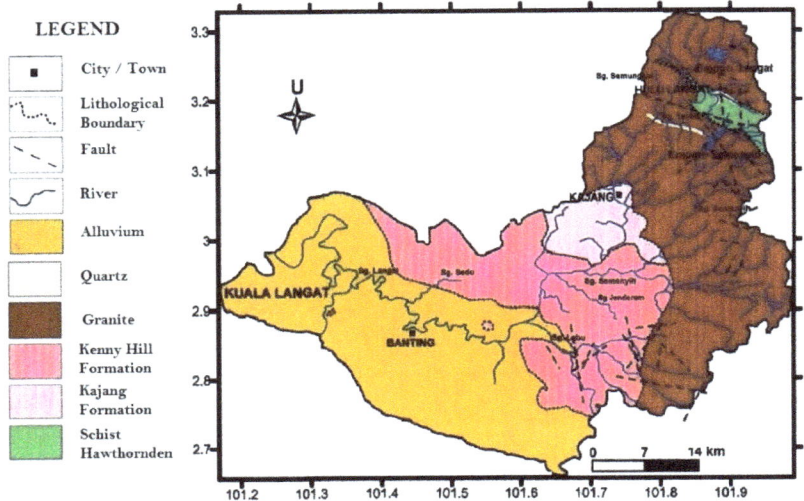

Figure 3. Geological map of Langat River Basin, Malaysia [4].

Table 5. Correlation of water quality and environmental parameters in Langat River.

	Parameters	Po-210	Salinity	DO	Conductivity	Temperature	Flood	Rainfall	Water Flow
Po-210	Pearson Correlation	1							
	Sig. (1-tailed)								
Salinity	Pearson Correlation	0.043	1						
	Sig. (1-tailed)	0.459							
DO	Pearson Correlation	0.244	−0.800 ***	1					
	Sig. (1-tailed)	0.280	0.009						
Conductivity	Pearson Correlation	0.016	0.995 ***	−0.811 ***	1				
	Sig. (1-tailed)	0.485	0.000	0.007					
Temperature	Pearson Correlation	0.161	0.819 ***	−0.852 ***	0.824 ***	1			
	Sig. (1-tailed)	0.352	0.006	0.004	0.006				
Flood	Pearson Correlation	0.542 *	−0.287	0.743 *	−0.318	−0.533	1		
	Sig. (1-tailed)	0.083	0.245	0.017	0.222	0.087			
Rainfall	Pearson Correlation	0.553 *	−0.546	0.900 ***	−0.556	−0.657 **	0.922 **	1	
	Sig. (1-tailed)	0.077	0.081	0.001	0.076	0.038	0.001		
Water Flow	Pearson Correlation	−0.370	0.838 ***	−0.867 ***	0.850 ***	0.815 ***	−0.609	−0.805 ***	1
	Sig. (1-tailed)	0.184	0.005	0.003	0.004	0.007	0.054	0.008	

*** Correlation is significant at the 0.01 level (1-tailed); ** Correlation is significant at the 0.05 level (1-tailed).
* Correlation is significant at the 0.10 level (1-tailed).

Moreover, human activities such as mining, aquaculture, agriculture, and industrial effluent discharged into the water also contribute to enhancing the levels of radionuclides in the water body [52]. Contrary, the inadequate collaboration among agencies has made the pollution management of river very complex since the river drains through three different constituencies [53,54]. Therefore, the lower Po-210 activity in the raw water at the upstream of Langat River might be due to higher DO as well as non-conservative characteristics of Po-210 [38,55]. Therefore, both the DO ($b = -0.95$, $p < 0.01$) and

Po-210 ($b = -0.09$, $p > 0.10$) show declining trends based on the linear regression (Figure 4, Table 4) from upstream to downstream at the Langat River. However, salinity ($b = 0.85$, $p < 0.01$) shows an increasing trend from upstream to downstream at the Langat River. It indicates that the Po-210 might have precipitated due to the increasing salinity towards downstream while mixing with the sea water.

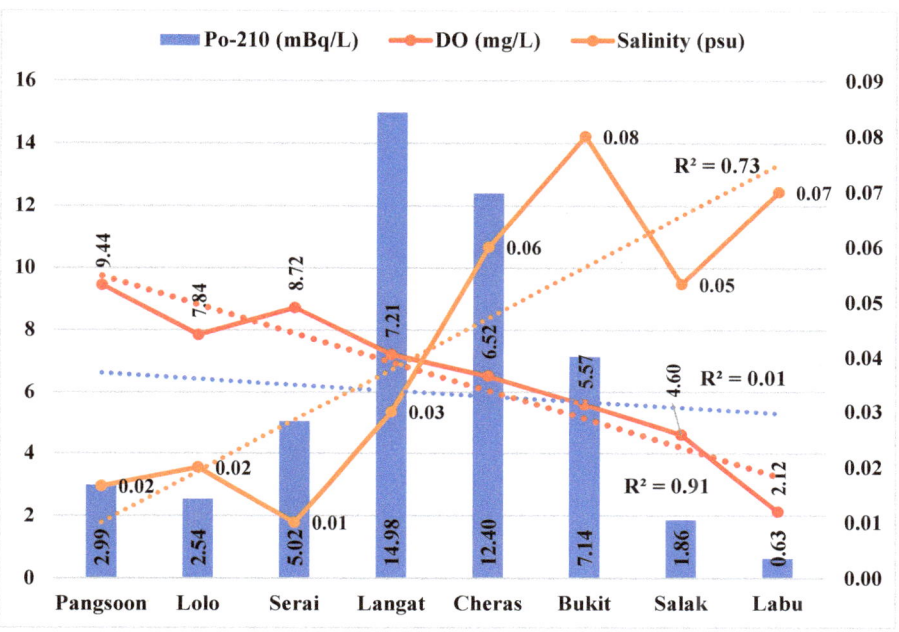

Figure 4. Po-210 activity in Langat River in relation with environmental parameters. Note: R^2 indicates the variance that is explained by the best-fit line from the upstream to the downstream of the Langat River.

Similarly, the increasing water flow ($b = 0.89$, $p < 0.01$) at the downstream (Figure 5, Table 4) might have also diluted Po-210 activity in dissolved phase. Moreover, Po-210 activity and water flow in the Langat River show a negative correlation ($r = -0.370$; Table 3). However, the declining rainfall trend ($b = -0.81$, $p < 0.01$) (Figure 6, Table 4) and flood incidents ($b = -0.74$, $p < 0.05$) (Figure 7, Table 4) trend towards downstream of Langat River indicates less atmospheric and terrestrial inputs to have lower Po-210 activity towards downstream than the upstream to midstream. Therefore, Po-210 activity shows a positive correlation (Table 5) with rainfall ($r = 0.553$; $p = 0.077$) and flood incidents ($r = 0.542$; $p = 0.083$) that means there will be lower Po-210 activity in Langat River if there are less rainfall and flood incidents.

Table 3 describes the influence of environmental and physiochemical parameters on the Po-210 activity in the Langat River. Significant positive correlations between Po-210 activity and rainfall ($r = 0.553$ *) as well as Po-210 activity and flood incidents ($r = 0.542$ *) are observed at the 0.10 level, respectively, in the Langat River, that might be because of their decreasing trends towards downstream. The decreasing trend of rainfall during 2005 to 2016 (Figure 6) and flood incidents during 2004 to 2016 (Figure 7) in the Langat River from upstream to downstream also supports the positive correlations between Po-210 and rainfall as well as Po-210 and flood incidents since there are less atmospheric and terrestrial inputs into the river. Accordingly, based on the geochemical behavior of Po-210, it precipitates toward downstream while mixing with the sea water [56]. Therefore, these findings indicate when there is less terrestrial runoff in Langat River, then there might be less attribution from natural and manmade sources to have lower Po-210 activity in raw water.

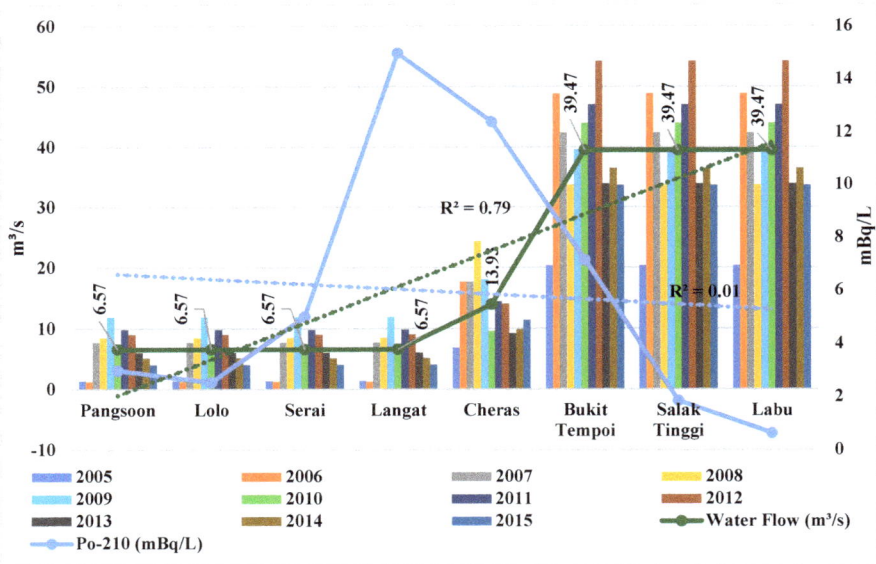

Figure 5. Po-210 activity in Langat River in relation with water flow in the Langat River. Note: Average water flow data (2005–2015) are from the Dept. of Drainage and Irrigation Malaysia. R^2 indicates the variance that is explained by the best-fit line from the upstream to the downstream of the Langat River.

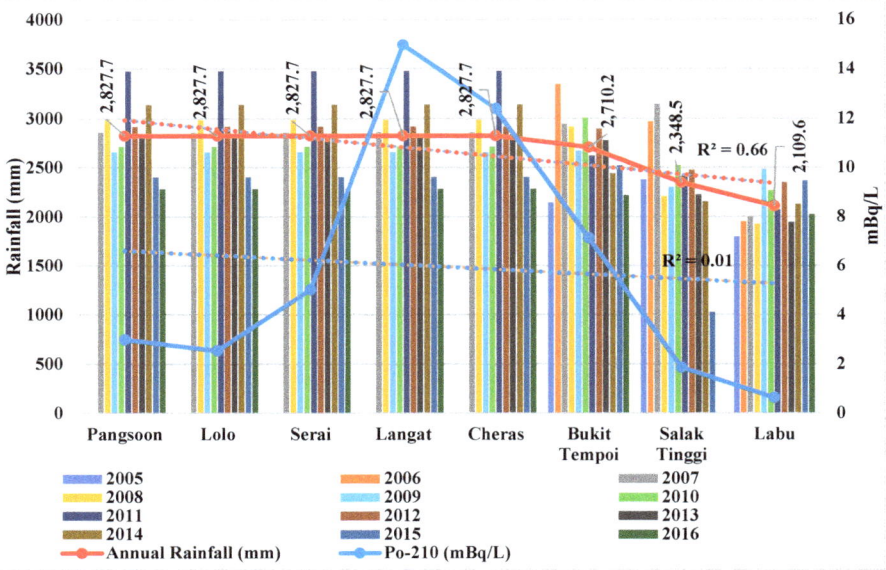

Figure 6. Po-210 activity in Langat River in relation with rainfall in the Langat Basin. Note: Mean rainfall data (2006–2015) from the Malaysian Meteorological Department. R^2 indicates the variance that is explained by the best-fit line from the upstream to the downstream of the Langat River.

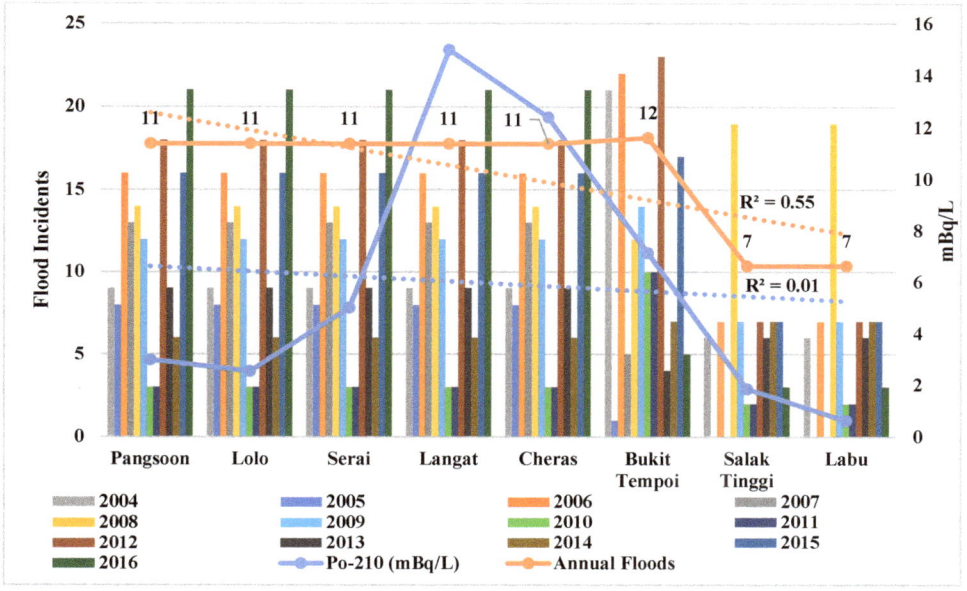

Figure 7. Po-210 activity in Langat River in relation with flood incidents in the Langat Basin. Note: Average flood Incidents data (2005–2016) from the Dept. of Drainage and Irrigation Malaysia. R^2 indicates the variance that is explained by the best-fit line from the upstream to the downstream of the Langat River.

The activity of Po-210, U-238 decay series progeny, i.e., 14.98 ± 1.18 mBq/L, in the Langat River is higher among many rivers around the world (Table 6); this might be because the river runs through a former tin mining area that can be the source of Naturally Occurring Radioactive Materials (NORM) [57,58]. The other reasons for the enhanced Po-210 activity in the Langat River might be due to the weathering process on the granitic formation of the river basin, the origin of the water, flow rate, flux of radionuclides, and geological characteristics of the area along with haze events in dry seasons [59,60]. The sources of radionuclide pollutants are also from fertilizers, tin mining, aquaculture feed [61] and industries [57]. Similarly, the higher Po-210 activity in the Vistula River, Poland 0.5 ± 0.1 to 9.8 ± 0.02 mBq/L, is mainly because of higher contamination from phosphate fertilizer and coal mining, along with natural sources [62].

However, the world average activity of Po-210 in the drinking water from private wells is 7 to 48 mBq/L [63]. In Malaysia, rivers provide about 98% of the drinking water sources [64,65] and in the case of the Langat River, it provides drinking water to over one-third of the population in the state of Selangor [47,66]. Therefore, the annual effective doses through ingestion of Po-210 by drinking water could be dangerous for human health.

Moreover, among the rivers of Malaysia, the annual effective dose of Po-210 from the Langat River is estimated the highest, i.e., 1.31×10^{-2} mSv/year (Table 7), because the river is located in a high rich uranium granite rock belt, although it is below the standard of 0.01 mSv/year. Comparison of the annual effective dose of Po-210 from the Langat River with other rivers around the world indicates that the Langat River is in the second position, while the Vistula River in Poland, i.e., 8.6×10^{-3} mSv/year, is in the first position [62].

Table 6. Activity of Po-210 (mBq/L) both in Malaysian and various rivers of the world.

River (Year)	Minimum	Maximum	References
Langat, Malaysia	0.63 ± 0.29	14.98 ± 1.18	*Present Study*
Langat, Malaysia (2015)	-	7.70 ± 0.60	[67]
Kuala Selangor, Malaysia (2010)	0.0002 ± 0.0001	0.014 ± 0.003	[38]
Kuala Selangor, Malaysia (2005)	0.22 ± 0.06	0.75 ± 0.28	[68]
Vistula, Poland (2004)	0.49 ± 0.09	9.80 ± 0.02	
Oder, Poland (2004)	0.60 ± 0.09	5.21 ± 0.19	[62]
Pomeranian, Poland (2004)	3.82 ± 0.24	5.50 ± 0.33	
Yellow, China (1999)	0.25 ± 0.08	1.55 ± 0.50	[69]
Tagus, Portugal (1997)	0.50 ± 0.36	0.67 ± 0.03	[70]

Table 7. Annual effective dose of Po-210 (mSv/year) based on river water globally.

Location (Year)	Minimum	Maximum	References
Langat, Malaysia	5.51×10^{-4}	1.31×10^{-2}	*Present Study*
Langat, Malaysia (2015)	-	6.8×10^{-3}	[67]
Kuala Selangor, Malaysia (2010)	0.0002×10^{-3}	0.01×10^{-3}	[38]
Kuala Selangor, Malaysia (2005)	0.2×10^{-3}	0.7×10^{-3}	[68]
Vistula, Poland (2004)	0.4×10^{-3}	8.6×10^{-3}	
Oder, Poland (2004)	0.5×10^{-3}	4.6×10^{-3}	[62]
Pomeranian, Poland (2004)	3.4×10^{-3}	4.8×10^{-3}	
Yellow, China (1999)	0.2×10^{-3}	1.4×10^{-3}	[69]
Tagus, Portugal (1997)	0.4×10^{-3}	0.6×10^{-3}	[70]

3.2. Po-210 Status in Household's Tap and Filtration Water

Po-210 activity ranges in tap water 1.05 ± 0.33 mBq/L to 22.35 ± 1.67 mBq/L and filtration water 0.49 ± 0.19 mBq/L to 7.30 ± 0.84 mBq/L at the household level in the Langat Basin were fairly within the maximum limit of drinking water quality standard of MOH and WHO i.e., $<0.1 \times 10^3$ mBq/L (Table 8). However, the higher mean Po-210 activity in tap water than the raw and treated water indicates contamination in the drinking water distribution pipeline. Terrestrial inputs might have elevated the Po-210 activity in the tap water through the heavy repairing activities of the water distribution pipeline while water was mixing with the soil at Hentian Kajang and UKM areas within the basin. The soil in the granite rock of Peninsular Malaysia including the Langat River Basin highly influences the radioactivity of naturally occurring radionuclides [2,4]. Similarly, the small number of water samples might be one of the reasons of higher Po-210 activity in tap and filtration water as well as the standard deviations. Fortunately, the effectiveness of the household water filtration systems to remove Po-210 from the drinking water in the basin is about 74% (Table 6). Among the commonly used household water filtration systems in the basin, the ultraviolet (UV) filtration system shows higher efficiency (93%) followed by distilled filtration system (69%) in removing Po-210 from drinking water and the Po-210 activity in drinking water at Langat River Basin is within both the national and international drinking water quality guidelines.

Table 8. Po-210 activity (mBq/L) in tap and filter water at Langat River Basin.

Location	Tap Water	Filter Type	Filtration Water	Efficiency Filter (%)	Weighted [1] Efficiency
Hentian Kajang	1.33 ± 0.25	Carbon	1.05 ± 0.33	21	0.66
UKM	1.57 ± 0.70	Distilled	0.49 ± 0.19	69	2.55
Hentian Kajang	22.35 ± 1.67	RO	7.30 ± 0.84	67	35.51
Serdang	1.05 ± 0.33	Alkaline	0.87 ± 0.28	17	0.42
UKM	16.08 ± 2.27	UV	1.13 ± 0.37	93	35.28
Mean	8.48 ± 10.10	Mean	2.17 ± 2.88	74	74.42 (Total)
t value	1.885	*t* value	1.684		
p value	1.32	*p* value	1.68		
MOH (2010)			$<0.1 \times 10^3$ mBq/L		
WOH (2017)			$<0.1 \times 10^3$ mBq/L		

Note: Reported Po-210 activity is in the sampling date (A_o) and Calculation of standard deviation is based on the radiochemistry method, not on the replicates [49]. [1] Sum of all the Po-210 activities in all the five-tap water has been taken as the basis of weighted average for each household water filtration system.

Ahmed et al. [67] reported that the Po-210 activity in the supplied water (1.7 mBq/L) in the Langat River Basin was slightly higher than the activity of the treated water 1.5 mBq/L at the outlet of water treatment plants might be due to the contamination in the pipelines of the drinking water supply system. Moreover, the activity of Po-210 in the supplied water in Malaysia is higher than many countries of the world such as 1.0 mBq/L in Italy [70], 2 to 15.2 mBq/L in Hungary [6], 0.48 mBq/L in Poland [71], 1.4 mBq/L in India [72], etc. (Table 9). On the other hand, Po-210 activity in the supplied water of USA 5 mBq/L [73], Italy 3.25 mBq/L [9] and Bombay, India 1.9 mBq/L [72] were higher than the Po-210 activity in the supplied water of Malaysia, 2015 (Table 7).

Table 9. Po-210 activity in household's tap water around the world.

Location (Year)	Activity (mBq/L)	Dose (mSv/Year)	References
Langat Basin	8.48	7.41×10^{-3}	*Present Study*
Bangi, Malaysia (2015)	1.7	1.5×10^{-3}	[67]
Italy (2009)	3.25	2.84×10^{-3}	[9]
Italy (2007)	1	0.9×10^{-3}	[70]
Hungary (2010)	2	1.75×10^{-3}	[6]
Poland (2001)	0.48	0.42×10^{-3}	[71]
India (2001)	1.4	1.2×10^{-3}	
Bombay, India (1977)	1.9	1.7×10^{-3}	[72]
Brazil (1992)	1	0.9×10^{-3}	
Portugal (1995)	0.21	0.2×10^{-3}	
Syria (1995)	1	0.9×10^{-3}	
Austria (2001)	0.4	0.35×10^{-3}	[74]
USA (2008)	5	4.4×10^{-3}	[73]

3.3. Human Health Hazard of Po-210 Ingestion

The annual effective doses of Po-210 through ingestion via drinking water are significant in terms of dose contributions. Although the radioactivity of Po-210 in drinking water is lower than the activity of the isotopes of uranium, however Po-210 is considered highly toxic. Moreover, Po-210 is the most important dose contributor through ingestion of drinking water. For instance, Jia et al. [9] investigated that the mean Po-210 activity 3.25 mBq/L and the Po-210 activity in drinking water remained in the last position in the series of U-238, Ra-228 and Pb-210, however in terms of annual effective dose 2.84×10^{-3} mSv/year Po-210 was the highest contributor in the same series of radionuclides (Table 9).

Unfortunately, the Po-210 activity in the drinking water and its annual effective dose exposure for a long time to human beings has not been studied extensively due the difficulties in determining the radioactivity [19].

Therefore, the calculated annual effective dose of Po-210 ingestion via tap water 7.41×10^{-3} mSv/year and household filtration water 1.90×10^{-3} mSv/year indicate an acceptable carcinogenic risk for the populations at the Langat River Basin, since the values are within the standard of UNSCAER < 0.12 mSv/year, WHO < 0.01 mSv/year, and ICRP < 1.0 mSv/year [36] and the Polish Ministry of Health < 0.01 mSv/year [75,76] (Table 10). Although the higher standard deviations might be due to the small number of environmental samples, however, the result indicates safe for human consumption. Similarly, the annual effective dose of river $5.20 \times 10^{-3} \pm 4.56 \times 10^{-3}$ mSv/year and treated water $2.14 \times 10^{-3} \pm 2.07 \times 10^{-3}$ mSv/year were significantly within the standard limit at 95% confidence level.

Table 10. Annual effective dose of Po-210 via drinking water at Langat River Basin.

Location	River (mSv/Year)	WTP (mSv/Year)	Location	Tap (mSv/Year)	Filter Type	Filtered (mSv/Year)
Pangsoon	2.62×10^{-3}	1.07×10^{-3}	Hentian Kajang	1.16×10^{-3}	Carbon Filter	9.18×10^{-4}
Lolo	2.22×10^{-3}	1.6×10^{-3}	UKM	1.37×10^{-3}	Distilled Filter	4.28×10^{-4}
Serai	4.39×10^{-3}	3.01×10^{-4}	Hentian Kajang	1.95×10^{-2}	RO Filter	6.38×10^{-3}
Langat	1.31×10^{-2}	2.50×10^{-3}	Serdang	9.18×10^{-4}	Alkaline Filter	7.61×10^{-4}
Cheras	1.08×10^{-2}	5.94×10^{-3}	UKM	1.41×10^{-2}	UV Filter	9.88×10^{-4}
Bukit	6.24×10^{-3}	4.53×10^{-4}	Average	7.41×10^{-3}	Average	1.90×10^{-3}
Salak	1.63×10^{-3}	7.35×10^{-4}	Std.	8.78×10^{-3}	Std.	2.52×10^{-3}
Labu	5.52×10^{-4}	4.43×10^{-4}	*t* value	1.886	*t* value	1.684
Average	5.20×10^{-3}	2.14×10^{-3}	*p* value	0.132	*p* value	0.167
Std.	4.56×10^{-3}	2.07×10^{-3}				
t value	3.223	2.926				
p value	0.015 *	0.022 *				

Note: * Significant at 95% confidence level. United Nations Scientific Committee on Effects of Atomic Radiation (UNSCAER) < 0.12 mSv/year. World Health Organization (WHO) < 0.01 mSv/year. International Commission on Radiological Protection (ICRP) < 1.0 mSv/year. Polish Ministry of Health < 0.01 mSv/year.

A few studies have predicted chronic human health risk of Po-210 ingestion via drinking water [9,10,42,71,77]. Although Zaga et al. [77] estimated Po-210 inhalation and lung cancer, however, there is no significant association study between ingestion of Po-210 via drinking water and types of cancer in human. Luckily, Scott [78] has estimated acute risk of Po-210 ingestion through experimenting on the animal. Scott [78] concluded that: (1) ingestion (or inhalation) of a few tenths of a milligram of Po-210 will likely be fatal to all exposed persons; (2) Lethal intakes are expected to involve fatal damage to the bone marrow which is likely to be compounded by damage caused by higher doses to other organs including the kidneys and liver; (3) Lethal intakes are expected to cause severe damage to the kidney, spleen, stomach, small and large intestines, lymph nodes, skin, and testes (males) in addition to the fatal damage to bone marrow; (4) The time distribution of deaths is expected to depend on the level of radioactivity ingested or inhaled.

Therefore, natural radioactivity ingestion is one of the main causes of human radiation exposure (i.e., global average is 2.4 mSv/year) and it should not exceed 0.1 mSv/year for drinking water according to the European Union Drinking Water Directives (DWD) 98/83/EC [79]. The naturally existing radionuclides in the U-238, Th-232 series, and K-40 are present everywhere in the Earth's crust. Ra-226, U-238 decay series progeny, and K-40 receive more attention due to their high solubility and mobility [80]. In fact, the radioactivity of radionuclides such as U-238, Th-232, and K-40 is very common in water, soil, and rocks [17]. Hence, it presents a serious threat of radiation to the population if ingested [23]. However, the amount of radioactivity of radionuclides in the surface water varies among different places in the world because of territorial and atmospheric sources [81] as well as man-made activities [16]. The proportion of natural and artificial radioactivity rates on earth is 85%:15% [69], whereas in Malaysia the proportion is 80%:20% [16].

4. Conclusions

Po-210 activity in the water supply chain of Langat Basin, Malaysia was within the drinking water quality standard of the Ministry of Health Malaysia and World Health Organization. However, Po-210 activity in the range of 0.63 ± 0.29 to 14.98 ± 1.18 mBq/L in the Langat River is higher than many countries around the world. The Langat River drains through the granite zone, an extension of the granite batholith series of Peninsular Thailand underneath the basin. Therefore, terrestrial sources are the main contributors of primordial radionuclides, such as U-238 and its progeny Po-210 along with the atmospheric and anthropogenic sources to elevate Po-210 activity in the Langat River. Moreover, the less efficiency i.e., an average 59% of conventional water treatment method to remove Po-210 entirely from the treated water might be the reason of higher annual effective dose of Po-210 ingestion via drinking water i.e., via tap water 7.41×10^{-3} mSv/year than many countries around the world, even though the limit is safe and the carcinogenic risk is acceptable for human beings. Previous studies have already reported Po-210 is 250,000 times more toxic than hydrogen cyanide, hence it can be carcinogenic to humans if ingested via drinking water for a long time. Moreover, the treated water might become contaminated in the long pipelines in between treatment plants and households. Therefore, a two-layer water filtration system (i.e., effective filtration system at the plants as well as at the household level) should be introduced in the basin to obtain the status of a developed nation by 2020 as well as to achieve the SDG target 6.1 of getting safe drinking water supply well before 2030.

Author Contributions: M.F.A. has solely prepared the manuscript under the guidance of the co-authors. The co-authors have edited the manuscript several times before submission for the journal publication. First, L.A. and C.A.R.M. conceived and designed the experiments; M.F.A. performed the experiments; M.F.A., C.A.R.M. and M.B.M. analyzed the data; Second, C.A.R.M., M.B.M. and G.C.T. contributed reagents/materials/analysis tools; and M.F.A. wrote the paper.

Funding: The study is supported by the grant: GUP-2017-069 and GUP-2015-029 of the Universiti Kebangsaan Malaysia.

Acknowledgments: The authors are grateful to the Department of Environment Malaysia, Department of Irrigation and Drainage Malaysia, and Malaysian Meteorological Department for the provided data and Information. The authors are also grateful to the Laboratory of Chemical Oceanography, Faculty of Science & Technology, Universiti Kebangsaan Malaysia for the analysis of water samples as well as to the water treatment plant authorities i.e., Puncak Niaga (M) Sdn. Bhd. and Konsortium Air Selangor Sdn. Bhd. to allow to collect water samples from the outlets of their plants. The authors are also thankful to the Institute of Climate Change, UKM to prepare the study area map through ArcGIS.

Conflicts of Interest: The authors declare no conflict of interest.

References

1. Yii Mei-Wo, P.; Assyikeen, M.J.N.; Ahmad, Z. Radiation Hazard from Natural Radioactivity in the Sediment of the East Coast Peninsular Malaysia Exclusive Economic Zone (EEZ). *Malays. J. Anal. Sci.* **2011**, *15*, 202–212.
2. Sanusi, M.S.M.; Ramli, A.T.; Wagiran, H.; Lee, M.H.; Heryanshah, A.; Said, M.N. Investigation of geological and soil influence on natural gamma radiation exposure and assessment of radiation hazards in Western Region, Peninsular Malaysia. Environ. *Earth Sci.* **2016**. [CrossRef]
3. Sanusi, M.S.M.; Ramli, A.T.; Gabdo, H.T.; Garba, N.N.; Heryanshah, A.; Wagiran, H.; Said, M.N. Isodose mapping of terrestrial gamma radiation dose rate of Selangor state, Kuala Lumpur and Putrajaya, Malaysia. *J. Environ. Radioact.* **2014**. [CrossRef] [PubMed]
4. Adnan, M.; Siti, N.S.B.; Yusoff, S.; Chua, Y.P. Soil chemistry and pollution study of a closed landfill site at Ampar Tenang, Selangor, Malaysia. *Waste Manag. Res.* **2013**. [CrossRef]
5. Alam, L.; Mohamed, C.A.R. Polonium. *Radionuclides in the Environment*; Atwood, D.A., Ed.; John Wiley & Sons Ltd.: Chichester, UK, 2010; pp. 149–154.

6.   Jobbágy, V.; Kávási, N.; Somlai, J.; Máté, B.; Kovács, T. Radiochemical characterization of spring waters in Balaton Upland, Hungary, estimation of radiation dose to members of public. *Microchem. J.* **2010**, *94*, 159–165. [CrossRef]

7.   Kurttio, P.; Salonen, L.; Ilus, T.; Pekkanen, J.; Pukkala, E. Auvinen, A. Well water radioactivity and risk of cancers of the urinary organs. *Environ. Res.* **2006**, *102*, 333–338. [CrossRef] [PubMed]

8.   Benedik, L.; Vasile, M.; Spasova, Y.; Wätjen, U. Sequential determination of 210Po and uranium radioisotopes in drinking water by alpha-particle spectrometry. *Appl. Radiat. Isot.* **2009**, *67*, 770–775. [CrossRef] [PubMed]

9.   Jia, G.; Torri, G.; Magro, L. Concentrations of 238U, 234U, 235U, 232Th, 230Th, 228Th, 226Ra, 228Ra, 224Ra, 210Po, 210Pb and 212Pb in drinking water in Italy: Reconciling safety standards based on measurements of gross α and β. *J. Environ. Radioact.* **2009**, *100*, 941–949. [CrossRef] [PubMed]

10.   Seiler, R. 210Po in drinking water, its potential health effects, and inadequacy of the gross alpha activity MCL. *Sci. Total Environ.* **2016**, *568*, 1010–1017. [CrossRef] [PubMed]

11.   Vasile, M.; Loots, H.; Jacobs, K.; Verheyen, L.; Sneyers, L.; Verrezen, F.; Bruggeman, M. Determination of 210Pb, 210Po, 226Ra, 228Ra and uranium isotopes in drinking water in order to comply with the requirements of the EU 'Drinking Water Directive'. *Appl. Radiat. Isot.* **2016**, *109*, 465–469. [CrossRef] [PubMed]

12.   Maguire, H.; Fraser, G.; Croft, J.; Bailey, M.; Tattersall, P.; Morrey, M.; Walsh, B. Assessing public health risk in the London polonium-210 incident, 2006. *Public Health* **2010**, *124*, 313–318. [CrossRef] [PubMed]

13.   Walsh, M.; Wallner, G.; Jennings, P. Radioactivity in drinking water supplies in Western Australia. *J. Environ. Radioact.* **2014**, *130*, 56–62. [CrossRef] [PubMed]

14.   Musa, S. Radioactive Level in Malaysia Still Safe and Low. 2011. UKM News Portal. Available online: http://www.ukm.my/news/arkib/index.php/en/extras/689-radioactive-level-in-malaysia-still-safe-and-low.html (accessed on 5 August 2018).

15.   Almayahi, B.A.; Tajuddin, A.A.; Jaafar, M.S. Measurements of natural radionuclides in human teeth and animal bones as markers of radiation exposure from soil in the Northern Malaysian Peninsula. *Radiat. Phys. Chem.* **2014**, *97*, 56–67. [CrossRef]

16.   Ahmad, N.; Jaafar, M.S.; Bakhash, M.; Rahim, M. An overview on measurements of natural radioactivity in Malaysia. *J. Radiat. Res. Appl. Sci.* **2015**, *8*, 136–141. [CrossRef]

17.   Almayahi, B.; Tajuddin, A.; Jaafar, M. Radiation hazard indices of soil and water samples in Northern Malaysian Peninsula. *Appl. Radiat. Isot.* **2012**, *70*, 2652–2660. [CrossRef] [PubMed]

18.   Tawalbeh, A.A.; Samat, S.B.; Yasir, M.S. Radionuclides level and its radiation hazard index in some drinks consumed in the central zone of Malaysia. *Sains Malays.* **2013**, *42*, 319–323.

19.   Ahmed, M.F.; Alam, L.; Ta, G.C.; Mohamed, C.A.R.; Mokhtar, M. A Preliminary Study on the Concentration of Po-210 in the Tap Water. In Proceedings of the 3rd International Conference Limit to Growth and Sustainability: Contemporary Issues and Perspectives, Kedah, Malaysia, 5–7 December 2015.

20.   Yap, C.K.; Ismail, A.; Tan, S.G.; Omar, H. Concentrations of Cu and Pb in the offshore and intertidal sediments of the west coast of Peninsular Malaysia. *Environ. Int.* **2002**. [CrossRef]

21.   Ta, G.C.; Meng, C.K.; Mokhtar, M.; Ern, L.K.; Alam, L.; Sultan, M.M.A.; Ali, N.L. Enhancing the regulatory framework for upstream chemicals management in Malaysia: Some proposals from an academic perspective. *J. Chem. Health Saf.* **2016**, *23*, 12–18. [CrossRef]

22.   Alina, M.; Azrina, A.; Yunus, M.A.S.; Zakiuddin, M.S.; Effendi, M.F.H.; Muhammad, R.R. Heavy metals (mercury, arsenic, cadmium, plumbum) in selected marine fish and shellfish along the straits of Malacca. *Int. Food Res. J.* **2012**, *19*, 135–140.

23.   Hamzah, Z.; Rosli, T.N.T.M.; Saat, A.; Wood, A.K. An assessment of natural radionuclides in water of Langat River estuary, Selangor. *AIP Conf. Proc.* **2014**, *1584*, 228. [CrossRef]

24.   Hamzah, Z.; Rahman, S.A.; Saat, A.; Agos, S.S.; Ahmad, Z. Measurement of 226 Ra in river water using liquid scintillation counting technique. *J. Nuclear Relat. Technol.* **2010**, *7*, 12–23.

25.   Bahari, I.; Mohsen, N.; Abdullah, P. Radioactivity and radiological risk associated with effluent sediment containing technologically enhanced naturally occurring radioactive materials in amang (tin tailings) processing industry. *J. Environ. Radioact.* **2007**, *95*, 161–170. [CrossRef] [PubMed]

26.   Department of Environment (DOE). *Malaysia Environmental Quality Report 2013*; Department of Environment: Putrajaya, Malaysia, 2013.

27. Juahir, H.H. Water Quality Data Analysis and Modeling of the Langat River Basin. Ph.D. Thesis, University of Malaya, Kuala Lumpur, Malaysia, 2009. Available online: http://repository.um.edu.my/1223/5/Chapter%203%20Revised.pdf (accessed on 07 February 2015).

28. Ashraf, M.A.; Maah, M.J.; Yusoff, I.; Wajid, A.; Mahmood, K. Sand mining effects, causes and concerns: A case study from Bestari Jaya, Selangor, Peninsular Malaysia. *Sci. Res. Essays* **2011**. [CrossRef]

29. Memarian, H.; Balasundram, S.K.; Talib, J.B.; Sood, A.M.; Abbaspour, K.C. Trend analysis of water discharge and sediment load during the past three decades of development in the Langat basin, Malaysia. *Hydrol. Sci. J.* **2012**. [CrossRef]

30. Lin, T.I. Regulatory Control of Milling of Minerals Containing Naturally Occurring Radioactive Materials (NORM) in Malaysia. At. Energy Licens. Board, Malaysia. 2015. Available online: https://www.iaea.org/OurWork/ST/NE/NEFW/Technical-Areas/NFC/documents/uranium/tr-darwin-2012/Presentations/46.Teng(Malaysia)_-_Regulatory_control_of_NORM_in_Malaysia.pdf (accessed on 1 February 2018).

31. JPN. Atomic Energy Licensing (Radioactive Waste Management) Regulations 2011. Jabatan Peguam Negera/Attorney General's Chambers of Malaysia. Federal Government Gazette, Part VIII, 13 (1b). 16 August 2011. Available online: http://www.aelb.gov.my/malay/dokumen/perundangan/P.U.(A)274.pdf (accessed on 7 August 2018).

32. MOH. Drinking Water Quality Standard. Ministry of Health: Malaysia, 2010. Available online: http://kmam.moh.gov.my/public-user/drinking-water-quality-standard.html (accessed on 28 February 2018).

33. Ahmed, M.F.; Lubna, A.; Choo, T.G.; Rahim, M.C.; Mazlin, M. A review on the chemical pollution of Langat River, Malaysia. *Asian J. Water Environ. Pollut.* **2016**, *13*, 9–15. [CrossRef]

34. Lim, W.Y.; Aris, A.Z.; Ismail, T.H.T.; Zakaria, M.P. Elemental hydrochemistry assessment on its variation and quality status in Langat River, Western Peninsular Malaysia. *Environ. Earth Sci.* **2013**. [CrossRef]

35. Mohamed, C.A.R.; Ahmad, Z.; Mon, G.C. Aktiviti 226Ra dalam sistem aliran sungai Lembangan Langat, Selangor. *Malays. J. Anal. Sci.* **2006**, *10*, 295–302.

36. Yussuf, N.M.; Hossain, I.; Wagiran, H. Natural radioactivity in drinking and mineral water in Johor Bahru (Malaysia). *Sci. Res. Essays* **2012**, *7*, 1070–1075. [CrossRef]

37. Amin, Y.B.M.; Jemangin, M.H.; Mahat, R.H. Concentration of Ra-226 in Malaysian Drinking and Bottled Mineral Water. *AIP Conf. Proc.* **2010**, *1250*. [CrossRef]

38. Mohamed, C.A.R.; Siang, T.C. Seasonal variation of Po 210 in different salinity: Case of Kuala Selangor river, west coast of peninsular Malaysia. (Special section: Ocean pollution). *Coast. Mar. Sci.* **2010**, *34*, 186–194.

39. International Atomic Energy Agency (IAEA). *A Procedure for the Determination of Po-210 in Water Samples by Alpha Spectrometry Vienna*; International Atomic Energy Agency: Vienna, Austria, 2009.

40. Saili, N.F.B.B. Aktiviti Polonium-210 (210Po) dan Plumbum-210 (210Pb) Dalam turus air di Sungai Mersing, Johor. Master's Thesis, Faculty of Science & Technology, Universiti Kebangsaan Malaysia, Bangi Selangor, Malaysia, 2012.

41. World Health Organization (WHO). *Guidelines for Drinking-Water Quality: Fourth Edition Incorporating the First Addendum*; World Health Organization: Geneva, Switzerland, 2017; Available online: http://apps.who.int/iris/bitstream/10665/254637/1/9789241549950-eng.pdf?ua=1 (accessed on 29 May 2017).

42. Jia, G.; Torri, G. Estimation of radiation doses to members of the public in Italy from intakes of some important naturally occurring radionuclides (238U, 234U, 235U, 226Ra, 228Ra, 224Ra and 210Po) in drinking water. *Appl. Radiat. Isot.* **2007**, *65*, 849–857. [CrossRef] [PubMed]

43. Department of Statistics (DOS). *Population Distribution by Local Authority Areas and Mukims 2010*; Department of Statistics: Putrajaya, Malaysia, 2013. Available online: http://newss.statistics.gov.my/newss-portalx/ep/epProductFreeDownloadSearch.seam (accessed on 25 November 2015).

44. Yamane, T. *Statistics: An Introductory Analysis*, 2nd ed.; Harper and Row: New York, NY, USA, 1967.

45. Alam, M.M. Linkages between Climatic Changes and Food Security among the Poor and Low-Income Households in the East Coast Economic Region (ECER), Malaysia. Ph.D. Thesis, Universiti Kebangsaan Malaysia, Bangi Selangor, Malaysia, 2014.

46. Poon, W.C.; Herath, G.; Sarker, A.; Masuda, T.; Kada, R. River and fish pollution in Malaysia: A green ergonomics perspective. *Appl. Ergon.* **2016**, *57*, 80–93. [CrossRef] [PubMed]

47. Juahir, H.; Zain, S.M.; Yusoff, M.K.; Hanidza, T.T.; Armi, A.M.; Toriman, M.E.; Mokhtar, M. Spatial water quality assessment of Langat River Basin (Malaysia) using environmetric techniques. *Environ. Monit. Assess.* **2011**, *173*, 625–641. [CrossRef] [PubMed]

48. Aris, A.Z.; Lim, W.Y.; Looi, L.J. Natural and Anthropogenic Determinants of Freshwater Ecosystem Deterioration: An environmental Forensic Study of the Langat River Basin, Malaysia. In *Environmental Management of River Basin Ecosystems*; Ramkumar, M., Ed.; Springer: Basel, Switzerland, 2015; pp. 455–476.

49. Ehmann, W.D.; Vance, D.E. *Radiochemistry and Nuclear Methods of Analysis*; John Wiley & Sons, Inc.: New York, NY, USA, 1991; p. 479. ISBN 0-471-60076-8 (c).

50. Shaheed, K.; Somasundaram, S.S.N.; Hameed, P.S.; Iyengar, M.A.R. A study of polonium-210 distribution aspects in the riverine ecosystem of Kaveri, Tiruchirappalli, India. *Environ. Pollut.* **1997**, *95*, 371–377. [CrossRef]

51. Alam, L.; Mokhtar, M.B.; Alam, M.; Bari, M.; Kathijotes, N.; Ta, G.C.; Ern, L.K. Assessment of environmental and human health risk for contamination of heavy metal in tilapia fish collected from Langat Basin, Malaysia. *Asian J. Water Environ. Pollut.* **2015**, *12*, 21–30.

52. United States Environmental Protection Agency (USEPA). *Radionuclides in Drinking Water: A Small Entity Compliance Guide*; United States Environmental Protection Agency: Washington, DC, USA, 2002. Available online: https://www.epa.gov/sites/production/files/2015-06/documents/compliance-radionuclidesindw.pdf (accessed on 12 August 2017).

53. Mokhtar, M.B.; Toriman, M.E.H.; Hossain, A.A. Social learning in facing challenges of sustainable development: A case of Langat River Basin, Malaysia. *Res. J. Appl. Sci.* **2010**, *5*, 434–443.

54. Mokhtar, M.B.; Toriman, M.E.H.; Hossain, M.; Abraham, A.; Tan, K.W. Institutional challenges for integrated river basin management in Langat River Basin, Malaysia. *Water Environ. J.* **2011**, *25*, 495–503. [CrossRef]

55. Seiler, R.L. 210Po in Nevada groundwater and its relation to gross alpha radioactivity. *Groundwater* **2011**, *49*, 160–171. [CrossRef] [PubMed]

56. Theng, T.L.; Mohamed, C.A.R. Activities of 210Po and 210Pb in the water column at Kuala Selangor, Malaysia. *J. Environ. Radioact.* **2005**. [CrossRef] [PubMed]

57. Yunus, S.M.; Hamzah, Z.; Wood, A.K.H.; Saat, A. Natural Radionuclides and heavy Metals Pollution in Seawater at Kuala Langat Coastal Area. *Malays. J. Anal. Sci.* **2015**, *19*, 766–774.

58. Lim, W.Y.; Aris, A.Z.; Zakaria, M.P. Spatial Variability of Metals in Surface Water and Sediment in the Langat River and Geochemical Factors That Influence Their Water-Sediment Interactions. *Sci. World J.* **2012**. [CrossRef] [PubMed]

59. Sabuti, A.A.; Mohamed, C.A.R. High 210Po Activity Concentration in the Surface Water of Malaysian Seas Driven by the Dry Season of the Southwest Monsoon (June–August 2009). *Estuaries Coasts* **2015**, *38*, 482–493. [CrossRef]

60. Yusoff, A.H.; Mohamed, C.A.R. Mini Review Uranium-Thorium Decay Series in the Marine Environment of the Southern South China Sea. *J. Geol. Geophys.* **2016**, *5*, 1–9. [CrossRef]

61. Vasukevich, T.A.; Nitievskaya, L.S. Application of deactivating properties of some sorbents in aquaculture feed production. *Radiats. Biol. Radioecol.* **2014**, *54*, 613–620. [PubMed]

62. Strumińska-Parulska, D.I.; Skwarzec, B.; Tuszkowska, A.; Jahnz-Bielawska, A.; Boryło, A. Polonium (210Po), uranium (238U) and plutonium (239+240Pu) in the biggest Polish rivers. *J. Radioanal. Nucl. Chem.* **2010**. [CrossRef]

63. Persson, B.R.R.; Holm, E. Polonium-210 and lead-210 in the terrestrial environment: A historical review. *J. Environ. Radioact.* **2011**. [CrossRef] [PubMed]

64. Leong, K.H.; Tan, L.B.; Mustafa, A.M. Contamination levels of selected organochlorine and organophosphate pesticides in the Selangor River, Malaysia between 2002 and 2003. *Chemosphere* **2007**, *66*, 1153–1159. [CrossRef] [PubMed]

65. Santhi, V.A.; Sakai, N.; Ahmad, E.D.; Mustafa, A.M. Occurrence of bisphenol A in surface water, drinking water and plasma from Malaysia with exposure assessment from consumption of drinking water. *Sci. Total Environ.* **2012**, *427*, 332–338. [CrossRef] [PubMed]

66. Alsalahi, M.A.; Latif, M.T.; Ali, M.M.; Magam, S.M.; Wahid, N.B.A. Distribution of surfactants along the estuarine area of Selangor River, Malaysia. *Mar. Pollut. Bull.* **2014**, *80*, 344–350. [CrossRef] [PubMed]

67. Ahmed, M.F.; Alam, L.; Ta, G.C.; Mohamed, C.A.R.; Mokhtar, M. A Preliminary Study on the Concentration of Po-210 in the Tap Water. In *In-House Seminar of the Chemical Oceanography Laboratory*; Chemical Oceanography Laboratory, School of Environmental Science and Natural Resources, Faculty of Science and Technology, Universiti Kebangsaan Malaysia: Kuala Selangor, Malaysia, 2016; Volume 1, pp. 34–38, ISBN 978-967-0829-22-7.

68. Hong, G.H.; Park, S.K.; Baskaran, M.; Kim, S.H.; Chung, C.S.; Lee, S.H. Lead-210 and polonium-210 in the winter well-mixed turbid waters in the mouth of the Yellow Sea. *Cont. Shelf Res.* **1999**. [CrossRef]

69. Carvalho, F.P. Distribution, cycling and mean residence time of 226Ra, 210Pb and 210Po in the Tagus estuary. *Stud. Environ. Sci.* **1997**. [CrossRef]

70. Desideri, D.; Meli, M.A.; Feduzi, L.; Roselli, C.; Rongoni, A.; Saetta, D. 238U, 234U, 226Ra, 210Po concentrations of bottled mineral waters in Italy and their dose contribution. *J. Environ. Radioact.* **2007**, *94*, 86–97. [CrossRef] [PubMed]

71. Skwarzec, B.; Strumińska, D.I.; Borylo, A. The radionuclides 234 U, 238 U and 210 Po in drinking water in Gdańsk agglomeration (Poland). *J. Radioanal. Nucl. Chem.* **2001**, *250*, 315–318. [CrossRef]

72. Kannan, V.; Iyengar, M.A.R.; Ramesh, R. Dose estimates to the public from 210Po ingestion via dietary sources at Kalpakkam (India). *Appl. Radiat. Isot.* **2001**, *54*, 663–674. [CrossRef]

73. Outola, I.; Nour, S.; Kurosaki, H.; Inn, K.; LaRosa, J. Investigation of radioactivity in selected drinking water samples from Maryland. *J. Radioanal. Nucl. Chem.* **2008**, *277*, 155–159. [CrossRef]

74. Irlweck, K. Determination of 210Pb, 210Bi and 210Po in natural drinking water. *J. Radioanal. Nucl. Chem.* **2001**, *249*, 191–196. [CrossRef]

75. Kozłowska, B.; Walencik, A.; Dorda, J.; Przylibski, T.A. Uranium, radium and 40K isotopes in bottled mineral waters from Outer Carpathians, Poland. *Radiat. Meas.* **2007**, *42*, 1380–1386. [CrossRef]

76. World Health Organization (WHO). *Polonium-210: Basic Facts and Questions*; World Health Organization: Grneva, Switzerland, 2018; Available online: http://www.who.int/ionizing_radiation/pub_meet/polonium210/en/ (accessed on 10 March 2018).

77. Zaga, V.; Lygidakis, C.; Chaouachi, K.; Gattavecchia, E. Polonium and lung cancer. *J. Oncol.* **2011**. [CrossRef] [PubMed]

78. Scott, B.R. Health risk evaluations for ingestion exposure of humans to polonium-210. *Dose-Response* **2007**, *5*, 94–122. [CrossRef] [PubMed]

79. Munter, R. Technology for the removal of radionuclides from natural water and waste management: State of the art Rein Munter. *Proc. Est. Acad. Sci.* **2013**. [CrossRef]

80. Yii, M.W.; Zaharudin, A.; Abdul-Kadir, I. Distribution of naturally occurring radionuclides activity concentration in East Malaysian marine sediment. *Appl. Radiat. Isot.* **2009**. [CrossRef] [PubMed]

81. Ramli, A.T.; Hussein, A.W.M.A.; Wood, A.K. Environmental 238U and 232Th concentration measurements in an area of high level natural background radiation at Palong, Johor, Malaysia. *J. Environ. Radioact.* **2005**. [CrossRef] [PubMed]

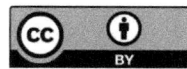

MDPI

St. Alban-Anlage 66

4052 Basel

Switzerland

Tel. +41 61 683 77 34

Fax +41 61 302 89 18

www.mdpi.com

International Journal of Environmental Research and Public Health Editorial Office

E-mail: ijerph@mdpi.com

www.mdpi.com/journal/ijerph

CPSIA information can be obtained
at www.ICGtesting.com
Printed in the USA
BVHW021424140419
545473BV00016B/301/P